Knottenbelt and Pascoe's

COLOR ATLAS

of

Diseases and Disorders of the Horse

Dedicated to
my greatly missed father,
Tom McAuliffe (RIP)

Content Strategists: Robert Edwards, Penny Rudolph
Content Development Specialist: Barbara Simmons
Project Manager: Lucía Pérez
Designer/Design Direction: Miles Hitchen
Illustration Manager: Jennifer Rose
Illustrator: Antbits Ltd

Knottenbelt and Pascoe's

COLOR ATLAS
of
Diseases and Disorders of the Horse

Edited by

Siobhan B. McAuliffe
MVB DipACVIM

Head of Internal Medicine
Kawell Equine Hospital and Rehabilitation Centre
Buenos Aires, Argentina

Foreword by

Derek Knottenbelt
OBE BVM&S DVMS DipECEIM MRCVS

Professor in Equine Internal Medicine
University of Liverpool
Liverpool, UK

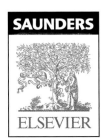

Edinburgh   London   New York   Oxford   Philadelphia   St Louis   Sydney   Toronto   2014

SAUNDERS
ELSEVIER

ISBN 9780723436607

British Library Cataloguing in Publication Data
A catalogue record for this book is available from the British Library

Library of Congress Cataloging in Publication Data
A catalog record for this book is available from the Library of Congress

Notices
Knowledge and best practice in this field are constantly changing. As new research and experience broaden our understanding, changes in research methods, professional practices, or medical treatment may become necessary.

Practitioners and researchers must always rely on their own experience and knowledge in evaluating and using any information, methods, compounds, or experiments described herein. In using such information or methods they should be mindful of their own safety and the safety of others, including parties for whom they have a professional responsibility.

With respect to any drug or pharmaceutical products identified, readers are advised to check the most current information provided (i) on procedures featured or (ii) by the manufacturer of each product to be administered, to verify the recommended dose or formula, the method and duration of administration, and contraindications. It is the responsibility of practitioners, relying on their own experience and knowledge of their patients, to make diagnoses, to determine dosages and the best treatment for each individual patient, and to take all appropriate safety precautions.

To the fullest extent of the law, neither the Publisher nor the authors, contributors, or editors, assume any liability for any injury and/or damage to persons or property as a matter of products liability, negligence or otherwise, or from any use or operation of any methods, products, instructions, or ideas contained in the material herein.

ELSEVIER your source for books,
journals and multimedia
in the health sciences
www.elsevierhealth.com

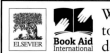

Working together
to grow libraries in
developing countries

www.elsevier.com • www.bookaid.org

The
publisher's
policy is to use
**paper manufactured
from sustainable forests**

Printed in China

FOREWORD

I am truly honored to be asked to write a foreword for the second edition of the *Color Atlas of Diseases and Disorders of the Horse*. I am only too aware of the work that it takes to bring such a vast project to fruition and so I am flattered enormously by the enthusiasm that the authors have put into it.

When Reg Pascoe and I started out with the idea of doing a color atlas that would provide a high quality pictorial reference, we had no idea what it would become. We collected and selected pictures, and then constructed a suitably brief and hopefully useful textural content. Of course it had to be comprehensive enough to satisfy veterinarians across the world and the pictures had to be the best available! Countless friends and colleagues were asked to contribute and, as a result, that edition contained possibly the best collection of equine disease and disorder pictures ever made. The first edition sold out quickly, and reprint after reprint was required to satisfy the demand for it. The book served as ready reckoner for veterinarians across all the continents (with translations into German and Russian) and rapidly became a means of demonstrating to owners what the diseases looked like. The book became a 'must have' for students and vets alike, and soon it was also acquired by lay horse owners and any others with an interest in horses. Dirty, well used copies can still be found in many practices and libraries across the world. When I visit other countries I am frequently asked 'where can I get a copy of the book?'.

Finally the publishers decided that enough was enough, and the first edition ceased publication. There was a need for a second edition, but that required a person or a team with the right dedication and determination. Siobhan McAuliffe decided to pick up the baton and this book is the result of the enthusiasm and hard work of her authoring team. Pictures do not age and diseases have not changed that much, but we now know so much more about them. The new book contains only a few of the original pictures, because communication and image quality and storage are far better now than in the days of slides and colour prints; and endoscopic and radiographic images are vastly better quality now than what they used to be. I am very pleased this edition represents an improvement from the last one, while still manages to retain the core values of high quality pictorial imaging and a comprehensive catalogue of the diseases and disorders of the horse. That's the mark of a good book!

Both Reg Pascoe and I commend this book to the reader with pride and satisfaction. It is no flattery to say that the value to the student, the practitioner, equine scientists and horse owners will be far greater now than the old version. We are proud to have provided the basis for such an amazing resource.

Derek Knottenbelt
April 2013

PREFACE

The first edition of this book was published in 1994. In today's technological world, where we all have cameras built into our telephones, taking pictures of our cases has become easy and widely used. However, looking back to the days of the first edition, where all the pictures were taken on cameras with film, I am repeatedly astounded not only at the quality but also the quantity of images that were compiled for its publication.

The idea of assisted learning through visualization, which Knottenbelt and Pascoe had in mind for this work, is continued here in the second edition. Wherever possible, images of clinical signs, diagnostics and post-mortems have been provided to give the reader step by step guidance for each one of the disorders. We have included a large number of diagnostic images that were simply not available at the time of the first edition, and information on disorders that were unknown or unclear at the time.

But this is not a definitive text of equine medicine. The aim of this book is to encourage interest in the field and stimulate readers to look through other texts for more in-depth information on particular diseases by helping them visually recognize the disorder in the first place.

Acknowledgements

Derek Knottenbelt is someone that I have looked up to not only as an excellent veterinarian, but also as an enormous contributor to veterinary learning. So when he asked me if I could put together the second edition of this book, I felt so honored that I could not refuse! He was on hand throughout the process to offer advice and has contributed a large number of images to this edition. Thank you Derek for giving me this project; I have thoroughly enjoyed working on it.

Putting together texts that incorporate a lot of images is an editorial nightmare for the production team, so a huge thanks goes to all those at Elsevier for their hard work, dedication and most especially patience throughout: Robert Edwards, Barbara Simmons, Penny Rudolph and Lucia Perez.

Special thanks go to the text contributors who worked hard to provide up to date information in such a concise format. Without the image contributors this book would not exist, so thank you to everyone all over the world who has provided images and patiently answered my questions on the cases.

Thanks also to Eric Swinebroad, who offered much assistance and advice on the skeletal chapter.

Noreen Galvin, a long time friend and sounding board, was called upon many times for her opinion from start to finish. I am sure I have not said it often enough but thank you so much, Noreen, for all your guidance. The biggest thanks have to go to my husband, best friend, fellow veterinarian and contributor, Fernando García-Seeber. He was always on hand to assist in the juggling act of work, kids and book.

Lastly, thanks to you, the reader. I hope you enjoy this second edition as much as I did the first.

Siobhan B. McAuliffe

CONTRIBUTORS

Chapters:

Noreen Galvin MVB, Cert EM(Int Med) DipECEIM MRCVS
The Phoenix Equine Group, Kildare Town, County Kildare, Ireland

Fernando García-Seeber MV
Private Practitioner, Hipódromo San Isidro, Buenos Aires, Argentina

Natasha Mitchell MVB DVOphthal MRCVS
Veterinary Ophthalmologist, Eyevet, Limerick, Ireland

Martin Nielsen DVM PhD DipEVPC
Assistant Professor, Gluck Equine Research Centre, Department of Veterinary Science, University of Kentucky, Lexington, Kentucky, USA

Karen Wolfsdorf DVM DACT
Hagyard Equine Medical Institute, Lexington, Kentucky, USA

Illustrations:

Sameeh M. Abutarbush BVSc MVetSc DipABVP DipACVIM
Associate Professor, Large Animal Internal Medicine and Infectious Diseases, Department of Veterinary Clinical Sciences, Faculty of Veterinary Medicine, Jordan University of Science and Technology, Jordan

Barbora Bezděková DVM PhD DipECEIM
Associate Professor, Equine Clinic, Faculty of Veterinary Medicine, University of Veterinary and Pharmaceutical Sciences, Brno, Czech Republic

Beatriz Buchinier Rodríguez BVM
University Alfonso X El Sabio, Madrid, Spain

Melissa Cordero DVM PhD
Equine Veterinarian, Stillwater, Oklahoma, USA

Carlos Dodera DVM
Triada Hospital Equino, Buenos Aires, Argentina

Waldemar H. Fink MV
Equine Veterinarian, Buenos Aires, Argentina

Genevieve L. Fontaine DMV MS DipACVIM
Field Care Associate, Hagyard Medical Institute, Kentucky, USA

Nicolás C. Galinelli MV
Veterinary staff member, Kawell Equine Hospital and Rehabilitation Centre, Buenos Aires, Argentina

Laurie Gallatin DVM DipACVIM
Gallatin Veterinary Services, Marysville, Ohio, USA

Facundo García Eyherabide MV
Private Practitoner, Buenos Aires, Argentina

Marta García Piqueres DVM
Equidinamia, Equine Rehabilitation Services, Madrid, Spain; Kawell Equine Hospital and Rehabilitation Centre, Equine Rehabilitation Consultant, Buenos Aires, Argentina

Alejandro Guglilminetti MV
Medical Director, Kawell Equine Hospital and Rehabilitation Centre, Buenos Aires, Argentina

Kristopher James Hughes BVSc FACVSc DipECEIM
Senior Lecturer in Equine Internal Medicine, Charles Sturt University, School of Animal and Veterinary Sciences, Charles Sturt University, Wagga Wagga, New South Wales, Australia

Michael Hurley BVSc CertEP GradDip Bus Studs MANZCVS MRCVS
Veterinary Surgeon, Hong Kong Jockey Club, Equine Hospital, Hong Kong

Philip J. Johnson BVSc (Hons) MS DipACVIM-LAIM DipECEIM MRCVS

Professor and Instructional Leader, Equine Medicine and Surgery, College of Veterinary Medicine, University of Missouri, Columbia, Missouri, USA

Gigi Rosalind Kay MA BVM&S MRCVS Cert AVP (Eq Med)

Director, American Fondouk, Fez, Morocco

Derek Knottenbelt OBE BVM&S DVMS DipECEIM MRCVS

Professor in Equine Internal Medicine, University of Liverpool, Liverpool, UK

Alan Thomas Loynachan DVM PhD DACVP

Assistant Professor, Veterinary Diagnostic Laboratory, University of Kentucky, USA

Andrew Matthews BVM&S PhD DipECEIM Hon Member ACVO FRCVS

Equine Practitioner, Ayrshire, UK

Alejandro Perón MV

Kawell Equine Hospital and Rehabilitation Centre, Buenos Aires, Argentina

Montague N. Saulez BVSc MS DipACVIM-LA DECEIM PhD

Specialist in Large Animal Medicine; European Specialist in Equine Internal Medicine; Associate Professor, Equine Medicine, Companion Animal Clinical Studies, Faculty of Veterinary Science, Onderstepoort, South Africa

Barbara Schmidt DVM

Equine Veterinarian, Kentucky, USA

Nathan Marc Slovis DVM DipACVIM CHT

Director, McGee Medical Centre, Hagyard Equine Medical Institute, Lexington, Kentucky, USA

Allison Jean Stewart BVSc (Hons) MS DipACVIM DACVECC

Professor of Equine Medicine, Department of Clinical Sciences, Auburn University, Auburn, Alabama, USA

Luis Vaudana Med Vet

Equine Medicine, Santa Fe, Argentina

Ricardo Videla DVM MS ACVIM

Clinical Assistant Professor, Large Animal Clinical Sciences, University of Tennessee, Knoxville, Tennessee, USA

Jamie Wearn BVSc DVCS MS DipACVIM

Associate Veterinarian, Bundall, Queensland, Australia

CONTENTS

CHAPTER 1

Gastrointestinal system

CHAPTER CONTENTS

Part 1: The mouth

Developmental disorders

Cleft palate (Figs. 1.1–1.3)

Cleft palate is an uncommon abnormality. When seen it most frequently involves the caudal aspect of the soft palate; however the hard palate, lips and external nares may also be affected. The degree to which it is heritable is not well defined. Foals with large clefts may show dramatic nasal regurgitation of milk during nursing. In some cases, particularly those with relatively small clefts or clefts in the soft palate, nasal return of milk becomes obvious only after feeding and may be relatively minor in amount. Small clefts may not always be easily visible or produce significant nasal return of food and, occasionally, some are only detected after some years, when nasal reflux of grass and more solid food material may be present. Consequent rhinitis and nasal discharges may not be immediately identifiable as resulting from a cleft palate. Occasionally the cleft is sufficiently small to produce no detectable evidence and these are sometimes identified incidentally during clinical or post-mortem examinations. Large palatal defects in young foals have profound effects including failure to ingest adequate amounts of colostrum, starvation and inhalation pneumonia.

Diagnosis
- In some cases, diagnosis can be made with a careful oral examination.
- Endoscopy should be performed via both nares. Oral endoscopy may also be required.
- Thoracic radiographs are useful to identify and characterize secondary pneumonia.

Treatment
- Treatment needs to be directed at two main areas, correction of the abnormality and treatment of secondary problems such as pneumonia.
- Treatment of the defect involves one of a variety of surgical techniques. Dehiscence of the surgical site is a common problem. In

severely compromised foals, surgery may need to be delayed while secondary problems (pneumonia, sepsis) are addressed. In these situations, feeding via a nasogastric tube or parenteral nutrition is required.
- The prognosis is better in foals with defects only involving the soft palate.

Cleft tongue and mandible (Fig. 1.4A,B)

This condition has been seen in a number of donkey foals. The condition is thought to be heritable. The condition is visually obvious with no differentials. None of the cases to date have been treated as the defects are usually extensive and frequently these foals present with severe secondary complications related to the inability to nurse.

Parrot mouth (brachygnathia) (Figs. 1.5–1.7)

Parrot mouth is a common congenital abnormality characterized by disparity of the lengths of the mandible and maxilla. The mandible is shorter than the maxilla and there is no occlusal contact between the upper and lower incisors. Males are more commonly affected. In the milder cases, the full extent of the discrepancy may not be obvious at birth, becoming more apparent as the permanent incisors erupt and grow into their normal occlusal positions. The failure of significant occlusion results in an increasing overgrowth of the upper incisors and impingement of the mandibular teeth into the soft tissues of the hard palate. Individuals with lesser degrees of inferior brachygnathia may be less affected but the lingual edges of the lower incisors may become sharp and lacerate the gums and hard palate. More commonly the lower incisors tend to prolong the line of the lower jaw and the labial margins of the upper incisors become long and sharp and may lacerate the lower lip. Simultaneously there is usually a discrepancy in the length of the lower molar arcade and a rostral hook will often develop on the first upper cheek teeth with an equivalent caudal hook on the last lower cheek teeth.

Sow mouth (prognathia) (Figs. 1.8 & 1.9)

Monkey, sow or hog mouth is more rarely encountered. Associated with it are projections (hooks) on the rostral edge of the first lower cheek teeth and the caudal edge of the last upper cheek teeth. Even

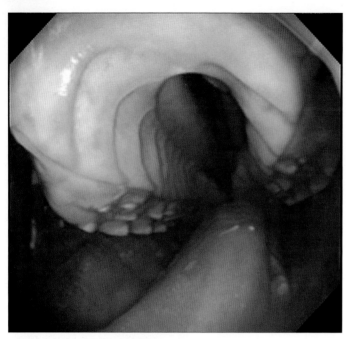

Figure 1.1 Cleft hard palate oroscopic view.

Differential diagnosis: Nasal/oral discharge of milk and/or dysphagia may also be seen with:
- Neurologic dysphagia (associated with hypoxic ischemic encephalopathy in foals)
- Esophageal obstruction
- Laryngeal/pharyngeal abnormalities
- Severe weakness/depression.

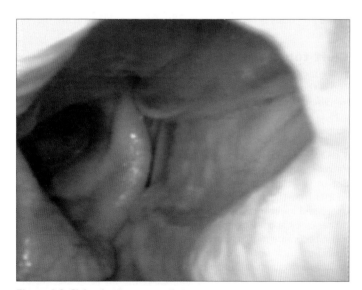

Figure 1.2 Cleft soft palate oroscopic view.

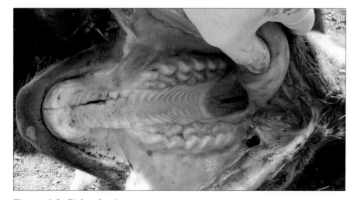

Figure 1.3 Cleft soft palate post-mortem.

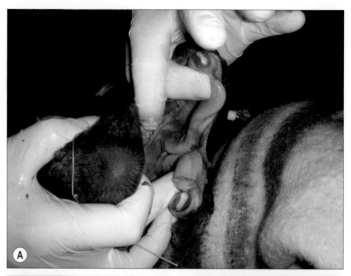

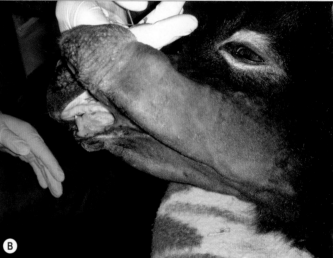

Figure 1.4 (A) Donkey foal with cleft mandible and tongue. (B) Donkey foal with cleft mandible and tongue (same as Fig. 1.3).

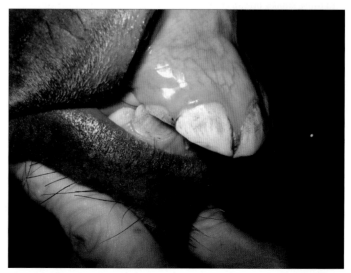

Figure 1.5 Inferior brachygnathism (parrot mouth). Marked disparity in lengths of maxilla and mandible in this young foal.

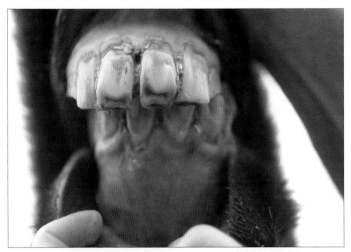

Figure 1.6 Inferior brachygnathism (parrot mouth). Cranial view in an adult horse.

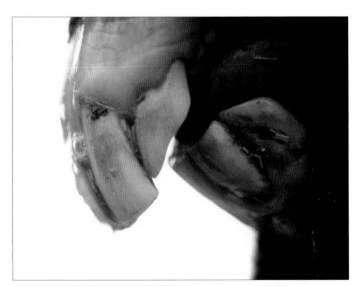

Figure 1.7 Inferior brachygnathism (parrot mouth) (same horse as in Fig. 1.6). Lateral view showing marked incisor overgrowth associated with the condition.

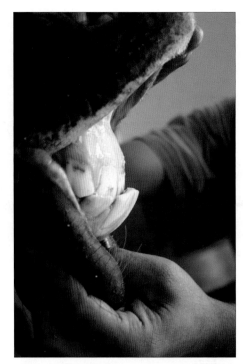

Figure 1.8 Superior brachygnathism (sow mouth, hog mouth).

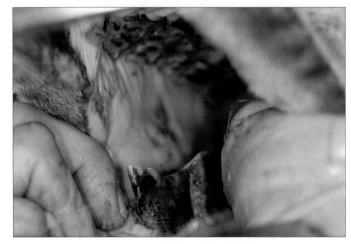

Figure 1.9 Superior brachygnathism (sow mouth) with resultant hook on first lower cheek tooth.

extensive overgrowth of either superior or inferior brachygnathism, where little or no effective occlusion is present, appears to cause little hindrance to prehension in many cases, with the cosmetic and aesthetic effects being of concern in the early years of life. Effects upon growth and condition are therefore unusual, provided that suitable forage is available. Short grazing however, makes prehension very unrewarding for the horse, and weight loss and poor growth are to be expected. Clearly, once the overgrowth becomes severe, difficulties with prehension are more likely.

Diagnosis and treatment of parrot mouth/sow mouth

- Diagnosis through oral examination.
- In many cases, these conditions are more of a cosmetic defect than a true medical problem. The treatment approach is dependent on the severity of the lesion and the age.
- Use of bite plates and surgical correction have been described for severe cases. Many affected horses will require more frequent dental care.

Shear mouth

Shear mouth (see also p. 10) arises when there is a discrepancy in the width of the upper and lower jaws. This disorder may be encountered in young horses as a result of developmental differences between the jaws.

Missing and malerupted teeth (Figs. 1.10–1.18)

Defects of the teeth relating either to genesis or eruption are relatively common.

Oligodontia

Oligodontia (absence of teeth) is a developmental disorder when one or more teeth are absent. The incisors are the most commonly affected but the molars may also be affected. In the latter cases the most common missing tooth is the first molar (fourth cheek tooth) which should erupt at around 1 year of age. In the case of the incisors, true

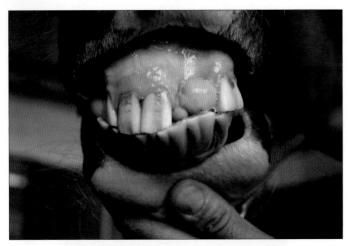

Figure 1.10 Oligodontia. Both central and left lateral incisor missing.

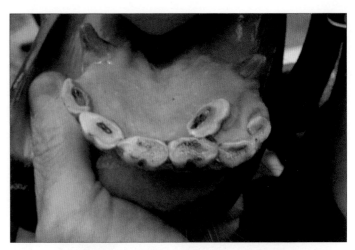

Figure 1.13 Maleruption (lingual) (permanent corner incisor). Permanent tooth erupted inside the temporary tooth resulting in persistence of the temporary corner incisor.

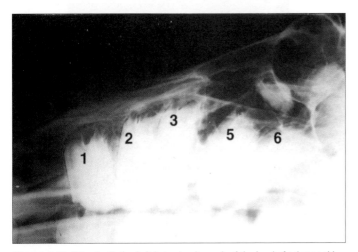

Figure 1.11 Oligodontia (molar). Lateral radiograph of the head of a 6-year-old Arabian gelding with a missing fourth cheek tooth. No dental surgery had ever been performed.

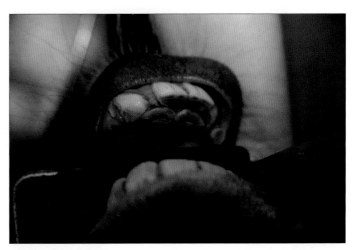

Figure 1.14 Persistent temporary incisors in a 3-year-old pony.

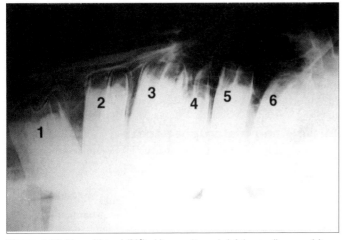

Figure 1.12 Normal lateral (30°) oblique radiograph (of the maxillary arcade). Roots of the maxillary teeth and their relationship to the sinuses.

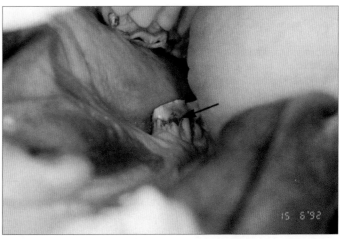

Figure 1.15 Premolar cap attached to erupting first cheek tooth in a 3-year-old Thoroughbred. The cap was easily dislodged.

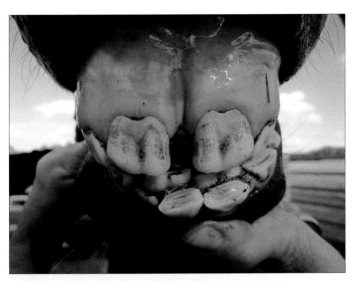

Figure 1.16 Oligodontia and persistent temporary dentition. This horse is missing right and left lateral incisors of the upper arcade and has persistent temporary central incisors on the lower arcade.

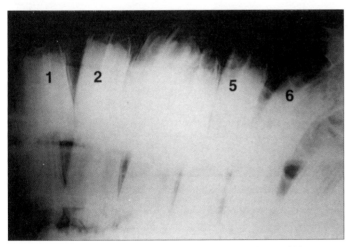

Figure 1.17 Lateral radiograph of the maxillary arcade of a 3-year-old hunter gelding, showing impaction of the third and fourth cheek teeth leading to maleruption.

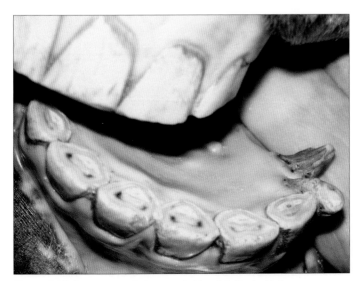

Figure 1.18 Extra incisor which was an incidental finding in this horse.

oligodontia is reflected in an absence of both temporary and permanent teeth, this being consistent with a complete absence of the dental germ cells. It may be associated with other epidermal defects such as maldevelopment of hair or hooves.

Maleruptions

Although the absence of teeth may be a true developmental defect, most frequently missing and malerupted teeth are due to previous traumatic damage to the dental germ buds or to systemic infections involving these during their maturation. The consequent maleruption of teeth may cause a significant deformity of the incisor dental arcades in particular. Maleruption of the molar teeth may, on occasion, only become apparent in later life, and most often affects the eruption of the fourth upper permanent premolar (third, upper cheek tooth), which is the last cheek tooth to erupt and may be identified at ages of 4 years and over.

Abnormalities of dental eruption may present with maxillary or nasal swelling associated with abnormal positioning or abnormal eruption of the permanent premolar and molar teeth. The third upper cheek tooth, being the last to erupt, is most likely to suffer from defects of eruption with gross deformity of the face over the site. Inability to erupt effectively results in considerable growth pressure within the associated rostral maxillary sinus. A discharging tract or enlarged sinus with a nasal discharge in a young horse should alert the clinician to the possibility of maleruption.

Persistent temporary dentition

Persistent temporary dentition may be accompanied by obvious or, occasionally, mild dental deviations of the permanent tooth, and most often affects the incisor arcade. Retained temporary incisors are usually firmly embedded in the gums and the permanent tooth usually erupts behind it rather than under it and so fails to occlude the blood supply to the temporary tooth or to push it out. They are, however, ordinarily loose and easily removed. Total retention of the temporary molars is much less common. In some cases, the temporary tooth creates a dental cap on the permanent tooth which may be so persistent as to make their identification difficult. However, as the first cheek teeth are most commonly affected, it is usually possible to see the cap on the erupted permanent tooth. Persistent, temporary premolar caps overlying the erupting permanent teeth may occasionally cause oral discomfort and masticatory problems. In the event that these caps rotate there may be associated cheek swelling and in this case the displaced temporary cap will be easily visible. Under such circumstances more significant abnormalities of mastication may be present with quidding (spitting out of partially chewed food material) and reluctance to eat. Most of these caps will resolve spontaneously but some will require removal.

Supernumerary teeth

Supernumerary incisors and molars (polyodontia) are not uncommon and develop as a result of multiple dental stalks from a single germ bud of a permanent tooth. In some cases there may be a complete double row of incisors but more often one or two extra teeth will be present. This polyodontia (dental duplication) may be restricted to one or more teeth, and affects incisors more often than premolar or molar teeth. Due to lack of wear by an opposing tooth, the extra tooth usually becomes elongated and may ultimately cause soft tissue injury to the opposing palate or tongue. Supernumerary molar teeth occasionally occur. Their position in the dental arcade is irregular; but they are frequently found caudal to the third molar tooth (sixth cheek tooth) in jaws which are longer than normal. Less often they are located either lingual or buccal to a normal molar and may in the latter case show obvious facial swelling. They often have a draining sinus onto the side of the face or into the maxillary sinus.

Diagnosis of missing/malerupted teeth

- Oral examination may be diagnostic for the majority of cases of missing or malerupted teeth.
- Radiographs may be required to differentiate supernumary teeth from persistent temporary dentition. A retained deciduous incisor has a more mature root and a shorter reserve crown than those of the adjacent permanent incisors.
- Radiographic examination and comparison with the normal arcade anatomy in cases of maleruptions show a variety of deformities ranging from complete absence of the tooth to an obvious tooth growing in an abnormal direction or position. Sometimes however, definite dental structure cannot be identified in a mass of abnormal tissue.

Treatment

- Regular dental examinations and care to prevent the development of unopposed dental elongations.
- In cases in which the supernumary or malerupted teeth have resulted in secondary complications such as sinusitis, the tooth may need to be removed and the complications treated.

Wolf teeth (Fig. 1.19)

The 'wolf teeth' are the vestigial first upper permanent premolar and, while many horses have these, some do not. In some cases their presence is blamed for a number of behavioral problems including head shaking, failure to respond to the bit and bit resentment. A wolf tooth is located just rostral to the first upper cheek tooth and may be in close apposition to this or may be somewhat removed from it. It is believed that the latter state is the more significant with respect to abnormalities.

They should not be confused with the normal canine teeth which occur in many (but not all) male horses and are located in the inter-dental space of both upper and lower jaw. Incomplete removal of the wolf teeth may result in persistent pain and fragments of enamel or root may be present. More usually, provided that the remains of the tooth are not exposed, there is little pathological effect.

Dentigerous cysts (Figs. 1.20 & 1.21)

Dentigerous cysts, also referred to as ear teeth, aural fistulae or het-erotropic polyodontia, are congenital defects characterized by an epithelium-lined cavity containing embryonic teeth. They are most commonly located adjacent to the temporal bone, but can be found in a variety of other areas of the head. Cysts contain a seromucoid fluid

and often fistulate. Dentigerous cysts may be recognized at any age, but are most commonly identified in horses less than 3 years of age.

The cyst-like structures may contain no obvious dental tissue or remnants and may then be described as a conchal cyst. These may be radiographically unconvincing, but consist of a cystic structure with a smooth lining and an associated chronic discharging sinus. Dental remnants may be identifiable in other sites including the maxillary sinuses.

Diagnosis and treatment

- Radiographs can confirm the presence of an aberrant tooth-like structure, which is either firmly attached to the cranium or loosely enclosed in a cystic structure and may in either case be surrounded by a collar of bone forming an apparent alveolus. A contrast fistu-logram can be used to delineate the mass and any draining tracts.

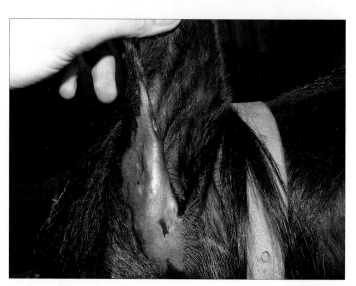

Figure 1.20 Dentigerous cyst. A discharging sinus is present on the anterior margin of the pinna. The tract leads to an obvious solid non-painful mass just rostral to the base of the ear. This is one of the typical clinical appearances of a dentigerous cyst.

Differential diagnosis:
- Abscess/seroma/hematoma
- Foreign body
- Sequestrum.

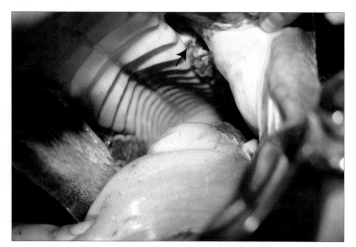

Figure 1.19 Normal wolf tooth (arrow).

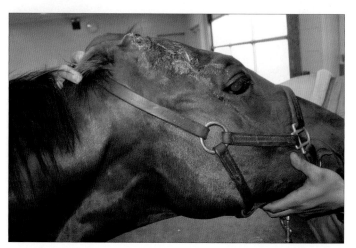

Figure 1.21 Dentigerous cyst. A discrete mass is evident at the base of the ear with a discharging tract.

- Surgical excision is required but may be difficult in some cases where the ectopic teeth are firmly attached. Prognosis following removal is good.

Non-infectious disorders

Dental tartar (Figs. 1.22 & 1.23)

Dental tartar commonly accumulates on any, or all, of the teeth and is most obvious on the lower canine. It is unusual for this to cause any significant gingival inflammation and/or alveolar infection. Extensive accumulations of tartar on the incisors and canine teeth may be an indication of underlying systemic disease (e.g. renal disease or equine motor neuron disease) but is commonly an incidental observation in healthy (particularly, old) horses.

Chronic gingival inflammation caused by dental calculus or other irritants may give rise to a benign inflammatory hyperplasia (epulis) of the gum. Again, the most obvious site for this is the buccal margin of the canine teeth but it may equally develop at any other site along the tooth–gum margin. It seldom reaches significant size although localized cheek swelling may be detected in severe cases. The subsequent development of neoplastic tissue, usually fibroma or fibrosarcoma but occasionally squamous cell (or undifferentiated) carcinoma, at these sites suggests that the inflammatory reaction may have longer-term significance.

Diagnosis and treatment
- Oral examination. Differentiation from other causes of dental tartar (EMND, see p. 427) or gum swelling.
- No treatment is usually required.

Ossifying alveolar periostitis (Fig. 1.24)

Swellings of the horizontal ramus of the mandible (chronic ossifying alveolar periostitis, pseudo-odontoma) are often encountered in young horses around the time of the eruption of the associated cheek teeth, and are probably due to alveolar periostitis around fluid-filled, active, dental sacs. In a few cases they may be associated with dental overcrowding and horizontally aligned unerupted teeth.

Diagnosis and treatment
- Although the apparent deformity of the mandibular bone may be obvious, radiographs of the area will demonstrate the presence, in young horses, of a normal dental sac, without any evidence of periapical inflammation or infection.
- Usually the extent of the defect improves somewhat with age, but persistence of some thickening and deformity are to be expected. Such swellings are totally benign and, in spite of apparently severe cosmetic changes, they are of little or no clinical significance and are in any case untreatable.

Lampas/inflammation of the hard palate (Fig. 1.25)

Lampas or inflammation/edema of the mucosa of the hard palate was historically regarded as a recognizable clinical disorder when swelling was sufficient to result in the mucosa of the hard palate being below the level of the incisor occlusal margin, warranting treatment. However, edema of the hard palate commonly occurs in young horses and is of no clinical significance. The disorder is occasionally reported to occur in older horses when irritant substances/foods are ingested.

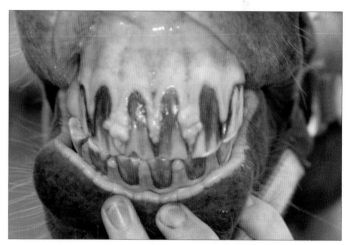

Figure 1.23 Epulis. Incidental finding in otherwise normal horse.

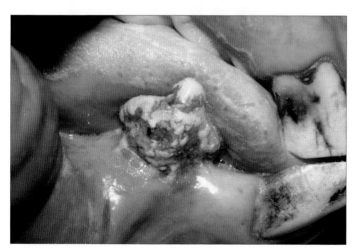

Figure 1.22 Dental tartar on a canine tooth.
Differential diagnosis:
- Incidental finding
- Chronic renal disease
- Equine motor neuron disease.

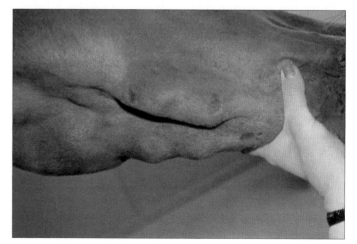

Figure 1.24 Benign dental lumps on the mandible of a 5-year-old mare. The lumps were cold, non-painful and remained in this form for the rest of the animal's life.
Differential diagnosis:
- Dental infection
- Dental maleruption
- Callus
- Neoplasia
- Soft tissue swelling.

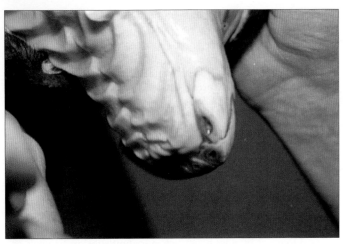

Figure 1.25 Edema of the hard palate (lampas) found incidentally in an otherwise healthy horse.

Diagnosis and treatment
- Diagnosis through oral examination.
- The main treatment is to ensure that diet is acceptable and causes no irritation.

Fractures of the maxilla and mandible (Figs. 1.26–1.30)

Fractures of the premaxilla or mandible are common, especially in young horses. The fractures may involve the whole premaxilla, but quite frequently only one or more of the incisor teeth are distracted and broken back from the alveolus. In the former cases the effect on dental eruption is likely to be minimal but the consequences of the fracture, if left untreated, are likely to be serious with little or no incisor occlusion possible after healing. The latter cases have more serious effects on eruption and less long-term serious effects on occlusion, although an individual tooth may be severely displaced or even fall out.

Diagnosis and treatment
- Usually obvious but radiographs are often required to determine the extent of the fracture and relationship to adjoining structures.
- Treatment is normally surgical; the method chosen is determined by the type of fracture involved. Antibiotic treatment is usually required as the mouth has a high bacterial load and there is usually contamination of the fracture site. In some cases of maxillary fractures secondary infections of the sinuses may occur and require separate treatment.

Dental disease

Dental disease is grouped into four basic types:

1) Abnormal wear patterns
2) Periodontal disease
3) Dental caries
4) Infection of the dental pulp.

All of these are interrelated, and horses with one type will also have, to varying degrees, the other types of disease.

Abnormal wear patterns (Figs. 1.31–1.38)

The horse is anisognathic, meaning that the bottom jaw is narrower (by about 25%) than the top jaw. The molar tables are sloped at a 10–15° angle. Lateral excursion of the jaw during mastication favors occlusal wear of the buccal aspect of the lower arcades and lingual aspects of the upper molar arcades.

The extent of lateral excursion of the mandible during normal mastication is affected by the length of stem or roughage in the horse's

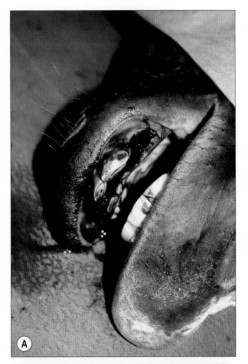

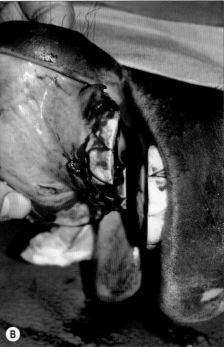

Figure 1.26 (A) Fracture of the premaxilla with obvious displacement of the incisors. (B) Placement of a cerclage wire for repair.

diet. Horses on pasture or hay have a wide area of mandibular excursion, whereas horses eating large amounts of concentrates have a more limited range of excursion with incomplete wear of the molar surface, predisposing the arcades to development of sharp edges or more pathological wear patterns.

Almost every normal horse, at some stage of its life, develops sharp enamel points along the lingual edges of the lower arcades and the buccal edges of the upper arcades. These enamel edges may result in

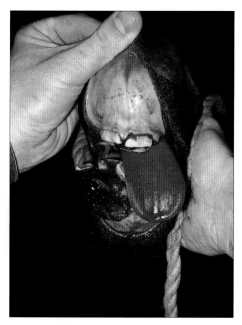

Figure 1.27 Fracture of the mandible in a young foal again with obvious displacement of the erupted incisor.

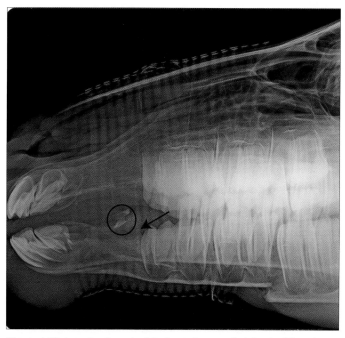

Figure 1.29 Lateral radiograph of the head of a young foal showing bilateral displaced fracture (arrow) of the mandible with bone fragments (circle).

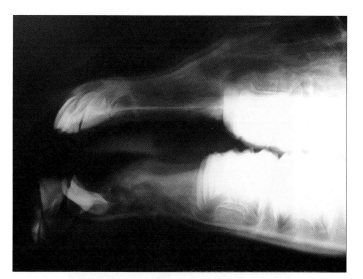

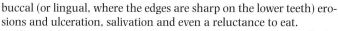

Figure 1.28 Radiograph of the head showing the displacement of the incisors that could be seen grossly (same foal as Fig. 1.27).

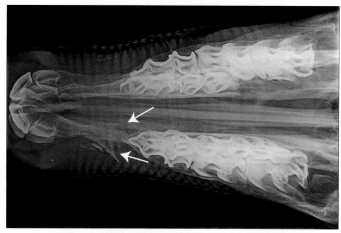

Figure 1.30 Dorsoventral radiograph of the head clearly showing displacement of the fracture (arrows) and bone fragmentation (same foal as Fig. 1.26).

buccal (or lingual, where the edges are sharp on the lower teeth) erosions and ulceration, salivation and even a reluctance to eat.

Abnormal wear patterns of the incisor and molar teeth may also be due to traumatic displacement or pathological softening of enamel. Painful or physical reasons for alteration of normal occlusal movements including oral ulceration, dental pain and/or abscesses, temporomandibular arthropathy, fractures of the mandible or soft tissue lesions, result in corresponding variations of wear pattern. Disorders inducing significant changes in the physical shape of the teeth have to be longstanding given the normal rate of wear of the cheek teeth being only approximately 3–5 mm per year.

Very old horses commonly have smooth occlusal surfaces even when they have no history of abrasive diets. In some cases the table of the molar teeth is completely smooth and concave and has almost

no enamel ridges. This severely limits the effective mastication of fibrous food and has debilitating effects.

- **Wave mouth.** Localized differences in the density of the occlusal surfaces of the molar teeth may also have marked effects upon the occlusal efficiency and the development of abnormal wear patterns. Alternate hard and soft areas in the structure of the cheek teeth or, more commonly, stereotyped chewing behavior, may result in the development of wave mouth in which either a series of waves develops on the occlusal surface or individual teeth wear faster or slower than their neighbors giving a much coarser irregularity of occlusal surfaces.

- **Step mouth.** In other cases, there may be one (or more) tooth which, often for inexplicable reasons, wears excessively. This

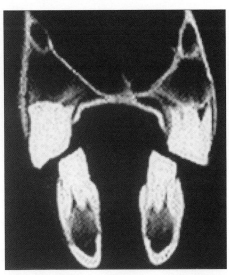

Figure 1.31 Computed tomographic image of a section of equine skull at the level of the first molars. Dorsal is at the top. Note that because the upper molars are offset laterally from the lower molars, the molar tables are sloped at a 10-15 degree angle from dorsal lingual to buccal ventral. Reproduced from Smith BP. *Large Animal Internal Medicine*, 4th edn. (2009), with permission from Elsevier.

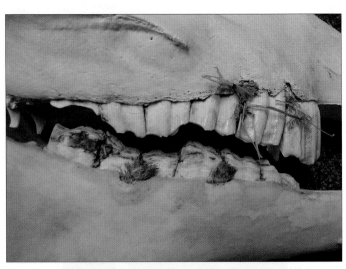

Figure 1.33 Step mouth: teenaged pony presented with a long history of quidding and salivation. The pony also had diarrhea with prominent long fiber fecal content. Euthanized because of the severity of the dental disease and the chronic sinusitis from alveolar infections extending to the caudal maxillary sinuses of both sides.

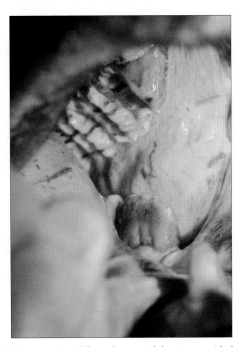

Figure 1.32 Wave mouth: middle-aged mare with long-term weight loss and slow mastication. Noted to have temporomandibular joint disease. This was assumed to be responsible for the abnormal wear pattern but the rostral hook was a longer-term conformational problem.

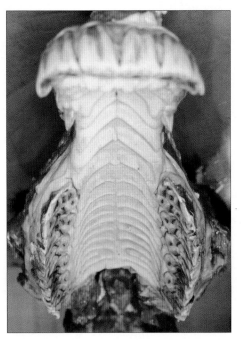

Figure 1.34 Shear mouth: 10-year-old Shire horse gelding with a long-term history of slow eating and weight loss. On clinical examination it was clear that he had restrictive mandibular movement: no lateral movement was possible. The horse had severe temporomandibular joint arthritis and it was likely that this had resulted in painful lateral movement over some years. The overgrowth was several cm in length over upper and lower cheek teeth.

results in gross variations in the height of the teeth (step mouth) and necessarily limits the occlusal efficiency. The full extent of the condition may only be apparent from lateral radiographs when gross variations in height and pyramid deformities of the crowns of the molar teeth may be present.

- **Shear/scissor mouth** (see p. 3). While the loss of lateral grinding movement of the molars, for any reason, will initially induce sharp buccal margins on the upper teeth, this may progress into a severe and debilitating **parvinathism** (shear/scissor mouth), in which lateral movement, which is essential for normal chewing, is prevented. These unfortunate horses are often noted to have an abnormally narrow lower jaw but, while under these circumstances it is regarded as a developmental deformity, the same dental deformity may develop as a consequence of a sensitive

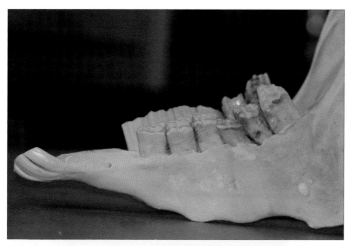

Figure 1.35 Overgrown cheek teeth. This skull was obtained from an equine slaughter house and was prepared because of the severe dental abnormalities.

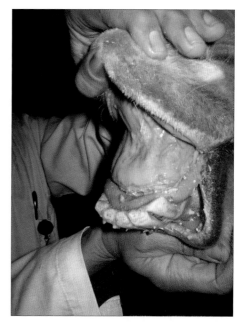

Figure 1.37 Severe crib biter with excessive wear of the incisors.

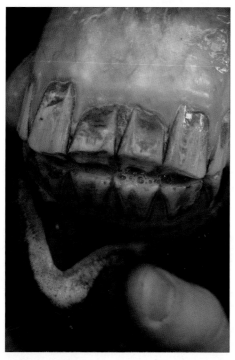

Figure 1.36 Mild (early) crib biter. Prominent wear on the rostral margin of the upper central incisors.

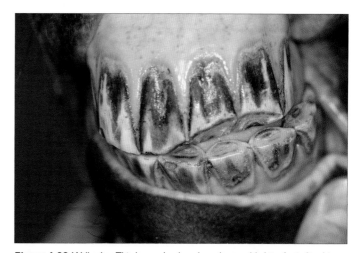

Figure 1.38 Wall raker. This horse developed an abnormal habit of grinding his teeth on the concrete edge of the stable wall resulting in an abnormal wear pattern.

molar tooth (or teeth) in the opposite arcade or from pain associated with the temporomandibular joints. This results in the upper molars becoming bevelled from the inside outwards with the lower molars worn in the opposite fashion. This deformity prevents further lateral movement of the teeth and seriously interferes with mastication. Under these circumstances extensive overgrowth or bizarre dental deformities may be encountered. This may itself induce secondary temporomandibular arthropathy as the animal attempts to chew with the sides of the molar teeth. It is, in most cases, impossible to identify whether the occlusal problem arose first and caused secondary joint degeneration, or whether the occlusal deformity is the result of abnormal jaw movement created by joint inflammation and degeneration. It represents one of the most serious deformities of the horse's mouth and carries a poor prognosis.

- **Sand mouth.** In areas where horses have, of necessity, to eat and chew large amounts of sharp sand or other abrasive substances the occlusal surface of the cheek teeth may become completely smooth and therefore ineffective as grinders of food. Failure to masticate efficiently results initially in difficulty with swallowing and slow eating. Weight loss, as a result of ineffective digestion, is commonly present. Under similar circumstances, because these horses are usually grazing very short pasture or having to find food in soil or sand the incisors may become severely worn down.

- **Overgrown cheek teeth.** Overgrown cheek teeth may arise from the absence of the opposite occlusal tooth. Such defects may follow either from normal old-age shedding, or from failure of normal eruption or, more often, from surgical extraction of one or more of the cheek teeth. Molar teeth with no occlusal pressure are likely to grow faster than normal teeth and in addition have no occlusal abrasion. The resultant loss of normal control of dental growth creates abnormal wear patterns which are usually visible as gross overgrowth. Pyramidal peaks on the tooth opposite the gap are common where the gap created by a missing cheek tooth is narrowed by angulation of the adjacent teeth but leaving a relatively small area of non-occlusion.

Normal shedding of molar teeth usually begins when the horse is over 25–30 years of age and the first molar tooth, being the oldest, would be expected to be lost first. Under these circumstances the scope for subsequent overgrowth in the opposite occlusal teeth is minimal and dental hooks, overgrowths or pyramids are usually of marginal significance.

The loss of any of the cheek teeth, except the first and last leaves a gap in the dental arcade, which may narrow significantly (and sometimes completely) with time as the adjacent teeth angle inwards. Although these defects may be less in size than the more dramatic overgrowth encountered in either the first or the last tooth the secondary consequences may be more significant and arise more quickly. Thus, limited overgrowth may result in gross discomfort and inability to chew effectively within months of the onset. Alternatively, overgrowth may continue unabated for years before any clinical effects may become apparent. Overgrowth impinges upon the opposing gingiva causing ulceration, necrosis and possibly infection of the ulcerated area.

- **Excessive incisor wear.** While severe incisor wear is sometimes encountered where grazing is short and large amounts of sand or other abrasive substances are ingested, the wear pattern of the incisors, in particular, may be influenced by behavioral factors. Crib-biting is a common vice (neurosis) developed by horses showing a characteristic wear pattern on the rostral margin of the upper incisor teeth which is variable in extent according to the severity and duration of the vice, and to some extent upon the structural character of the teeth. The earliest indications of the vice may be gained from close examination of the rostral margin of the upper central incisors where a worn edge will be detected. The persistence and severity of the effort involved in cribbing is often enough, even in young horses, to cause severe wear of the central incisors, often down to gingival level.

    Habitual grinding of the teeth on metal rails or concrete walls results in wear patterns involving, usually, the corner and lateral incisors. The pattern is usually such that it is hard to visualize any normal behavior pattern which could produce them. Usually only one side is affected.

Periodontal disease (Figs. 1.39–1.41)

Periodontal disease (alveolar periostitis) is a common significant dental disorder. The molar teeth are more commonly affected. Most cases are the result of food material and infection gaining access to the dental alveolus. Food of poor quality may be a predisposing factor. Horses in which the molar teeth are separated from each other by a gap and those in which gum recession and/or inflammation/infection of the periodontal tissues develops are predisposed. Gingival and alveolar infection results in progressive loosening of the dental ligaments, gum recession and potential penetration infection. Localized periodontal disease (alveolar periostitis) may result in localized abscesses within or adjacent to the affected alveolus. This may have secondary effects, particularly where the affected tooth is situated within the maxillary sinuses.

Secondary infective sinusitis or focal abscessation onto the face or into the nasal cavity are common effects of periodontal disease. Loosening of the cheek teeth may also be the consequence of degenerative disorders of the alveolar ligaments, such as occur in nutritionally deprived horses or in those ingesting relatively large amounts of

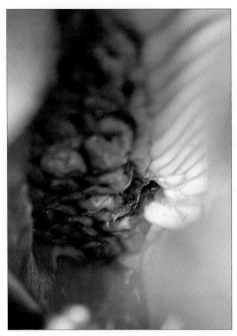

Figure 1.39 Periodontal disease. Young adult pony gelding presented with a fetid unilateral nasal discharge. Oral examination revealed a discharging sinus tract on the lingual margin of the first molar tooth. A fluid–air interface was present in the maxillary sinuses in lateral radiographs.

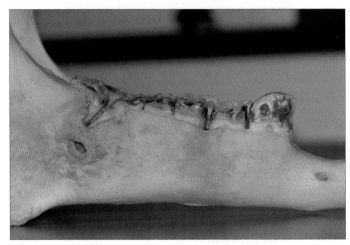

Figure 1.40 Periodontal disease. This skull was obtained from an equine abattoir. Note the area of bone lysis and new bone formation around the last cheek tooth. No external abnormality was detected in the live horse.

phosphate in their diet (see p. 220). Horses affected by pituitary adenoma (see p. 227) commonly suffer from degenerative changes within the dental alveoli and consequent loosening of teeth. Old horses have a natural slowly progressive loosening of the teeth which ultimately results in shedding but the process of natural shedding is seldom accompanied by prolonged or serious alveolar infection.

Dental caries (Fig. 1.42)

Dental caries is a localized, progressively destructive, decay of the teeth which originates in the enamel. Dental decay in the horse is not common although, where it exists, the consequences may be severe.

Incisor caries is particularly unusual and may be secondary to defects of enamel, fluorosis or other defects of dental structure. In

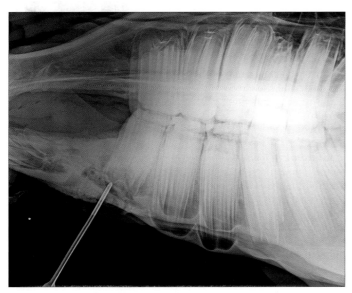

Figure 1.41 Periodontal disease. Radiograph showing probe placed in draining tract.

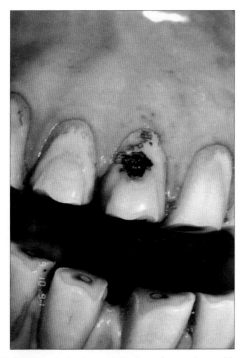

Figure 1.42 Dental caries in the central incisor of an aged mare. No alveolar infection was present and the mare was not apparently affected with either pain or discomfort.

some cases it arises from previous trauma, including cracks or abnormal wear patterns. Where caries develop in the temporary teeth, infection of, or damage to, the underlying germinal cells of the permanent teeth may result in a complete absence or deformity of the permanent structure.

Caries in the cheek teeth is much more commonly encountered, but is, initially, much less obvious, with the long-term secondary consequences of discharging sinus tracts or maxillary sinus infections being, usually, the major presenting signs. Infection within the pulp cavity of the molar teeth may arise from cement hypoplasia of

the maxillary teeth, and caries arising from the fermentation and decay of food material impacted within a patent infundibulum. The infundibulum is normally filled with cement, and when this is either not present, or is defective or eroded, food material may be forced into the cavity under occlusal pressure. The decay of this material produces organic acids and provides an ideal environment for bacterial multiplication. As the upper cheek teeth have prominent infundibuli these are most often affected by such necrosis. The defective infundibulum is often very small and difficult or impossible to visualize directly.

Infection of the dental pulp

This occurs most commonly in horses 4–10 years of age and is usually secondary to dental caries, fractures or splitting of the enamel layers from the sides of the cheek teeth. The two deep and prominent infundibular cavities of the upper cheek teeth provide a potential line of weakness in the sagittal plane along which fractures may occur. Sagittal or other fractures of the lower teeth are much less common, as they have no infundibular cavities and are in any case much narrower and denser than the corresponding upper teeth.

Horses with infection of the pulp are usually presented for signs associated with inflammation of the apex of the tooth. These clinical signs may vary depending on the involvement of local structures.

The second and third cheek teeth in the lower jaw and the third and fourth in the upper jaw are the most frequently diseased teeth in the horse. The first maxillary molar (fourth cheek tooth) is the oldest tooth in the mature horse and the most often diseased. The position of the upper teeth in relation to the rostral and caudal maxillary sinuses and their respective drainage pathways result in the characteristic clinical features of dental infections or defects of eruption/location in the upper arcade.

The rostral root of the third upper cheek tooth and the two more rostral premolars usually have roots which are not related directly to the sinuses, and infections in these induce focal facial swellings and discharging sinus tracts at the appropriate site. More unusually these drain into the nasal cavity, producing a purulent, unilateral nasal discharge and a characteristic fetid breath without any apparent deformity of the face.

Where the caudal root of the third upper cheek tooth (fourth premolar) or any of the upper molars are involved, sinusitis will generally develop. The rostral and caudal maxillary sinuses drain independently into the nasal cavity by separate drainage ostia. The bony barrier separating the caudal and rostral sinuses is seldom disrupted except by trauma or persistent sinus infection and a common drainage channel is only then available.

Most often the rostral sinus becomes infected and while drainage into the nasal cavity continues, appearing as a unilateral nasal discharge, distortion of the face just above the rostral half of the facial crest, will gradually develop.

Enlargement of the caudal maxillary sinus is usually less obvious as the drainage is more efficient and less liable to occlusion as a result of localized inflammation or physical obstruction from purulent material.

Lower arcade defects induce less extensive secondary effects and those involving even the most caudal teeth produce firm circumscribed swellings, usually on the ventro-lateral aspect of the mandible which may, or may not, be associated with an innocuous-looking, discharging sinus tract. The amount of discharge is often deceptively small.

Diagnosis
- History and clinical signs are frequently indicative.
- Individuals with occlusal difficulties of all types which result in poor mastication exhibit an inordinately high long-fiber content of feces.

- As a result of dental pain, or inefficient mastication (or as a consequence of some neurological deficits of sensation within the oral cavity), food material may become impacted between the cheek and the cheek teeth. In some cases this might pass unnoticed but in others an obvious lump may be visible.
- In almost every case of sinusitis with underlying dental disease there is an offensive necrotic odor on the breath, which will be restricted to the affected nostril.
- Many of the deformities of wear pattern are directly visible on oral examination. Radiography may be required to identify the site, etiology and extent of the defect.
  - Radiography with a probe inserted into draining sinus tracts will usually enable accurate identification of the diseased tooth. Usually there is some degree of radiolucency around the offending root and variable degrees of rarefaction of the root itself.
  - Radiographic examination of horses with purulent material in the sinuses as a result of periapical (or other dental or localized) conditions shows the presence of an obvious air–fluid interface.
  - Longstanding apical infection in the more rostral teeth may result in moderate or severe bone erosion and the laying down of soft, diffuse new bone around the area.
- Endoscopic examination of the contents of the sinus, and the roots of the associated teeth following trephination.
- Advanced diagnostic methods such as computed tomography (CT) may help to identify abnormalities of individual teeth.

Treatment

- Abnormal wear patterns require more frequent dental care.
- Delaying the progression of infundibular caries which predisposes to the development of many abnormal wear patterns can be done by cleaning, packing and sealing of abnormally large infundibular channels.
- Treatment of secondary complications such as sinusitis may involve trephination of the affected sinus.
- Use of antibiotics has been successful in the treatment of horses with apical infections in the early stages but frequently dental removal is required with subsequent treatment of associated bone and sinus infections.

Equine protozoal myeloencephalitis (see p. 436), **guttural pouch mycosis** or localized neurological damage following trauma can cause neurological deficits associated with cranial nerves IX, X and XII, which result in an inability to move the tongue and jaw effectively. Partially masticated food material accumulates between the teeth and the cheeks and there may be a loss of oral sensation if the sensory functions of the trigeminal nerve (cranial nerve V) are also impaired. Horses lacking in oral co-ordination and/or sensation frequently bite their cheeks and the tongue along its buccal margin.

Bilateral trigeminal neuritis of central origin with loss of motor function results in an inability to close the mouth effectively, and the tongue is seen protruding from the mouth. Other muscles innervated by the trigeminal nerve, including the temporalis muscle, and the distal portion of the digastricus muscle undergo rapid atrophy. Additional signs which may accompany damage to the trigeminal nerve include enophthalmos and a slight but obvious drooping of the upper eyelid on the affected side(s). Unilateral atrophy of the masseter muscle mass occurs when unilateral neuritis or damage to the peripheral course of the trigeminal nerve has been sustained or subsequent to local myopathies affecting specific muscle masses. Unilateral neuropathies involving the motor innervation of the tongue may be detected by careful palpation of the musculature of the body of the tongue. Unilateral atrophy of the affected side may be detectable.

Equine protozoal myeloencephalitis (see p. 436) and **polyneuritis equi (cauda equina neuritis)** (see p. 422) are also, on occasion, responsible for unilateral trigeminal neuropathies which are manifested by unilateral atrophy of the masseter and temporal muscles.

Vitamin E deficiency resulting in **nutritional myodegeneration (white muscle disease)** occurs in foals as a cardiac or skeletal form. In some foals the only sign that is seen is dysphagia with muscles of the tongue affected. There can also be severe swelling of the masseter muscles. There is marked local pain and resistance when the jaws are opened, and affected horses are understandably anorectic.

Tetanus (see p. 438) also results in a marked resistance to jaw movement but in all cases of this condition there are other signs which are usually more prominent.

Part 2: The tongue

Position and function

The position of the tongue (Figs. 1.43 & 1.44) may reflect abnormalities of function and/or local damage or disease.

Fracture/dislocation of the mandible and/or *fracture of the stylohyoid bone* usually manifest as a dropped jaw with dysfunction of the tongue, and abnormalities of mastication and deglutition. Where the condition has been present for a considerable time there may be obvious concurrent masseter atrophy which in these cases is usually bilateral.

Excessive tension on the tongue during examination may induce severe tearing of the frenulum or, sometimes, even fracture of the hyoid bone. In the former case healing is usually rapid and complete with minimal scarring and disability although some tongue flaccidity is commonly present for months. In the latter there may be moderate or severe, transient or permanent, neurological damage as a result of traumatic disruption of the cranial nerves within the guttural pouch. In both cases, loss of tongue tone and dysphagia might be encountered, particularly if there are concurrent neurological deficits.

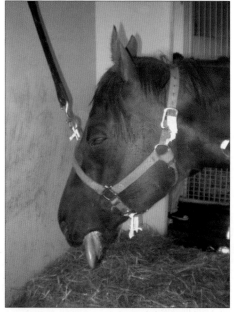

Figure 1.43 Protrusion and swelling of the tongue due to infection secondary to a wire foreign body.

Hypoxic ischemic encephalopathy in foals can result in tongue protrusion as a clinical sign. It may occur as the only clinical sign or be accompanied by other signs. In some cases the tongue cannot be withdrawn into the mouth or has a noticeably poor withdrawal tone when pulled gently. If accompanied by pharyngeal paralysis inhalation pneumonia is a possible sequel.

Tongue sucking is a well-recognized behavioral problem of adult horses and usually occurs without concurrent dysphagia in spite of the tongue having an apparently flaccid character. No overt neurological or physical disorder can usually be established and the condition is usually without serious clinical significance. Racing horses fitted with tongue ties frequently protrude the tongue during and after racing and this is, again, usually of no importance.

Botulism results in tongue flaccidity which is regarded as a cardinal sign of the disease. The disorder has few other pathognomonic signs and horses of all ages suffering from an apparent tongue paralysis should be carefully assessed for this possibility.

Encephalomyelitides, including the Togaviral encephalitides, heavy metal poisoning (such as lead and mercury), yellow star thistle poisoning (nigropallidal encephalomalacia) and leukoencephalomalacia (moldy corn poisoning/aflatoxicosis), may all have marked effects upon the function of the tongue and the ability of the affected horse to prehend and masticate effectively. Most of these are characterized by a flaccid paralysis of the tongue with saliva accumulations and overflow.

Diagnosis and treatment of abnormal tongue position/function

- Clinical signs and physical examination. In many instances it may be necessary to rule out each condition individually before a diagnosis can be reached.
- Localization of neurological lesions may be difficult in many cases. Radiographs/ultrasonography or advanced imaging techniques are required to detect fractures or dislocations.

Treatment will depend on the underlying cause with some having a better prognosis for full recovery than others.

Traumatic lesions involving the tongue (Figs. 1.45 & 1.46)

These occur relatively commonly in the horse. The blood supply to the tongue and the buccal mucosa is good and rapid healing is usual with these, and other oral lesions. Although the trauma may be extensive, the function of the tongue may still be adequate after the wounds have healed.

Hyperkeratinized oral mucosa (Fig. 1.47)

This is an unusual inflammatory response to oral insults. The changes are usually most prominent in the sublingual tissue but the reasons for it are not clear. Once the insults are removed and the mouth is allowed to heal, the abnormal mucosa is gradually replaced

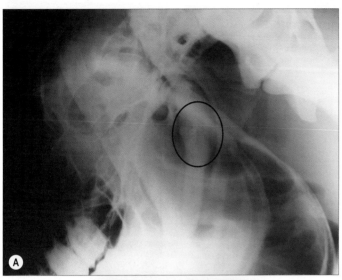

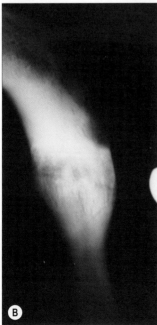

Figure 1.44 Fractured hyoid. (A) This lateral radiograph shows a fractured hyoid bone (circle) in a pony presented with an abnormal tongue position and dysphagia. This fracture shows marked callus formation and was assumed to be associated with a severe fall some months previously. (B) A radiograph of the hyoid bone removed during necropsy and shows the extent of the callus and the malunion/non-union fracture that is commonly a feature of this type of injury.

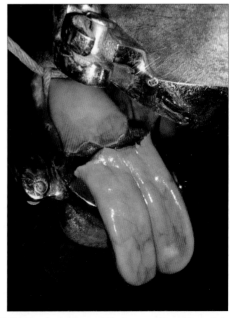

Figure 1.45 This 2-year-old Thoroughbred unseated its rider and then stepped on the reins, resulting in a severe tongue laceration. This laceration was sutured and the horse made an uneventful recovery.

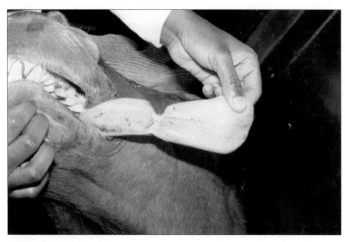

Figure 1.46 Some 5 years previously this horse had been restrained by the application of a tongue twitch. In spite of the severe constriction the tongue was mobile and showed no atrophy of the distal portion. The horse showed no apparent ill-effect.

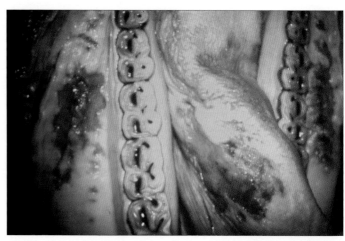

Figure 1.48 Oral ulceration: Chronic overgrowth of the enamel points on the buccal margin of the upper cheek teeth and the lingual margin of the lower cheek teeth commonly results in ulceration of the buccal and lingual mucosa respectively. In this case the ulceration was severe.

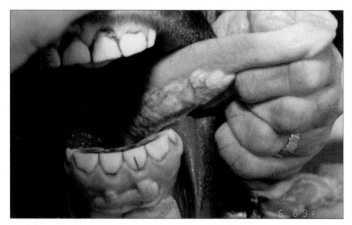

Figure 1.47 Chronic oral irritation accompanied by repeated episodes of salivation and dysphagia had been present in this case. Marked hyperkeratosis of the sublingual mucosa and the buccal surface of the lower lip became thickened and hyperkeratotic. A change in diet resulted in a gradual improvement until no abnormality could be found after 6 months.

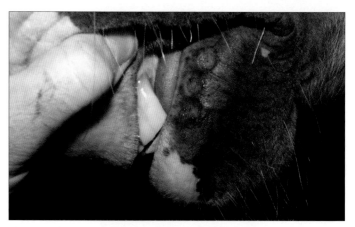

Figure 1.49 Viral (vesicular) stomatitis. Numerous ulcerated lesions were present over the lips, gums and muzzle.

and returns to normal. Affected horses should be carefully examined to determine the cause of the chronic or repeated inflammation.

Stomatitis (Figs. 1.48–1.50)

Oral ulceration and/or diffuse inflammation (stomatitis) may arise from ingestion of caustic or irritant chemicals such as organo-phosphate anthelmintics and including some medications such as enrofloxacin given orally. Diffuse, multiple oral ulceration occurs occasionally after, or during, medication with non-steroidal anti-inflammatory drugs. Oral ulceration may also be related to systemic disease such as chronic liver or renal failure. More focal inflammatory lesions may also arise from coarse or sharp food materials such as plant awns. The ulcerations and erosions which are seen in these disorders may appear to be similar but recognition of the underlying cause is very important when considering the treatment and prognosis.

- ***Bullous pemphigoid*** (see p. 321) is very rare but may result in severe ulcerative glossitis and stomatitis.

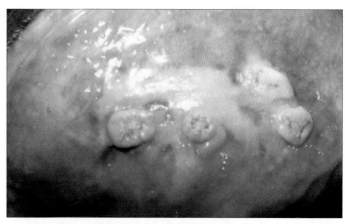

Figure 1.50 Typical lesions on the mucosa of the upper lip caused by the larval stages of *Gastrophilus intestinalis* (Bot fly).

- *Viral (vesicular) stomatitis* occurs rarely and there are usually large numbers of ulcers and vesicles over the oral mucosa, although in many cases these are limited to the dorsum of the tongue and the lips. The udder of mares and the prepuce of males are also frequently involved. The condition may be confused primarily with the appearance of stomatitis caused by irritant chemicals.
- *Gasterophilus spp. flies* (see p. 339) in the larval stages migrate through and within the tissues of the tongue, gingivae and dental alveoli, where they cause significant inflammation of the margin of the gums and the formation of characteristic circular raised ulcer-like lesions on the lips, tongue, palate and buccal mucosa. Similar lesions may also be caused by focal irritations from sharp grass awns.

Diagnosis and treatment
- History and thorough clinical examination are frequently sufficient to reach a diagnosis.
- Supportive care is the most important aspect of therapy. Severe ulceration/irritation may preclude ingestion of food and nutritional/fluid support may be required in addition to anti-inflammatory therapy.

Part 3: The salivary glands and ducts

Significant pathological disorders of the salivary glands of the horse are not often recognized.

Developmental disorders

Salivary mucocele (Fig. 1.51)
A salivary mucocele is an accumulation of salivary secretions in a single or mulitloculated cavity adjacent to a ruptured salivary gland. These may be congenital resulting from defects in the salivary duct or the integrity of the gland and can reach considerable size.

A more frequent cause of salivary mucocele is trauma to the associated duct(s) or to the glands themselves. These cysts are commonly noted to vary in size from day to day but ultimately they become large pendulous bags of skin which fill with saliva at irregular intervals.

Diagnosis and treatment
- Clinical signs are suggestive.
- Needle aspiration from these structures produces a viscid, saliva-like substance which may be slightly blood-tinged when of recent origin. Measurement of electrolyte concentration is useful to distinguish from hematomas. Salivary potassium and calcium concentrations are higher than plasma.
- Ultrasound examination may reveal obstructions in the salivary ducts as well as differentiating mucoceles from other masses.
- There are two treatment options: creating a salivary fistula into the oral cavity and/or removing the affected portion of the duct or chemical ablation of the gland.

Non-infectious disorders

Idiopathic sialadenitis (Fig. 1.52)
Idiopathic sialadenitis is encountered relatively commonly in grazing horses in particular, and occurs either sporadically or in outbreaks. Affected horses show a bilaterally symmetrical enlargement of either the parotid or the submandibular salivary glands. In some cases all the glands may be involved. The non-painful, firm, glandular swelling, which often develops within a few hours of being turned-out into the pasture and which may reach alarming proportions, resolves equally quickly when the affected horse is brought back into a stable. Salivation is not a prominent feature and this further suggests that it arises from direct inflammation of the gland rather than as a result of oral irritation.

Diagnosis and treatment
- History and clinical signs can be used for diagnosis.
- Treatment involves removing the horses from the offending pasture.

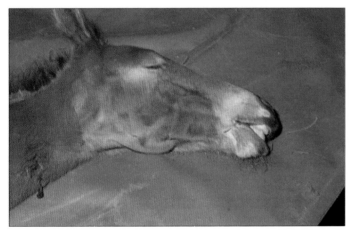

Figure 1.51 Salivary mucocele in a young foal. The lesion in this case was present from birth and fluctuated in size from day to day. Aspiration revealed a fluid with all the characteristics of saliva. The lesion is clinically indistinguishable from acquired salivary cysts.
Differential diagnosis:
- Sialadenitis
- Sialolithiasis
- Other causes of soft tissue masses: abscess/seroma/hematoma.

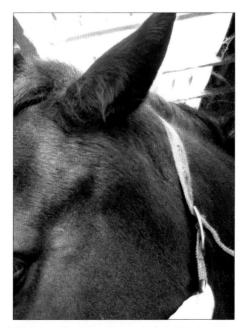

Figure 1.52 Parotid swelling (idiopathic parotitis) that develops in grazing horses (usually bilaterally) is a common event associated with some particular pastures. The condition is not well understood but it is assumed to be some form of parotid inflammation. Remarkably the swelling can be large but usually resolves within a few hours when the horse is removed from the pasture.

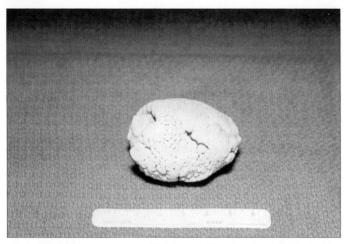

Figure 1.53 Salivary calculus removed surgically from the parotid duct.

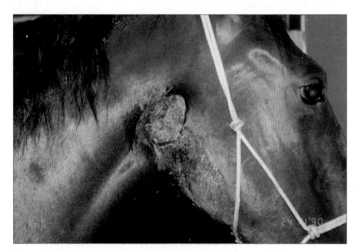

Figure 1.54 Acute obstruction of a major branch of the parotid duct by a calcium carbonate calculus (which was identified by radiography and ultrasonography) resulted in a gross, painful and hot swelling of the parotid salivary gland. The swelling burst onto the surface of the skin discharging a quantity of blood-stained saliva. The lesion failed to heal, becoming progressively larger and discharging saliva over 8 months without any sign of healing.

Sialoliths (Figs. 1.53 & 1.54)

Obstructive disorders of the salivary ducts are usually restricted to the superficial (Stenson's duct) and intraglandular portions of the parotid duct. Obstructions are most often due to sialoliths lodged within the common duct, often in the more distal portion where it passes along the anterior border of the masseter muscle. Sialoliths are usually spherical or oval and consist of calcium carbonate deposited around a nidus created by a foreign body or inflammatory cells originating in the gland or duct. Their size is very variable. The actual size may, or may not, relate to the extent of the obstruction. Thus, some very small calculi may cause more severe obstructions than the obvious larger ones and this may be more a reflection of the speed of onset of the obstruction and the rate of development of the calculus. Continuous enlargement of sialoliths occurs over some years, as more and more mineral content is laid down. Most longstanding cases are those in which the obstruction is partial and saliva continues to pass around the mass. In these circumstances the secondary effects upon the gland are minimal. However, where there is abrupt and complete obstruction a dramatic and painful enlargement of the associated gland is usually induced. Occasionally there may be localized obstructions within the substance of the gland itself. Obstructions sufficiently severe to cause rupture of the duct or traumatic disruption of the

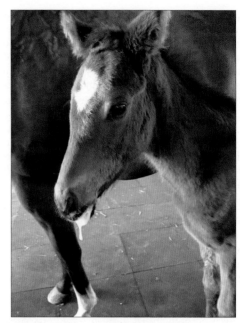

Figure 1.55 Ptyalism in a foal with severe gastric ulceration and marked bruxism.

associated gland result in the release of saliva into the adjacent tissue producing an acquired salivary mucocele.

Diagnosis and treatment

- Some will be evident clinically while others, especially those involving obstructions within the gland itself, may require radiographic or ultrasonographic examination for diagnosis.
- Treatment depends on the location of the obstruction. Surgical removal can be attempted through a buccal or external approach; frequent complications include permanent stenosis of the duct at the surgical site, chronic distension and mucocele formation. Alternatively the affected part of the gland may be removed or the gland can be chemically ablated.

Ptyalism (Fig. 1.55)

Ptyalism (excessive salivation) is seen in normal horses under a variety of circumstances such as excitement, oral irritation and when coarse food is fed. Horses which mouth persistently on the bit may produce large amounts of foamy saliva at the mouth. This is seldom of any clinical importance.

Differential diagnosis

- Feeding on preserved grass products that contain the fungus *Rhizoctonia leguminicola*. The extreme salivation which is seen under these conditions is particularly severe immediately after feeding and usually ceases after withdrawal of the offending foodstuff.
- The migration of larvae of *Gastrophilus* spp. through the tissues of the mouth and esophagus.
- **Parasympathetic stimulation** induces a profuse but short-lived salivation, while parasympatholytic drugs and plants such as *Belladona atropina* reduce the extent of salivation and produce a dryer than normal mouth.
- **Grass sickness** (see p. 58) and any alteration in the function of the cervical sympathetic trunk (such as might occur in Horner's syndrome) might also influence the function of the salivary glands.
- Foals (and occasionally adult horses) which have **gastric ulceration** often salivate significantly associated with bruxism (see p. 61).
- Salivation may also be present in horses with **stomatitis or traumatic injuries** but this is most often accompanied by malodorous breath, sanguineous saliva and/or a swollen tongue.

- Conditions which result in dysphagia and/or pharyngeal paralysis, such as **grass sickness**, **lead poisoning**, **rabies**, **African horse sickness** and several others, may show significant overt salivation and pooling of saliva in the mouth and pharynx. The extent of salivation in many of these cases may be marked and attempts at swallowing may be accompanied by profuse nasal reflux of saliva and food material.

Diagnosis and treatment

- The aim is to establish the cause and should include an oral examination and examination of feedstuffs. Endoscopic examination of the pharynx, esophagus and stomach. Testing for grass sickness and neurological abnormalities.
- Treatment will vary depending on the inciting cause.

Infectious disorders

Sialadenitis

Active inflammation of the salivary glands associated with infection is uncommon as a primary disorder but may be seen secondary to trauma. The condition is painful and often accompanied by fever and anorexia. The presence of abnormal amounts of saliva should be differentiated from an inability to swallow normal amounts, such as might occur where a pharyngeal foreign body or intraluminal esophageal obstruction is present.

Diagnosis and treatment

- Physical examination reveals an enlarged edematous gland which can be confirmed by ultrasonography. Culture and cytological evaluation of aspirates may also be useful for diagnosis. If secondary to trauma it is important to try to determine whether there is duct obstruction.
- Usually consists of anti-inflammatories and antibiotics where indicated by culture results.

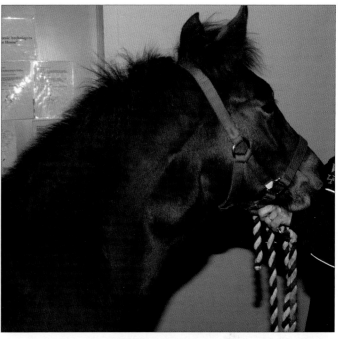

Figure 1.56 This 14-month-old Welsh pony gelding was presented with weight loss and some difficulty eating. The owners had noticed a fluctuant swelling in the right upper neck. Aspiration revealed a clear, mucoid ("saliva-like") fluid but no salivary enzymes were present. A diagnosis of an esophageal cyst was made. Surgical reduction was attempted but was not possible and he was euthanized.

Differential diagnosis:
- Esophageal obstruction
- Megaesophagus
- Laryngeal/pharyngeal dysfunction
- Esophageal stricture
- Extra-esophageal soft tissue mass such as an abscess or hematoma.

Part 4: The esophagus

Developmental disorders

Congenital disorders of the esophagus are rare but may include: intramural and esophageal duplication cysts, stenosis and strictures, persistent right aortic arch and idiopathic megaesophagus.

Congenital intramural and esophageal duplication cysts (Figs. 1.56 & 1.57)

These cysts are usually located in the proximal third of the cervical esophagus. The clinical signs associated with these include dysphagia and regurgitation. While most affected foals are not unduly distressed by their presence, weight loss and inhalation pneumonia are serious complications. Nasogastric intubation may prove difficult with marked resistance at the site.

Diagnosis and treatment

- Clinically many of these foals may be difficult to differentiate from cases of esophageal obstruction.
- Endoscopy may reveal compression of the esophageal lumen and in some cases a communication with the cyst. Ultrasonography may be the most useful form of diagnosis if the cyst is in the cervical esophagus. Plain or contrast radiography which reveals a filling defect proximal to the cyst. Aspirates from the cysts usually reveal keratinized squamous cells.
- Where they are causing esophageal obstruction surgical treatment is indicated. Complete resection or marsupialization of the cyst have been performed with fewer complications associated with the latter.

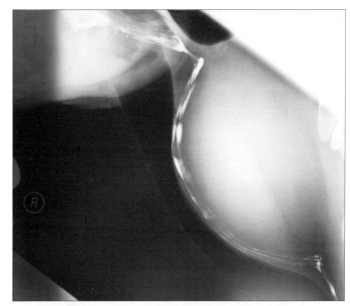

Figure 1.57 Contrast radiography of the esophagus, used to delineate the esophageal cyst. The esophagus is evidenced by the presence of contrast within its lumen. The radiograph demonstrates ventral deviation and compression of the esophagus.

Non-infectious disorders

Intraluminal obstruction (Figs. 1.58–1.63)

Intraluminal obstruction ('choke') is probably the commonest disorder involving the esophagus of the horse. The most common causes of obstruction are the ingestion of food of abnormal consistency, and foreign bodies. Even small amounts of dry feed, such as (dry) sugar beet or cubed/pelleted feed, may cause intraluminal obstruction. Greedy feeders, horses which are poorly fed at irregular intervals, horses with prior esophageal trauma and those with dental disease are particularly liable to the condition. The condition is also relatively

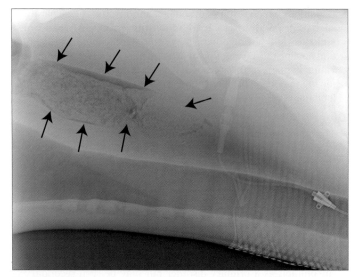

Figure 1.60 Radiographic image of the proximal esophagus demonstrating an esophageal impaction (arrows). Note also the distension of the esophagus at the site of impaction.

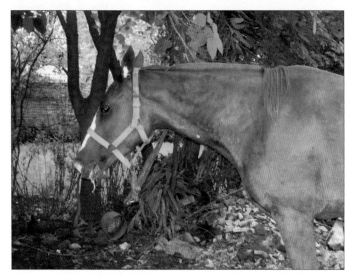

Figure 1.58 Horse with esophageal impaction (choke). Note the mixture of feed and saliva present at the mouth. Note also the extension of the neck and swelling ventrally in the mid cervical area of the neck consistent with the location of the impaction.

Differential diagnosis:
- Other causes of dysphagia
- Neurologic disorders
- Laryngeal/pharyngeal dysfunction
- Megaesophagus
- Esophageal strictures
- Intramural/extramural cysts
- Other causes of bilateral nasal discharge:
- Cleft palate in foals
- Oral foreign body.

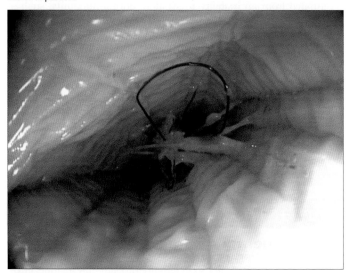

Figure 1.61 Esophageal foreign body as a cause of esophageal obstruction.

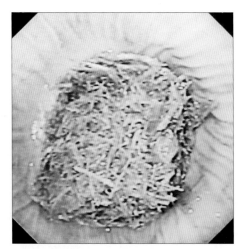

Figure 1.59 Endoscopic image of esophageal impaction with feed material.

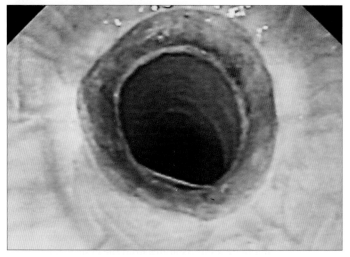

Figure 1.62 Endoscopic image of esophageal ulceration post clearance of an esophageal obstruction in a 6-month-old. This area of ulceration led to stricture formation. The foal was treated with sucralfate and corticosteroids and made a complete recovery over a 3-month period.

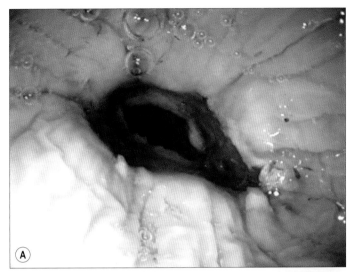

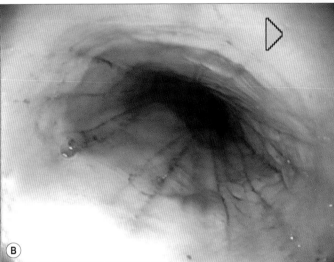

Figure 1.63 (A) Cranial esophageal circular ulceration; 2-year-old Thoroughbred mare presented with a history of episodes of esophageal obstruction. (B) Sulfonamides and phenylbutazone were given and the lesion healed completely within 3 weeks.

frequently seen in horses that are fed while exhausted or dehydrated (e.g. after a long ride) or those that are weakened by chronic disease.

Secondary impactions are caused by intramural or extramural abnormalities that prevent the passage of food. Examples include diverticula, strictures, tumors, cysts and vascular ring anomalies.

Some horses affected by complete intraluminal obstruction continue to eat, particularly where the obstruction is situated in the thoracic or distal cervical esophagus.

In some cases the obstruction is, at first, incomplete and results in proximal dilatation of the esophagus which, over time, may become complete with the proximal accumulation of fluid, saliva and food material. Repeated refluxing of this liquid-based material as a result of muscular contractions of the esophagus results in marked nasal regurgitation of non-acidic material which is salivary in appearance, but which may not contain any obvious food material. Sometimes, particularly in those animals with continued access to food, the esophagus may become filled with food material up to the pharynx. In these cases, and more rarely in the milder forms of choke, food material and saliva may be inhaled into the trachea.

Obstructions due to firm foreign bodies such as corn cobs, rough straw, wood shavings, potatoes, apples, carrots, etc. are potentially more serious than the diffuse type of obstruction associated with dry roughage or beet pulp. These obstructions may be partial or complete, and the firm nature of most such objects results in significant local spasm of the esophagus around the foreign body. Variable degrees of mucosal ulceration develop. Limited depth (mucosal), longitudinal or linear ulceration is relatively common and may take the form of a single broad ulcer or multiple, finer, short, linear lesions. These shallow, mucosal ulcers have little long-term consequence and heal rapidly. Circumferential ulceration involving the mucosa only, or the mucosa and the superficial muscular layers, or more severe lesions affecting the deeper layers of the wall of the esophagus may be visualized endoscopically, and occurs particularly with rough or sharp foreign bodies. The circumferential nature of these lesions makes their long-term consequences more serious than the longitudinal ulcers. Fibrous (scar tissue) strictures commonly develop some days or weeks later. Acquired strictures may be sufficiently severe to cause repeated episodes of choke which are usually progressive in severity.

Usually there is an acute onset of clinical signs which include anxiousness and standing with the neck extended. Gagging and retching may be noted as may repeated attempts at swallowing, especially with proximal obstructions.

Pain appears to be most severe with foreign body obstruction as opposed to the more diffuse impactive condition caused by dry feeds. Profuse salivation and the nasal regurgitation of saliva mixed with food particles is usually present, particularly after swallowing attempts. Rarely, some blood may be present in the regurgitated food and saliva. The esophagus may be visibly distended or the obstruction may be palpable. Crepitus or cellulitis may be evident in some cases suggesting esophageal rupture. Longstanding cases may have an unpleasant, fetid breath. Inhalation pneumonia may be evident in some adult cases and is frequently encountered in foals with choke.

Diagnosis

- In addition to history and clinical signs the proximal extent of the obstruction can frequently be located by passage of a nasogastric tube or by endoscopy, or by contrast radiography.
- The full length of the esophagus of all horses which have suffered from any 'choke' should be carefully examined endoscopically. This is particularly important in cases caused by foreign bodies.
- Ultrasonographic examination of the cervical region is useful not only to help determine the location, nature and extent of the impaction but also the esophageal wall thickness and integrity.
- Endoscopic examination of the trachea is also important to determine whether any feed material or milk has been aspirated.

Treatment

- The primary goal of treatment is to relieve the obstruction.
- Parenteral administration of sedatives and/or oxytocin and/or intraesophageal instillation of lidocaine may help relieve the muscular spasm associated with the obstruction.
- Physical dispersal of the material is usually required and may involve physical massage if the obstruction is in the cervical region combined with gentle use of a nasogastric tube.
- Lavage via a nasogastric tube is often required and depending on the case and individual clinician's preference this may be done with a single cuffed/uncuffed tube and the head maintained in a lowered position (normally under sedation), a double tube method with a tube placed into the esophagus from either nares or by combined use of a nasogastric tube and cuffed endotracheal tube under general anesthesia.
- If the obstruction has been longstanding intravenous fluids may be required to correct electrolyte and acid–base abnormalities.

• The rate of re-obstruction is high and feed should be withheld for 24–48 hours following resolution and a softened diet fed for a further 48–72 hours.

Esophageal strictures (Figs. 1.64–1.70)

Esophageal strictures may be congenital or acquired following esophageal injury. Congenital web strictures usually occur in the upper third of the cervical esophagus and are seen most frequently in Haflinger ponies, although they have been reported in other breeds.

Cases of acquired strictures usually have a history of severe or longstanding esophageal obstruction, esophagitis from gastroesophageal reflux, trauma (internal or external) or esophageal surgery. Circumferential esophageal lesions are more likely to cause strictures than linear lesions. Acquired strictures may occur in the thoracic or cervical esophagus. In young foals, clinical signs of stricture may not be apparent until solid feed is ingested.

A developmental hypertrophy of the esophageal musculature (particularly that of the distal third) results in an unusual form of functional esophageal stricture. Clinical signs of esophageal obstruction typically develop only once the foal starts to ingest solid food but some foals with severe strictures may present with nasal reflux of milk shortly after birth. Recurrent esophageal obstruction is the main clinical sign. With chronic recurrent obstructions, megaesophagus may develop proximal to the site of stricture.

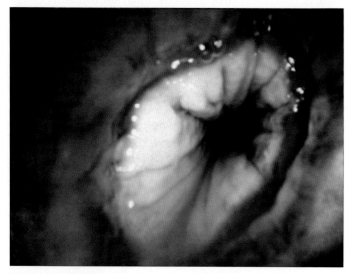

Figure 1.64 Esophageal necrosis in a 2-year-old WB colt. This necrosis occurred following a prolonged episode of 'choke'. The endoscopy image was obtained immediately following resolution of the obstruction. A stricture subsequently formed at the site and the horse was euthanised 40 days later.

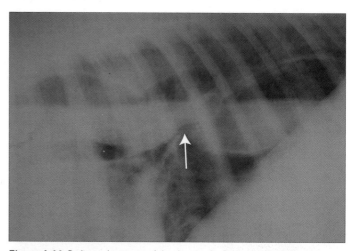

Figure 1.66 Radiographic image of the thorax of a 3-month-old foal with a thoracic esophageal stricture (arrow) and related esophageal dilatation.

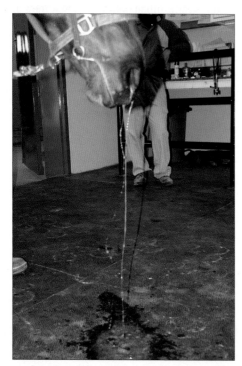

Figure 1.65 Feed material at the nostrils of this 3-year-old TB colt. He was presented for pneumonia which was secondary to an intrathoracic esophageal stricture.

Differential diagnosis: recurrent esophageal obstruction may also be seen with:
• Megaesophagus
• Neurological disorders
• Cervical/mediastinal mass
• Persistent aortic arch.

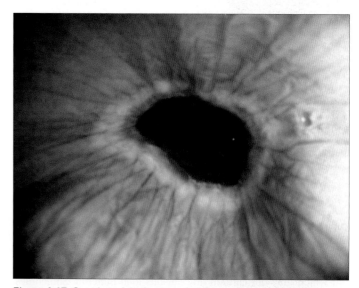

Figure 1.67 Cranial esophageal stricture in 1.5-year-old Friesen colt, which occurred subsequent to obstruction induced ulceration. This picture was taken after 27 days of medical treatment. Following initial medical therapy bougienage, balloon dilatation and esophageal ring resection were performed, but the stricture recurred and the colt was finally euthanized.

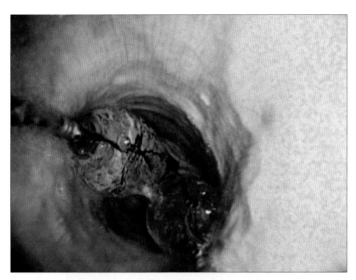

Figure 1.68 Balloon dilation of the esophageal stricture in Fig. 1.67.

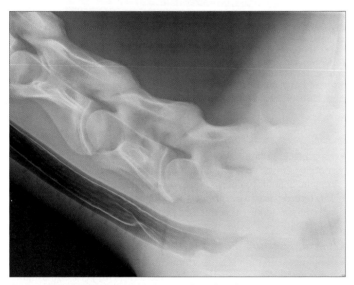

Figure 1.69 Contrast radiographic image of esophageal stricture.

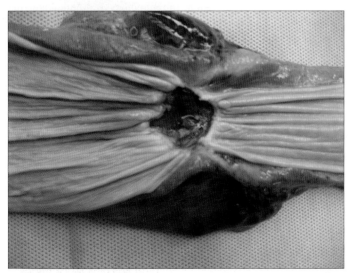

Figure 1.70 Post-mortem image of an esophageal stricture with ulceration.

Diagnosis

- History is important for identification of situations that may have led to stricture development such as previous obstruction ingestion of caustic substances, etc.
- Esophageal dilation may be evident proximal to the stricture on plain or contrast radiographs.
- With contrast radiography, an area of narrowing of the esophagus may be identified, however it may be difficult to differentiate stricture from peristalsis. Repeated contrast radiographs can be useful for differentiation. Double contrast radiography or negative contrast (using air) can confirm the presence of a stricture and may assist in determining the width.
- Endoscopic examination of the esophagus is important to visualize the extent and character of the stricture and identify concurrent problems (i.e. esophagitis, gastric ulceration).

Esophageal dilatation/megaesophagus
(Figs. 1.71–1.74)

Esophageal dilatation or megaesophagus in the cervical and/or the thoracic esophagus occurs occasionally and in spite of marked local changes the defects may only become apparent when dysphagia and inhalation pneumonia are present. The disorder can be congenital or more commonly acquired and generally only becomes apparent when the affected animal begins to eat significant amounts of solid food from ground level. The normal nursing foal may be regarded as being posturally fed in its early life, with liquid feed passing easily into the cervical esophagus.

Causes/differential diagnosis

- **Esophageal hypomotility** is the most common motility dysfunction resulting in esophageal dilatation.
- Acquired cases are due to **primary or secondary esophageal obstruction**. Primary esophageal obstructions result in a proximal dilatation which is normally reversible. If the obstruction is longstanding then the motility of the esophagus may be permanently affected. Longstanding obstructions are also more likely to result in esophageal strictures with a secondary dilatation. Extraesophageal obstructions include **tumors, abscesses or vascular ring anomalies.**

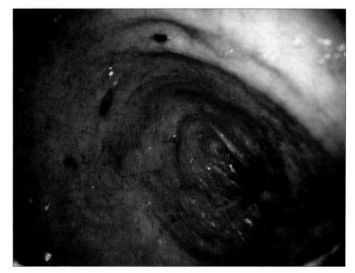

Figure 1.71 Megaesophagus endoscopic image. This 2-year-old Friesian horse was admitted with choke. He was treated medically with esophageal lavage. The initial esophageal dilation found during endoscopy was considered to be post-obstructive megaesophagus.

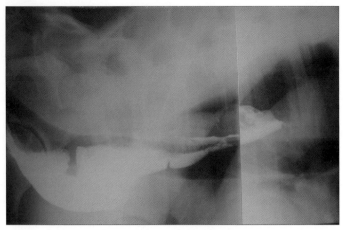

Figure 1.72 Contrast radiography of the horse in Fig. 1.71 clearly demonstarting a megaesophagus. The radiograph was taken 30 min after administration of barium contrast. The horse was readmitted to the hospital for another episode of choke two weeks later; at that time, a functional or anatomical cause of the choke was suspected. The horse is now managed by elevated feeding, and at a four year follow up was doing well.

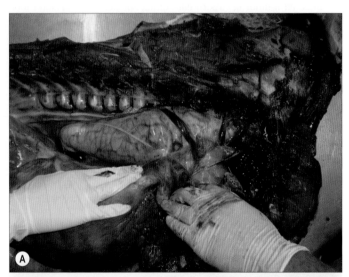

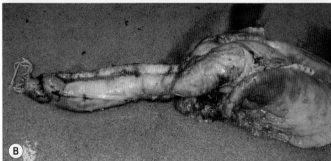

Figure 1.73 (A, B) Post-mortem images of an intrathoracic megaesophagus.

- **Pleuropneumonia** can also result in a **vagal neuropathy** resulting in megaesophagus.
- Neurologic disorders such as EPM, equine herpesvirus myeloencephalopathy, botulism, equine dysautonomia and idiopathic vagal neuropathy.

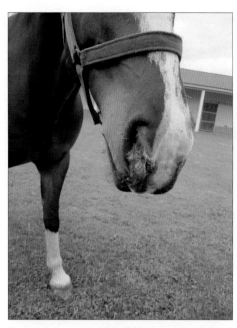

Figure 1.74 Feed at the nostrils of this adult horse with esophageal dysfunction of unknown origin. This horse did not show any pain associated with swallowing and plain radiographs of the esophagus were normal. Transit studies were not performed due to financial restrictions. Endoscopic examination of the guttural pouches and esophagus did not reveal any obvious abnormalities. The owner reported that the condition had occurred suddenly. The horse was treated with anti-inflammatories and elevated feeding and made a complete recovery over a 2-month period.

- Esophageal inflammation, such as **reflux esophagitis**, may affect motility. However, as hypomotility may cause relux esophagitis it may be difficult to differentiate cause and effect.
- **Iatrogenic megaesophagus** may occur with the use of the α_2-adrenergic agonist detomidine. This is usually reversible but may complicate diagnostic studies.

Clinical signs and diagnosis

- Esophageal dilation is a functional obstruction and as such clinical signs are similar to esophageal obstruction with ptyalism, dysphagia and nasal discharge of saliva and food material.
- Endoscopic and radiographic examinations of the cervical and thoracic esophagus may reveal intraluminal or extraluminal obstructions, esophagitis or strictures.
- Demonstration of hypomotility requires transit studies. Transit time of a bolus from the cervical esophagus to the stomach can be measured using contrast radiography or fluoroscopy. Pooling of contrast material and absence of peristaltic constrictions also indicate esophageal dilatation.

Treatment

- Therapy is aimed at the underlying cause with dilatation secondary to strictures carrying a poor prognosis.
- Cases occurring secondary to esophagitis usually respond well to therapy with antiulcer medication and promotion of gastric emptying through the use of prokinetics.
- Other therapies include dietary modification through the use of slurries and feeding from an elevated position.

Esophagitis (Figs. 1.75 & 1.76)

Esophageal inflammation occurs in a variety of conditions and may or may not be ulcerative. Causes include trauma (foreign bodies, nasogastric tubes), infections which in many cases are secondary to prior

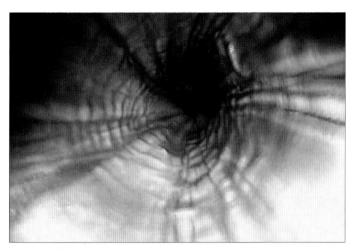

Figure 1.75 Endoscopic image of esophagitis in a foal with severe gastric ulceration and duodenal stricture.

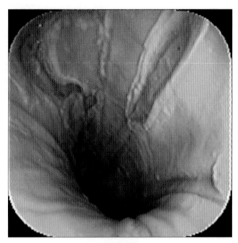

Figure 1.76 Endoscopic image of another foal with esophagitis as a result of gastric reflux associated with severe gastric ulceration. Note in this case that the esophagitis is associated with more discrete ulceration of the esophageal mucosa.

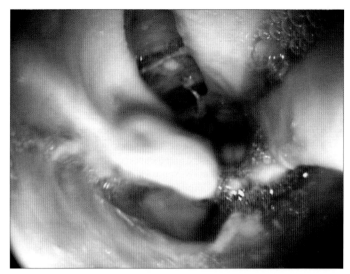

Figure 1.77 Esophageal diverticulum. 13-year-old Shetland pony presented with signs of abdominal pain and inappetence. Longitudinal ulceration (dorsal) and diverticulum (ventral) of the distal esophagus were present. The pony was treated initially with parenteral nutrition prior to re-institution of feeding, and antimicrobials and anti-inflammatory medications. The lesions healed over a period of 4 weeks.

ulceration or trauma, and chemical injury such as caused by some medications, toxic plants and irritant chemicals. **Chillagoe horse disease** in Australia, and '**dunsiekte**' in South Africa are associated with the ingestion of hepatotoxic plants of the *Crotalaria* spp. In these as with ingestion of irritant chemicals and medications, esophageal ulceration is particularly severe at the proximal end in contrast to the similar ulcerative esophagitis encountered at the distal end as a result of gastroesophageal reflux such as occurs in **grass sickness, gastric ulcer disease, motility disorders, increased gastric volume from gastric outflow obstructions, intestinal ileus** or **impaired lower esophageal sphincter function**.

Diagnosis

- Endoscopic examination of the entire length of the esophagus with critical assessment of the extent of the inflammation/ulceration.
- Endoscopic examination of the stomach should also be performed as esophagitis is frequently accompanied by gastric ulceration.
- Contrast radiography and transit studies are useful for assessing motility disorders.
- In instances where the esophagitis is related to ingestion of toxic plants there may be other more obvious cranial or hepatic signs.

Treatment

- The goals of therapy are control of gastric acidity, mucosal protection and correction of any underlying disorders such as hypomotility.
- Reduction of gastric acidity is achieved through the use of H2 histamine receptor blockers such as ranitidine or proton pump blockers such as omeprazole.
- Sucralfate is often used for mucosal protection although its efficacy in the esophagus has not been proven.
- Prokinetics can be used in horses with hypomotility. Bethanechol or metaclopramide can be used but many horses are sensitive to the extra-pyramidal effects of metaclopramide.
- Judicial use of anti-inflammatories is warranted in some cases, especially those secondary to trauma or pressure injury.
- Dietary modification may be required with frequent small well-moistened feeds.

Esophageal diverticula (Fig. 1.77)

There are two types of esophageal diverticula:

- **Traction (true) diverticula** which probably arise as a result of peri-esophageal scarring and subsequent scar contraction although some of these appear to develop without any apparent instigating factor. They may be encountered anywhere along the length of the esophagus, and some may be a result of a longitudinal developmental defect in the integrity of the muscular layers, particularly in the distal, smooth-muscle portion of the organ.
- **Pulsion (false) diverticula** arising from focal muscular or mucosal damage are potentially more serious, and present with progressive (variable) swellings in the cervical esophagus. Secondary effects such as local occlusion of the jugular vein and fistulation are more common with pulsion diverticula. In both types of diverticulum clinical evidence of 'choke' may be present and both may sometimes be seen to enlarge, momentarily, when the animal swallows. Nasogastric intubation is sometimes easy, suggesting that there is no obstructive lesion, while at other times the procedure may be difficult or even impossible.

Diagnosis and treatment

- Diagnosis of esophageal diverticula may be frustrating. Combinations of ultrasound, endoscopy and contrast radiography may confirm the diagnosis. Endoscopic examination will usually identify the site and extent of the lesion. Contrast radiography can be used to differentiate the type of diverticula. Traction appears as a dilatation with a broad neck while pulsion appears to be flask-shaped with a narrow neck.
- ***Differential diagnosis***: Any cause of recurrent esophageal obstruction (see above, p. 20).
- Treatment depends on the size and location of the lesion in addition to the presenting clinical signs. Some lesions may be surgically corrected but post-surgical complications are common.

Esophageal perforation (Figs. 1.78–1.81)

Perforation of the esophagus most often occurs in the cervical region secondary to external trauma or rupture of an esophageal lesion such as an impacted diverticulum. Iatrogenic perforation can occur as a result of excessive force with a nasogastric tube against an obstruction or in an area of pre-existing damage.

The esophagus is most vulnerable in the distal third of the cervical region as it is only protected by a thin layer of muscle at this point. Perforations may be open or closed to the exterior but both result in extensive necrosis as saliva and feed materials enter fascial planes. Bacterial contamination with anaerobic organisms is usual and, where this occurs in the cervical esophagus, the tissues surrounding the esophagus become emphysematous, hot and very painful. Closed perforations may result in extension of discharge as far as the mediastinum, resulting in a fatal mediastinitis and pleuritis. In general the prognosis is poor but some cases have recovered. In those that recover the incidence of sequelae such as diverticula and fistulas is high.

Diagnosis

- Diagnosis is usually obvious in horses with open perforations. Closed perforations will usually present with heat pain and swelling in the area. Crepitus may be palpated over the area.
- Ultrasound can be used to determine the site and extent of the perforation as well as determining the extent of associated cellulitis.
- Radiographic examination can be used to detect the presence of gas and tissue swelling.
- ***Differential diagnosis***: internal ruptures resulting in pleuritis may be confused with primary pleuritis; esophageal obstruction; esophageal diverticula; other soft tissue swellings (abscesses/seroma/hematoma); esophageal fistula.

Treatment

- Closed perforations should be converted to open perforations wherever possible.
- Extensive debridement, lavage of affected tissues, broad-spectrum antibiotics and tetanus prophylaxis.

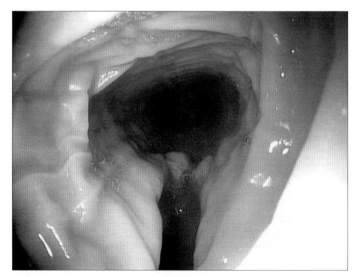

Figure 1.79 Esophageal rupture endoscopic view (same horse as Fig. 1.78).

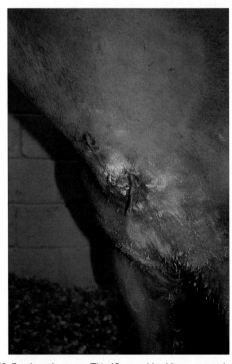

Figure 1.78 Esophageal rupture. This 15-year-old gelding presented with a swelling involving the caudo-ventral aspect of the neck which had been lanced by the referring veterinarian, revealing purulent material consistent with abscessation. On presentation, the pony was pyrexic and ingesta was observed to be draining from the incisions over the swelling. Endoscopic examination of the esophagus and contrast radiography using iohexol confirmed esophageal rupture and accumulation of ingesta, saliva and exudate in the surrounding soft tissues. The cause of the esophageal rupture was not determined, however external trauma was suspected. The pony was euthanised.

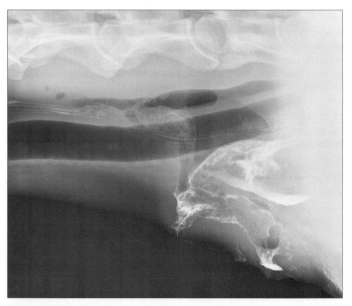

Figure 1.80 Esophageal rupture contrast radiography (same horse as Fig. 1.78).

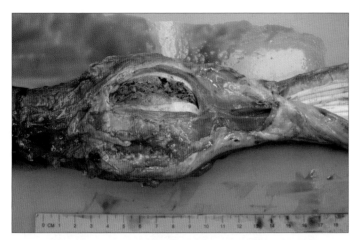

Figure 1.81 10-year-old Warmblood that had been treated for esophageal impaction over a 3-day period with repeated nasogastric intubation. On admission to a referral hospital there was copious discharge of food and saliva from both nostrils and crackles on lung auscultation. Post-mortem examination confirmed the esophageal rupture and subsequent pneumonia.

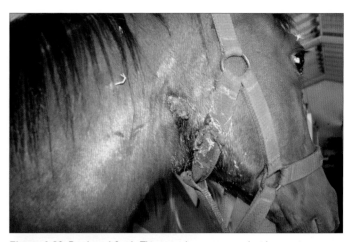

Figure 1.82 Esophageal fistula. This young horse presented with a previous history of strangles. The referring vet had reportedly lanced a number of retropharyngeal abscesses but in so doing had inadvertently incised into the esophagus.

Differential diagnosis: esophageal rupture.

- Esophageal rest is also required and can be achieved by placing a small-diameter nasogastric tube or directly through the hole in the esophagus in the early stages.
- Monitoring for acid–base abnormalities during the course of treatment is required due to the extensive presence of electrolytes and bicarbonate in saliva.

Esophageal fistulae (Figs. 1.82 & 1.83)

Fistulae which may discharge saliva and food material during swallowing are effectively restricted to the cervical esophagus. Most are sequels to internal ulceration, mural or peri-esophageal abscesses or necrosis; they may also arise from traumatic rupture of the esophagus. Where the fistula develops from lesions within the esophageal wall (such as a diverticulum) fistulation is usually preceded by local abscess formation in the esophageal wall and subsequent rupture onto the skin surface, with minimal subcutaneous involvement. In either case the persistent food and saliva contamination prevent healing of the defect.

Diagnosis and treatment

- Clinical signs: usually the fistulae are obvious but endoscopic or radiographic visualization allow assessments of length, diameter and proximity to local structures.
- Ideally, treatment will be surgical closure, but in some cases this may be difficult or impossible depending on the location of the fistula and proximity to local structures. There is also a high likelihood of stricture formation at the surgery site.

Infectious disorders

Oropharyngeal necrosis (Fig. 1.84)

Oropharyngeal necrosis with clostridial infection of the pharynx and esophagus is sometimes encountered following the use of long-term, in-dwelling, nasogastric and feeding tubes and is characterized by the development of extensive local myonecrosis and infiltration of the pharyngeal tissues with gas. Depending upon its severity and proximity to the pharynx, severe limitations to swallowing and, often life-threatening, pharyngeal swelling may accompany this condition.

Diagnosis and treatment

- In addition to history and clinical signs ultrasound and radiographic examinations reveal the presence of gas within the tissues and soft tissue swelling.

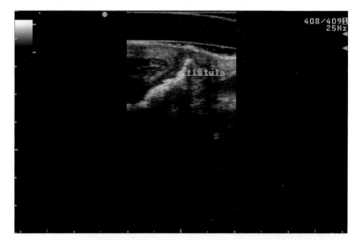

Figure 1.83 Ultrasonographic image of esophageal fistula (same horse as Fig. 1.82). Note the hyperechoic feed material occupying the fistula. The image was obtained from the right side caudal to the mandible directly over the cutaneous opening of the fistula.

- Treatment depends on the severity of the condition, underlying problems and secondary complications.
- Antibiotic and anti-inflammatory therapy are mainstays. The presence of gas within the tissues is suggestive of clostridial infection and if samples for culture cannot be obtained, therapy for *Clostridium* spp. (metronidazole, penicillin) should be included in the antibiotic regimen. If infection has spread into the subcutaneous tissues fenestration may be required to improve drainage.
- Esophageal rest may be required and would involve the placement of an esophagotomy tube.
- Secondary complications should be treated individually.

Esophageal abscesses (Fig. 1.85)

Esophageal abscesses are unusual but are associated with foreign bodies such as brush bristles or twigs. These present as focal solid or fluctuating swellings in the wall and may be sufficiently large to cause jugular obstruction. Other effects are usually minimal.

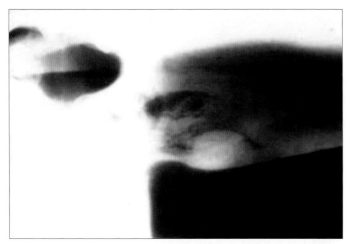

Figure 1.84 Esophageal necrosis. A long-term, in-dwelling, nasogastric (feeding) tube resulted in necrosis and clostridial infection (gas in peri-esophageal tissue). A large abscess developed at the site.

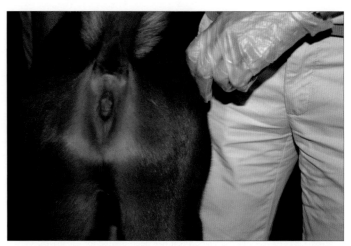

Figure 1.86 Atresia ani. Fortunately in this foal it was only the external opening of the anus that was absent and surgical creation of an opening yielded a good result.

Differential diagnosis: other causes of progressive abdominal distension with failure to pass feces:
• Meconium impaction
• Lethal white syndrome.

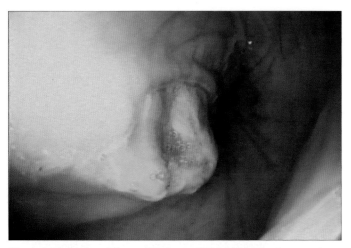

Figure 1.85 Esophageal abscess. This 4-year-old Polish Warmblood presented with a 2-week history of dysphagia. An intramural abscess was found within the lateral part of the esophagus. The abscess was treated with marsupialization and antibiotic therapy. This case had a good short-term follow up.

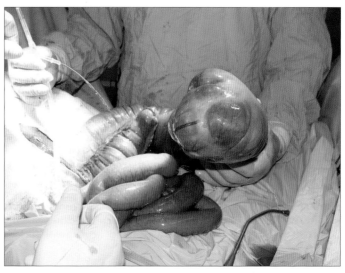

Figure 1.87 Atresia coli. The large colon in this case ends in a blind sac with subsequent enlargement in size due to failure of passage of contents.

Diagnosis and treatment
• They are difficult to differentiate clinically from a diverticulum or a mural neoplasia and the use of ultrasonography and endoscopy is essential.
• Treatment is usually not required but large abscesses may require internal endoscopically guided drainage.

Part 5: The gastrointestinal tract

Congenital/developmental disorders

Intestinal atresia: atresia ani (Fig. 1.86) / atresia coli (Fig. 1.87)

Both disorders are uncommon congenital abnormalities. Atresia coli, although rare, is the most common type of intestinal atresia and may be related to vascular accidents during intestinal development; it usually occurs in the region of the pelvic flexure, that is between the left ventral and left dorsal colon, but may affect any site in the large or small colon. Foals affected by either condition are born normally and appear to be normal for the first 24 hours of life. As feces and gas accumulate proximal to the blind-ended anus or section of colon, progressive signs of abdominal pain and distension develop. Atresia coli is associated with more severe and earlier onset signs than atresia ani. In some fillies with atresia ani, development of rectovaginal fistula will be associated with some relief of pain, depending on the amount of feces and gas that can be passed. In cases of atresia coli in which intestinal rupture occurs, there may be a transient period of improvement, based on lessening of intraintestinal pressure, followed by rapid deterioration within hours as septic peritonitis ensues.

Diagnosis:
• **Atresia ani.** The perineum should be examined for evidence of a normal anus. In some cases, the anus is absent. In others, an external anus is visible but not patent. If feces are present in or around

the vulva, vaginal examination for a rectovaginal fistula should be performed. If an external anus is present, a blind-ended structure may be palpable within the rectum. Proctoscopy can be used to confirm that a palpable obstruction is indeed atresia ani. Foals should be examined for other congenital abnormalities. Rarely, deformities (or absence) of the tail or vagina may also be present.

- **Atresia coli**. Diagnosis is more difficult because the lesion is not evident grossly; meconium impaction is often suspected initially because of the failure to pass feces and progressive abdominal pain and distension. Digital rectal examination may be highly suggestive as there will be no fecal 'staining' of the glove and only mucus evident in the rectum. A blind-ended lesion may be evident with proctoscopy/colonoscopy. Distension of the proximal intestine may be evident radiographically. Contrast radiographs (barium enema, barium series) can confirm an obstruction but not necessarily atresia coli. Exploratory laparotomy may be required for definitive diagnosis. Thorough examination for other congenital problems that may accompany atresia coli (i.e. renal aplasia or hypoplasia, hydrocephalus, cerebellar dysplasia) should be performed.

Treatment and prognosis

- **Atresia ani**. Prompt surgical correction is required, and has been successful in some cases. The prognosis with surgery is dependent, in part, on the amount of intestine involved and whether concurrent abnormalities are present. The prognosis is better when the anal sphincter is normal and the obstruction is only a thin, bulging layer of tissue. Affected horses should not be bred because of the possibility of a genetic basis.
- **Atresia coli**. This condition should be regarded as fatal. Intestinal motility problems or failure of the anastomosis have resulted in poor outcomes in cases in which surgical correction has been attempted.

Inguinal hernia (see also p. 48) (Figs 1.88 & 1.89)

Most congenital inguinal hernias are indirect, with the intestines passing through an intact vaginal ring and contained within the parietal layer of the vaginal tunic. Indirect hernias are usually reducible, are not life-threatening and usually resolve with manual reduction within a few days. A direct hernia occurs when the parietal vaginal tunic or the peritoneum in the vaginal ring region tears and the intestines become positioned under the skin. Direct hernias are normally

irreducible, contain large amounts of intestine, are life-threatening and regarded as a surgical emergency.

An uncomplicated hernia is any type of hernia which either does not contain intestine or contains non-incarcerated intestine. A complicated hernia is any type of hernia which contains incarcerated or strangulated intestine.

Diagnosis and treatment

- Hernias are usually apparent visually or detected by palpation. Individual loops of small intestine may be apparent under the skin in foals with direct inguinal hernias. The inguinal skin is thin and associated stretching may result in tearing of the skin or disruption of dermal circulation.
- Signs of colic are often but not always observed when strangulation has occurred but will develop as intestinal compromise progresses and intestinal distension develops.
- Direct inguinal hernias and complicated hernias are regarded as a surgical emergency. Indirect hernias depending on their size may be managed conservatively with frequent reduction or bandaging to facilitate reduction although bandage sores are a frequent complication.

Lethal white syndrome (Figs. 1.90 & 1.91)

Also known as *ileocolonic aganglionosis*, lethal white syndrome is an inherited, congenital condition that occurs in foals that are homozygous for the lethal white gene. It is an autosomal recessive condition that means that if two carriers (heterozygotes) are bred approximately 1 in 4 of their offspring will be homozygous or affected. Heterozygotes usually have the Overo color pattern, which is most common in American Paint horses but may also be found in Quarter Horses, Pintos and Saddlebreds. Most affected foals are entirely white with white irises, but some may have small areas of pigmentation on the forelock and tail. Within 4–24 hours of life, abdominal distension and pain develop. These signs are progressive and become very severe. Minimal feces are passed.

Diagnosis and treatment

- A white foal born to an Overo–Overo mating with progressive abdominal distension and minimal fecal production is highly

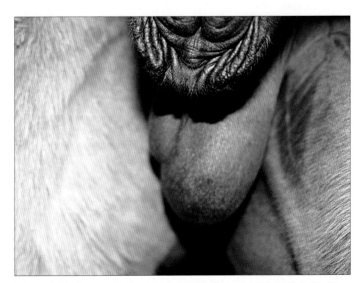

Figure 1.88 Congenital indirect inguinal hernia. Reproduced from McAuliffe SB, Slovis NM (eds), *Color Atlas of Diseases and Disorders of the Foal* (2008), with permission from Elsevier.

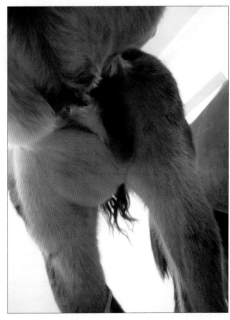

Figure 1.89 Congenital direct inguinal hernia. This foal had its entire colon herniated through the inguinal ring and was lying in a subcutaneous position.

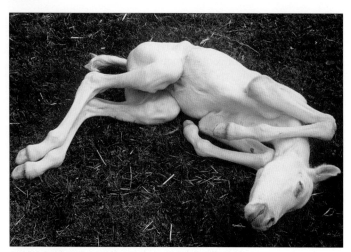

Figure 1.90 Lethal white foal showing early signs of colic.

Differential diagnosis: other causes of progressive abdominal distension with passage of little or no feces:
• Atresia ani/coli
• Impending enteritis
• Peritonitis
• Meconium impaction.

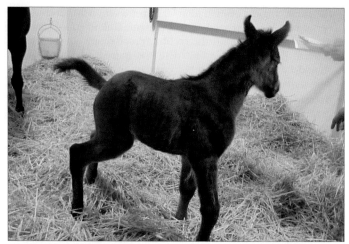

Figure 1.92 Meconium impaction. Foal showing typical attempts to defecate interspersed with signs of colic.

Differential diagnosis: other causes of progressive abdominal distension with passage of little or no feces:
• Atresia ani/coli
• Impending enteritis
• Peritonitis
• Lethal white.

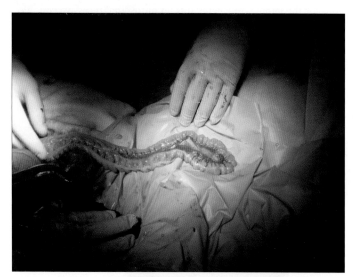

Figure 1.91 Colonic hypoplasia. No histopathology was performed in this case but it was believed that the etiology may have been some form of ileocolonic aganglionosis (similar to that found in lethal white foals). This was a 2-day-old TB foal that presented with early colic signs (at 24 h). Serial ultrasound examinations showed progressive small intestinal distension with no intestinal motility detectable on ultrasound or auscultation.

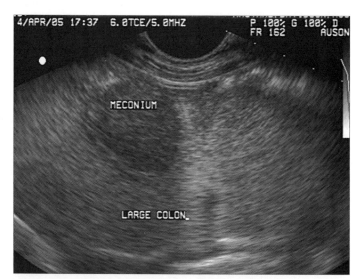

Figure 1.93 Ultrasonographic image of meconium within the large colon of a foal with meconium impaction. Reproduced from McAuliffe SB, Slovis NM (eds), *Color Atlas of Diseases and Disorders of the Foal* (2008), with permission from Elsevier.

suggestive. This history and progression of clinical signs is typically used to make a diagnosis. It should not be confused with colic in white foals born to non-Overo parents.
• Diagnostic imaging (ultrasound, radiography) demonstrates gaseous intestinal distension.
• Genetic testing can determine whether the foal is homozygous for the condition but is impractical considering the time delay.
• There is currently no treatment; this is an invariably fatal condition and affected foals should be promptly euthanized.

Meconium impaction (Figs. 1.92–1.95)

Normally, meconium is passed within a few hours of birth. Incomplete passage of meconium can result in abdominal pain and

distension in foals ranging from <1 to 2 days of age. Meconium may be impacted anywhere from the large colon to the rectum. Colts are more commonly affected as they have a narrower pelvis than fillies. Signs of abdominal pain, including dorsal recumbency, rolling, flank watching, anorexia, tail swishing, tail raising, and tenesmus are common.

Diagnosis

• Signalment and a history of minimal or no passage of meconium is often used for a subjective diagnosis. A history of passing a small volume of meconium does not rule out meconium impaction.
• Meconium impactions can often be visualized with abdominal radiographs.

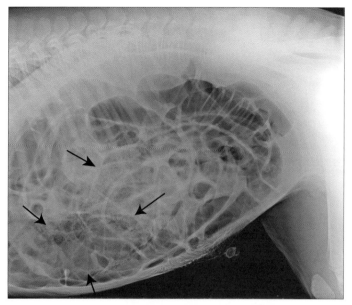

Figure 1.94 Radiographic image of meconium impaction demonstrating gaseous distension of the colon and meconium (arrows).

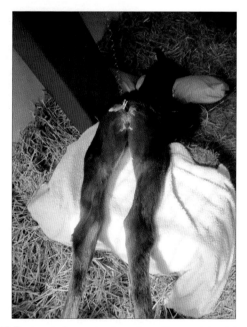

Figure 1.95 Treatment of meconium impaction with an acetyl cysteine enema. Sedation of the foal and elevation of the hindquarters allows for more cranial access of the enema; it is important however to ensure that ventilation is not compromised. Administration of N-butylscopoammonium bromide (Buscopan^R) decreases colonic spasm and allows the enema to work more effectively.

- Abdominal ultrasound is useful to rule out other causes of colitis, but may not consistently confirm an impaction.

Treatment
- In mild cases, a single enema (mild soap and water, light lube and water, commercial enema) may resolve the impaction. Intestinal relaxants may decrease colonic spasm and aid in passage of the meconium. Low-level exercise (paddock turnout) may also aid passage of the meconium following the administration of an enema. If there is no gastric reflux and a surgical lesion is not

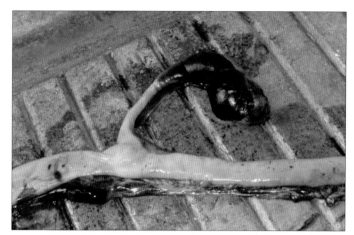

Figure 1.96 Meckel's diverticulum (at proximal ileum). Strangulated distal end of diverticulum which contained impacted food material and had been responsible for obstruction of jejunum and ileum.

suspected, allowing the foal to nurse may be useful to help stimulate intestinal motility.
- If there is poor response to a routine enema, an acetylcysteine enema is indicated. Concurrently, water or mineral oil can be given via nasogastric tube. Analgesics and spasmolytics may be required.
- If nursing is restricted, fluid and nutritional support may be required. Conservative over-hydration with intravenous fluids may also be useful in cases that are refractory to initial treatment.
- Occasionally, surgical intervention is required because of severity of pain or poor response to medical treatment.

Meckel's diverticulum (Fig. 1.96)
Meckel's diverticulum, which is formed from the persistent remnants of the vitelline (omphalomesenteric) duct, is also a possible cause of colic deriving from developmental defects. Although in many cases it never causes any problem, most affected horses are adult. The structure, whose lumen is continuous with that of the ileum, usually takes the form of a finger-like projection extending from the antimesenteric border of the ileum. Severe, strangulating colic as a result of this developmental defect is sometimes encountered in adult (often old) horses and the extent of the strangulated intestine is variable. Furthermore, impaction of the diverticulum with food material may result in recurrent non-strangulating colic. Rupture of the impacted and distended organ may cause fatal peritonitis.

Mesodiverticular bands (Fig. 1.97)
Persistent mesodiverticular bands, which are also possibly related to the vestigial vitelline artery, have also resulted in strangulating and non-strangulating obstructions of the small intestine. These present as small bands extending from the mesentery onto the antimesenteric border of the intestine. The band forms a potential cavity or hiatus into which small intestine may pass. Once entrapped through the space, strangulating and obstructive colic may develop at any stage and the extent of the entrapped bowel may be limited, or may include considerable lengths of jejunum.

Herniation of bowel through the umbilicus (Fig. 1.98)
This is occasionally encountered and can occur following natural or assisted deliveries. It is associated with traumatic rupture or excessive tension on the umbilical cord at birth. The extent to which this can be classed as a developmental problem is variable. Some foals may have particularly tough cords and natural separation may then be

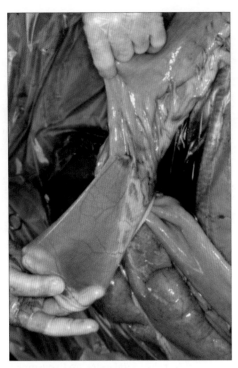

Figure 1.97 Mesodiverticular band.

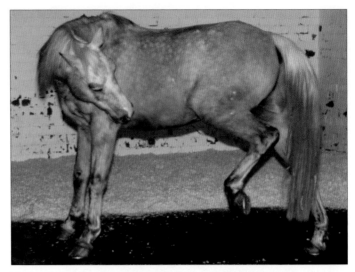

Figure 1.99 Colic. Flank watching and kicking at abdomen.

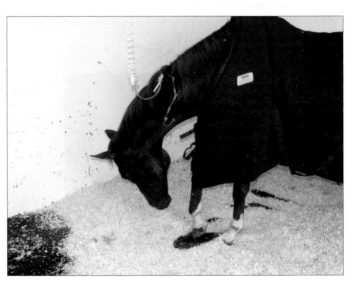

Figure 1.100 Colic. Pawing.

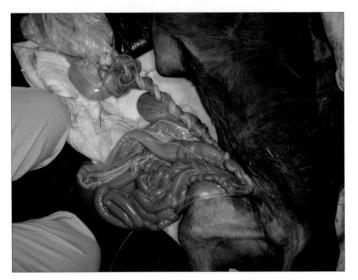

Figure 1.98 Herniation of bowel through umbilicus in newborn foal. Note uncut umbilicus.

inhibited. However, most are considered to be of traumatic origin relating to excessive tension or to abnormal parturient behavior by the mare, or both.

Diagnosis and treatment
- The diagnosis is obvious.
- Surgical replacement and closure of the abdomen is the only treatment option but in many cases there is severe contamination of the intestine and/or abdominal cavity resulting in severe post-surgical peritonitis.

Congenital diaphragmatic hernias

These may be very small or may be extensive and result in major interference at a very early age (or even in utero) and are possible

causes of colic in young foals. Lesions which are presumed to be congenital defects in the diaphragm are sometimes found incidentally at post-mortem examination of adult horses. Occasionally, however, they become clinically significant when loops of jejunum pass into the thorax and then may result in dangerous strangulating colic.

Non-infectious disorders

Colic (Figs. 1.99–1.117)

Colic is not a specific disease but is the name given to the syndrome of abdominal pain. This abdominal pain is most commonly related to disorders of the gastrointestinal tract, but also can be related to other organs or body systems giving rise to abdominal pain and even to pain elsewhere which may be interpreted as abdominal pain. A wide variety of intestinal obstructive and vascular disorders are diagnosed in horses and while many are of interest and occur commonly it is not within the scope of this book to provide a definitive description of them all. Horses showing colic as a result of abdominal pain exhibit a variety of clinical signs in combination.

Critical examination of cardiovascular and respiratory status is of vital importance in assessing the severity of abdominal diseases and

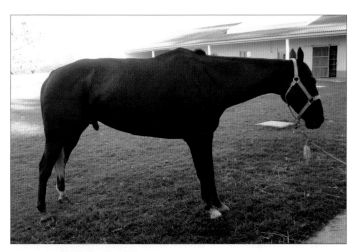

Figure 1.101 Colic. Stretching.

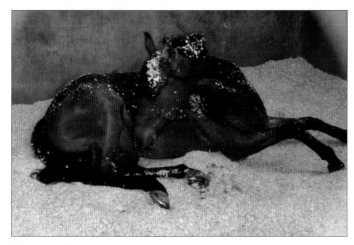

Figure 1.102 Colic. Lying down repeatedly.

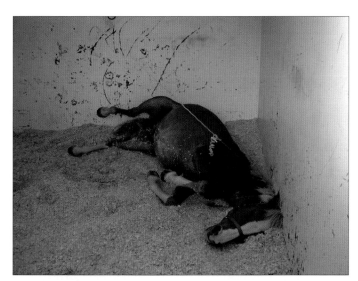

Figure 1.103 Colic. Rolling.

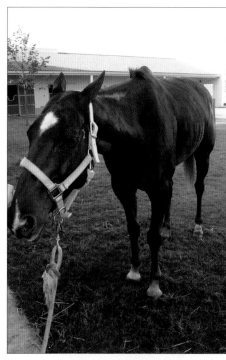

Figure 1.104 Colic. Generalized patchy sweating; may have cold extremities or other signs of shock.

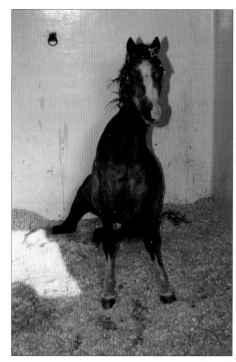

Figure 1.105 Colic. Dog-sitting.

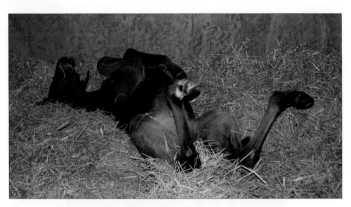

Figure 1.106 Colic. Repeated dorsal recumbency.

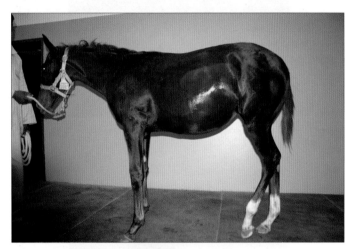

Figure 1.107 Colic. Abdominal distension.

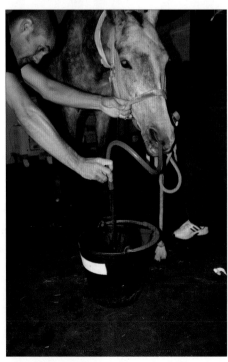

Figure 1.108 Colic. Gastric reflux.

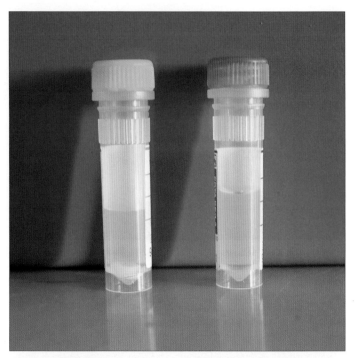

Figure 1.109 Normal peritoneal fluid is straw-colored and is usually present in limited volumes such that it may be difficult to obtain a sample.

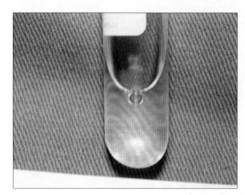

Figure 1.110 Clear peritoneal fluid. May be indicative of a ruptured bladder or ascites (accumulation of serous fluid in the peritoneum) which can occur with circulatory, hepatic or hypoproteinemic disorders.

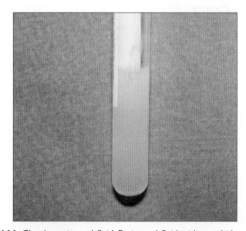

Figure 1.111 Cloudy peritoneal fluid. Peritoneal fluid with a turbid appearance (which may be slightly red or orange in color) is usually indicative of a high cell content and may be associated with peritonitis (either localized or generalized). In these cases the protein content of the fluid is also markedly raised and close examination of the cells will usually identify active and degenerate neutrophils.

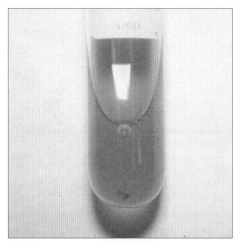

Figure 1.112 Blood-stained peritoneal fluid. Horses suffering from strangulating lesions of the intestine frequently have blood-stained peritoneal fluid.

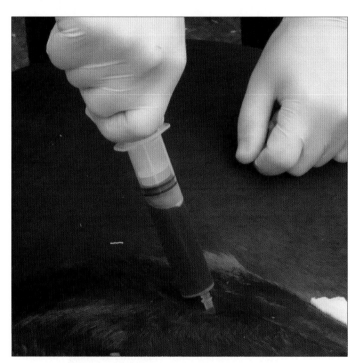

Figure 1.113 Cloudy blood-stained peritoneal fluid.

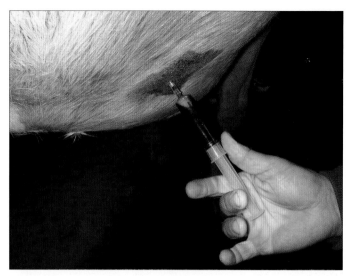

Figure 1.114 Hemorrhagic peritoneal fluid is indicative of intraperitoneal bleeding, such as might occur in horses suffering from verminous arteritis or rupture of the middle uterine artery at foaling. In these cases the hematocrit of the fluid obtained is usually slightly higher or lower than circulating blood (depending upon the duration and extent of the bleeding and its consequences upon circulating volume).

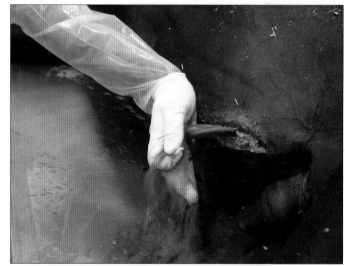

Figure 1.115 Contaminated peritoneal fluid. An abdominal paracentesis (which produces a fluid which is contaminated with food material) may arise from inadvertent puncture of an abdominal viscus (usually the cecum or ventral colon), or when an abdominal viscus has ruptured (usually the stomach, cecum or colon). The latter are invariably associated with severe, rapidly deteriorating colic with dramatic cardiovascular compromise.

disorders (see Figs. 4.39–4.45). The color and content of free **peritoneal fluid** is an important diagnostic aid in the investigation of colic and other abdominal disorders. Other important diagnostic aids are rectal examination, nasogastric intubation and ultrasonography.

For all practical purposes causes of gastrointestinal colic may be divided into:

1) **Obstructive disorders**
   - *Simple obstruction* (those lesions which obstruct the lumen but, initially, do not interfere with intestinal blood supply)
   - *Non-strangulating obstruction* (those lesions which result in extraluminal obstruction, but also initially, do not interfere with intestinal blood supply).
2) **Ischemic disorders**
   - *Strangulating obstruction* (in which the blood vessels are compromised, as well as the lumen of the bowel)

   - *Non-strangulating infarction* (in which blood supply is occluded without the intestinal lumen being obstructed).

The extent of vascular compromise in cases of gastrointestinal colic appears to be one of the most vital factors in the pathophysiology of the colic complex.

Obstructive disorders: Simple non-strangulating obstructive lesion

Simple obstructions can arise in all segments of the intestinal tract as a result of intraluminal obstructions, or pressure from outside the bowel itself, or from lesions within the bowel wall. Vascular compromise is not usually prominent in most of these cases. Initially the

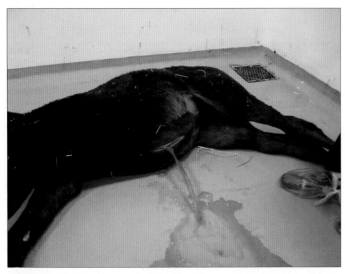

Figure 1.116 Cloudy/green/yellow peritoneal fluid is associated with rupture of a proximal viscus such as the duodenum.

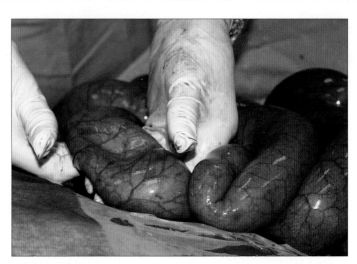

Figure 1.118 Ileal impaction.

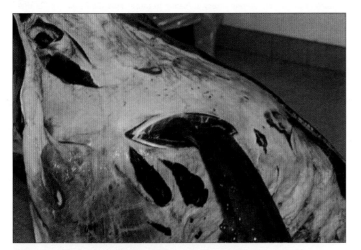

Figure 1.117 Brown peritoneal fluid. Very large volumes of brown/red peritoneal fluid with a high cell content (including abdominal cells) are usually a result of abdominal neoplasia such as mesothelioma.

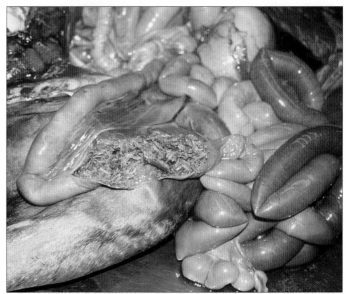

Figure 1.119 Ileal impaction at post-mortem.

mucosal barrier remains effective and affected horses are usually therefore in good metabolic condition, at least in the early stages. As the obstruction progresses bowel distension in the small intestine and increased intraluminal pressure in the large intestine may result in localized vascular compromise.

Obstructions within the small intestine are less frequent than those of the large bowel, due to the fluidity of the contents, although the ileum may become severely impacted.

The severity of the clinical signs and their rate of progression depend largely upon the location of the obstruction, with more proximal obstructions being more acute and more severe. However, even very distal obstructions, such as those occurring at the ileum, may induce a rapidly deteriorating and acutely painful colic.

Obstructions may be partial, allowing some food material (particularly the wetter and smaller particulate matter) to pass into the distal segments of the intestine.

Ileal impaction (Figs. 1.118–1.120)

Ileal impaction is an infrequent cause of moderate or severe colic. Gross distension of the proximal small intestine and, ultimately, the

stomach, with gas or fluid is usually encountered. Many cases have no apparent etiology but ileal hypertrophy or inflammatory swelling of the ileo-cecal opening are possible predisposing causes. Affected horses have frequently had a change of diet in the immediate past. The ingestion of poor-quality forage, or inadequate mastication of coarse fibrous foods, or water deprivation may be important factors in the disorder. Large accumulations of tapeworms (*Anoplocephala* spp.), at or near the ileo-cecal opening, may cause sufficient inflammation to result in narrowing and may be partially responsible for some cases of ileal impaction, particularly when this is accompanied by one or more of the other predisposing factors (see Fig. 1.239). Recent anthelmintic treatment in young horses carrying heavy burdens of ascarids (*Parascaris equorum*) may result in knots of dead worms obstructing the ileum.

Diagnosis

Rectal examination may identify a solid, distended ileum with proximal gas distension of the jejunum but more often there is little palpable evidence of the condition. The cecum and large colon are usually empty and few feces are passed.

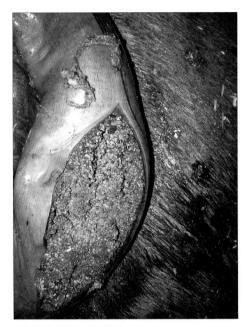

Figure 1.120 Ileal impaction with sand.

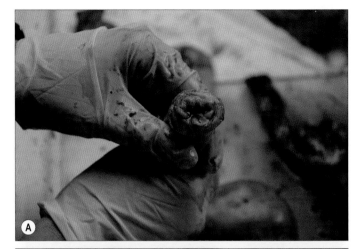

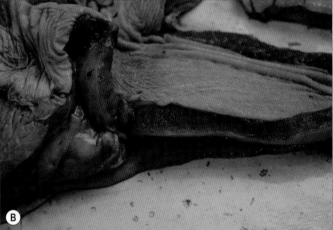

Figure 1.121 (A, B) Ileal hypertrophy in a middle-aged Friesian mare with a history of chronic colic and weight loss. The primary finding was chronic gastric impaction (stomach plus its content: 43 kg); there was distal esophageal hypertrophy present in the same case.

Ileal hypertrophy (Fig. 1.121)

Ileal hypertrophy results from persistent or longstanding partial obstruction of the ileum, either as a result of motility abnormalities or more usually as a result of ileo-cecal stenosis of inflammatory, neoplastic or neurogenic origin, ileo-ileal intussusception or parasitic lesions. While in most cases the extent of this muscular thickening is limited to the ileum itself, considerable secondary hypertrophy may be found in the distal segments of the jejunum, extending a considerable distance proximally. The presence of such a finding should alert the clinician to the possibility of chronic ileal or ileo-cecal obstructions.

Large intestine simple obstruction (Figs. 1.122 & 1.123)

Simple obstructions of the large intestine tend to have a more gradual onset than those of the small intestine. Ingesta impactions of the large intestine occur at areas of reduced luminal diameter such as the pelvic flexure and right dorsal colon. These impactions are a common cause of persistent, mild or moderate colic. Occasional cases may be more severely affected, particularly where there is gaseous distension of the colon and cecum proximal to the obstruction. The disorder sometimes follows ingestion of coarse, indigestible foods, poor mastication or reduced water intake (or combinations of these), or a sudden restriction in exercise which is frequently accompanied by a change in diet; but some cases apparently occur without any obvious etiological factor.

Diagnosis and treatment

- Most cases have a marked reduction in fecal output over the previous 2 days. Only occasional, very longstanding cases have significant small intestinal or gastric distension.
- Rectal examination is usually characteristic, with palpation of a firm mass in the colon. Significant impaction results in the displacement of the pelvic flexure into the pelvic inlet where the impaction is palpable as a firm doughy mass.
- The extent of the impaction may be severe in some cases but seldom, even then, warrant surgical interference. Cases are normally treated with a combination of oral and intravenous fluid therapy. The quantity of each administered depends on the size and severity of

the impaction, cardiovascular status of the patient and in many cases economics of the owners.

Sand impactions of the large colon (Fig. 1.124)

The persistent ingestion of large volumes of sand occurs commonly in horses with accesss to sandy soils and can be seen in some individuals as an indication of dietary inadequacies or idiosyncratic behavior patterns. Mineral deficiencies are often blamed for capricious appetites but there is little evidence to support most such claims. Occasional horses persist with the eating of sand and soil in spite of the availability of adequate forage. Fine sand tends to accumulate in the ventral colon with coarser sand accumulating more commonly in the dorsal colon. Distension from the impaction itself or gas proximal to the impaction leads to abdominal pain. Moderate persistent colic with an insidious onset is characteristic but some horses may show more acute colic signs. The mucosal surface of the affected bowel is also usually acutely inflamed and the motility of the affected portions is often first increased and then reduced. Fecal output is commonly normal in the early stages but becomes reduced and may ultimately cease altogether.

Diagnosis and treatment

- The presence of sand in the feces is usually of diagnostic help, and can be demonstrated by suspending a quantity of feces in water, when the sand will form an obvious sediment. In some cases,

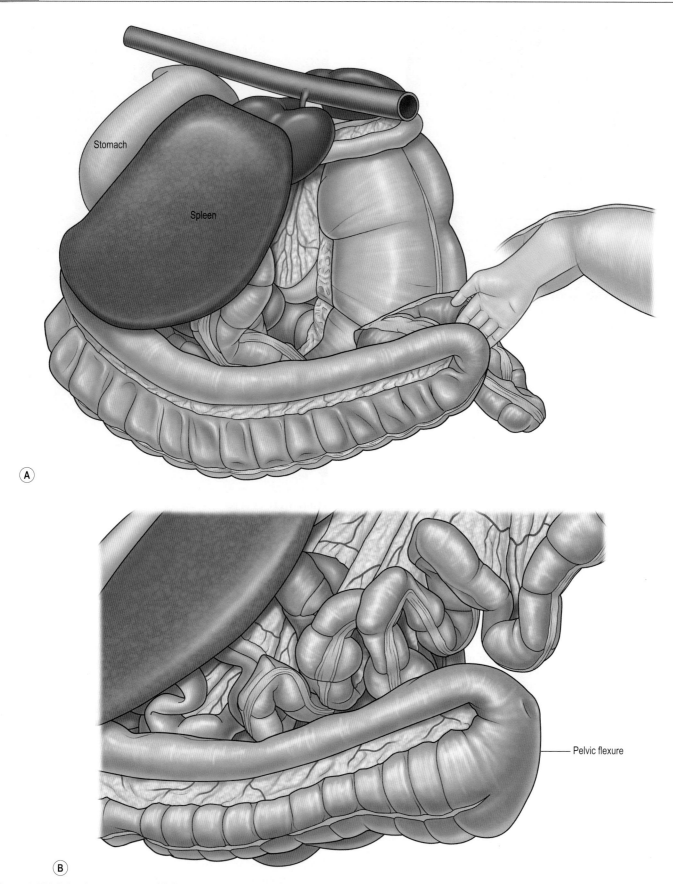

Figure 1.122 Pelvic flexure impaction. (A) Schematic representation of position of the examiner's hand when palpating the normal position and size of pelvic flexure. (B) Schematic representation of an impaction of the pelvic flexure. Note that the exact location of the pelvic flexure may change when impacted.

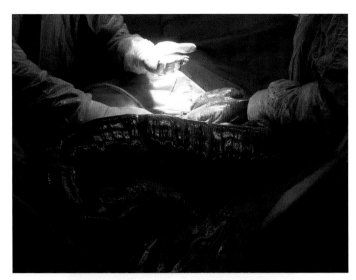

Figure 1.123 Pelvic flexure impaction.

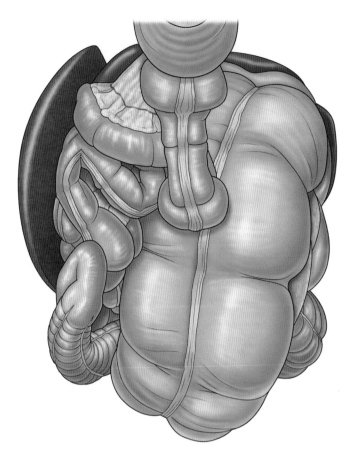

Figure 1.125 Cecal impaction.

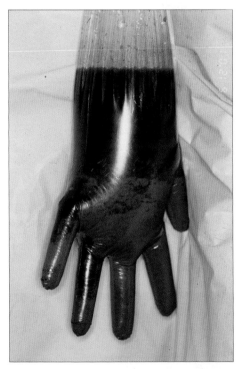

Figure 1.124 Sand impaction of large colon. Placement of feces in a glove and mixing with water allows for separation of sand contents to the bottom of the glove. While this is a useful test it may not always yield a positive result and abdominal radiographs should also be taken.

however, the feces may contain no detectable sand particles and in others the presence of sand may be incidental.

- The decision to choose medical or surgical therapy is largely dependent on the clinical condition of the horse, laboratory indicators of intestinal compromise and the size of the impaction as determined by radiography. Medical therapy frequently involves the administration of psyllium (0.25–0.5 kg/500 kg) either mixed with water or mineral oil and then followed by water administered by nasogastric tube. If mixed with water it forms a viscous gel and should be

administered rapidly to avoid blocking the nasogastric tube. It can alternatively be administered with 2 L of mineral oil and then followed by 2–4 L of water. Administration of intravenous and oral fluids may also be required. There is much debate as to the usefulness of psyllium but many anecdotal reports of its usefulness.

- Many authors advocate early surgical intervention and it is likely that the treatment plan chosen will be based on a combination of factors including economics.

Cecal impactions (Figs. 1.125 & 1.126)

Cecal impactions can be divided into two types:

- **Primary cecal impactions** that result from accumulation of ingesta or sand with an insidious onset of pain similar to colon impactions. Despite the insidious onset of signs, cecal impactions may result in cecal rupture prior to the onset of severe clinical signs of systemic deterioration.
- **Secondary cecal impactions** typically have a more fluid consistency to the contents but the cecum fails to evacuate these contents in a normal fashion. This type of cecal impaction has been particularly associated with hospitalization for another reason or unrelated surgical procedures that result in postoperative pain. Frequently there is a delay in diagnosing this type of impaction as the decrease in fecal output as a result of the impaction is often attributed to post-operative depression and the operative procedure itself and not to a cecal impaction. It is proposed in these cases that cecal muscular activity is abnormal but this has yet to be demonstrated. There is a subsection of this group of horses that have been shown to have hypertrophy of the circular muscle layer in the cecal base.

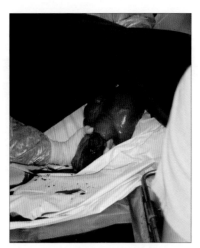

Figure 1.126 Surgical evacuation of the cecum through a typhlotomy. This horse developed a secondary cecal impaction following an unrelated surgical procedure, and was unresponsive to medical therapy for the impaction.

Diagnosis and treatment
- Rectal palpation is essential with primary impactions detectable as a firm mass. In some cases it may be difficult to differentiate cecal impaction from impaction of the large colon. Differentiation is based on the inability to move the hand completely dorsal to the impacted viscus because of the attachment of the cecum to the body wall. Secondary impactions are detectable as greatly distended masses with semifluid contents.
- Treatment of primary impactions may include initial medical therapy with aggressive intravenous fluids, nasogastric administration of fluids with or without magnesium sulfate, mineral oil or dioctyl sodium succinate and judicious use of analgesics. Feed should also be restricted until the impaction has been cleared. However, if the cecum is greatly distended or medical therapy has no significant response in a reasonable timeframe surgical evacuation via a typhlotomy is indicated. The exact length of a suitable timeframe is difficult to define as much depends on the cardiovascular status of the horses and presence of other related or unrelated complications. However, most clinicians would advocate surgical intervention if there is little palpable change in the impaction after 3 days of medical therapy. An ileocolostomy to bypass the cecum is also frequently indicated as post-operative cecal motility dysfunction results in a high incidence of re-impaction.
- Secondary impactions usually require a more rapid surgical intervention as the cecum is frequently greatly distended when diagnosed. However, unlike primary impactions, cecal bypass is not always indicated as long as the cecum looks healthy and the inciting cause (such as orthopedic pain) can be controlled.

Foreign body impactions (Fig. 1.127)
Ingestion of foreign bodies such as nylon carpeting or fibers from nylon-belt fences also affects the patency and progressive motility of the large and small colon in particular and may lead to obstruction. There are few pathognomonic features of these forms of colic but an accurate history may assist.

Fecaliths and enteroliths (Figs. 1.128–1.132)
Concretions of fecal material known as fecaliths (a hard mass of inspissated feces) or enteroliths (intestinal calculi formed of layers surrounding a nucleus of some hard indigestible substance) may be found in the colon of horses. Fecaliths are frequently formed when foreign bodies such as baler twine, rubber or nylon string/fibers are

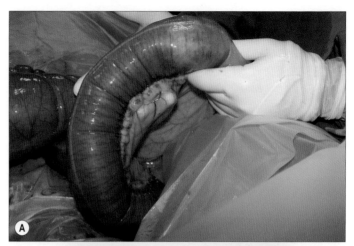

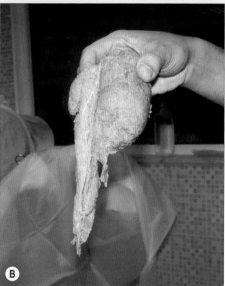

Figure 1.127 (A, B) Foreign body impaction of small colon. This Arabian cross mare was presented with acute abdominal distension and pain that was non-responsive to pain killers. The foreign body consisted of small ropes and rags.

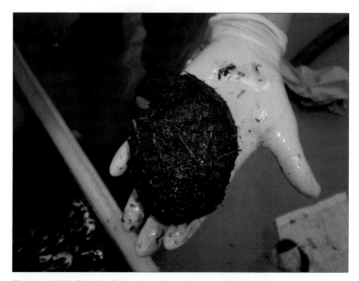

Figure 1.128 Fecalith. Relatively uniform shape and obvious fecal nature; very hard and difficult to break up.

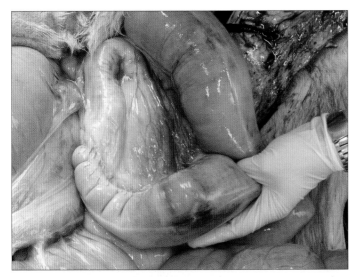

Figure 1.129 Fecalith within the bowel showing pressure necrosis of the bowel wall.

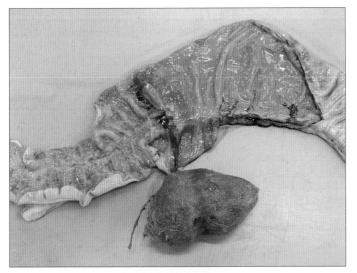

Figure 1.130 Fecalith (same horse as Fig. 1.129).

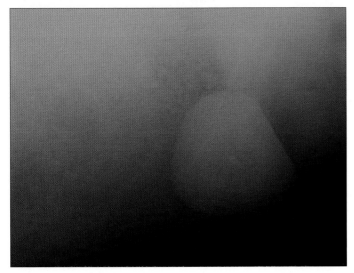

Figure 1.131 Enterolith. Radiograph taken prior to surgery clearly showing the presence of an enterolith.

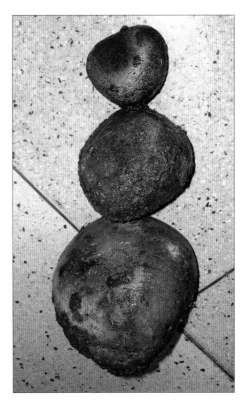

Figure 1.132 Enteroliths removed (same horse as Fig. 1.131).

ingested with fecal material accumulating around the object to form large obstructing masses. They are usually formed in the large colon and most often result in simple luminal obstruction within the transverse or small colon. The more solid, rock-like concretions (**enteroliths**) are usually composed of ammonium and magnesium phosphate complexes and, although they are smoother, they may also cause intraluminal obstructions in the large and small colon. They have been associated with diets with elevated levels of magnesium and proteins. The Arabian breed appears to be at particular risk with cases also reported in donkeys, Morgans and Saddlebreds.

Enteroliths are much slower to develop than fecaliths and may be found in any part of the colon although there is a predilection for right dorsal and transverse colon. The shape and location of the developing mass largely dictates the associated clinical signs. Thus, roughened and irregular enteroliths occurring in the cecum or large colon may have little or no pathological effect or may produce mild, recurrent episodes of colic associated with local bowel-wall irritation. The commoner larger, smoother enteroliths and fecaliths characteristically cause obstructions in the narrower portions of the large bowel including the pelvic flexure, transverse colon and small colon. Rarely, enteroliths may be multiple and smooth with flat sides. Some masses of limited size may be passed normally in the feces. Obstructions caused by enteroliths or fecaliths may be complete, when acute clinical signs associated with the gross proximal accumulation of gas and ingesta may be seen but are more usually incomplete. In the latter cases the clinical signs are similar to those of impactions at the relevant anatomical sites. Intermittent impactions may be associated with slow and intermittent movement of the object through the colon. Rough objects located within the cecum or large colon may not, however, have any obstructive effects but may cause quite extensive intermittent (and sometimes persistent) inflammation of these organs and each episode might be accompanied by significant colic symptoms.

Diagnosis and treatment

- Rectal examination may or may not detect the presence of these objects depending on their location and weight.
- Abdominal radiography may help diagnose some cases but exploratory laparotomy is required in many cases.
- Typically, surgery is required or the diagnosis is made during a laparotomy. Removal of the fecalith or enterolith is normally through a pelvic flexure enterotomy but frequently a separate enterotomy may be required to prevent colon or cecal rupture.

Intramural lesions and abdominal abscesses (Figs. 1.133–1.138)

A variety of intramural lesions such as **abscesses**, **neoplasia** and **hematomas** may also result in significant obstructive colic, which may be a combination of simple and non-strangulating obstruction. Abscesses may arise from luminal insults or may more commonly extend from the mesentry or mesenteric lymph nodes and commonly result from systemic spread of respiratory infections. Most are due to *Streptococcus equi*, *Streptococcus zooepidemicus*, *Rhodococcus equi* and *Corynebacterium pseudotuberculosis*.

Although few cause any significant bowel disorders, some result in intermittent, recurrent colic associated with chronic weight loss. The commonest obstructive conditions caused by these lesions are adhesions between loops of bowel or between bowel and other peritoneal organs.

Cecal abscesses may reach considerable size and involve extensive portions of the jejunum and ileum and other abdominal structures. There is little known about their pathogenesis, but they are most often centered around the ileo-cecal or ceco-colic openings. The clinical signs are insidious in onset and only when peritonitis and/or bowel obstruction occur are acute signs of colic presented.

Diagnosis and treatment

- The diagnosis is frequently made at post-mortem following abscess or intestinal rupture.
- In many cases, if detected ante-mortem, treatment is difficult due to involvement of other sections of intestine. Depending on the size and extent of the abscess, intraluminal drainage, resection or long-term antibiotics individually or combined may be used as therapy.

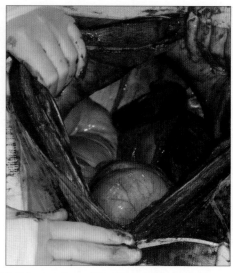

Figure 1.134 Abdominal abscess. This 15-year-old Arabian gelding presented for investigation of pyrexia and laminitis. Abdominocentesis yielded a purulent fluid exudate. Abdominal ultrasound examination revealed a large abscess in the cranioventral abdomen on the left side adjacent to the spleen and liver. The mass was surgically resected via flank incision. Although no bacteria were isolated from the abscess, the laminitis was suspected to be associated with release of inflammatory mediators and bacterial toxins.

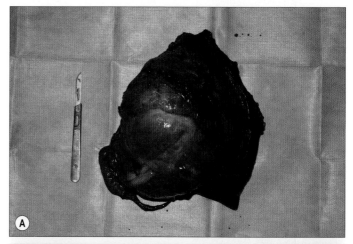

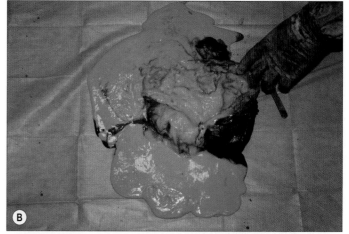

Figure 1.135 (A, B) Abdominal abscess following removal and opening (same as Fig. 1.134).

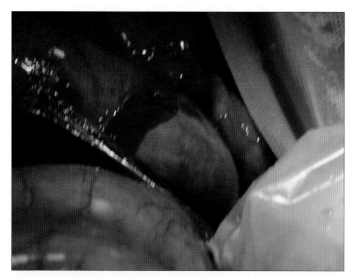

Figure 1.133 Duodenal abscess. This horse presented with a history of repeated bouts of colic. Abdominal ultrasonography revealed no abnormalities, but gastroscopic examination demonstrated delayed emptying of the stomach. An exploratory laparotomy was performed and an abscess of the duodenum was discovered.

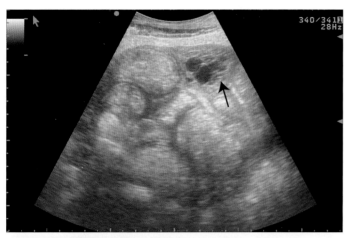

Figure 1.136 Ultrasonography of abdominal abscesses frequently reveals a loculated mass that may or may not involve a portion of the abdominal or intestinal wall depending on the inciting cause. In some cases single or multiple air–fluid interfaces may be seen. In this case there is a small abscess in the cranioventral abdomen with a thick fibrous wall (arrow).

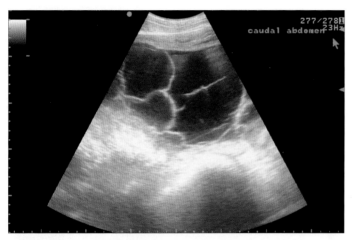

Figure 1.137 A large abscess in the caudal abdomen which is clearly loculated (same horse as Fig. 1.136). This abscess developed in this case secondary to peritonitis.

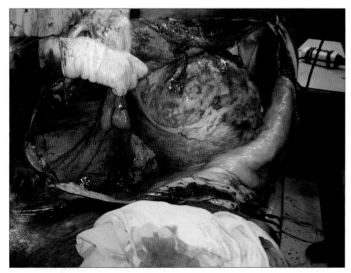

Figure 1.138 Large ovarian abscess that occupied much of the peritoneal cavity.

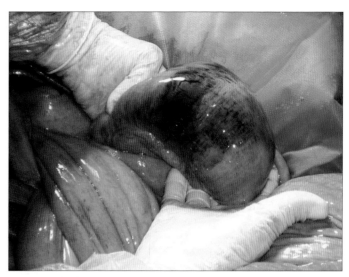

Figure 1.139 Bowel wall hematoma.

Submucosal hematomas (Fig. 1.139)

Submucosal hematomas occur in the wall of the small colon and exert the same effect as other obstructions. They are often large and result in partial or complete luminal obstruction. Chronic ulceration of the small colon at the site of the hematoma, iatrogenic damage following rectal examination, parasitism, foaling injuries and other as yet unidentified factors may be responsible for their development. The pain associated with this obstruction is usually inordinately severe when compared to that due to other forms of small colon obstruction and this is possibly due to the tension created by the swollen mass on the visceral peritoneum.

Diagnosis and treatment

- Diagnosis may in some cases be made by transrectal ultrasonography but frequently is made during exploratory laparotomy.
- If they result in complete obstruction the treatment of choice is surgery which involves evacuation of the hematoma and resection and anastomosis of the affected segment of small colon.

Obstructive disorders: Non-strangulating obstructions (Figs. 1.140–1.143)

Non-strangulating obstructions of the small intestine (or other segments of the intestinal tract) may arise from alterations in the ability of the gut to move naturally and to propel ingesta distally.

There are many proposed theories related to neurogenic ileus. Among these is the theory that inflammatory mediators released within the intestinal wall as a result of inflammation (enteritis/colitis, septicemia or bowel handling) inhibit smooth muscle contractility. The secretory and absorptive functions are typically maintained and under these conditions the proximal (secretory) organs (stomach and small bowel to the level of the distal jejunum) continue to fill, while in the ileum, large colon and cecum the sustained absorptive functions continue to render the contents progressively more desiccated. This type of disorder would result in a physiological obstruction to bowel function.

Another common cause of non-strangulating obstruction is the development of adhesions between adjacent areas of bowel. These loops frequently become adherent to each other in response to peritonitis and/or areas of infarction (ischemia or necrosis) within the bowel wall. Adhesions between different sections of the intestine or between the intestine and other abdominal organs, including the spleen and the parietal peritoneum, are common sequels to

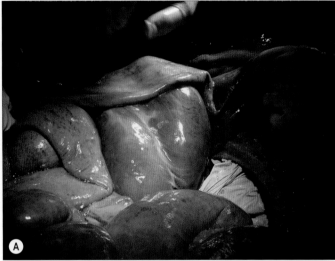

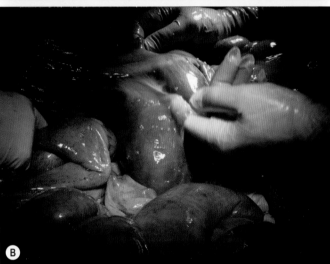

Figure 1.140 (A, B) These adhesions formed following a previous colic surgery.

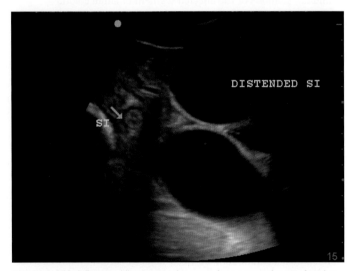

Figure 1.141 Adhesions. Ultrasonographic image from a mare that was found to have adhesions on exploratory laparotomy. The mare had had a previous colic surgery 3 weeks before. The image shows a distended loop of small intestine adjacent to a thickened collapsed loop of small intestine (arrow). The adhesion prevented propulsion of ingesta, resulting in proximal distension, and distal collapse of the small intestine.

DISTENDED SI

SI

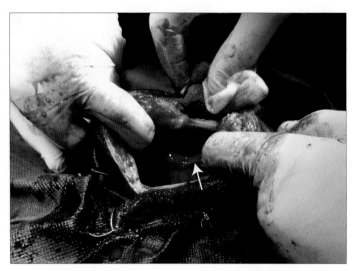

Figure 1.142 Adhesions. Adhesions can occur between sections of intestine or between intestine and the abdominal wall. This horse had a previous colic surgery and developed an adhesion between intestine and the abdominal wall at the incision site (arrow).

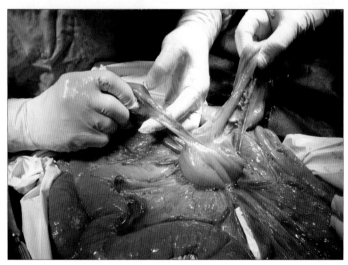

Figure 1.143 Adhesions. Fibrinous adhesion between loops of ileum.

peritonitis or surgical interference, particularly where vascular compromise is present. The organization of these may lead to the development of non-elastic scar tissue bands which may create partial or complete, non-strangulating obstructions in any segment of the tract although the small intestine appears to be most commonly involved. While there may be no obstruction to the passage of food in the early stages, the impaired mobility and motility of the affected loops result in either a physical obstruction through narrowing or kinking or a functional obstruction with little or no ability to propel food onward. Post-prandial colic caused by intermittent partial obstruction of the jejunum and/or ileum is a common feature of developing or mature adhesions. Most cases affected by this type of disorder have a history of recurrent episodes of drug-responsive, mild or moderate, colic with a single, more acute, persistent episode, with signs typical of intraluminal small intestinal obstruction. It is unusual to find signs of active peritonitis. One of the more serious consequences of these adhesions, which may become densely fibrosed as scarring matures within them, is their liability to cause secondary strangulating obstructions.

Diagnosis and treatment

- History and clinical signs; many affected horses have a history of recent abdominal surgery or abdominal incident. Exploratory laparotomy or laparoscopy is frequently required to characterize the extent of the adhesions and organs involved.
- Treatment options are limited as surgical intervention may lead to further adhesion formation.

Large colon displacements

Large colon displacements occur relatively commonly. The relatively mobile anatomical character of the ascending colon (except the right dorsal and ventral portions) and its relatively high gas content make a wide range of displacements possible. Any impairment or alteration of motility (commonly associated with the feeding of high-grain diets and the parasitic infestations) can result in gaseous distension causing the colon to migrate from its normal position.

Displacement of whatever type partially obstructs the lumen, resulting in accumulation of gas and/or digesta leading to distension. This distension which may be exacerbated by increased fluid secretion is an important source of the pain associated with the condition. In some cases, displacement has no compromising effect upon the blood supply in the early stages but the size and weight of the organ, especially when filled to capacity, makes some compromise inevitable in almost all cases.

Displacements of the colon are divided into three types:

1) **Left dorsal displacement of the colon (LDD)** (Figs. 1.144–1.147). The ascending colon becomes entrapped in the nephrosplenic space. It is theorized that excess gas accumulation, perhaps in some cases combined with abnormal motility, causes the left colon to displace lateral to the spleen and then dorsally into the nephrosplenic space. In addition the colon is often rotated through 180° such that the left ventral colon is in a more dorsal position relative to the left dorsal colon. The entrapped portion may be only the pelvic flexure or involve a large portion of the ascending colon. Gastric distension is also thought to predispose to left dorsal displacement by pushing the spleen into a more medial than normal position thus allowing easier migration of the colon along the abdominal wall. While in most cases there is little vascular compromise, the progressive accumulation of food material in the right ventral colon, and progressive gas accumulation in the entrapped

distal colon, result in continuous though frequently mild colic. Fecal output is reduced. Few cases show gross distension of the abdomen but cecal tympany is common and gastric distension may be present

2) **Right dorsal displacement (RDD)** (Fig. 1.148). Displacement may occur clockwise or anticlockwise. The former is more common and occur when the pelvic flexure is displaced between the cecum and body wall in a cranial to caudal direction. This may then progress with further medial and cranial movement of the pelvic flexure with the result that the pelvic flexure comes to lie near the diaphragm. Anticlockwise displacements occur when the pelvic flexure travels in a caudal to cranial direction; in this case the pelvic flexure may also come to lie close to the diaphragm.

3) **Retroflexion.** Retroflexion of the ascending colon occurs by movement of the pelvic flexure cranially without movement of the sternal or diaphragmatic flexures

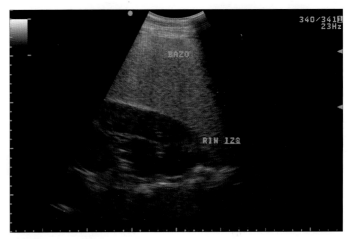

Figure 1.145 Ultrasound image demonstrating the normal relationship between the spleen and left kidney.

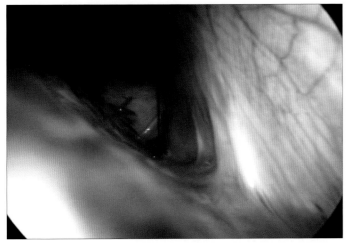

Figure 1.144 Normal laparoscopic view of nephrosplenic space. Note the stomach cranially, kidney to the right of the image and the spleen to the left of the image.

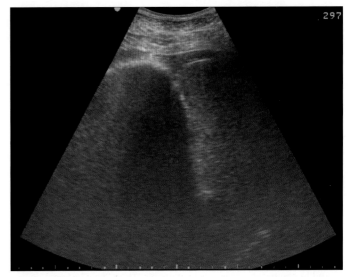

Figure 1.146 Ultrasound of nephrosplenic entrapment demonstrating the spleen on the right of the image and gas filled colon on the left which is obstructing the normal image of the kidney.

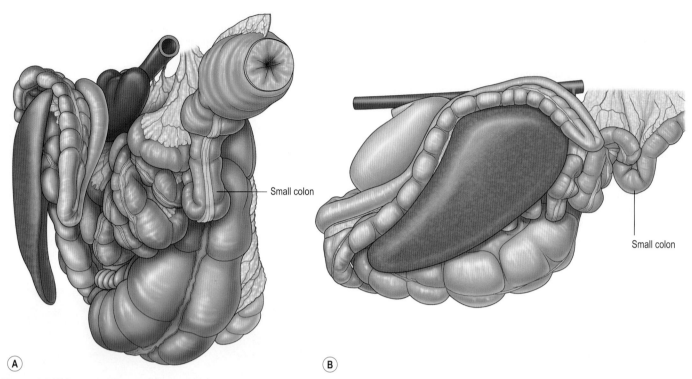

Figure 1.147 Diagram of left dorsal displacement (nephrosplenic entrapment).

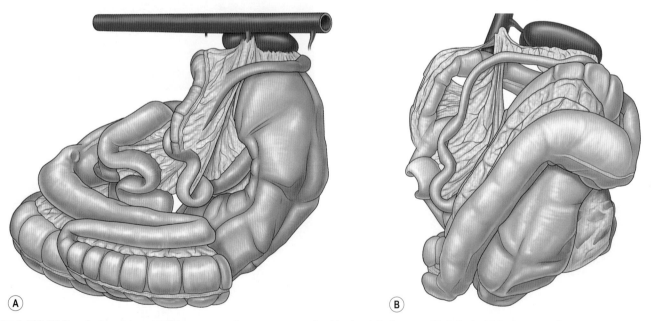

Figure 1.148 (A) Retroflexion of the colon. This may occur alone or may preceed a right dorsal displacement. (B) Right dorsal displacement of the colon in an anticlockwise direction as seen from a rectal view.

Diagnosis

- LDD: rectal examination can be diagnostic, when converging tenial bands can be easily identified and the displaced colon is obviously in the nephrosplenic space. The spleen may be displaced medially and in some cases may not be palpable. There may be some degree of vascular compromise at the site of the entrapment with the more distal portion (the pelvic flexure) becoming edematous.

- RDD: rectal examination is diagnostic in most cases and regardless of the path the colon actually takes, rectal examination findings are the same: the taenia of the colon run transversely across the pelvic inlet and difficulty is encountered when an attempt is made to palpate the ventral cecal band.

- Ultrasonographic examination may assist the diagnosis. In LDD the spleen will be visible on the left side but the gas-filled colon will obstruct the image of the kidney. In RDD the pelvic flexure cannot be imaged in its normal position and may be replaced by small intestine. However, false positives and false negatives can occur so ultrasound should be used as a diagnostic aid and not the sole means of diagnosis.

- In some instances a definitive diagnosis can only be reached during exploratory laparotomy. Peritoneal fluid may increase in amount but the color, protein concentration and white cell count are usually normal. With the passage of time developing edema in the bowel wall results in serosal leakage of proteins, resulting in an increased protein concentration in the peritoneal fluid.

Treatment

- Retroflexion and RDD: horses which have severe pain, significant large-colon distension or severe secondary impactions are candidates for surgical intervention. In cases which are presented early with normal parameters and minimal-to-mild abdominal pain medical therapy can be attempted. This involves administration of intravenous fluids, retention of food and sequential monitoring for resolution.
- LDD: in cases with mild-to-moderate pain, medical therapy can be attempted. Options for medical therapy include intravenous fluid therapy with retention of food, exercise with or without the use of vasopressor agents or rolling under general anesthesia with or without the use of vasopressor agents.

Ischemic disorders: Strangulating obstructions

Strangulating obstructions of the bowel form an extremely important group of disorders in the horse and occur when the intestinal blood supply and the lumen of the bowel are obstructed simultaneously. Strangulating lesions are much more common in the small intestine than in other segments of the gut. The extent and significance of these disorders depend largely on the degree of vascular compromise, but most of them are life-threatening. The affected portion of the intestine is often devitalized rapidly. Initially, the venous drainage of the affected portion is impaired and localized swelling and edema cause progressively more severe arterial obstruction. Ischemia of the gut then results in localized spasm of the affected length and there is a consequent accumulation of gas and fluid proximal to the obstruction. Severe gastric distension is a common sequel which develops rapidly. Gross, intraluminal distension of the bowel results in further ischemia and disruption of the protective mucosal layers. Loss of protein-rich fluid into the lumen and passage of endotoxins into the peritoneal fluid and bloodstream occur early.

The systemic consequences of these changes are profound. Hypovolemic and endotoxic shock accompanied by electrolyte and acid–base deviations occur and are responsible for the continuing metabolic collapse of the patient. Vascular compromise and capillary necrosis result in the loss of high-protein fluid containing both red and white cells into the abdomen. Peritoneal fluid is usually blood-stained and has a high protein concentration and raised total leucocyte count. Typically, affected horses have an acute onset of severe and unrelenting, non-drug-responsive abdominal pain. Where the lesion occurs in the proximal segments of the small intestine, progression is particularly rapid and is usually accompanied by gastric distension resulting from reflux of alkaline intestinal fluid into the stomach. Lesions occurring further down the small intestine have a somewhat slower course but all have a characteristically rapid progression over 1–12 hours. The extent of pain shown by these cases finally becomes less severe due to devitalization of the distended and damaged intestine. Critical clinical assessment confirms that the apparent improvement is not a result of resolution of the underlying problem, and that cardiovascular compromise and terminal shock

are imminent. Most affected horses will die within 24–36 hours unless treated effectively.

Small intestinal strangulation

Strangulating lesions caused by entrapment through a natural body opening or acquired hernia or through internal openings, or as a result of fibrous mesenteric bands or from strangulating pedunculated lipomas, cause a complete luminal obstruction and result in considerable vascular compromise. The location of the proximal and distal viable or undamaged segments of the intestine is of paramount importance and in these cases this is usually evident as a sharp demarcation in the bowel wall. The prognosis for survival in horses with small intestinal strangulating lesions is much lower than other types of colics in part because of long-term complications such as adhesions.

Umbilical hernia entrapment (Figs. 1.149–1.152)

Developmental umbilical hernia is very commonly encountered in foals. Small or large hernias generally appear as soft, fluctuant, reducible swellings in the umbilical region. In most cases the defect is of little immediate importance but rarely may be a source of bowel incarceration. Smaller hernias are considered more dangerous as bowel is more likely to become entrapped than in larger hernias where it can

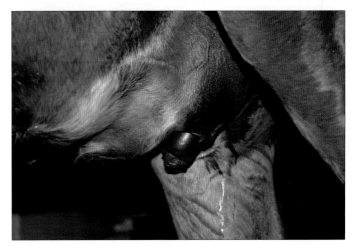

Figure 1.149 Umbilical hernia. Swelling and edema of the umbilicus and ventral abdomen associated with an incarcerated umbilical hernia.

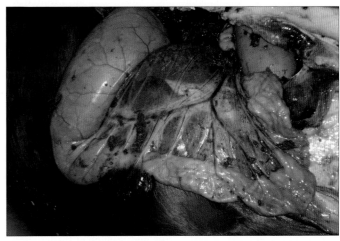

Figure 1.150 Umbilical hernia (Richter's hernia) (same foal as Fig. 1.149). A section of the anti-mesenteric surface of ileum had become incarcerated within this hernia, resulting in proximal distension of the small intestine and eventual gastric rupture. The entrapment necrosed area of intestine is clearly demarcated.

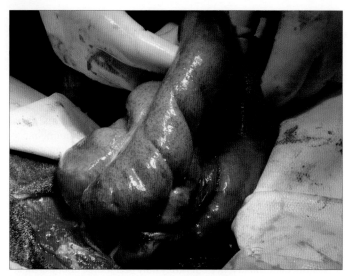

Figure 1.151 Umbilical hernia. Herniation of the colon through the umbilicus.

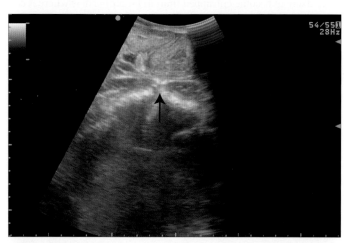

Figure 1.152 Ultrasonographic image of an umbilical hernia. Note the break in the abdominal wall (arrow) and the incarcerated edematous small intestine

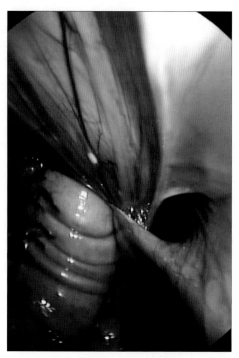

Figure 1.153 Laparoscopic image of normal inguinal ring.

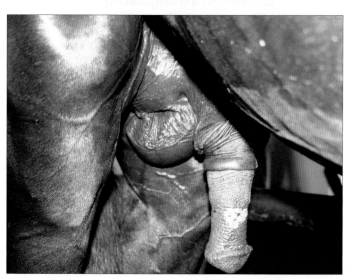

Figure 1.154 Inguinal hernia in a stallion. This hernia developed spontaneously while the horse was in a rehabilitation facility for treatment for a tendon lesion.

move more easily in and out of the hernial ring. Clinical signs of bowel entrapment include increased swelling of the hernia, heat, pain and difficulty in reduction. Small intestine is most commonly involved but cecum or colon can also become incarcerated within the hernia. In some cases, only a portion of the bowel wall may be affected; these are known as Richter's hernias and may lead to the development of enterocutaneous fistulas.

Inguinal hernia entrapment (Figs. 1.153–1.157)
In entire stallions (and rarely in geldings) loops of small intestine may become incarcerated in the inguinal canal or scrotum. The disorder is common and of relatively minor significance in the neonatal foal which often has significant lengths of small bowel herniated through the inguinal canal and lying within the enlarged scrotum. Lesser or greater lengths of intestine appear to have considerable freedom to move in and out of the inguinal canal and the condition usually resolves spontaneously over the first few weeks of life. In some foals, and in adult horses, the disorder is, however, extremely serious. Severe strangulating colic may result with gross asymmetrical enlargement of the scrotum associated with edema and swelling of the ipsilateral testicle. Open castration of horses affected by inguinal hernias or those with an abnormally wide inguinal canal may result in serious herniation of variable lengths of small intestine.

Epiploic foramen entrapment
Entrapment of jejunum and/or ileum through naturally occurring internal anatomical openings, such as the epiploic foramen, occurs relatively frequently and the incidence of this particular disorder increases with age as the foramen increases in size in older horses. Rectal examination of horses suffering from epiploic foramen entrapment is often somewhat disappointing but it is the ileum and terminal portions of the jejunum which are usually involved early in the disorder. Tension applied to the ventral tenial band of the cecum per rectum will often elicit a sharp pain response in these cases.

Intussusceptions (Figs. 1.158–1.163)
Intussusception of a length of small intestine and its associated mesentery most commonly involves the more distal jejunum or the ileum, and is most often encountered in young horses. A history of

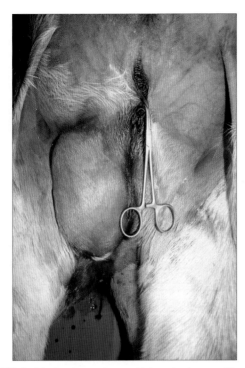

Figure 1.155 Foal in dorsal recumbency with large inguinoscrotal hernia.

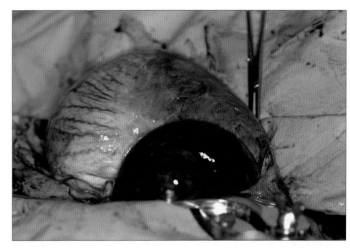

Figure 1.157 Inguinal hernia. Incarcerated and necrotic bowel is imaged beside the testicle in this stallion.

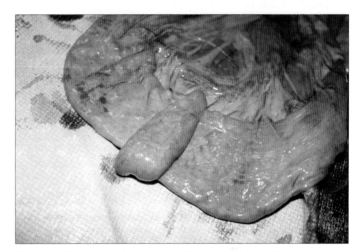

Figure 1.158 Ileo-ileal intussusception. This horse was undergoing an exploratory laparotomy for another reason and a section of ileum spontaneously developed an intussusception during the course of the surgery.

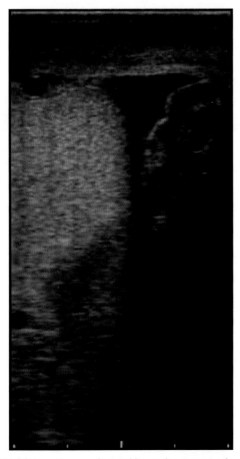

Figure 1.156 Ultrasound image of inguinal hernia demonstrating the testicle to the left and small intestine to the right.

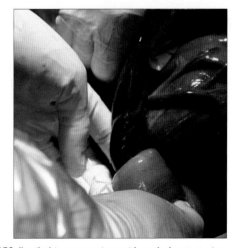

Figure 1.159 Ileo-ileal intussusceptions, with marked compromise and necrosis of the intussusceptum.

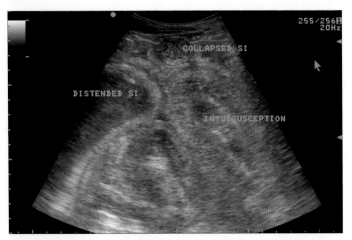

Figure 1.160 Ultrasonogram of the ventral abdomen demonstrating a long-axis view of an ileo-ileal intussusception.

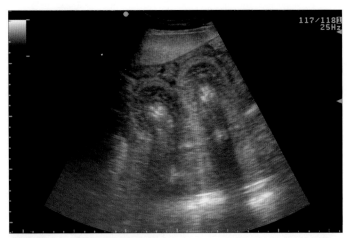

Figure 1.161 Ultrasonogram of the ventral abdomen illustrating a short-axis view of an ileo-ileal intussusception with the typical clown face appearance.

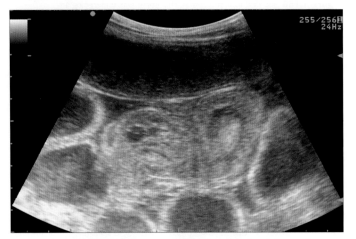

Figure 1.162 Small intestinal intussusception. Note the adjacent loops of distended small intestine

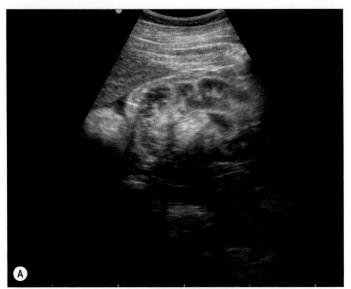

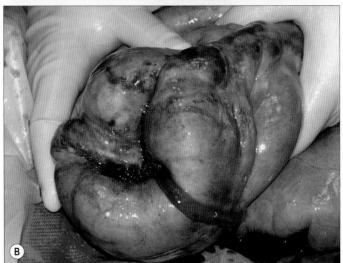

Figure 1.163 (A) Transabdominal ultrasonographic image obtained from the right mid ventral abdomen, demonstrating a ceco-cecal intussusception. Note the marked edema of the cecal wall. (B) Ceco-cecal intussusceptions.

diarrhea may be present, particularly in foals, although the onset of the intussusception and related colic signs is acute. Parasitism may be an instigating factor (see below). Intussusception of the jejunum into itself, or into the ileum or cecum, results in few changes in the peritoneal fluid as the length of damaged bowel (intussusceptum) is firmly enclosed in the distal segment (intussuscipiens). However, the proximal small intestine rapidly becomes significantly distended and gastric distension with its attendant dangers may also develop.

In some cases the obstruction created by an intussusception (particularly ileo-ileal intussusceptions) may not be complete with limited amounts of food material able to pass the site and, under these conditions, the severity of the clinical signs may be less. Intussusception of the ileum (and variable lengths of jejunum) into the cecum is potentially very dangerous as the ileum has a particularly poor collateral circulation. There is little or no alteration in the peritoneal fluid in these cases, so that diagnosis may be difficult and is often dependent on rectal examination or laparotomy. The detection, per rectum, of distended small intestine and a large, sausage-shaped, solid object within the cecum is usually pathognomonic. Ileo-cecal intussusceptions usually induce a complete obstruction and the clinical features are correspondingly more severe than the partial obstructions often found in ileo-ileal or jejuno-ileal intussusceptions.

Ceco-cecal intussusception probably arises from impaired, or altered, motility of the organ and in these cases the degree of circulatory compromise is much less than in the small intestine, as there is little strangulation and vascular impairment. Also, there is insignificant hindrance to the passage of food material into the large colon and, although affected horses are anorexic and have mild, recurrent or persistent colic, feces of normal consistency usually continue to be passed. These may, however, contain evidence of intestinal bleeding. The clinical signs of colic in these animals are therefore less severe and slower in progression, but the long-term consequences are no less dangerous. Rectal examination is often unremarkable but the presence of melena (dark tarry feces containing changed blood) may be a significant finding for this and other types of intussusception.

Acquired (or developmental) defects in the diaphragm or mesentery (Figs. 1.164–1.166)

These may also be responsible for the development of strangulating lesions. In the acquired defects, such as mesenteric tears or rents, incarceration probably occurs at the time of the damage to the mesentery. Most of these probably arise from physical tearing during falls, or from blows, but many have no such history.

Mesodiverticular bands (see Fig. 1.97) and pedunculated lipomas (Figs. 1.167–1.169)

These may arise from the mesentery or from the serosal surface of the small intestine, and are common causes of incarceration and

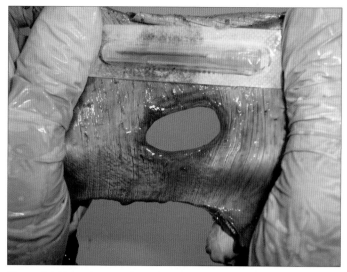

Figure 1.165 Diaphragmatic hernia. Post-mortem specimen showing a diaphragmatic hernia through which bowel herniated. Frequently these lesions are small, which results in rapid strangulation of the bowel after it passes through.

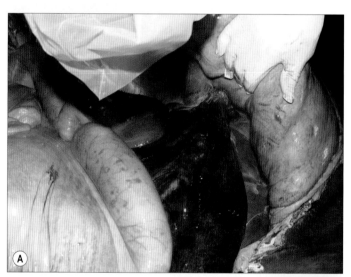

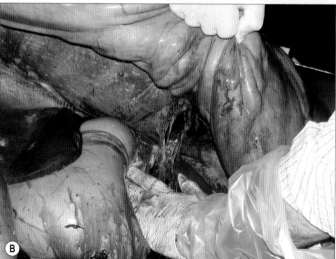

Figure 1.164 (A) Intestine passing through a diaphragmatic hernia; the marked compromise and congestion of the bowel is evident. (B) Defect in the diaphragm following removal of the incarcerated bowel.

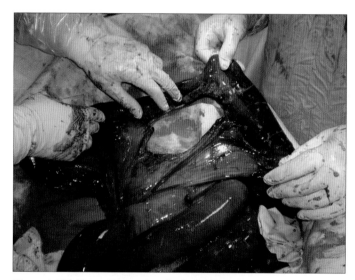

Figure 1.166 Mesenteric tear through which a large portion of small intestine had passed and become strangulated.

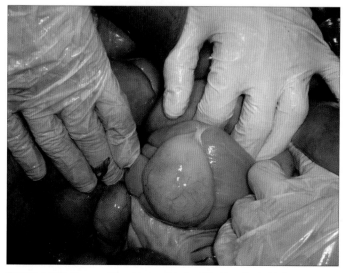

Figure 1.167 Lipoma with a short pedicle found incidentally during laparotomy.

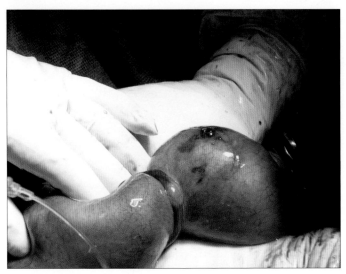

Figure 1.168 Pedicle of lipoma (lipoma not visible) resulting in strangulation of a section of small intestine.

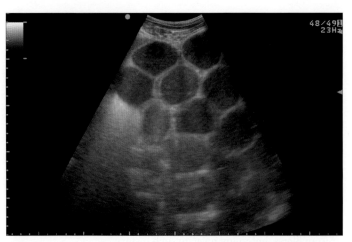

Figure 1.170 Ultrasonographic image of small intestinal volvulus secondary to adhesions in this mare that have had previous colic surgery. The volvulus in this case is in the early stages as sedimentation of contents cannot yet be seen.

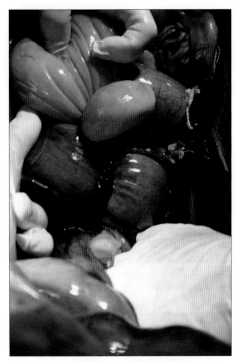

Figure 1.169 Lipoma with a long pedicle that resulted in bowel strangulation.

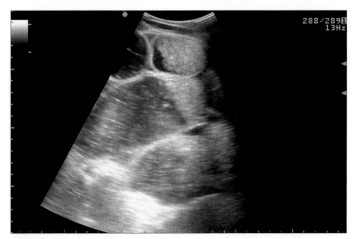

Figure 1.171 Ultrasonographic image of small intestinal volvulus with sedimentation of intestinal contents.

strangulation of small intestine or small colon. Lipomas of significant size are most often encountered in horses over the age of 15 years, but while many horses have large and/or numerous lipomas without any untoward effect, some small and relatively innocuous-looking masses have serious consequences. Younger horses may also be affected. The most dangerous forms of lipoma are those with long pedicles and while in some cases this may cause extreme and complete strangulation of small intestine or small colon, others may have a lesser effect from tension within the pedicle. The latter are more commonly associated with large lipoma masses with relatively long pedicles. The body condition of the horse is not reliably related to the presence of lipomas with some horses in moderate body condition

having large masses while some inordinately fat horses may have no, or a few, small lipomas.

Rotation of segments of jejunum or ileum (Figs. 1.170–1.173)

Rotations through more than 180°, along the long axis of the mesenteric attachment (volvulus), initially result in impairment of blood supply and, later, obstruction of the lumen of the affected portion. These lesions often occur secondarily to some other obstructive or incarcerative condition such as Meckel's diverticulum, adhesions, infarctions or mesenteric rents. Continued twisting of the affected loop results in progressive vascular compromise and luminal obstruction. The loop becomes devitalized, while the segments proximal to the obstruction become filled with gas and fluid. Where the affected loop of jejunum or ileum becomes knotted rather than merely twisted upon itself, the term volvulus nodosus is applied. These strangulating obstructive lesions are easily recognized but it is difficult to understand how they are formed. It is presumed that the underlying cause is basically a defect of motility. The clinical features are typical of severe and complete strangulating obstruction with proximal distension and distal emptying of the bowel. Peritoneal fluid is usually indicative of strangulation lesions (see p. 54). Again, there is a considerable risk of gastric distension and consequent gastric rupture.

Rotation of the mesenteric root about its axis

This results in a severe vascular obstruction to the entire small intestine. The progression of colic signs is rapid and relentless. This stage is often followed by a period when less pain will be shown associated with intestinal devitalization and impending death. Gross abdominal distension may not, however, be a major feature of the disorder, although in some cases this may be present. Rectal examination is usually diagnostic, and will at least identify that a large number of loops of small intestine are grossly dilated, tense and, in the early stages, painful to the touch. In this condition the loops of distended jejunum will be felt lying next to each other as can be demonstrated clearly at post-mortem examination.

Torsion of the cecum (Fig. 1.174)

Torsion of the cecum alone is much less common than small intestinal torsion and entrapments; most being related to large colon torsion. As there is a poor collateral blood supply, vascular compromise occurs rapidly. The amount of distension of the organ may be limited. Peritoneal fluid usually provides evidence of a strangulating obstruction but fecal output may be little affected. Rectal examination is often disappointing but a distended cecum with an edematous wall may be identifiable.

Strangulating displacements (torsion) of the large bowel (Figs. 1.175 & 1.176)

These are variable in their extent and effect upon the horse. The degree of rotation and consequent vascular and luminal obstruction largely dictates the rate of onset and progression and the severity of the clinical signs. Thus, rotations of less than 90° may present with no apparent vascular obstruction, and relatively minor luminal interference. Such displacements are best regarded as physiological and probably occur frequently. Rotations of between 90° and 180° cause increased, but often insignificant, luminal obstruction. Under these conditions it may be impossible to identify the disorder except by careful examination of the position and appearance of the colon at laparotomy. Torsion of 180–270° will obstruct the lumen and impair blood supply (and venous drainage, in particular), while degrees of rotation greater than this probably represent the most rapidly

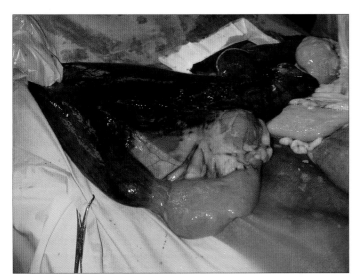

Figure 1.172 Volvulus of small intestine. Note section of intestine with marked vascular compromise to the left of the image.

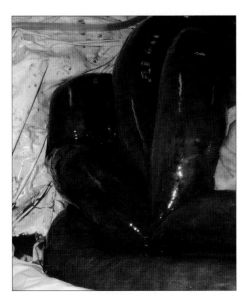

Figure 1.173 Mesenteric root volvulus.

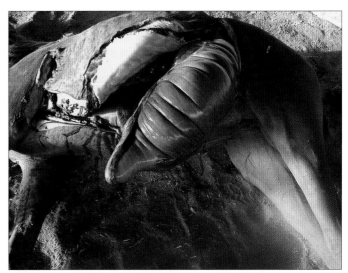

Figure 1.174 Cecal torsion. This aged arabian had a concurrent severe sand impaction of the colon.

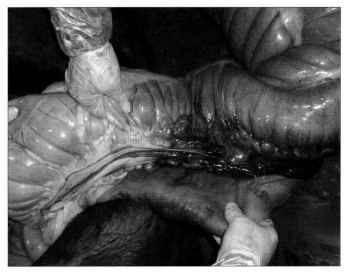

Figure 1.175 Colon torsion showing clear demarcation between area of vascular compromise and normal at site of the torsion.

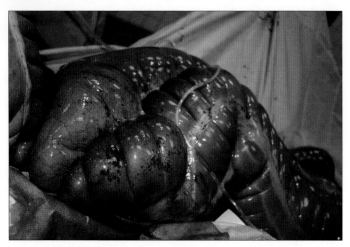

Figure 1.176 Colon torsion with multiple hemorrhages evident throughout the colon wall as a result of vascular compromise.

progressive and dangerous forms of colic. The latter cases are extremely serious, and there is a dramatic buildup of gas within the large colon and the cecum, sufficient to result in an obvious bloating of the abdomen.

Rectal examination of horses suffering from serious degrees of large colon torsion is often impossible due to the massive gaseous distension. A tense, gas-filled viscus occluding the pelvic inlet is strongly suggestive of colonic torsion, but the metabolic effects may make further exploration unnecessary. Torsion of the large colon usually occurs in a clockwise direction, when viewed from the back of the standing horse, and is most often centered around the right colon just forward of the cecum. Some involve the origin of the large colon and some even include the cecum. Vascular compromise is always severe, with gross edema and congestion of the colon and its mesenteric vasculature. Black or dark-purple mucosa, identified during surgery in cases of large colon torsion, is a grave prognostic sign. The dramatic progression of these cases is a result of a combination of serious endotoxic shock arising from massively compromised mucosal layers of the colon, and to gross distension and consequent circulatory compromise. Rupture of the grossly distended large colon (or the cecum) represents the ultimate progression of the disorder, but most cases die before this can occur.

Diagnosis

- Diagnosis of strangulating obstructions is frequently based on a combination of clinical and laboratory data. These horses show rapid marked cardiovascular compromise and frequently present in cardiovascular shock with elevated heart rates, injected mucous membranes and delayed capillary refill time.
- Severe unrelenting pain frequently unresponsive to analgesics is also characteristic of strangulating lesions.
- Abdominal ultrasonography may help identify the specific section of bowel involved.
- Normal peritoneal fluid can contain up to 10 000 WBC/μl (although usually <3 000 WBC/μl) for adult horses and up to 3 000 RBC/μl. There is normally a 2:1 ratio of neutrophils to mononuclear cells. With strangulating lesions or obstructive lesions severe enough to cause bowel ischemia, cell concentrations in the peritoneal fluid will rise. RBCs exceeding 20 000/μl indicate a severe intestinal injury, total WBC numbers will rise and the percentage of neutrophils will also rise with degeneration of neutrophils becoming apparent with more severe injury.
- Increasing blood or peritoneal lactate levels indicate inadequate tissue perfusion. Normal levels for adults are 0.2–0.7 mmol/L.

Typically, in horses with visceral ischemia, the first increases in lactate concentration occur in peritoneal fluid, after which a gradual increase is seen in the systemic circulation.

- Increases in peritoneal lactate concentrations greater than blood levels have been shown to be an indicator of strangulating bowel lesions.

Treatment

- Surgical correction is required in all cases but resuscitative measures should be instituted prior to surgery. The most important aspects of pre-surgical treatment are:
- *Cardiovascular support.* Dehydration and hypovolemia are commonly found in horses presented for colic. Fluid administration to provide cardiovascular support is required in all cases and in most instances can be instituted in the field prior to referral. Crystalloids are usually administered first but administration of hypertonic saline prior to crystalloid fluid therapy can also be considered for rapid expansion of intravascular volume. The shock dose for crystalloids is 60–80 ml/kg as fast as possible (30–40 L/500 kg). The shock dose for 10% pentastarch is 10–15 ml/kg (5–7.5 L/500 kg) and for 10% Hetastrach is 10 ml/kg (5 L/500 kg). The dose for hypertonic saline is 2–4 ml/kg (1–2 L/500 kg). It should be followed by half the shock dose of crystalloids and should not be administered to foals. If administering crystalloids or colloids half the shock dose is administered first and then the animal should be reassessed before administering the second half.
- *Pain relief* is administered to prevent the horse injuring itself or others and in many cases to facilitate early treatment and transportation. A combination of sedative-analgesic can be used or flunixin meglumine. For sedative-analgesic combinations most commonly an α2-adrenergic agonist such as xylaxine (0.5–1.0 mg/kg IV) or detomidine (0.01–0.04 mg/kg IV) is given in combination with the opioid butorphanol (0.01–0.02 mg/kg IV). Flunixin meglumine is commonly given not only for its analgesic effects but also for its antiendotoxic properties. A single dose is generally safe in terms of neprotoxic effects even in moderately dehydrated horses.
- *Gastric decompression* is an absolute must in any horse that is confirmed with gastric distension prior to transport. However, even in field situations where confirmation of gastric distension by ultrasonography may not be available, passage of a nasogastric tube to check for reflux or gaseous distension should be regarded as a priority in any treatment or pretransport plan. If reflux is present the nasogastric tube should be left in place during transportation so that decompression can be repeated. Not only does gastric decompression reduce the risk of gastric rupture but also provides significant pain relief.

Prolapse of the rectum (Figs. 1.177–1.179)

This is usually the consequence of persistent, intense tenesmus (straining) and it may, therefore, be a sequel to intestinal disorders (diarrhea, constipation, enteritis, parasitism or other factors which result in local inflammation), or other urinary or genital tract disorders in which straining is a prominent feature. Horses which ingest manmade, fibrous material such as carpeting, nylon twine or fiberglass may develop a severe and protracted proctitis which is sufficient to result in rectal prolapse. It may also occur secondary to an increase in intra-abdominal pressure such as occurs during parturition.

There are four different forms of the disorder (see Table 1.1). Type I with mucosal prolapse alone has a characteristic appearance and represents the simplest form. These vary from mild partial or intermittent prolapses, to severe, complete prolapses with extensive mucosal edema. Necrosis, drying and laceration of the prolapsed mucosa are a frequent complication of prolonged or neglected cases. In this type there is usually no serious compromise of the underlying rectal wall. The more severe type IV, complete prolapse with invagination of the

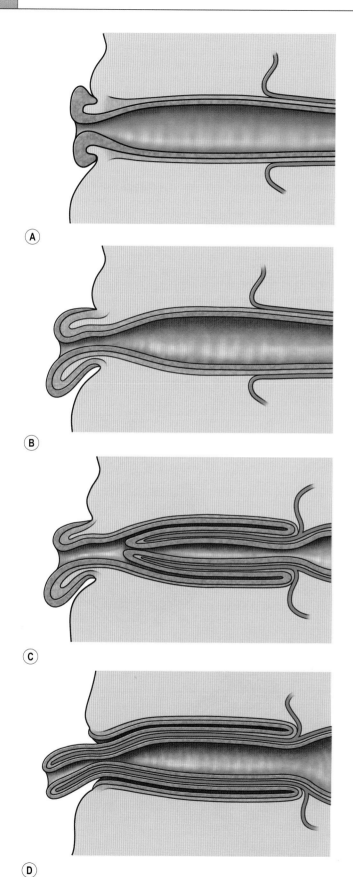

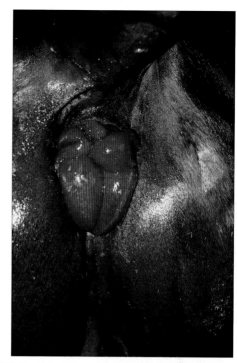

Figure 1.178 Type 1 rectal prolapse from chronic rectal irritation in a horse with salmonellosis and diarrhea.

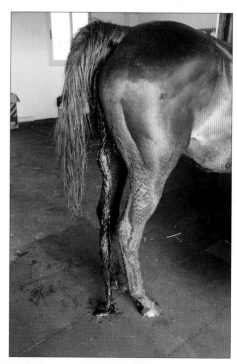

Figure 1.179 Type 4 rectal and small colon prolapse in a mare following dystocia.

Figure 1.177 Grades of rectal prolapse. (A) Type 1: the rectal mucosa alone is prolapsed. (B) Type 2: all or a portion of the ampulla recti is everted. (C) Type 3: all or a portion of the ampulla recti is everted, and the peritoneal portion of the rectum or colon is intussuscepted. (D) Type 4: the peritoneal portion of the rectum or colon is intussuscepted through the anus.

Grade	Description	Prognosis
Table 1.1 Classification of rectal prolapse		
I	Prolapse of rectal mucosa	Good
II	Prolapse of full thickness rectum	Fair to good
III	Prolapse of full thickness rectum with additional protrusion of small colon	Guarded
IV	Intussusception of rectum and small colon through anus	Poor

colon, may be complicated by intussusception of the peritoneal rectum or colon through the anus. This is the type most commonly seen in mares post foaling or associated with dystocia. This type is almost always fatal because of stretching and tearing of mesenteric vasculature with subsequent infarction of sections of bowel.

Diagnosis and treatment

- Rectal prolapse is visually obvious. Differentiation of small colon intussusception and rectal prolapse can be made by detailed examination of the mucosal reflection at the anal ring. In the former case a probe (finger) can be inserted a considerable distance between the anus and the prolapsed organ whereas in the latter, the reflection occurs at the anal ring or just inside it. A probe (finger) cannot be inserted beyond this reflection. Ultrasound can be useful to detect intussusceptions within the prolapse.

- In type I and type II, the prolapsed portion of the rectum should be replaced. It should be thoroughly cleaned and application of osmotic agents solution to decrease edema to minimize the risk of iatrogenic damage is required in all but the most recent cases. The prolapsed section should be lubricated well and gently replaced using the fist rather than fingers to provide pressure. Topical application of lidocaine solution or gel may also aid in reducing tenesmus and facilitate treatment. In most cases it is necessary to provide epidural anesthesia to prevent straining while attempting to replace the prolapse mucosa and to help prevent repeated tenesmus and avoid a recurrence of the prolapse.

- In type III, the affected section of small colon should be replaced. In some cases this may be done manually or a laparotomy may be required. Abdominocentesis should be first performed to determine if there is peritonitis present. If a laparotomy was not performed and the small colon not directly evaluated, serial abdominocenteses may be required to detect necrosis of bowel.

- In type IV, determination of bowel viability is frequently made during laparotomy and if evidence of compromise of mesenteric vasculature is present, euthanasia is generally recommended.

Rectal tears (Figs. 1.180–1.185)

Rectal tears are a relatively common occurrence and while most are certainly iatrogenic, occurring during rectal examination, some occur spontaneously. Nervous and young horses are more often affected, possibly as a result of the difficulties these create with respect to rectal examination. The most common initial presenting sign of damage is the presence of fresh blood on the rectal sleeve of the operator or fresh blood in the feces of spontaneous cases. However caused, most tears are located in the dorsal rectal wall and are classified according to their depth into four grades. The extent of the damage varies (see Fig. 1.180) from mucosal tears only (grade I), to complete disruption of the wall (grade IV) with consequent contamination of the surrounding tissues. Where the tear occurs in the retroperitoneal part of the rectum the consequences are likely to be somewhat less severe than those occurring in the more anterior portions. In the former cases the consequences include retroperitoneal abscessation or generalized

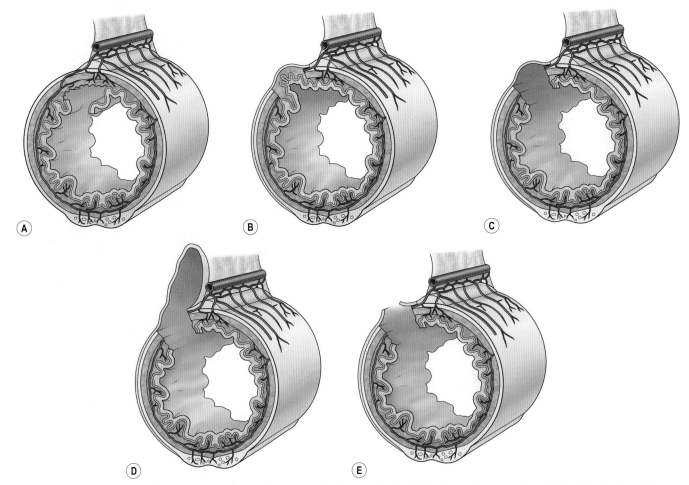

Figure 1.180 Degrees of rectal tear. (A) Grade I: involves only the mucosa and submucosa. (B) Grade II: involves only the muscularis. (C) Grade IIIa: involves all layers except the serosa. (D) Grade IIIb: dorsal tear involving all layers and extending into the mesocolon/mesorectum. (E) Grade IV: involves all layers and extends into the peritoneal cavity.

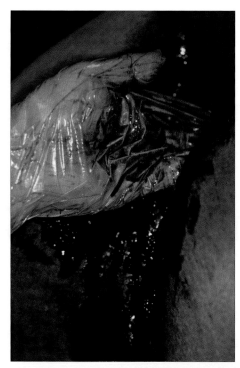

Figure 1.181 Rectal tear. Blood on a rectal sleeve following palpation; indicative of a rectal tear.

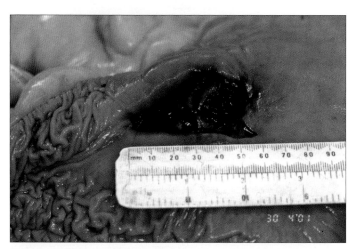

Figure 1.182 Rectal tear. Post-mortem showing full-thickness rectal tear.

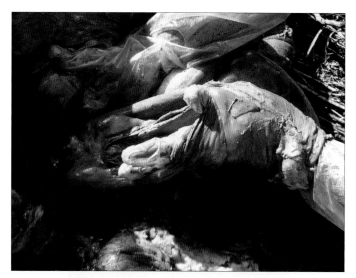

Figure 1.183 Rectal tear. Post-mortem showing large rectal tear with hand placed inside the rectum.

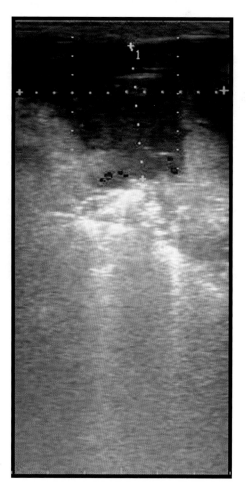

Figure 1.184 Rectal abscess (ultrasonographic view).

intrapelvic infection. In the latter, peritoneal contamination usually occurs particularly rapidly and these cases carry a grave prognosis even when identified early. Affected horses usually strain heavily within a few minutes (or hours) of the initial incident. Peritoneal contamination (as evidenced by rising neutrophil counts in peritoneal fluid) or gross peritoneal contamination results in peritonitis and abdominal guarding (indicative of parietal pain). Colic within a few hours of rectal examination should alert the clinician to the possibility of rectal tears, even if blood was not seen on the sleeve at the time of the examination.

Diagnosis and treatment

- Diagnosis of rectal tears should be made with the aid of careful rectal examination and endoscopy, accurate location and characterization of the tear will enable the clinician to make the appropriate therapeutic decisions. Frequently a combination of sedation, spasmolytics and/or epidural anesthesia may be required in order to perform a through examination without worsening the condition. Blood on a sleeve following rectal examination should never be ignored.

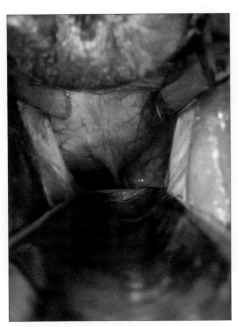

Figure 1.185 Rectal abscess (vaginal view).

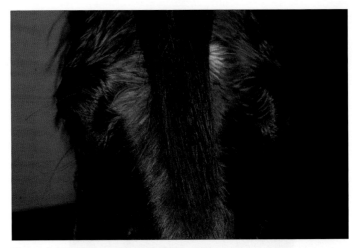

Figure 1.187 Acute grass sickness. Eyelid ptosis.

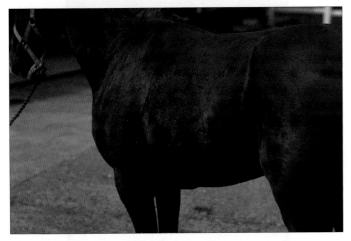

Figure 1.186 Acute grass sickness. Patchy sweating.

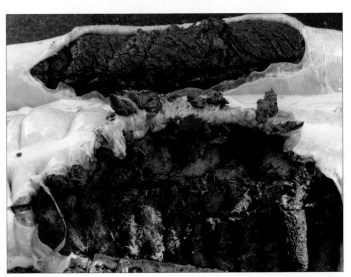

Figure 1.188 Acute grass sickness. Colon impaction.

- Grade I and II tears rarely require surgical treatment. Medical management includes dietary adjustment to soften feces, laxatives such as mineral oil, antibiotics and antiinflammatories.
- Grade III tears usually require surgical intervention though there have been reports of successful medical treatment.
- Full-thickness tears into the retroperitoneal space are treated with manual evacuation of feces several times daily, antibiotics and stool softeners. Many develop secondary abscesses which can be drained into the rectum/vagina or perirectally.
- Surgical techniques described for repair of rectal tears include colostomy, insertion of a temporary rectal liner and direct suturing. These techniques may be used alone or in combination.

Grass sickness (Figs. 1.186–1.193)

Equine grass sickness is an acquired degenerative polyneuropathy that predominantly affects the neurons of the autonomic and enteric nervous systems. Cases of grass sickness are presently largely restricted to limited areas of Europe and more specifically to the United Kingdom, although a clinically and histopathologically similar disease, mal seco,

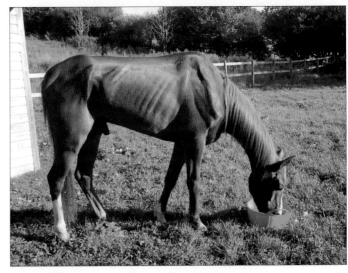

Figure 1.189 Chronic grass sickness. Typical tucked up appearance.

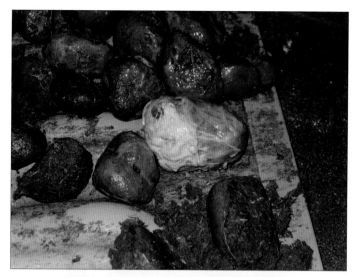

Figure 1.190 Chronic grass sickness. Hard mucus-covered feces.

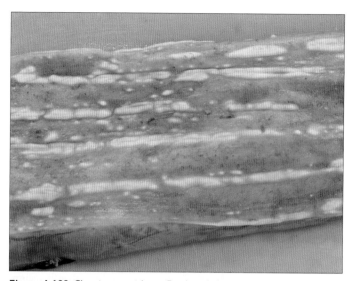

Figure 1.192 Chronic grass sickness. Esophageal ulceration.

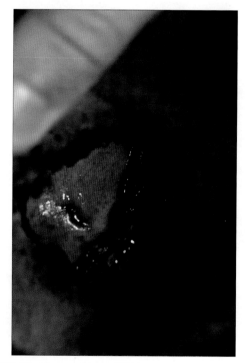

Figure 1.191 Chronic grass sickness. Rhinitis sicca.

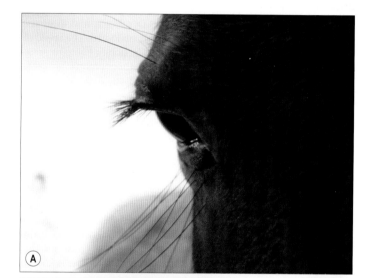

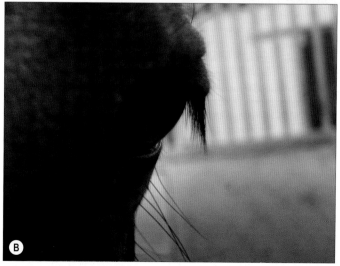

Figure 1.193 Phenylephrine test for acute grass sickness. Phenylephrine has been applied to the right eye (A) and not to the left (B); notice the ptosis evident in the left eye compared to the right.

occurs in southern Argentina. While most cases are encountered in grazing horses between 2–10 years of age, in spring or early autumn, rare cases occur in older horses, stabled horses and during the winter months.

The etiology of the disease is unknown, but currently toxic infection with *C. botulinum* type C is thought to be involved in combination with other trigger factors. Cases are encountered more commonly when warm wet weather has prevailed over a few days, and both outbreaks involving several horses and single sporadic cases are recognized. Specific fields seem to be particularly associated with grass sickness, but many cases occur in isolated places without any apparent reason and sometimes when pasture has had no previous horse contact.

The disease has a wide range of clinical manifestations which are largely dependent upon the speed of onset and the extent of the characteristic alimentary paralysis.

1) **Acute form**. Clinical signs are related to acute onset of gastrointestinal ileus. Signs of abdominal pain may be severe. Spontaneous nasal regurgitation of greenish, acidic fluid is common and indicative of dramatic, dangerous gastric distension and impending gastric rupture. Patchy sweating and triceps fasciculations are regular signs. Other clinical signs include pyrexia, dysphagia and bilateral ptosis. Horses affected with the acute form invariably die within 24–48 hours of onset, in spite of the best nursing efforts.

2) **Subacute form**. These horses do not develop gastric and small intestinal distension but have marked large colon impactions. They have intermittent colic and patchy sweating and may have rhinitis sicca. The clinical course is usually 3–7 days.

3) **Chronic form**. The course of the chronic form is weeks to months. Progressive desiccation of the contents of the hypomotile colon results in dramatically reduced fecal output and hard, black, pelleted feces are characteristic. These are often covered with a slimy mucus, indicative of prolonged small colon transfer time. Although colonic hypomotility is the usual finding, occasional cases of grass sickness develop profuse diarrhea (presumably as a result of the deranged motility). Paralysis of the esophagus and consequent dysphagia are also common features. Dysphagia and dramatic weight loss result in a boarded, tucked-up abdomen. The speed of development of this typical appearance, in horses living in areas where the disease is endemic, is almost pathognomonic for grass sickness. Most chronic cases have rhinitis sicca.

Diagnosis, treatment and prognosis

- Most cases in endemic areas are diagnosed on the basis of clinical signs with the diagnostic accuracy of clinicians in these areas being reported as high as 100%.
- A definitive ante-mortem diagnosis is currently based on histopathological examination of the intrinsic myenteric plexus in the ileum, while post-mortem diagnosis can be made with certainty from examination of the mesenteric autonomic ganglia. The finding at laparotomy of a markedly reduced or an obvious hypermotility (without any apparent co-ordination of movement of the bowel) in an animal without any other apparent cause for this should be treated as suspicious in areas where the disease is known to exist.
- Post-mortem examination in the acute cases reveals the grossly distended stomach which contains a greenish mucoid fluid, while the contents of the cecum and colon, in cases surviving for more than 48 hours and in a few of the more acute cases, will be desiccated and scanty.
- The acute and subacute forms of the disease carry a poor prognosis. The reported survival rate with the chronic form of the disease is up to 49% with appropriate nursing care. It may reach 70% if cases are carefully selected.

Infiltrative bowel diseases (Figs. 1.194 & 1.195)

Infiltration of the intestinal tract with inflammatory or neoplastic cells results in malabsorption of nutrients and frequently protein-losing enteropathies. Clinical signs may be similar regardless of the cells involved and include weight loss, lethargy, diarrhea and in some cases dependent edema. The cause of invasion of inflammatory cells can be determined in some cases and may be related to parasitism, mycobacterial infections or neoplasia. However, in many cases the cause cannot be determined and these cases are collectively referred to as chronic inflammatory bowel disease (CIBD). In the horse there are four types of CIBD recognized:

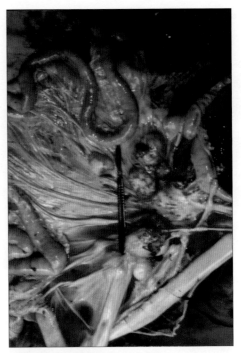

Figure 1.194 Malabsorption. Intestinal tuberculosis.

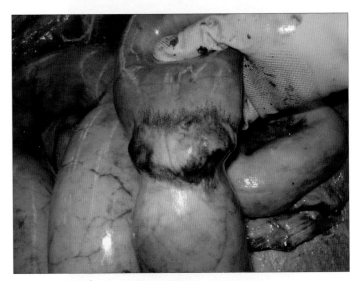

Figure 1.195 Malabsorption. Intestinal lymphosarcoma.

- granulomatous enteritis (GE)
- lymphocytic-plasmacytic enteritis (LPE)
- multisystemic eosinophilic epitheliotropic disease (MEED)
- and idiopathic focal eosinophilic enterocolitis (IFEE).

Diagnosis

- While definitive diagnosis in most cases of CIBD relies on histological examination of a biopsy specimen some special considerations should be borne in mind.
- Normal populations of inflammatory cells vary in number between individuals, segment of intestine and species. Therefore it is important to have a pathologist who is very familiar with reading equine intestinal biopsies.

- Lymphoid and plasma cells can be found in the rectal tissue of horses with a variety of intestinal disorders and their presence can rarely be used to support a diagnosis of LPE.
- As there is often involvement of the liver in MEED, liver biopsies can be useful for aiding diagnosis. However, IFEE can be difficult to diagnose by biopsy due to its focal nature.

Granulomatous enteritis

GE has been reported in many breeds of horse but appears to be over-represented in Standardbreds in which there is a suggested genetic predisposition to development of the condition. Most affected horses are young and present with a history of weight loss and poor appetite. Some cases may also have skin lesions of the head and limbs (especially coronary band).

The most consistent clinicopathological features are hypoalbuminemia and anemia. Glucose or xylose absorption testing reveals abnormal absorption which is attributed to the severe villous atrophy that is normally present. Early cases may retain normal absorption.

The disease is histologically similar to Crohn's disease in humans and Johne's disease in cattle but horses have not responded to drugs used to treat Crohn's disease in humans. The cause is undiagnosed in many cases although it has been linked to possible *Mycobacterium* infection in a few individuals and aluminum toxicosis in a farm outbreak. There have been a few reports of successful short-term treatment by surgical removal of the most severely affected areas of bowel or dexamethasone therapy. However, there are no reports of long-term successful treatment and any therapy undertaken should bear in mind the usually diffuse and advanced nature of the disease at diagnosis.

Lymphocytic-plasmacytic enterocolitis

LPE is rarely reported in horses but in the cases reported there appears to be no predilection of age, sex or breed. These horses usually present for weight loss but may also present for chronic diarrhea or recurrent colic. Anemia or hypoalbuminemia are not consistent features of the disease but most have abnormal carbohydrate absorption tests. Some cases have responded to treated with dexamethasone (0.02 mg/kg IM q 48 h) but the majority were euthanized due to lack of response to therapy and/or poor body condition.

Multisystemic eosinophilic epitheliotropic disease

This disease is characterized by eosinophilic infiltration of not only the bowel but also other organs. Similar to GE it is overrepresented in young Standardbreds. Affected horses usually have an exudative dermatitis of the face, limbs and ventral abdomen along with ulcerations of the coronary band and mouth. Anemia is rarely present, unlike GE. White cell counts may be normal but some cases have a marked eosinophilia. The liver is also commonly affected and γ-glutamyl transferase measurements are often high. Most horses with MEED have normal carbohydrate absorption tests as lesions are more likely to involve the large intestine.

Treatment of affected horses with antimicrobials, anthelmintics and corticosteroids has in many cases been unsuccessful. Proposed treatments include cytotoxic drugs such as vincristine or hydroxyurea; or immunomodulating drugs such as cyclosporine or interferon-α. These proposals are based on treatment of human patients with hypereosinophilic syndromes.

The causes of most cases are unknown but in one horse was related to concurrent lymphosarcoma and in another to T-cell lymphoid hyperplasia. Unresponsive cases in humans are often related to a chromosomal mutation that results in T-cell proliferation and as such it is suggested that affected horses should be tested for underlying T-cell proliferation as it may indicate a poorer prognosis.

Idiopathic focal eosinophilic enterocolitis

In some horses eosinophilic infiltration is restricted to the bowel. These horses are given a different classification to MEED as they have a better prognosis and usually present with different clinical signs. Affected horses are unlikely to be anemic or hypoalbuminemic and most present with a history of colic rather than weight loss. The small intestine or large intestine can be affected. When the former is affected distended loops of small intestine can be palpated per rectum and peritoneal fluid has a high protein concentration but normal white cell count. When the latter is affected there may be a soft impaction of the pelvic flexure palpable per rectum and peritoneal fluid is turbid or sanguineous with a high concentration of proteins and a high white cell count.

Surgical treatment is generally required and can involve resection of the affected segment of bowel or decompression and post-operative treatment with prokinetics with or without corticosteroids. Survival rates are reported as being better with fewer post-surgical complications if decompression without resection is performed.

Intestinal lymphoma

The intestinal form of lymphoma can occur as a single or multiple solid tumors, or as a diffuse infiltrate of neoplastic cells. Weight loss is the most common clinical sign but fever, dependent edema, diarrhea and recurrent colic can all be seen. Those horses with small intestinal involvement may have abnormal carbohydrate absorption tests. Rectal examination may reveal diffuse thickening of the bowel or enlargement of lymph nodes. Neoplastic cells can on occasion be found on examination of peritoneal fluid. Treatment with corticosteroids may prolong the survival time and there are various reports of treatments with chemotherapy. Treatment with progesterone is also thought to retard the growth of some lymphomas due to the presence of progesterone receptors in some cases.

Prognosis

All these disorders carry a guarded or poor prognosis but some cases may improve or reach a satisfactory level with treatment. The specific requirements of the owner in terms of use of the horse, life expectancy and medication compliance should be discussed. It is important to try to differentiate the cases with a poor outlook from those conditions with similar general clinical signs, but which are resolvable, such as heavy parasitic infestation, dental disease and diet-related digestive disturbances.

Gastric and gastroduodenal ulceration

(Figs. 1.196–1.206)

Gastric and gastroduodenal ulceration occur frequently in very young foals, particularly when subjected to stressful circumstances and/or non-steroidal anti-inflammatory drugs. Even those foals subjected to relatively minor stresses, such as transportation or minor surgery, are prone to the disorder. It may develop in individual foals which have no apparent stress or other inciting cause.

There are four distinct clinical syndromes recognized in foals; silent or subclinical ulcers; active or clinical ulcers; perforating ulcers and pyloric strictures caused by resolving ulcers.

- *Silent (subclinical) ulcers*. These are usually found in the non-glandular mucosa along the greater curvature bordering the margo plicatus but may be found in the glandular mucosa. They are commonly found in foals less than 4 months of age and may heal spontaneously.
- *Active (clinical) ulcers*. These are most frequently found in the non-glandular mucosa along the greater or lesser curvature bordering the margo plicatus, but may also be found in the glandular mucosa. These foals are those that have the typical clinical signs associated with gastric ulceration. Frequently there is persistent

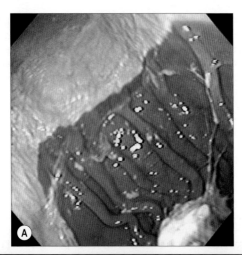

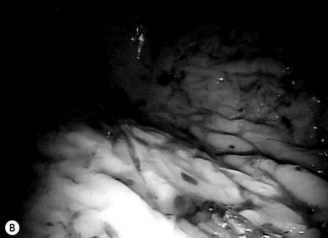

Figure 1.196 Normal gastric mucosa. (A) From a foal with a liquid diet in which the mucosa appears 'clean'; (B) from an adult with a solid diet. It is frequently necessary to clean the gastric surface with water in order to examine it fully.

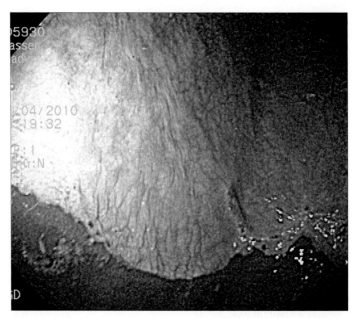

Figure 1.197 Gastric ulceration. Grade 1. Intact mucosa with areas of redding or hyperkeratosis.

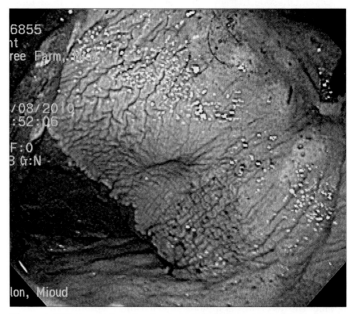

Figure 1.198 Gastric ulceration. Grade 2. Small single or multifocal lesions.

grinding of the teeth (bruxism) which results in a foamy saliva-tion. Affected foals spend long periods in dorsal recumbency. They are depressed and frequently show interrupted nursing pat-terns and, sometimes, overt post-prandial colic.

• ***Perforating gastric or duodenal ulcers***. These can occur in the glandular or non-glandular mucosa or in the proximal duode-num. Perforation is followed in most cases by a diffuse peritonitis with progressive signs of abdominal distension and endotoxemia. Rare cases may develop a more localized peritonitis and recover with intensive therapy. Many of these foals have no or few clinical signs prior to rupture.

• ***Pyloric or duodenal ulcers***. While this syndrome is less common than the others it is regarded as significant due to the related formation of pyloric strictures and restriction of gastric outflow. Foals from 3–5 months are most typically affected and clinical signs include: bruxism, salivation, drooling of milk, colic and low-volume diarrhea or scant feces. These foals may also present with a variety of secondary complications such as aspiration pneumonia, cholangitis, erosive esophagitis, gastroesophageal reflux and severe secondary gastric ulceration.

Gastric ulcers

Gastric ulceration in horses over 3–4 months of age has been shown to occur frequently and again is most often encountered in

stressed horses and in association with non-steroidal administration. Horses in training seem particularly prone to ulceration whilst pasture-rested animals and brood mares are probably less affected. Similar to foals, silent ulcers are perhaps the most common but all of the syndromes seen in foals can also occur in adults. However, in contrast to foals, adults have ulceration of the glandular mucosa much less frequently and most ulcers are found in the non-glandular mucosa along the margo plicatus and may be on the greater or lesser curvatures.

Gastric ulcers are consistently more severe in horses with clinical signs as opposed to those without clinical signs but the degree of clini-cal signs is not consistent with the degree of ulceration. Gastric ulcers may be focal or diffuse, single or multiple.

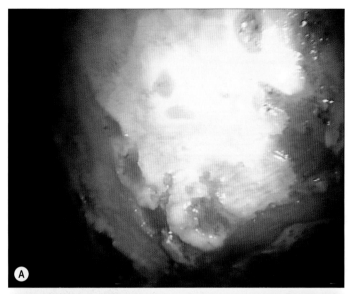

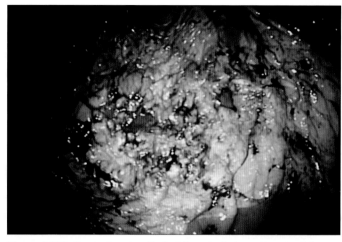

Figure 1.200 Gastric ulceration. Grade 4. Extensive lesions with areas of deep ulceration.

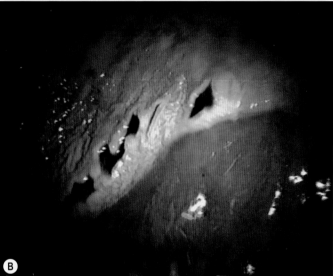

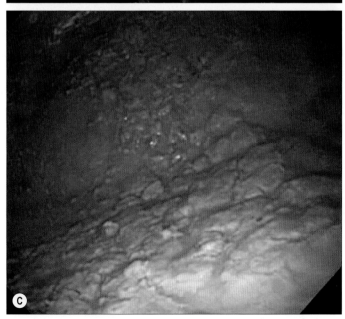

Figure 1.199 (A, B, C) Gastric ulceration, Grade 3. Large single or multifocal lesions or extensive superficial lesions.

A number of other conditions can result in diffuse erosions of the gastric mucosa. Severe generalized inflammation and variable hemorrhage characteristic of the caustic epithelial necrosis caused by **arsenic compounds**, **blister beetle toxicity** and by other irritant chemicals (including organophosphate anthelmintics). A similar syndrome may also be associated with salmonellosis, colitis and a number of other systemic disorders. Clinical signs of extreme pain and depression with dramatic generalized organ failure and circulatory collapse are typical, with the extent of the signs largely dependent upon the extent of the damage, and the specific toxicity of the inciting cause. The pathological changes encountered in the stomach from large doses of arsenic compounds are repeated throughout the gastrointestinal tract and the clinical signs are associated with massive caustic burning of the intestinal mucosa. The entire tract is intensely hyperemic and massive fluid loss occurs.

Diagnosis

- Diagnosis of gastric ulceration in both young and adult horses is largely reliant upon gastroscopy and this necessarily limits the number of cases in which the condition can be diagnosed definitively.
- Supportive evidence for its existence can be gained from the effects of specific anti-ulcer therapy, including the use of H₂-receptor-blocking drugs.
- If other conditions are suspected such as blister beetle toxicosis, specific diagnostic tests should be performed. Cantharidin can be assayed in the urine and stomach contents from affected horses. Arsenic concentration can be measured in urine ante-mortem and often exceeds 2 ppm. Post-mortem the liver, kidney, stomach and intestinal contents should be evaluated for arsenic content. Blood and milk can also be tested with levels >10 ppm confirming arsenic toxicosis.

Treatment

- Reduction of gastric acidity is the main goal of therapy and can be achieved through the use of a number of different drugs such as antacids, H₂-receptor antagonists (ranitidine and cimetidine), sucralfate, prostaglandin analogs and proton pump inhibitors (omeprazole). The mode of action of some of these drugs is illustrated in Fig. 1.201.
- Administration of omeprazole is now the preferred choice for many practitioners with greater efficiency of treatment shown in many

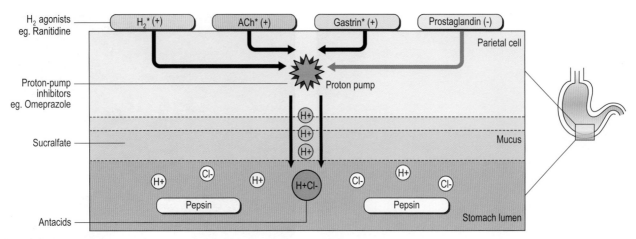

*Acid-stimulating receptors

Figure 1.201 Schematic image of gastric gland and mode of action of common anti-ulcer medications. Reproduced from McAuliffe SB, Slovis, NM (eds). *Color Atlas of Diseases and Disorders of the Foal* (2008), with permission from Elsevier.

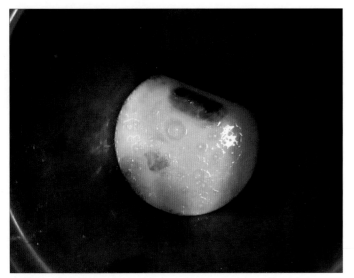

Figure 1.202 Gastric ulceration with secondary duodenal stricture. This foal presented with bruxism, ptyalism and gastric distension. Passage of a nasogastric tube resulted in spontaneous reflux of milk with fresh blood.

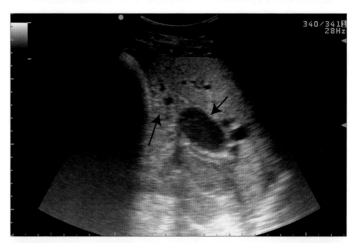

Figure 1.204 Ultrasonographic image demonstrating a section of duodenal thickening (arrow) and an adjacent section of duodenal distension (arrowhead), suggestive of a duodenal stricture.

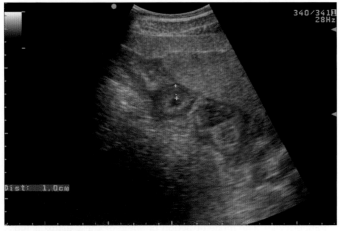

Figure 1.203 Ultrasonographic image of duodenal thickening (same foal as Fig. 1.202).

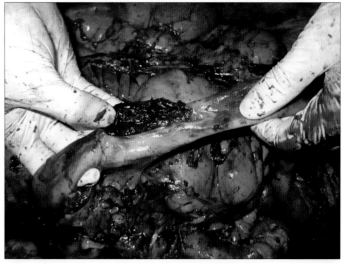

Figure 1.205 Post-mortem image of duodenal rupture.

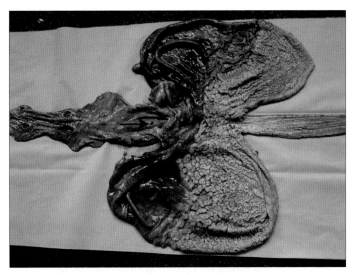

Figure 1.206 Post-mortem image of stomach and duodenum showing gastric and duodenal ulceration with duodenal perforation (arrow).

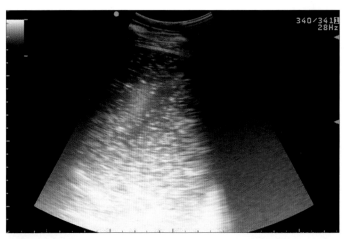

Figure 1.208 Ultrasonographic image of gastric distension (same foal as Fig. 1.202). A gas fluid interface is not evident due to the large amount of fluid present (7 L).

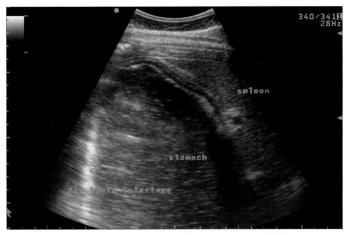

Figure 1.207 Ultrasonographic image of gastric distension. The stomach is markedly distended with gas and fluid; the interface between gas and fluid is seen as a vertical hyperechoic line.

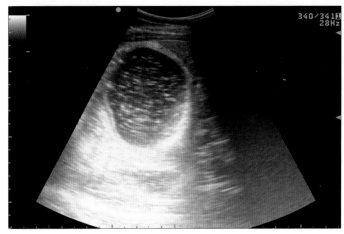

Figure 1.209 Ultrasonographic image showing marked distension of the duodenum (same foal as Fig. 1.208). Duodenal distension is frequently recognized with gastric distension.

clinical trials and increased availability of more economical generic forms.

- It is also important to remember that foals with gastric outflow obstruction cannot be treated with oral medications and require intravenous administration of either H$_2$-receptor antagonists or proton pump inhibitors.

Gastric distension (Figs. 1.207–1.210)

Acute gastric distension is one of the most painful and dangerous conditions of the horse and affected horses show prominent signs of colic with characteristically elevated heart and respiratory rates. The anatomical location of the stomach means that even severe distension is unlikely to produce any abdominal enlargement, although splenic displacement may be discernible during rectal examination. Horses, after racing or other heavy exercise, occasionally engorge sufficient amounts of cold water to create a painful and dangerous gastric distension. It is possibly the result of a pyloric spasm which prevents onward progression of gastric contents.

Gastric distension arising primarily from solid food material (grain overload) or secondarily to disorders of gastric motility/emptying is a serious and difficult disorder to diagnose definitively. Engorgement with, or accumulation of fibrous food or dry food which expands within the stomach are the commonest causes of primary gastric impaction. A chronic form of gastric distension is also recognized in which there is a progressive accumulation of fibrous food material in the stomach and while this becomes larger and firmer, more liquid material may pass over it and into the duodenum. Feces continue to be passed in small amounts and the horse develops a pot-bellied appearance which is not due to fluid accumulation within the peritoneal cavity. This form is likely to be a result of failure of the intrinsic gastric motility and while starvation may eventually result in some resolution, the condition recurs once feeding starts again.

A second somewhat similar gastric impactive syndrome has been described as a result of chronic ingestion of *Senecio* spp. plant poisoning, but a more significant consequence of this is chronic hepatic failure. Horses with the more common acute impactive gastric

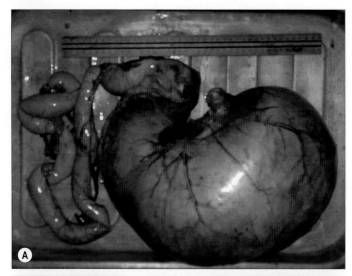

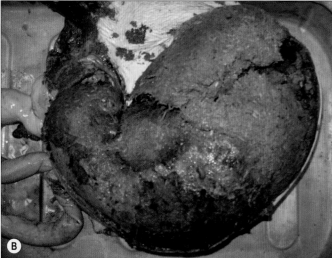

Figure 1.210 Gastric impaction secondary to chronic hepatic failure.

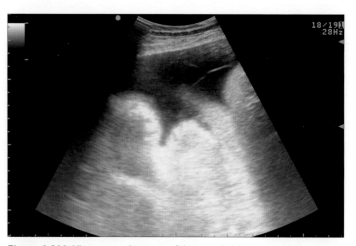

Figure 1.211 Ultrasonographic image of the ventral abdomen revealing copious amounts of fluid of a mixed echogenicity. Abdominocentesis yielded fluid contaminated with feed material and a gastric rupture was confirmed at post-mortem examination.

distension syndromes are presented with mild or moderate, progressive colic. They are often severely acidotic and may progress to hypovolemic shock. Chronic and recurrent gastric distension arising secondarily to pyloric obstructions is rare in adult horses but heavy accumulations of parasites such as *Gastrophilus* spp. larvae (Bots) may induce sufficient gastritis and pyloric swelling to cause recurrent gastric distension.

Physical and functional obstructive disorders of the small (and to a lesser extent the large) intestine are common causes of gastric distension. This is frequently seen with small intestinal ileus either from a proximal jejunitis/ileitis or a post-operative ileus. It can also be seen with some colon displacements that result in obstruction of the duodenum. Under these circumstances there may be spontaneous reflux of gastric fluid and large amounts of gastric reflux can usually be released by the passage of a nasogastric tube. The clinical signs are otherwise similar to gastric distension due to other causes. Significant gastric distension may, also, be due to the accumulation of gas/air in horses affected by the neurosis, windsucking (aerophagia), although in these the stomach is usually chronically distended and non-painful. Horses subject to this vice are often not hungry in spite of poor condition and show no other evidence of disease. They seldom show colic as a result of gastric distension but gross swallowing of air may result in clinically significant, recurrent, and occasionally acutely painful distension in the more distal alimentary tract.

Diagnosis

- Clinical signs of colic with elevations of heart and respiratory rates.
- Ultrasound examination reveals an enlarged stomach with a visible gas–fluid interface and caudal displacement of the spleen.
- Rectal palpation may reveal caudal displacement of the spleen.
- Passage of a nasogastric tube invariably results in relief in acute distensions which is usually complete in cases of water engorgement. It may however be unrewarding in cases of impaction with solid feed material.
- Gastroscopy or laparotomy may be required for diagnosis of chronic impactions with feed material.
- Assessment of gastric fluid pH. Primary gastric disorders usually have large volumes of fluid having a very low pH. Distension of the stomach arising secondarily to intestinal obstructions, however, shows elevation of the pH of gastric contents due to reflux of strongly alkaline duodenal secretions. The pH is, however, seldom actually alkaline.
- In cases of suspected aerophagia history and physical evidence of windsucking may aid diagnosis.

Treatment

- Depends on the cause but nasogastric intubation and reflux of gastric contents may be all that is required in acute distensions.
- Motility disorders require specific treatment depending on the section of the bowel affected.
- Obstructions resulting in secondary distension require specific treatment which may in many cases be surgical.

Gastric rupture (Figs. 1.211 & 1.212)

Gastric rupture usually occurs along the greater curvature of the stomach and is commonly associated with neglected or untreated cases of excessive gastric distension. It is also a frequent complication of grass sickness. Grain overload may also result in rupture but in these cases slow progressive hydration and swelling of the contents is responsible. Imminent rupture is accompanied by a dramatic rise in heart rate and sometimes an acidic, green, nasal reflux will be seen, although the latter is usually in small amount. Rupture is associated with an apparently dramatic cessation of pain and a further small amount of reflux, often containing some blood, may occur spontaneously.

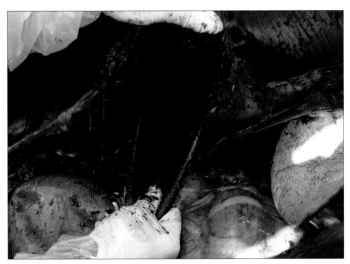

Figure 1.212 Gastric rupture along greater curvature.

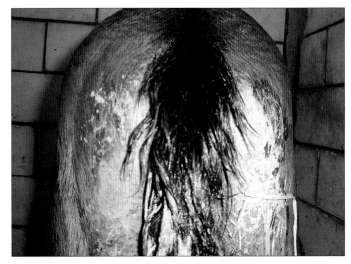

Figure 1.213 Foal with rotavirus diarrhea.

Diagnosis

- Clinically, the patient is obviously in a very critical condition with deteriorating cardiovascular parameters and the rapid development of endotoxic and hypovolemic shock.
- Rectal examination of horses affected by gastric (or other viscus) rupture has a very characteristic granular or gritty feel.
- Abdominal ultrasonography reveals large amounts of free fluid. The echogenicity of the fluid depends on the duration and cause of the rupture in addition to the diet of the horse.
- Abdominal paracentesis of such a case will reveal contaminated brown or reddish fluid which contains a high cell content and a sediment of food particles. Gastric rupture usually occurs as a result of excessive pressure within the organ; most cases show extensive and severe abdominal contamination.

Infectious disorders

Viral disease

Infections with enteric pathogens are relatively uncommon in horses when compared to other species of large animals. However, several viral and bacterial infections are significant causes of disease.

Rotavirus (Fig. 1.213)

Rotavirus is probably the commonest cause of infectious enteritis in foals. While most affected horses are between 1–6 months old, foals as young as 1 day old can be affected and outbreaks are common. Adult horses are usually solidly immune following previous challenge but foals, particularly those stressed by environmental or other factors, are susceptible. A profuse, watery diarrhea is typically present and affected foals are mildly febrile and anorectic. However, many cases show only limited, transient diarrhea without any other systemic effects. The disease is more severe in foals receiving heavy challenges of virulent strains of the virus or that have concurrent bacterial infections. The source of infection is thought to be adult carriers or the environment. A few foals show a persistence of diarrhea and chronic ill-thrift following the disease, possibly due to more severe and persistent changes in the mucosal structure of the intestine, which in some cases is related to lactose intolerance.

Diagnosis and treatment

- A presumptive diagnosis can usually be made on clinical and epidemiological features but specific identification of the virus particles by ELISA (enzyme-linked immunosorbent assay) or electron microscopy are definitive means of diagnosis.
- Rotaviral diarrhea is usually self-limiting and typically resolves within 3–5 days but supportive therapy, especially in very young or very severely affected foals, including intravenous fluid therapy and nutritional support may be required.
- Lactase supplementation may be useful, especially in cases with a more prolonged course.
- Affected foals and their dams should be regarded as infectious and appropriate measures should be taken to prevent spread to other foals.

Equine coronavirus

Equine coronavirus (ECoV) has been found in the feces of both healthy foals and those with enteric disease. It is not generally associated with outbreaks of diarrhoea in the foal; when present in diseased foals, it appears to be present concurrently with other pathogens.

Recent ECoV related outbreaks in adults have been reported in Japan and USA. Clinical signs included anorexia, lethargy, fever and diarrhea. In a recent report, there were four fatalities from 59 affected horses; in two of these cases, septicaemia was suspected on postmortem (most likely from bacterial translocation).

Diagnosis and treatment

- Diagnosis is currently based on fecal PCR, supported by clinical signs.
- Hematological abnormalities may include leukopenia due to neutropenia/lymphopenia.
- Data from the recent outbreaks would suggest that ECoV is a self-limiting disease in adults with clinical signs lasting from 1–4 days. Supportive care including fluid replacement and NSAIDs for pyrexia may be warranted in some cases. In cases where there are secondary complications, such as septicaemia, further intensive treatment will be warranted.
- In diarrheic foals, currently ECoV is unlikely to be the only aetiological agent, therefore treatment regimes will be determined by the clinical signs and other aetiological agents present.
- The epidemiology and pathophysiology of ECoV is not fully understood, but from recent outbreaks, ECoV appears to be highly contagious. Transmission is thought to be via fecal-oral route.
- Strict biosecurity measures should be in place in properties with confirmed or suspect cases to help prevent the spread of viral particles to other animals.
- There are currently no prophylactic strategies available.

Bacterial diseases (Figs. 1.214–1.216)

Bacterial enteritis in foals is usually the result of Gram-negative pathogens such as *Escherichia coli* and *Salmonella* spp. Very young foals, or those suffering from stress, or those affected by immunocompromising disorders (including failure of passive transfer of colostrally derived antibodies), are most likely to suffer from bacterial enteritis. The infections are usually septicemic and this group of organisms is responsible for most cases of the neonatal septicemia syndrome in which clinical signs of enteritis may or may not be prominent. In most cases the origin of the infection is likely to have been the alimentary tract or the umbilicus. Septicemic foals are dull, febrile and anorectic. Diarrhea, which often contains blood and/or shreds of mucous membrane, may be seen.

Acute equine colitis

Acute colitis is characterized by diarrhea with varying degrees of dehydration, toxemia and abdominal pain. It is a frequent and important cause of death in horses. It is estimated that a definitive diagnosis of the cause of the colitis is only made in 20–30% of cases. A variety of organisms may be involved, but *Salmonella* spp., *Clostidia* spp., and *Neorickettsia risticii* are among the more common ones.

Salmonellosis

Adult carriers of *Salmonella* spp. organisms may develop a fulminating and highly fatal diarrhea syndrome shortly after they are subjected to stress. Even short transportation or apparently minor surgical procedures may be sufficient to allow the organisms to multiply and invade the mucosa of the large intestine with serious consequences including profuse, dark diarrhea, often containing shreds of mucosa and blood, dullness, and in many cases, rapid death. Compromised animals (young, concurrently ill or hospitalized for other reasons) may be infected with much lower doses.

Equine intestinal clostridiosis

Clostridial infections within the gut may cause severe enterocolitis in both adults and foals. *Clostridium perfringens* and *Clostridium difficile* are most commonly recognized but other *Clostridium* spp. may also cause intestinal infections in horses. In horses of all ages it is a common antibiotic-associated and nosocomial cause of diarrhea.

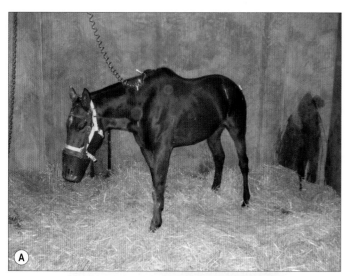

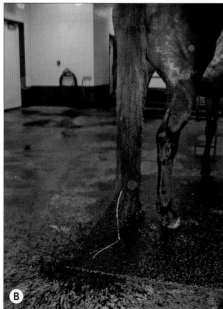

Figure 1.214 (A) Salmonellosis in an adult horse with profuse watery diarrhea. (B) Hemorrhagic colitis.

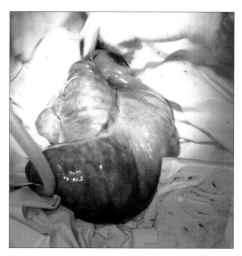

Figure 1.215 Salmonellosis in this yearling resulted in multifocal necrosis of the cecum.

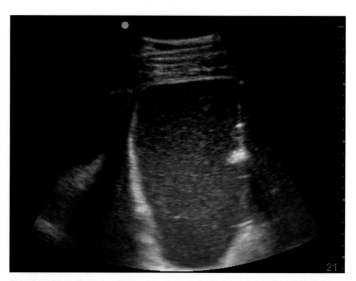

Figure 1.216 Ultrasound image of cecum and colon demonstrating fluid-filled contents typical of a typhlocolitis.

Table 1.2 Diagnostic testing for *Clostridium difficile*-associated colitis

Test	Positive result	Negative result	Comment
Culture	Also found in normal horses and detects nontoxigenic strains. Poor PPV	Good NPV if performed in laboratory accustomed to handling samples	Not useful for diagnosis unless combined with other tests
Antigen ELISA	Indicates presence of toxigenic or non-toxigenic strains, which can both occur in normal horses	Good NPV	Useful initial screening test with positives selected for toxin testing
Cell cytotoxicity assay	Considered true positive but not readily available	Considered true negative	**Gold standard that tests for Toxin B**
Toxin A/antigen ELISA	Combined positive antigen/toxin has good PPV	Paired negative good NPV	Antigen positive, toxin negative, should be tested for Toxin B by alternate method
Toxin A ELISA	PPV is likely good but there may be variability between tests	NPV is not good as A−/B+ strains will give a negative result	Will miss clinically relevant A−/B+ strains
Toxin A/B ELISA	PPV is likely good but there may be variability between tests	NPV better than Toxin A tests but overall sensitivity is unclear	Reasonable clinical option but combined with antigen testing or detection of toxin genes strengthens diagnosis
PCR for toxin genes	Poor PPV as toxigenic strains may occur in healthy horses	Not useful	Unvalidated and not useful alone but may add strength to positive ELISA

Adapted from Weese JS. Clostridial Disease. In Robinson NE, Sprayberry KA (eds) (2009) Current Therapy in Equine Medicine, 6th edn. WB Saunders, St. Louis, MO, USA.

Clostridium perfringens

The virulence of a given strain of *C. perfringens* is thought to be based on exotoxin production. There are five types of exotoxin: A, B, C, D and E. Type A is the most common isolate from healthy horses worldwide. Types A–D have been isolated from foals with hemorrhagic enteritis, with type C being the most common in the United States. The primary toxin of type A is an α-toxin which interferes with glucose uptake and energy production in the enterocyte. The β-toxin of types B and C is a cytotoxin that causes enterocyte necrosis and ulceration. Virulent strains may also produce an enterotoxin which results in altered cell permeability leading to cell necrosis.

C. perfringens is commonly found in the feces of healthy horses, especially foals, and, as with *C. difficile*, the clinical presentations and clinical pathology findings seen are very variable. Although historically regarded as producing a more severe hemorrhagic diarrhea than *C. difficile*, this has been clearly proven.

Clostridium difficile

This *Clostridium* species produces several toxins but only types A and B are thought to be significant. Type B is a potent cytotoxin in vitro but its role in vivo is less clear. Type A, on the other hand, induces a marked vasodilatory and secretory response in the intestine. The colitis caused is most often sporadic but outbreaks can occur especially in foal populations. *C. difficile* is reported as being present in up to 42% of antibiotic-associated diarrheas. The clinical presentation seen is quite variable, ranging from mild diarrhea with no apparent systemic illness to a peracute fatal necrohemorrhagic enterocolitis with signs of severe endotoxemia. Clinical pathology results are also variable and non-specific for clostridial infection. Leukopenia with neutropenia, hypo- or hyperproteinemia and prerenal azotemia are commonly seen.

Neorickettsia risticii (Potomac horse fever)

This obligate intracellular organism causes a seasonal (July-October) colitis that is most frequently encountered in the US mid-Atlantic states, but has been reported sporadically in other states in addition to isolated cases in Canada and Europe. The exact pathogenesis remains unknown. High fevers (up to 41.70°C/1070°F) may precede the onset of diarrhea and a high percentage develop peracute laminitis.

Diagnosis

- *Salmonella* spp. can be identified by bacterial culture and, in some cases, polymerase chain reaction (PCR).
- The diagnostic tests and their usefulness for *Clostridia* spp. are outlined in Table 1.2.
- PCR testing of blood and feces for *Neorickettsi risticii* is the most rapid diagnostic test; although a rise in antibody titer can be used, it is generally too slow to guide antibiotic therapy. Both feces and blood should be tested as early as possible in the disease, as both may be negative later in the disease.

Treatment

- Supportive care is the mainstay of therapy regardless of cause, and involves variable amounts of intravenous fluids (crystalloids and colloids), nutritional support and anti-endotoxin therapy.
- Metronidazole is the drug of choice for clostridial infections, although there have been reports of rare cases of metronidazole resistance. It is important to remember that a failure to respond to metronidazole therapy may not actually be an indication of resistance, but rather an indicator of the severity of the disease.
- Oxytetracycline (6.6 mg/kg iv. q12h for 3–5 days) is indicated in cases confirmed or suspected of Potomac horse fever. A response is normally seen within 12 hours, with an abatement of fever and subsequent improvement in attitude and appetite. Judicious use of this antibiotic is required, as it is associated with the production of drug induced colitis.
- Other adjunct therapies include Di-Tri-octahedral smectite (1.5 kg loading dose then 450 g PO q4–6h), which binds toxins in vitro, although its efficacy in vivo is not as clear. The administration of probiotics and the yeast *Saccharomyces boulardii* may shorten the course of the disease but has not been shown to improve the overall survival rate.

Public health

C. difficile is an important pathogen in humans and pathogenic strains found in horses are often indistinguishable from those found in horses. Although direct transfer has not yet been shown it is wise to regard the disease as potentially zoonotic and take all suitable precautions.

Lawsonia intracellularis *infection* (Figs. 1.217–1.220)

Proliferative enteropathy caused by *L. intracellularis* typically affects 4–7-month-old weaned foals. The characteristics of the condition are chronic wasting, severe hypoproteinemia and markedly thickened small intestine. Multiple animals on the farm may be affected. The

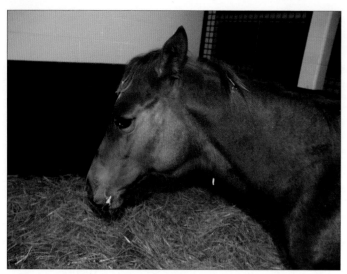

Figure 1.217 *Lawsonia intracellularis* infection. Weanling foal with typical submandibular edema.

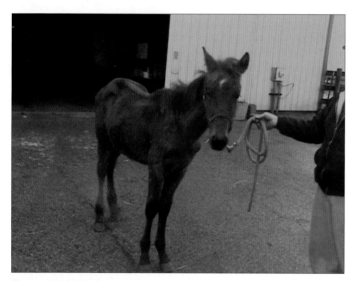

Figure 1.218 Weanling with *Lawsonia intracellularis*, showing typical poor body condition and some limb edema.

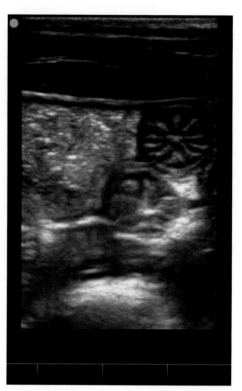

Figure 1.219 Ultrasonographic image of small intestine showing marked thickening and edema (cart-wheel appearance) typical of *Lawsonia intracellularis* infection.

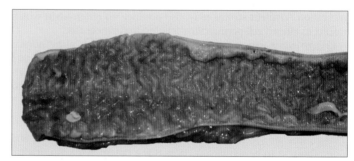

Figure 1.220 *Lawsonia intracellularis* infection. Post-mortem specimen showing marked thickening of small intestine giving it a 'corrugated' appearance. Note also the presence of *Anoplocephala perfoliata* in this image.

onset is often insidious and abnormal signs may not be identified until disease is advanced. Weakness, depression, ill thrift, poor body condition and submandibular edema are most common. Diarrhea is not present in all cases and the hypoproteinemia is often more severe than would be expected considering the duration and severity of diarrhea.

Diagnosis
- Diagnosis is often presumptively made on the basis of ultrasonographic findings of intestinal thickening and edema, hypoproteinemia and classical clinical signs.
- Indirect fluorescent antibody testing is useful but currently there is limited availability. Titers >1 : 30 are considered to be diagnostic of infection in foals.
- Detection of *L. intracellularis* in feces via PCR is diagnostic and commonly used but there is a high incidence of false-negatives.

Treatment
- Tetracyclines (docycline, oxytetracycline) are now considered the treatment of choice although macrolides have been used with good success.

- Supportive therapy in the way of plasma administration is required in many cases.

Miscellaneous disorders

Intestinal hyperammonemia
Hyperammonemia not associated with hepatic dysfunction has been reported in a number of adult horses and foals. Histories frequently include some type of abdominal disturbance such as enterocolitis or neoplasia. Most are suspected of having hyperammonemia on the basis of the presence of neurological signs which can vary from mild depression to manic behavior and seizures.

Diagnosis
- Diagnosis of hyperammonemia is based on detection of elevated serum ammonia levels but diagnosis of the cause of this elevation

may be somewhat more challenging. Hepatic dysfunction should first be ruled out based on determination of hepatic enzymes and if necessary hepatic function tests.

- Further diagnostics including abdominal ultrasonography, radiography or biopsies of specific organs may then be required.

Treatment

Treatment is largely dependent on treatment of the primary disorder in addition to treatment for the hyperammonemia (see p. 89). A recent study put the survival rate of horses presenting with intestinal hyperammonemia at 39%.

Peritoneal disorders

Peritonitis (Figs. 1.221–1.227)

Peritonitis may result from septic causes (either acute or chronic) or from chemical causes. Acute septic peritonitis is usually a result of intestinal rupture (i.e., gastric or duodenal perforation) or secondary to intestinal inflammation, e.g., *Clostridium* diarrhea and/or ischemia. It may also be seen in relation to uterine or bladder rupture. Chronic septic peritonitis is usually caused by abscesses within the peritoneal cavity. These are usually a sequel to either bacteremic conditions, such as *Rhodococcus equi*, *Streptococcus equi* abdominal abscessation, tuberculosis, or penetrating wounds from the abdominal wall or from

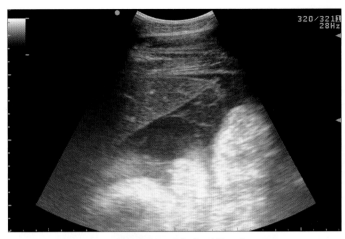

Figure 1.223 Peritonitis. Free abdominal fluid and fibrin formation.

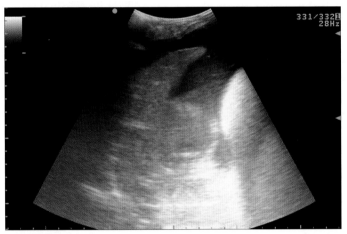

Figure 1.221 Peritonitis. Ultrasonographic image showing copious amounts of hypoechoic peritoneal fluid. The ultrasonographic findings of peritonitis can be very variable depending on the inciting cause and the duration of the peritonitis.

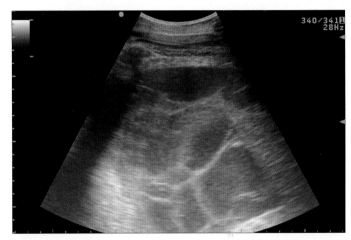

Figure 1.224 Peritonitis. Loculated appearance as continued fibrin formation results in septation of sections of fluid. This is typical of longstanding cases of peritonitis.

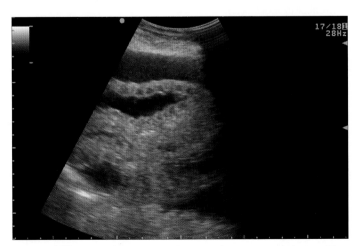

Figure 1.222 Peritonitis. Ultrasonographic image demonstrating thickening and edema of the small intestine in response to peritonitis.

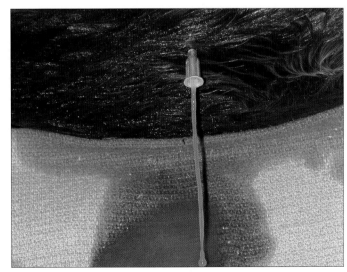

Figure 1.225 Copious amounts of dark peritoneal fluid associated with peritonitis.

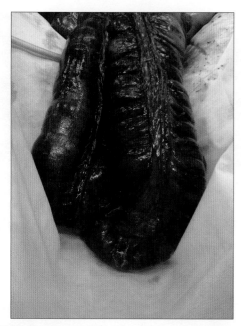

Figure 1.226 Inflammation of the bowel (colon) in response to peritonitis.

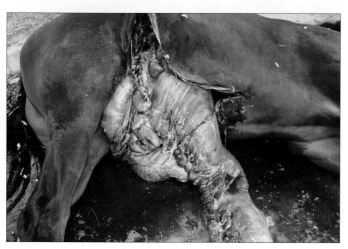

Figure 1.227 Fibrinous peritonitis.

penetrations of the gut, such as occurs after cecal perforations and rectal tears, or from surgical interferences such as castration. Chemical/mechanical peritonitis may occur secondary to uroperitoneum, hemoabdomen, parasite migration or surgical handling of the bowel.

Focal peritonitis or **diffuse fibrinous peritonitis** are relatively common and where the inflammation extends to the parietal peritoneum affected horses show a characteristic reluctance to move, stretching, a tense 'boarded' abdomen and pain and resentment on abdominal palpation. Signs of acute septic peritonitis include depression, abdominal distension, signs of shock and colic. Clinical signs of chronic peritonitis include weight loss, poor hair coat, diarrhea, colic and 'pot belly' appearance. There may also be evidence of multi-organ disease especially in foals with swollen joints, uveitis and pneumonia.

Most abdominal abscesses remain discrete and may reach considerable size. The clinical signs of peritoneal abscesses are usually vague and ill-defined. Rupture of peritoneal abscesses causes either a focal or diffuse peritonitis and unless intestinal contents are involved the former are more common.

Diagnosis

- The tentative diagnosis of peritonitis is based upon history and clinical findings and ultrasound examination of the abdomen.
- Ultrasound examination is particularly useful for detection of increased fluid associated with peritonitis and for identification of abdominal abscesses.
- Abdominocentesis should be performed to confirm the diagnosis and look for a causative organism. The white cell count and protein will be increased in the peritoneal fluid and bacteria may be observed or cultured, depending upon how focalized the peritonitis is. With acute septic peritonitis such as seen with *Clostridium perfringens*, type C bacteria are usually seen on cytological exam. If the peritonitis is due to intestinal leakage, a mixed bacteria population may be observed.
- Rectal examination of acute peritonitis cases reveals a granular, gritty feel, with an impression of abnormal freedom of movement within the abdominal cavity.
- Rectal examination of infected or longstanding cases of peritonitis gives an impression of lack of abdominal mobility, probably due to the extensive adhesions which develop between the loops of small intestine and extensive binding-down of the large colon to the abdominal wall.
- Abdominal abscesses may be detected by rectal examination and they frequently involve the cecal head and/or the spleen. A detectable lack of mobility of a normally mobile organ within the peritoneal cavity may indicate the presence of adhesions between it and other organs or to the parietal peritoneum and, in some cases, this arises from abscesses in the wall of the intestine, the cecum or other abdominal organs.

Treatment

- Treatment of both acute and chronic peritonitis is often unrewarding.
- Attempts to treat acute peritonitis following rupture of an abdominal viscus with surgery to repair or remove the affected bowel, in addition to medical support (fluids and antibiotics), have been largely unsuccessful. Acute peritonitis following uterine or bladder rupture carries a better prognosis and warrants aggressive therapy.
- Primary septic peritonitis in which bacteria are sequestered into the cavity from the blood has been treated successfully with abdominal lavage and parenteral antibiotics.
- Chronic peritonitis secondary to abdominal abscess(es) is usually treated with appropriate antibiotics based upon etiologic agent. Surgical drainage can be considered depending upon the size and number of abscess(es).

Omental prolapse

Following abdominocentesis (usually with a teat canula), horses with increased abdominal pressure/distension may prolapse the omentum through the centesis site.

Treatment

Any disorder causing abdominal distension should be treated appropriately. The protruding omentum should be severed at the body wall and a bandage applied around the abdomen. Application of a small amount of antibiotic ointment to the bandage where it overlies the omentum prevents the omentum adhering to the bandage.

Parasitic diseases

Diagnostic methods

Parasitic diagnostic information can be collected for three different purposes and it is important to recognize that the techniques currently available are not equally reliable for all three. The three purposes are as follows:

1) Clinical diagnosis in an individual horse suspected of suffering from a parasitic clinical condition
2) Surveillance of parasite levels on the herd level as part of a parasite control program
3) Screening for anthelmintic resistance with the fecal egg count reduction test (FECRT).

Clinical diagnosis

While information about present intestinal parasite burdens can be obtained by performing fecal egg counts, it is not as straightforward to diagnose parasitic disease as one may assume. There are several reasons for this, but foremost it is important to recognize that the mere presence of parasites such as strongyles, ascarids or tapeworms does not necessarily lead to disease. These parasite categories should be considered ubiquitous in equine establishments world-over, but parasitic disease is the rare event rather than the rule. In other words, parasites are likely to be present in a horse with colic or diarrhea without a causal relationship. Second, the adult egg-shedding parasites are not necessarily the stages causing disease in the horse. A couple of examples are cyathostomin larvae causing larval cyathostominosis or migrating stages of *Strongylus vulgaris* causing thromboembolic colic. The adult stages of strongyle are only considered mild pathogens, while there currently are no diagnostic methods available for detecting the larval stages.

Moreover, strongyle-type eggs cannot be told apart by size or morphological characteristics. In principle, a strongyle egg could represent any of the over 50 different strongyle species described infecting horses. The large strongyles (including *Strongylus vulgaris*, *S. edentatus* and *S. equinus*) can be diagnosed by culturing fecal samples and subsequently identifying the third-stage larvae to the species level. Recent validations using retrospective data have shown that egg counts and larval cultures generally have high positive predictive values (>0.90) but that the negative predictive values were more moderate (about 0.75). This underlines the fact that a horse with a negative fecal egg count or larval culture may still harbor adult strongyle parasites. The same study illustrated that horses in the 0–500 strongyle egg count range had significantly smaller worm burdens compared to horses with higher egg counts. This supports the use of fecal egg counts for treatment decisions.

Parasite surveillance (Figs. 1.228 & 1.229)

Fecal egg counts are generally useful for performing routine parasite surveillance on a farm and designing a parasite control program based on the findings. Several studies have illustrated that adult horses are capable of maintaining their level of strongyle egg shedding over time, even with little or no anthelmintic treatment (Nielsen et al, 2006; Becher et al, 2010). Each horse can be said to possess a certain strongyle contaminative potential (SCP), and a few egg counts performed over time will allow classification of any given herd into low (often <200 EPG), medium (often 200–500 EPG) and high shedders (>500 EPG). This knowledge can then be used to treat horses according to their SCP. It should be noted that in any given herd of mature horses, the large majority of horses will belong to the low or moderate category.

Fecal egg counts will also generate useful information about the occurrence of *Parascaris equorum* in young horses. Given the levels of ivermectin and moxidectin resistance often encountered in *P. equorum*, it has become crucial to know whether this parasite is present or not in order to select the most appropriate drug for treatment (see Table 1.3).

Anthelmintic resistance

The most important reason for performing fecal egg counts is to screen for anthelmintic resistance. Resistance to anthelmintic drugs in equine parasites has been described since the late 1950s. Today, levels of resistance have reached a point, where some degree of

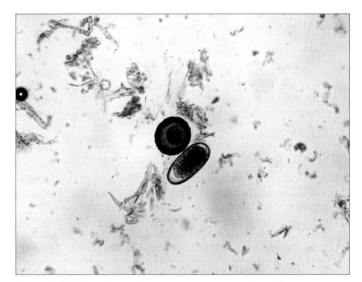

Figure 1.228 Egg of *Parascaris equorum* next to a strongyle egg. Photo courtesy of Tina Roust.

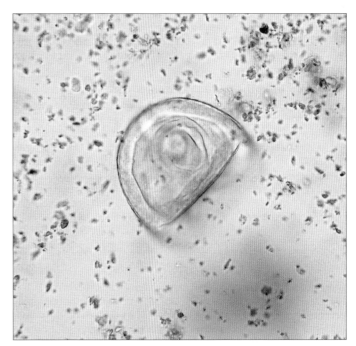

Figure 1.229 Egg of the tapeworm *Anoplocephala perfoliata*.

Table 1.3 Guideline thresholds for classifying anthelmintic resistance on farms based on the fecal egg count reduction test. Percent fecal egg count reductions (FECR) should be calculated across a group of horses in each farm

Anthelmintic	No signs of resistance	Suspect resistance	Clear signs of resistance
Benzimidazoles	>95%	95-85%	<85%
Pyrantel	>90%	90-80%	<80%
Macrocyclic lactones	>95%	95-85%	<85%

Table 1.4 Current levels of resistance by major nematode parasites to three anthelmintic classes in managed horse herds

Drug class	Cyathostomins	Large strongyles	P. equorum
Benzimidazoles	Widespread	None	None
Pyrimidines	Common	None	Early indications
Avermectin/ milbemycin	Early indications	None	Widespread

reduced anthelmintic efficacy is to be expected on every managed horse establishment. Therefore, it is of paramount importance to routinely evaluate the efficacy of the anthelmintic treatments applied to ensure that the parasite control program is working satisfactorily.

For cyathostomin parasites, benzimidazole resistance has been reported to be widespread over several continents, while pyrantel resistance appears to occur at a somewhat lower level, but also on multiple continents. Most recently, there have been reports of early signs of resistance to ivermectin and moxidectin. The egg reappearance period (ERP) is defined as the number of weeks from the day of treatment till strongyle eggs can again be detected in the feces. For ivermectin and moxidectin, the ERP has been found markedly reduced compared to when the drugs were initially introduced, and this has been associated with survival of immature luminal stages of cyathostomin. A summary of current occurrences of anthelmintic resistance in equine parasites is presented in Table 1.4. All types of resistance are not necessarily present on every farm, but the table can be used as a guide to which parasites are most likely to be resistant to which drug on any given farm.

Detection of anthelmintic resistance

The only practical method currently available for determining anthelmintic efficacy is the fecal egg count reduction test (FECRT). There are several ways to perform this test, but the basic principle is to measure the percent reduction of fecal egg counts after anthelmintic treatment. FECRTs can only be performed on the farm level, where an average anthelmintic efficacy is calculated across a group of horses. Based on this result the farm can be classified as having no signs of resistance, suspect resistance or convincing signs of resistance. The percent reductions are calculated with the following formula:

$$\%FECR = \left(\frac{FECpre - FECpost}{FECpre} \right) \times 100\%$$

Individual FECRs are calculated for each horse, and the farm FECR is then reached by averaging these values. There are no internationally accepted general guidelines for classifying farms based on these findings, but a guideline committee has been formed and useful thresholds for determining resistance can be expected in the relative near future. In the meantime, guideline thresholds for determining resistance are provided in Table 1.3. Among other things the selected thresholds depend on the efficacy the drug had when it was first introduced to the market. It should be noted that due to levels of variability known to occur in FECR data, it is recommended to include a 'gray zone', where farms are categorized as suspect resistance and results are inconclusive. If a farm gets classified as suspect resistance, it is recommended to repeat the test or collect more data by including more horses.

On a given farm, a minimum of six horses should be chosen for the test. It is preferable to use horses with moderate to high fecal egg counts, and pre-treatment egg count levels below 200 EPG should generally be avoided. Similarly, the choice of egg counting technique is critical. The key feature is the detection limit of the technique. Detection of early reduction in efficacy requires a technique capable

of detecting low numbers of eggs in the post-treatment samples, and this is especially important when pre-treatment egg counts are not overly high (i.e. above 500 EPG). However, the large majority of adult horses will have egg counts below this level. For this reason, a technique with a minimum detection limit of 50 EPG or above is not useful for the FECRT. It is generally recommended to use egg count techniques with detection limits of 25 EPG or below, but lower is always better. The lower detection limit, however, comes with a cost in terms of more time and effort required to perform the egg counts. This is most often because of one or more centrifugation steps involved with these methods.

Tapeworm diagnosis

Diagnosing tapeworm infections remains a challenge despite the availability of several techniques. Fortunately, tapeworm diagnostic methods have been well-validated, so their weaknesses and strengths can be evaluated precisely.

Fecal examination for tapeworm eggs

Any qualitative or quantitative fecal examination technique is capable of detecting tapeworm eggs. However, cestode eggs are distributed unevenly in feces as proglottids disintegrate, which makes the sensitivity of most techniques too low to make a reliable diagnosis. If eggs are found, they should be regarded as the tip of the iceberg, and many more could be recovered with a modified technique.

The basic modification employed for detecting tapeworms is to increase the amount of feces examined. Whereas a routine McMaster procedure typically uses 4 g of feces, 30–40 g of feces are examined to increase the likelihood of finding tapeworm eggs. Furthermore, the more effective tapeworm methods use enhanced flotation with coverslips sitting on top of centrifuge tubes. This often requires a centrifuge with a closed swing-bucket rotor to prevent coverslips from being dislodged. Some studies have reported that examination of fecal samples 24 hours after tapeworm treatment yielded higher *Anoplocephala* egg counts and a higher percentage of positive samples. Presumably, segments from dead tapeworms disintegrate within the host gut and release eggs into the feces. The highest diagnostic sensitivity reported for an egg counting technique for detection of tapeworm eggs is 61%. This, however, means that the method has a 39% chance of a false-negative result. However, these findings were based on detection of cestode burdens of all sizes. If this threshold were adjusted to detect 20 or more tapeworms, the diagnostic sensitivity increases to about 90%. In other words, only 10% of tapeworm burdens of 20 or more worms would be missed with this method. The choice of 20 tapeworms as a cutoff level is supported by the fact that no or very little mucosal pathology is observed with tapeworm burdens of fewer than 20 worms.

In summary, the modified egg count method has proven useful for diagnosing moderate and large tapeworm burdens, while the smaller worm burdens may go undetected. The method is relatively easy to perform in most laboratories, but does require a centrifuge and is more time-consuming than the simple McMaster.

Tapeworm serum ELISA

An ELISA method is commercially available for detection of antibodies against 12/13 kDa excretory/secretory (ES) antigens of *Anoplocephala perfoliata*. This assay has been thoroughly validated, with determination of diagnostic sensitivity and specificity as well as correlation with worm burdens. However, interpretation of the results can still be somewhat complicated due to the high incidence of both false negatives and false positives.

These shortcomings indicate that antibody titers reflect exposure rather than contemporaneous infection. The serum ELISA remains a very useful test for investigating historical *Anoplocephala* exposure in a herd, but a positive result for an individual animal may not be a reliable indicator of current infection.

Manifestations of parasitic disease

The large majority of parasitic infections go unnoticed and parasitic disease is the exception rather than the rule. When disease occurs, symptoms are often nonspecific and no pathognomonic findings occur. When the limitations of the diagnostic methods are taken into account, diagnosing parasitic disease remains a challenge.

The classical manifestations of parasitic disease include stunted growth, pot belly appearance and general signs of unthriftiness. This can then be found combined with loose or diarrheic feces and/or colic. However, several other conditions can present with similar symptoms. Bloodwork can provide additional information, but findings are not parasite specific. Plasma protein and albumin levels are perhaps the most useful parameters as horses with cyathostominosis are often hypoproteinemic.

Taken together, diagnosing parasitic disease is based on pattern recognition rather than definitive diagnostic tools or pathognomonic signs. The typical parasitic case is a young horse with a history of inadequate anthelmintic treatment. The horse can present with some of the signs described above. Inadequate treatment can either be in terms of no or too few anthelmintic treatments or treatment with a drug against which resistance has developed. In some cases, anthelmintic treatment can even trigger parasitic disease, and this will be explained further below. Thus, a parasitic diagnosis is best reached by collecting good history information about the patient and performing a good clinical examination. This can be supported by bloodwork and fecal analysis. In the following some distinct and well-characterized parasitic syndromes are described further.

Ascarid impaction (Figs. 1.230–1.232)

Verminous small intestinal impactions with *Parascaris equorum* are by far the most serious parasitic condition in foals. Impactions in the small intestine are associated with a guarded prognosis for survival, and surgical intervention is not unusual. The condition can be further complicated by intestinal rupture.

Ascarid impactions are most often encountered in foals and weanlings aged 4–10 months.

Apart from the size of the worm burden, other identified risk factors include the age of the horse and its deworming history. Ascarid worms are known to increase in size with age, so a certain worm burden in foals aged 2 months will take up less space than a worm burden of the same size in a 4-month-old. Treatment of a large intestinal ascarid burden with a paralytic drug has been identified as a significant risk factor. Drugs with paralytic modes of action include ivermectin, moxidectin and pyrantel salts. Taken together, a late first anthelmintic treatment performed at about 4–8 months of age is associated with a considerable risk of inducing an ascarid impaction. Therefore, it is recommended to perform the first anthelmintic treatment at around age 2–3 months and to use a benzimidazole drug as these do not appear to be associated with the same risk of impaction. It should be noted that ascarid impactions can also occur in the absence of anthelmintic treatment.

Diagnosis

- Patients typically present with obvious colic manifestations, elevated heart rates and normo- to hyperperistalsis. Gastric reflux

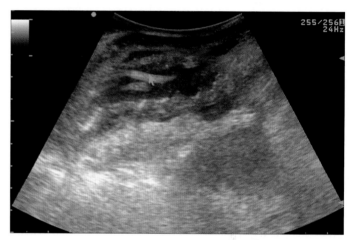

Figure 1.231 Ultrasonographic image of ascarids within the bowel.

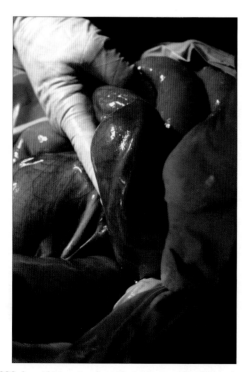

Figure 1.230 Ascarid impaction. Ascarids can be seen through the intestinal wall in this foal that presented with an ascarid impaction and associated intussusceptions.

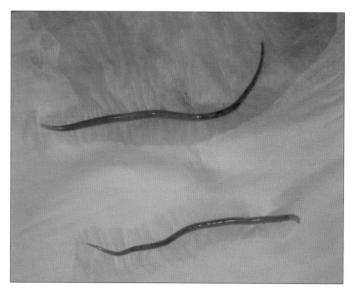

Figure 1.232 Ascarids following removal (same foal as Fig. 1.230).

can be positive and sometimes worms are recovered via the nasogastric tube.

- Transabdominal ultrasound is very useful for diagnosing the condition. Ascarid worms are very echogenic large-moving objects located in the intestinal lumen. Typical adult worms measure about 1 cm in width and 10–20 cm in length. Impacted horses can harbor several hundreds of these worms.

Treatment and prognosis

- Choice of treatment approach will depend on the horse's general condition and response to the general palliative colic treatment and pain management. If pain manifestations are uncontrollable, surgery remains the only option.
- Impactions are most often located in the ileum and in the absence of complications such as rupture, volvulus or intussusceptions, two approaches can be taken: (1) the verminous impaction is gently massaged into the cecum without enterotomy; (2) enterotomy with manual removal of worms.
- Although risks of contamination are considerable with the latter approach, massaging of the serosal surface of the intestine is associated with a risk of serosal damage and subsequent formation of abdominal adhesions. Regardless of the surgical approach taken, the prognosis for complete recovery should be guarded.
- In case of less dramatic colic symptoms and more controllable pain manifestations, a medical approach can be attempted. This includes administration of a single dose of fenbendazole (5 mg/kg), which can be combined with about 1 liter of mineral oil. In addition, the horse should be given fluid therapy and analgesics, when needed. The horse should be monitored closely for the next 24–48 hours with passing of nasogastric tube with gastric decompression at 3–4-hour intervals. More mineral oil can be administered on subsequent occasions. In this case, the prognosis is still guarded, but is greatly improved if the horse makes it through the first 24 hours without further complications.

Larval cyathostominosis (Figs. 1.233–1.235)

Larval cyathostominosis is considered the primary parasitic disease in juvenile and adult horses. It should be borne in mind, however, that cyathostomins are virtually ubiquitous in grazing horses but that this clinical disease complex occurs very rarely. The condition is triggered by mass emergence of encysted cyathostomin larvae from the large

intestinal mucosa. This is associated with an inflammatory reaction in the intestinal walls which causes diarrhea.

In its acute form patients often present with a profuse diarrhea, which can sometimes contain fresh blood. However, the fecal consistency can vary from a loose cowpat texture to watery diarrhea. Ventral edemas are common but not always present, and horses sometimes present with fever. Hyperperistalsis is often encountered and patients frequently present dehydrated. Invariably, several signs of cardiovascular shock are present. Blood work typically reveals absolute neutrophilia and anemia as well as hypoproteinemia and hypoalbuminemia.

The literature tends to focus on the acute form described above, but it should be noted that the condition exists in milder forms as well. In the milder versions, the degree of diarrhea, dehydration and cardiovascular shock is less pronounced, but horses can present with a history of a variable fecal consistency with weight loss and malthrift

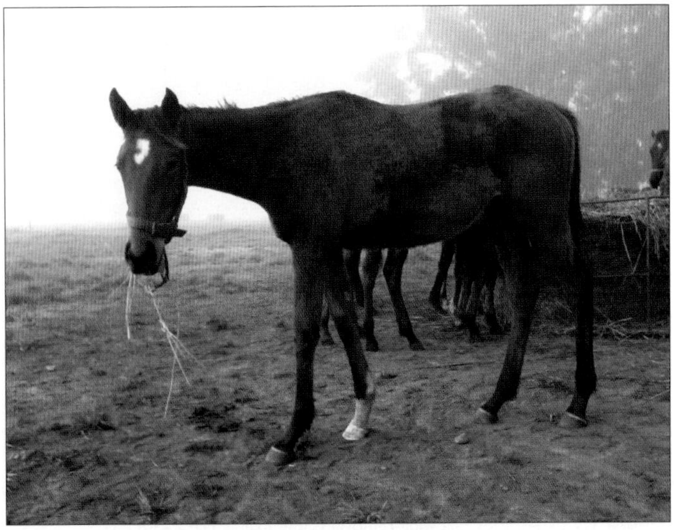

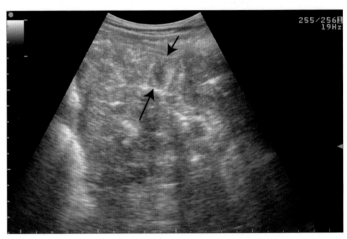

Figure 1.234 Ultrasonographic image from weanling with chronic cyathostomiasis showing marked thickening of colonic walls (arrows).

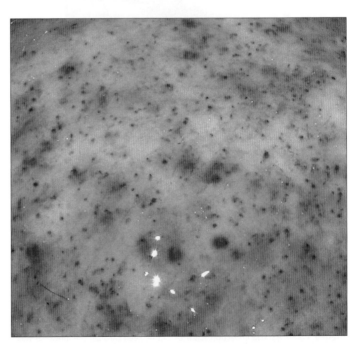

Figure 1.235 Colonic mucosa with large numbers of encysted cyathostomins. Each red dot represents an encysted larva. Photo courtesy of Tetyana Kuzmina.

Figure 1.233 Yearling with chronic cyathostomiasis.

over several weeks or months. Blood work often reveals hypoprotein-emia and hypoproteinemia.

Three significant risk factors for development of larval cyathos-tominosis are:

1) Age: horses less than 4 years of age are at higher risk. The condition is only very rarely seen in foals, so the high-risk age range appears to be 1–4 years.

2) Season: in a northern temperate climate, most cases tend to occur during the winter or early spring months. In a more subtropical climate the dynamics are markedly different, and arrested development of cyathostomins appears to occur more during the summer.

3) Anthelmintic treatment: treatment with a non-larvicidal drug such as ivermectin or pyrantel has been identified as a significant risk factor for triggering the disease. Although the evidence is limited, treatment with a larvicidal drug such as moxidectin may be less associated with this risk.

Diagnosis

- No simple diagnostic measures exist.
- Larval cyathostominosis is diagnosed based on patient history, clinical examination, and blood work. Key history features are the three risk factors mentioned above.
- Clinical findings leading to a suspicion of this condition include the fecal consistency, the plasma protein and albumin levels, and neutrophilia.
- Fecal egg counts have no diagnostic significance in relation to larval cyathostominosis, but a Baermann test can be performed for identification of recently emerged cyathostomin larvae in the feces. Identification of premature stages of strongyle requires some expertise.

Treatment and prognosis

- In the acute form, the chance for recovery is about 50%. The case–fatality rate is much lower for the milder forms of the condition.
- The acute cases require intensive fluid therapy, both crystalloid and colloid.
- The anthelmintic of choice for larval cyathostominosis is moxidectin due to its longevity within the host, and the effect against encysted cyathostomins. In addition, recent findings suggest that the inflammatory reaction is less pronounced with moxidectin treatment compared to other drugs.
- Some treatment protocols include oral supplementation of prednisolone to reduce the intestinal inflammation. Broad-spectrum antibiotics should be considered to prevent potential secondary infection with bacterial pathogens.

Thromboembolic colic (Figs. 1.236–1.238)

Thromboembolic colic is the most dramatic parasitic syndrome described in horses. It is caused by migration of larval stages of *Strongylus vulgaris*, the bloodworm. This parasite was once reported present in 80–100% of horses but has now become extremely rare in managed horse populations. As a result, thromboembolic colic is rarely encountered nowadays. However, it can still occur if parasite control is inadequate.

S. vulgaris larvae migrate to the cranial mesenteric artery (CMA), where they dwell for about 4 months. During this time, they eventually molt to the fifth stage and subsequently travel by the bloodstream to the large intestine where they penetrate the intestinal wall to finally reach the intestinal lumen. The life cycle is complete after about 6.5 months, when the female worms start shedding eggs in the intestine. In the CMA, the larvae cause a verminous endarteritis with roughened intima and thrombus formation. Despite these pronounced alterations, most horses with these lesions show no clinical

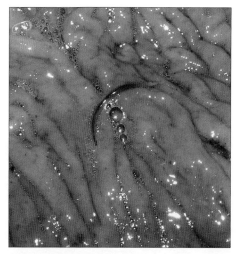

Figure 1.236 Adult female Strongylus vulgaris attached to the cecal mucosa. Photo courtesy of Tetyana Kuzmina.

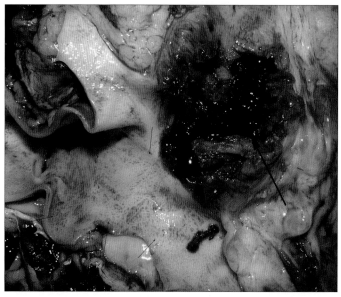

Figure 1.237 Aorta with the cranial mesenteric artery (CMA) branching off. The aortic intima has extensive migratory tracts caused by *Strongylus vulgaris* larvae (small arrows). A verminous thrombotic endarteritis can be seen with visible larvae in the CMA (large arrow). Photo courtesy of Martin K. Nielsen.

symptoms. Thromboembolism, however, can be the cause of serious disease. Small thrombi can detach from the main thrombus and will be carried down the vessel tree by the bloodstream. Here, they can eventually occlude an artery or arteriole, which can cause ischemia and infarction in larger or smaller segments of the intestinal tract. Infarction is painful and most descriptions of thromboembolic colic depict a very painful colic with heart rates often around 100 beats per minute, cyanotic mucous membranes, profuse sweating and signs of cardiovascular shock. Abdominal taps will often reveal elevated measures of protein content and white blood cell counts as signs of the inflammatory condition in the intestinal wall. In some cases, the infarcted area will eventually rupture with the characteristic finding of intestinal contents in the abdominal tap. Milder forms of the disease complex exist, with some horses showing a slowly progressing quiet colic, which initially appears to respond well to standard colic management, but recurs when the effect of the analgesics wears off. As

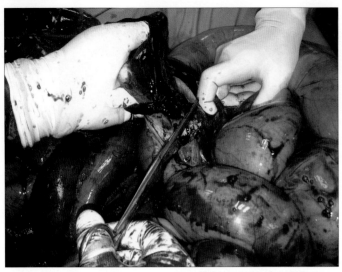

Figure 1.238 Verminous arteritis of a mesenteric artery has resulted in thrombus formation and necrosis of the related section of bowel.

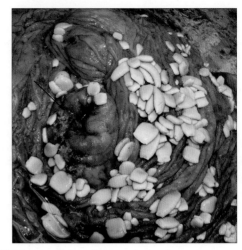

Figure 1.239 *Anoplocephala perfoliata* attached to the cecal mucosa surrounding the ileo-cecal valve (arrow). Photo courtesy of Tetyana Kuzmina.

the peritonitis develops, the clinical condition will gradually worsen. In some horses, localized lesions with fibrotic adhesions or strictures are occasionally encountered without any history of violent colic.

Diagnosis

- No good diagnostic methods exist for diagnosing thromboembolic colic. Performing fecal egg counts has no clinical significance. A larval culture can diagnose presence of adult *Strongylus vulgaris* in the intestine, but does not yield any information about larvae in the mesenteric arteries.

- Although it could be argued that horses with adult *S. vulgaris* are likely to also harbor larval stages, it takes about 14 days to culture third-stage strongyle larvae for identification, by which time the results are likely to be irrelevant for the clinical case. In addition, most horses harboring *S. vulgaris* will not develop thromboembolic colic.

- Transrectal ultrasonography has been described to be useful for measuring the dimensions of the CMA and possibly detecting the presence of a thrombus mass. However, this may not be possible in larger horses, and there are no published normal ranges for vessel thickness and artery dimensions for the CMA.

- A definitive diagnosis of thromboembolic colic can only be reached during exploratory laparotomy or on the necropsy table.

Treatment and prognosis

- The full-fledged version of acute thromboembolic colic described above is associated with a very poor prognosis for survival, and even the milder forms are associated with a guarded prognosis.

- Treatment should include pain management and fluid therapy and follow general principles for colic management.

- There is no additional benefit from administering anthelmintic treatment to a horse with thromboembolic colic.

Tapeworm-associated colic (Fig. 1.239)

Anoplocephala perfoliata is generally a mild parasitic pathogen, but it has been incriminated with some defined colic types, which can all be associated with their predilection site for attachment near the ileocecal valve. A number of case reports associate tapeworms with surgical conditions such as intussusceptions and cecal invaginations. One study has convincingly associated *A. perfoliata* with ileal impactions, and a few studies have found a similar association with spasmodic

colics. However, other studies have been unsuccessful in associating colics with tapeworm measures, so there still appears to be some controversy over the role of tapeworms in colic.

Diagnosis

- Tapeworm infection can be diagnosed with the methods described above, but diagnosing tapeworms in a colicking horse does not equate a causal relationship.

- A definitive diagnosis of tapeworm-associated colic can only be reached during explorative laparotomy or on the necropsy table.

- Ultrasonography may be helpful in some cases but the cecum and ileum are usually difficult to visualize and worms are not easy to identify.

Treatment and prognosis

- In the absence of complications such as intussusceptions and invaginations, a tapeworm-associated colic should have a good prognosis for full recovery.

- Ileal impactions may require surgical intervention, which is of course associated with a somewhat guarded prognosis.

- Colic management should be following general principles, and the tapeworms can be treated with either praziquantel or pyrantel following the manufacturers' recommendations.

Principles for equine parasite control

Recommendations given for equine parasite control used to consist of relatively simple calendar-based recommendations with anthelmintic treatments administered with regular intervals year-round. There is no doubt that this has led to the current levels of anthelmintic resistance, and it is now recommended to decrease the treatment intensity to further delay the development of resistance as much as possible, while still achieving satisfactory control over relevant parasites. Parasite control recommendations should be tailored to the conditions on each farm, and a 'one-size-fits-all' program no longer exists. However, it is possible to identify and define a number of elements, which should always be part of any parasite control program. These elements should be implemented taking into account farm-specific conditions, such as climate, length of grazing season, stocking rate, age range of horses, etc. The following section presents the major elements to include in a parasite control program.

Evaluation of drug efficacy. No matter the anthelmintic treatment regimen, drug efficacy should be evaluated every year with the Fecal Egg Count Reduction Test (FECRT). It is of utmost importance to perform the FECRT in foals and weanlings as they are likely to harbor both strongyles and ascarids capable of developing resistance to different anthelmintic drug classes.

Basic foundation of treatments. A majority of adult horses appear to maintain low egg count levels over time, despite no or very few anthelmintic treatments. For these horses, one or two yearly treatments will be sufficient to avoid re-emergence of large strongyle parasites, particularly *S. vulgaris*. All drugs work against large strongyles at the intestinal stage, but it is preferred to use a drug with efficacy against migrating larvae as well. This would include ivermectin, moxidectin or the 5-day regimen of double-dose fenbendazole. If there is evidence of tapeworm transmission in the area, these foundation treatments could be combined with praziquantel or pyrantel.

Targeting high strongyle egg shedders. Fecal egg counts will identify horses that are prone to return to higher levels of egg shedding after anthelmintic treatment, and it will be beneficial to target these with some additional treatment, while the constant low shedders should be covered by the foundation treatments defined above. Options for additional treatment include moxidectin, which suppresses egg shedding for a longer time period post treatment compared to other drugs. An alternative is daily in-feed supplementation of pyrantel, which can be used if there is no sign of resistance to this drug. With this approach an adult high strongyle shedder (>1 000 EPG) can receive three or four yearly treatments at most.

Defining the grazing seasons. Most geographical and climatic locations feature a distinct grazing season with a clearly defined off-season where horses are instead fed roughage in barns and/or paddocks. In a northern temperate climate, the off-season will occur during the colder winters, while in subtropical and tropical climates, the summers may be too hot for grazing. During such off-seasons, there will be very little or no parasite transmission, and there is no justification for rigorous anthelmintic treatments during this period. Some climates allow year-round transmission, where no off-season can be defined.

Anthelmintic treatments during the horse's first year of life. When a foal hits the ground, there is a certain order of parasites that it encounters during its first year of life. As each parasite category requires its own treatment considerations, it is worth keeping this order of appearance in mind:

1) *Strongyloides westeri*. Foals acquire this parasite through the mother's milk during the first weeks of life. However, it is rarely encountered nowadays and there is little evidence that suggests any pathogenic effects. Therefore it is not recommended to treat foals or mares for *S. westeri*.

2) *Parascaris equorum*. This is the primary parasitic pathogen of foals. Treatments should be carried out at 2–3 months of age with a benzimidazole drug to minimize the risk of small-intestinal impaction.

3) *Cyathostomins*. Foals start grazing during the first months of life, and will begin to acquire a strongyle burden. The first time to consider treatment of this burden is around the time of weaning, which is often at the age of 6 months. However, *P. equorum* can still be predominating at this age, so fecal samples are recommended to investigate the presence of this parasite. Ivermectin is often the drug of choice for strongyles, but other drug classes can be used, if there are no signs of resistance against them. Benzimidazoles are still the recommended drug type for *P. equorum*, but they cannot be expected to work against strongyles without performing a FECRT clearly showing a satisfactory efficacy.

4) Tapeworms. Foals are likely to encounter tapeworms when they start grazing, but there may be considerable differences in the level of exposure between individual farms. It is most often recommended to include tapeworm treatment once or twice yearly.

In summary, the foundation treatment for a foal during its first year of life would be four treatments: (1) 2–3 months targeting *P. equorum*; (2) about 6 months targeting *P. equorum* and/or strongyles; (3) about 9 months targeting strongyles and possibly tapeworms; and (4) about 12 months targeting the same parasite groups. Local circumstances, such as clinical problems due to parasites, high stocking rates, high levels of traffic in and out of the farm, etc. can justify including more than four treatments, but in a large majority of cases it will not be needed. It is very important to routinely monitor anthelmintic efficacy against both strongyles and *P. equorum* using the FECRT.

Horses in the age group of 1–4 years of age are likely to harbor larger worm burdens and have higher egg counts than adult horses. In addition, this age group is more likely to develop clinical disease due to parasite infection. Therefore, they should receive more treatments than the adult horses. The decision regarding the number of treatments will depend on conditions on the given farm, but 3–4 annual treatments should be the guideline foundation. It can be recommended to include a larvicidal treatment towards the end of the grazing season to reduce the size of the encysted worm burden. It is of utmost importance to routinely monitor anthelmintic efficacy in this age group.

Part 6: Neoplastic disorders

The mouth (Figs. 1.240–1.245)

Neoplastic lesions of the mouth and associated structures are rare. Oral neoplasms can be divided into three basic types: **odontogenic**, **osteogenic** and **secondary** (soft tissue).

Odontogenic neoplasms are derived from the remnants of dental epithelium. The five types that have been described in the horse are: ameloblastomas, ameloblastic odontomas, complex odontomas, compound odontomas and cementomas.

Ameloblastoma (adamantinoma) is the most common of the five. Most occur in the incisor region of the mandible and are highly infiltrative, rapidly involving the underlying bone of the mandible.

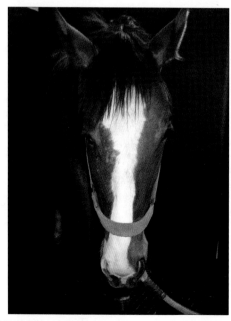

Figure 1.240 Odontoma. This young horse presented with unilateral facial swelling and epiphora.

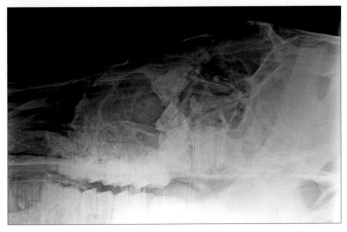

Figure 1.241 Radiograph of the odontoma in the maxillary sinus (same horse as Fig. 1.240).

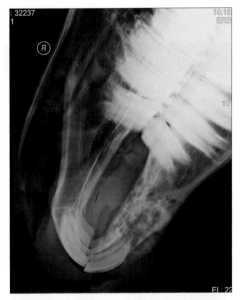

Figure 1.242 A middle-aged Shire cross mare had a large exophytic mass on the incisive region of the mandible. This was diagnosed by biopsy as an ameloblastoma. The radiograph shows the extensive bone destruction. An attempt to perform a rostral mandibulectomy was unsuccessful and she was euthanized.

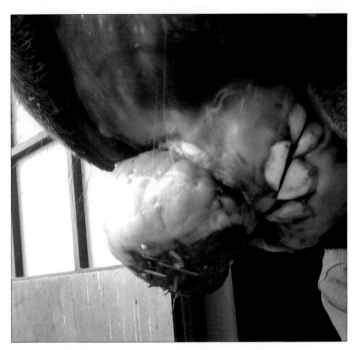

Figure 1.243 This ameloblastoma was successfully removed from the upper incisive region of a young horse. Radiation was also required to ensure non-recurrence.

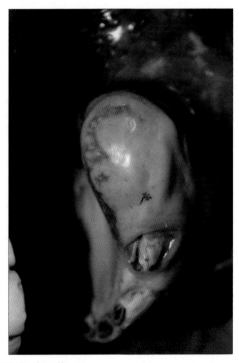

Figure 1.244 Ossifying fibroma.

Teeth included in the proliferating mass may become loose or displaced. Most occur in mature horses without sex or breed predilection. A congenital ameloblastoma which may include teeth and tooth-like material is exceptional.

Osteogenic neoplasms are rare and most (osteoma, ossifying fibroma), although unsightly, are often slow-growing or static. They are sometimes associated with defects of dental eruption or trauma. More than 80% of equine osteosarcomas occur in the head region.

Secondary neoplasms of the oral cavity include squamous cell carcinoma, lymphosarcomas, papillomas and melanomas that have reached the oral cavity from local extension or metastasis from a distal site. Other reported tumors of the tongue are multiple myeloma, rhabdomyosarcoma and paraneoplastic bullous stomatitis.

Squamous cell carcinoma is the most prevalent neoplastic lesion of the oral cavity of the horse and affects either the tongue or the buccal mucosa. In some cases the lesion is large, resulting in facial deformity. The tumor may infiltrate the cheek and ulcerate onto the side of the face. A similar ulcerative appearance may be seen with fibrosarcomas involving the cheek. Involvement of local lymph nodes in horses affected with either squamous cell carcinoma or fibrosarcoma is uncommon but the parotid lymph node is usually hyperplastic if not infiltrated with neoplastic tissue.

Diagnosis

- Physical examination usually allows for a preliminary diagnosis of neoplasia, although histopathological examination of biopsy specimens is usually required to determine the type of neoplasia.

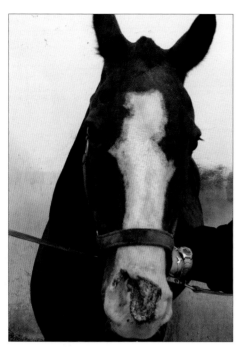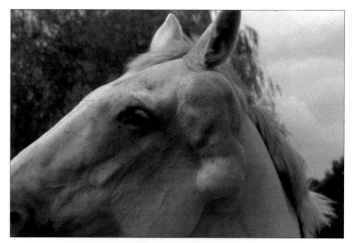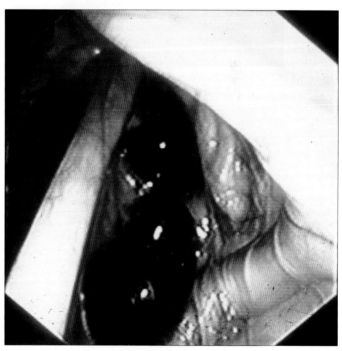

Figure 1.245 Squamous cell carcinoma of the muzzle showing extensive local tissue destruction.

Figure 1.246 Melanoma. This middle-aged gray mare had a bilateral parotid region swelling, typical of parotid (salivary gland and lymph node) melanoma.

Figure 1.247 Melanoma. Melanomas are commonly found within the guttural pouches of gray horses in particular. They vary in their clinical appearance from small "splashes" of melanosis to obvious spherical or multinodular masses. They are far more common in the lateral wall of the pouch where they can be associated with the external maxillary artery.

Odontogenic and osteogenic neoplasms may be difficult to classify histologically.

- Diagnosis of ossifying fibromas is by occlusal radiographic examination which usually establishes the true character of the mass.

Treatment

There are a number of treatment options depending on the type of tumor involved, stage of development and involvement of other tissues or organs. These include: radiotherapy, hyperthermia, chemotherapy, cryosurgery, immunotherapy, autogenous vaccines, photodynamic therapy, laser therapy and surgical resection.

Salivary glands (Figs. 1.246 & 1.247)

Neoplastic disorders of the salivary glands are effectively restricted to melanoma and melanosarcoma in gray horses. The often gross enlargement in the parotid area of gray horses suffering from melanoma masses is sometimes due to the presence of the tumor masses in the adjacent lymph nodes but tumors in lymphoid tissue within the salivary glands may reach massive proportions. The existence of these lesions in the salivary glands and adjacent structures may or may not be accompanied by the presence of tumors elsewhere.

Diagnosis and treatment

- The character of the solid tumors is usually simply assessed clinically. Needle aspirates from the mass contain black cells which are very characteristic. Surgical biopsy is not necessary and indeed may be contraindicated.
- For treatment see p. 3.51.

The esophagus

Intramural space-occupying lesions of neoplastic nature are very rare but may be sufficiently large to affect food transit. Lesions of sufficient size to obstruct the esophagus in the cervical region would be expected to be palpable but may not affect the endoscopic appearance of the mucosa except in the case of squamous cell carcinoma. Masses within the thorax, such as lymphosarcoma, may result in an extraluminal esophageal obstruction with proximal dilatation and present the characteristic signs of recurrent choke. Several episodes of obstruction without any endoscopic lesion should alert the clinician to this possibility. The clinical effects on the esophagus are usually of relatively minor importance in these cases.

Lower gastrointestinal tract (Figs. 1.248–1.251)

Table 1.5 outlines the frequently encountered neoplasms of the gastrointestinal tract. Clinical signs are related to tumor location and organ involvement. Gastric neoplasia is associated with anorexia, weight loss, chronic colic, abdominal distension, intermittent pyrexia, and in some cases abnormal chewing or swallowing. Abdominal neoplasia may result in chronic colic, weight loss, ventral edema, altered

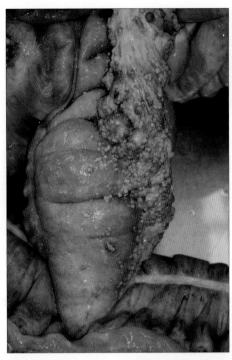

Figure 1.248 Intestinal adenocarcinoma (same horse as Fig. 1.250).

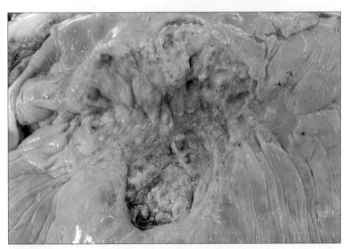

Figure 1.249 Intestinal adenocarcinoma.

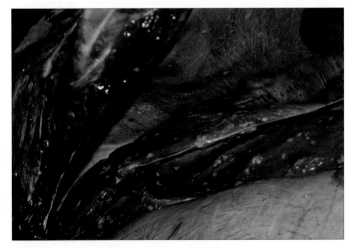

Figure 1.250 Intestinal adenocarcinoma with metastasis to the liver.

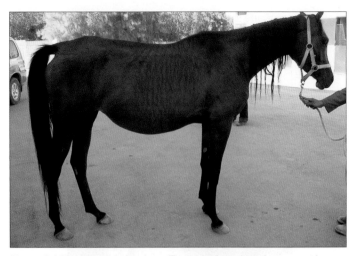

Figure 1.251 Multicentric lymphoma. This mare showed rapid recent weight loss. Ultrasonographic examination of the abdomen revealed masses associated with the liver, spleen and other unidentified masses which at necropsy were revealed to be enlarged mesenteric lymph nodes.

Table 1.5 Neoplasia of the gastrointestinal tract

Location	Type of neoplasm
Esophagus	Squamous cell carcinoma
Stomach	Gastric polyp
	Leiomyosarcoma
	Lymphoma (lymphosarcoma)
Small intestine	Adenocarcinoma
	Adenomatous polyposis
	Ganglioneuroma
	Intestinal carcinoid
	Leiomyoma
	Leiomyosarcoma
	Lipoma
	Lymphoma (lymphosarcoma)
	Neurofibroma
Cecum	Adenocarcinoma
	Intestinal myxosarcoma
	Stromal tumor
Large colon	Adenocarcinoma
	Lipomatosis
	Lymphoma (lymphosarcoma)
	Neurofibroma
Small colon	Leiomyoma
	Lipoma
	Lipomatosis
Rectum	Leiomyosarcoma
	Lipoma
	Polyps
	Lymphoma (lymphosarcoma)
Peritoneum	Disseminated leiomyomatosis
	Mesothelioma
	Omental fibrosarcoma

Adapted from Reed and Bayly (2004) Equine Internal Medicine, 2nd edn. Elsevier, St. Louis, MO, USA; pp. 938.

fecal consistency and intermittent pyrexia. Paraneoplastic syndromes are also frequently encountered associated with abdominal neoplasms; these can include cancer cachexia, anemia, leucocytosis, thrombocytopenia, hypocalcemia, ectopic hormone production and various skin conditions.

Diagnosis
- Diagnosis is often challenging and frequently a presumptive diagnosis is reached, based on exclusion of other causes of presenting clinical signs.
- Serum biochemical analysis, complete blood count, urinalysis and rectal examination may all support a diagnosis but do not confirm it.
- Ultrasonography can be used to assist diagnosis in some cases but many tumors that affect the wall of the gastrointestinal tract are not routinely visible on echographic examination. It is perhaps more useful for tumors that can be palpated rectally and for detecting enlargement of mesenteric lymph nodes in horses with intestinal lymphosarcoma.
- Definitive diagnosis is based on biopsy results which may be obtained ante-mortem or more frequently at post-mortem.

References and further reading

Beccati, F., Pepe, M., Gialletti, R., et al., 2011. Is there a statistical correlation between ultrasonographic findings and definitive diagnosis in horses with acute abdominal pain? Equine Vet J 43 (Suppl. 39), 98–105.

Becher, A., Mahling, M., Nielsen, M.K., Pfister, K., 2010. Selective anthelmintic therapy of horses in the Federal states of Bavaria (Germany) and Salzburg (Austria): An investigation into strongyle egg shedding consistency. Vet Parasitol 171, 116–122.

Breuer, J., Schmoll, F., Uhlig, A., Schusser, G.F., 2011. A follow up study on antibodies against Lawsonia intracellularis in mares and foals from two breeding farms in Germany. Berl Munch Tierarztl Wochenschr 124 (7–8), 337–342.

Delesalle, C., Dewulf, J., Lefebvre, R.A., et al., 2007. Determination of lactate concentrations in blood plasma and peritoneal fluid in horses with colic by an Accusport analyzer. J Vet Intern Med 21, 293–301.

Dunkel, B., Chaney, K.P., Dallap-Schaer, B.L., et al., 2011. Putative intestinal hyperammonaemia in horses: 36 cases. Equine Vet J 43 (2), 133–140.

Frazer, M.L., 2008. Lawsonia intracellularis infection in horses: 2005–2007. J Vet Intern Med 22 (5), 1243–1248.

Kaplan, R.M., 2004. Drug resistance in nematodes of veterinary importance: a status report. Trends Parasitol 20 (10), 477–481.

Kaplan, R.M., Nielsen, M.K., 2010. An evidence-based approach to equine parasite control: It ain't the 60s anymore. Equine Vet Educ 22, 306–316.

Lyons, E.T., Tolliver, S.C., Collins, S.S., 2009. Probable reason why small strongyle EPG counts are returning "early" after ivermectin treatment of horses on a farm in Central Kentucky. Parasitol Res 104, 569–574.

Lyons, E.T., Tolliver, S.C., Kuzmina, T.A., Collins, S.S., 2010. Critical tests evaluating efficacy of moxidectin against small strongyles in horses from a herd for which reduced activity had been found in field tests in Central Kentucky. Parasitol Res 107, 1495–1498.

Mair, T., Divers, T., Ducharme, N., 2002. Manual of Equine Gastroenterology. WB Saunders, Edinburgh, UK.

Mair, T.S., Couto, C.G., 2006. The use of cytotoxic drugs in equine practice. Equine Vet Educ 8 (3), 149–156.

McAuliffe, S.B., Slovis, N.M., 2008. Colour Atlas of Diseases and Disorders of the Foal. WB Saunders, Philadelphia, PA, USA.

Moore, J.N., Owen, R.R., Lumsden, J.H., 1976. Clinical evaluation of blood lactate levels in equine colic. Equine Vet J 8, 49–54.

Nielsen, M.K., Baptiste, K.E., Tolliver, S.C., et al., 2010. Analysis of multiyear studies in horses in Kentucky to ascertain whether counts of eggs and larvae per gram of feces are reliable indicators of numbers of strongyles and ascarids present. Vet Parasitol 174, 77–84.

Nielsen, M.K., Haaning, N., Olsen, S.N., 2006. Strongyle egg shedding consistency in horses on farms using selective therapy in Denmark. Vet Parasitol 135 (3–4), 333–335.

Page, A.E., Slovis, N.M., Gebhart, C.J., et al., 2011. Serial use of serologic assays and fecal PCR assays to aid in identification of subclinical Lawsonia intracellularis infection for targeted treatment of Thoroughbred foals and weanlings. J Am Vet Med Assoc 238 (11), 1482–1489.

Page, A.E., Stillst, H.F., Chander, Y., et al., 2011. Adaptation and validation of a bacteria-specific enzyme-linked immunosorbent assay for determination of farm-specific Lawsonia intracellularis seroprevalence in central Kentucky Thoroughbreds. Equine Vet J Suppl 40, 25–31.

Patton, K.M., Peek, S.F., Valentine, B.A., 2006. Gastric adenocarcinoma in a horse with portal vein metastasis and thrombosis: a novel cause of hepatic encephalopathy. Vet Pathol 43 (4), 565–569.

Peek, S.F., Divers, T.J., Jackson, C.J., 1997. Hyperammonaemia associated with encephalopathy and abdominal pain without evidence of liver disease in four mature horses. Equine Vet J 29 (1), 70–74.

Perez Olmos, J.F., Schofield, W.L., Dillon, H., et al., 2006. Circumferential mural bands in the small intestine causing simple obstructive colic: a case series. Equine Vet J 38 (4), 354–359.

Pusterla, N., Mapes, S., Wademan, C., et al, 2013. Emerging outbreaks associated with equine coronavirus in adult horses. Vet Microbiol 162 (1), 228–231.

Reed, S.M., Bayly, W.M., Sellon, D.C., 2009. Equine Internal Medicine, third ed. WB Saunders, St. Louis, MO, USA.

Reid, S.W., Mair, T.S., Hillyer, M.H., Love, S., 1995. Epidemiological risk factors associated with a diagnosis of clinical cyathostomiasis in the horse. Equine Vet J 27, 127–130.

Robinson, N.E., Sprayberry, K.A. (Eds.), 2009. Current Therapy in Equine Medicine, sixth ed. WB Saunders, St. Louis, MO, USA.

Sharkey, L.C., DeWitt, S., Stockman, C., 2006. Neurologic signs and hyperammonemia in a horse with colic. Vet Clin Pathol 35 (2), 254–258.

Slovis, N.M., Elam, J., Estrada, M., Leutenegger, C.M., 2013. Infectious agents associated with diarrhoea in neonatal foals in Central Kentucky: A comprehensive molecular study. Equine Vet J 2013 Jun 17. doi: 10.1111/evj.12119. [Epub ahead of print]

Stratford, C.H., McGorum, B.C., Pickles, K.J., Matthews, J.B., 2011. An update on cyathostomins: Anthelmintic resistance and diagnostic tools. Equine Vet J 43, 133–139.

Watson, T.D., Sullivan, M., 1991. Effects of detomidine on equine oesophageal function as studied by contrast radiography. Vet Rec 129, 67.

Conditions of the liver, spleen and pancreas

Developmental disorders

There are no clinically significant common congenital splenic, pancreatic or peritoneal abnormalities of the horse. Congenital hepatic abnormalities include rarely reported portosystemic shunts, biliary atresia and hyperammonemia of Morgans. Increases in liver enzymes and bilirubin concentration without overt hepatic insufficiency can frequently be seen in septicemic neonates.

Hepatic disorders

Portosystemic shunt

Congenital portosystemic shunts in foals are rare. Clinical signs are most commonly seen at 2–6 months of age when the foals have a higher dietary intake of protein, but in some cases may be noted soon after birth. Shunts may be single or multiple, intrahepatic or extrahepatic. The vascular shunts allow blood within the portal system to bypass the liver and drain into the systemic circulation. The signs seen are mostly a result of hepatoencephalopathy and include depression, recurrent seizures, ataxia and cortical blindness. These signs may wax and wane and affected foals are often unthrifty.

Diagnosis and treatment

- The diagnosis may be difficult in some cases since liver enzymes and serum bilirubin are usually normal and any condition resulting in abnormal behavior and poor growth is a differential. Markedly elevated serum bile acids and blood ammonia with normal serum hepatic enzymes are highly supportive of the diagnosis. The diagnosis can be confirmed by a portogram or by nuclear scintigraphy.
- *Differential diagnosis:* The main clinical signs are abnormal behavior and poor growth. Therefore any condition producing this combination of signs could be considered as a differential. This would include: brain abscesses, mesenteric/lung abscesses, microencephaly or hydrocephalus and chronic intestinal inflammation. Morgan foals with hyperammonemia can also have similar signs.
- Surgical repair has been performed in one foal. Single extrahepatic shunts would have a better prognosis than multiple or intrahepatic shunts.

Biliary atresia

A number of cases of extrahepatic biliary atresia have been documented. These foals present at a young age with a variety of nonspecific signs including anorexia, depression, poor weight gain, colic, pyrexia and icterus. Polydipsia and polyuria may also be present. Serum biochemical profiles may be consistent with biliary obstruction.

Diagnosis

- Ante-mortem diagnosis has not been made in any reported cases but hepatobiliary scintigraphy has been used in other species for diagnosis.

- It may be clinically impossible to differentiate from acquired obstructions in biliary outflow.
- Post-mortem of the affected foals revealed a large firm liver with abscence of the main bile duct with intrahepatic biliary hypertrophy. There are no treatment options.

Hyperammonemia of Morgan foals

This is presumed to occur because of an inherited abnormality in hepatic ammonia metabolism. Based on abnormal serum and urine amino acid concentrations it is theorized that this condition is similar to the hyperornithinemia, hyperammonemia and homocitrullinemia (HHH) syndrome in man. HHH is a rare autosomal recessive disorder that results in abnormal ornithine transport into mitochondria with subsequent ornithine accumulation and a reduced ability to clear ammonia through the urea cycle.

Affected Morgan foals are usually 4–7 months old and have an acute onset of signs caused by cerebral dysfunction. These signs include blindness, head pressing, circling and seizures. In some cases, there is hemoglobinuria.

Diagnosis and treatment

- The diagnosis is based upon signalment and clinical signs in addition to measurement of blood ammonia.
- Blood ammonia levels are often very high (300–600 µmol/L). If blood ammonia is to be measured, it should be performed either 'in house' with a control sample or, if it is sent to a laboratory, serum should be immediately collected and frozen and a control sample handled in the identical way.
- Although the disease has been uniformly fatal, some cases will improve for several days with supportive therapy only to have a second onset of severe neurological signs later.

Hepatic insufficiency

Hepatic disease in the horse is a relatively common occurrence, but only those with either biliary obstruction or extensive hepatic parenchymal disease (or both) will exhibit easily identifiable signs of hepatic failure.

The wide range of disorders of the liver reflects the diversity of its metabolic functions and the clinical signs of hepatic failure may, in turn, reflect the loss of one or more of these. In some cases, specific metabolic processes are deranged and this results in conspicuous clinical signs which may not immediately be attributable to the liver.

The onset of clinical signs attributable to liver disease is invariably acute, as the liver has a large functional reserve and normally greater than 75% of the liver mass must be functionally lost before clinical signs are apparent (see Table 2.1). Thus when signs of hepatic failure become obvious damage is usually severe, whether this is of chronic or acute onset. The organ does, however, have some regenerative

Table 2.1 Clinical signs associated with hepatic insufficiency

Common	Less common	Infrequently reported
Icterus	Photosensitization	Acites
Hepatic encephalopathy	Diarrhea	Dependent abdominal edema
Depression	Bilateral laryngeal paralysis	Steatorrhea
Anorexia	Hemhorragic diathesis	Tenesmus
Colic		Generalized seborrhea
Weight loss		Pruritis
		Endotoxic shock
		Polydipsia
		Hemolysis

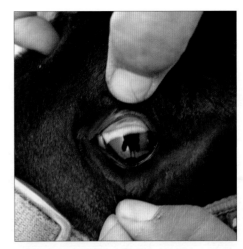

Figure 2.1 Icterus (jaundice) of the sclera. This can be seen with acute or chronic hepatic insufficiency in addition to biliary obstruction.

capacity and may regain some, if not all, of its complex functions even after severe acute insults. Acute hepatic damage therefore provides the clinician with therapeutic opportunities while chronic severe changes are usually frustratingly unmanageable.

Icterus (Figs. 2.1 & 2.2)

Icterus (jaundice) is caused by hyperbilirubinemia with subsequent deposition of the pigment in tissues causing a yellow discoloration. It is most apparent in the mucous membranes and non-pigmented skin. It may be particularly difficult to assess accurately in the horse; 10–15% of normal horses have slightly yellow discoloration of mucous membranes and inherently high blood concentrations of natural, harmless carotenes can be found in some grazing horses.

Hyperbilirubinemia may result from:

1) Increased production of bilirubin
   - Hemolysis (such as equine neonatal isoerythrolysis or equine babesosis) or intracorporeal hemorrhage (uterine artery hemorrhage) with subsequent reabsorption of heme from RBCs results in an elevation of unconjugated bilirubin, although occasionally there may be elevations in conjugated bilirubin as well, due to hepatic spillover.
2) Impaired hepatic uptake or conjugation of bilirubin result in increased levels of unconjugated bilirubin.
   - Acute or chronic hepatocellular disease. (Conjugated bilirubin may also increase in hepatocellular disease.)
   - Administration of certain drugs. Steroids inhibit bilirubin uptake in all species. Heparin may also impair bilirubin uptake.
   - Anorexia frequently causes icterus in horses and is believed to be related to reduced stores of lignadin, a hepatic enzyme responsible for extracting unconjugated bilirubin from albumin in the sinusoidal blood.
   - Premature and neonatal foals are more susceptible to retention icterus than adults and this is also believed to be related to lower stores of ligandin in neonates.
3) Impaired excretion of bilirubin through a blockage of bile flow results in regurgitation icterus with an increase in the conjugated bilirubin (>25%). This can be seen with:
   - Cholangitis
   - Hepatitis
   - Cholelithiasis
   - Neoplasia
   - Fibrosis or hyperplasia of the bile ducts
   - Colonic displacements.

The establishment of the cause of icterus is obviously important and biochemical analysis of the proportions of conjugated and non-conjugated bilirubin in circulating blood may be required to

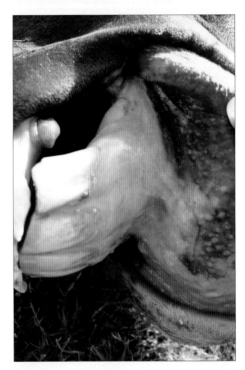

Figure 2.2 Icterus of mucous membranes.

Non-hepatic differential diagnosis:
- Hemorrhage
- Hemolysis
- Starvation
- Colonic displacements
- Cholelithiasis
- Neoplasia
- Duodenal stricture.

accurately identify the type of icterus which is present and thereby provide indications as to its origin.

Hepatic encephalopathy (HE) (Figs. 2.3–2.6)

This is a complex syndrome of abnormal mental status resulting from increased neuronal inhibition that accompanies severe hepatic insufficiency. There are no specific features of HE that allow it to be distinguished from other causes of cerebral dysfunction and a diagnois is usually made based on abnormalities of serum liver enzymes or the accompaniment of other clinical signs of liver disease. HE has been divided into four clinical stages (Table 2.2).

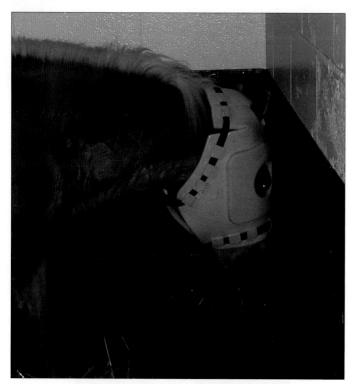

Figure 2.3 Hepatoencephalopathy (head pressing). This horse had serum sickness (Theilers disease, see p. 93). Although head pressing may rarely be seen in a number of other neurological conditions, it is very characteristic of hepatic insufficiency.

Differential diagnosis of abnormal behavior patterns: neurological disorders.

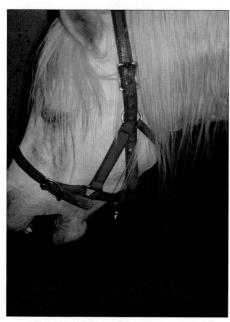

Figure 2.4 Hepatoencephalopathy (abnormal behavior: repeated yawning).

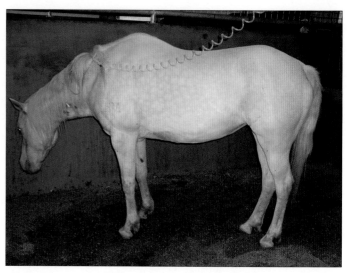

Figure 2.5 Hepatoencephalopathy (abnormal behavior: compulsive circling). Repeated circling can be seen in some horses as a vice and in other nervous horses especially on movement to a new location. Those which have hepatoencephalopathy will usually have other indicators of hepatic insufficiency, such as icterus.

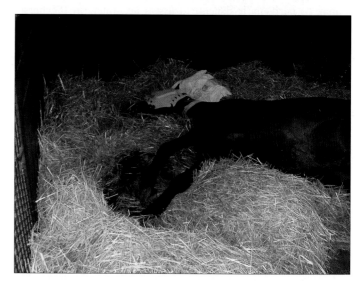

Figure 2.6 Hepatoencephalopathy terminal seizures.

Table 2.2 Stages of hepatoencephalopathy		
Stage	Mental status	Clinical signs/mental status
I	Mild confusion. Decreased attention and irritability	This stage is often missed as the signs are very subtle
II	Drowsiness, lethargy, inappropriate behavior and disorientation	Head-pressing, circling, aimless walking, mild ataxia, yawning and lethargy
III	Somnolent but rousable, marked confusion, amnesia, aggressive uncontrolled behavior	Somnolence with either minimal or hyperresponsiveness to external stimuli. Aggressive or violent behavior
IV	Coma	Coma +/− seizures

The pathogenesis of HE is most likely multifactorial and has not been clearly defined. Proposed mechanisms which may all play a role to a greater or lesser degree are:

1) Gastrointestinal-derived neurotoxins, e.g. ammonia
   - Ammonia has a toxic effect on the cell membrane of neurons by inhibiting Na$^+$, K$^+$-ATPase causing a depletion of adenosine triphosphate.
   - Hyperammonemia also causes disturbances in CNS energy production by altering the tricarboxylic acid cycle.
   - Detoxification of ammonia by brain astrocytes leads to accumulation of glutamate and glutamine. Glutamine accumulation in astrocytes then results in cell swelling and death.
   - Prolonged exposure of neuronal tissue to ammonia also results in downregulation of glutamate receptors resulting in decreased excitatory transmission.

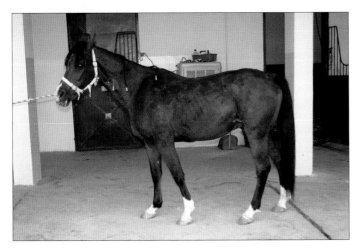

Figure 2.7 Chronic weight loss. This is more commonly associated with chronic hepatic insufficiency but can obviously occur with a variety of non-hepatic conditions.

Differential diagnosis of chronic weight loss:
- Starvation
- Intestinal disease
- Renal failure
- Neoplasia
- Chronic pulmonary conditions.

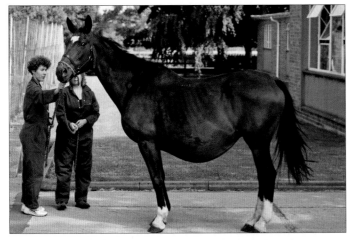

Figure 2.8 Ascites (distended, pot-bellied abdomen), poor body condition.

2) False neurotransmitter accumulation following plasma amino acid imbalance
   - During liver failure false neurotransmitters such as octopamine and phenylethanolamine increase while true neurotransmitters such as norepinephrine and dopamine decrease with a net effect of reduced neuronal excitation and increased neuronal inhibition.
3) Augmented activity of γ-aminobutyric acid (GABA) in the brain
   - Binding of GABA to pre-synaptic neurons results in generation of an inhibitory post-synaptic potential. The GABA receptor has interactive binding sties for benzodiazepines and barbiturates. Improvement in clinical signs is seen when patients are treated with the benzodiazepine receptor antagonist flumazenil.
4) Increased permeability of the blood–brain barrier.

Weight loss (Fig. 2.7)
Weight loss and ill thrift are more commonly associated with chronic hepatic insufficiency. Anorexia and impaired hepatocellular metabolic functions contribute to weight loss. However, chronic liver disease can be present without significant weight loss.

Colic, diarrhea, edema, tenesmus, ascites and steatorrhea (Fig. 2.8)
Abdominal pain associated with hepatocellular disease may result from acute hepatic swelling or biliary obstruction.

Diarrhea may occasionally accompany chronic hepatic insufficiency. The pathogenesis of this diarrhea is thought to include alterations in intestinal microflora, portal hypertension and deficiency of bile acids.

Failure of the anabolic functions of the liver is reflected in a depression of glucose and albumin synthesis. While the reduced blood glucose shows few specific signs, reductions in circulating albumin have distinctive clinical signs. Significant hypoalbuminemia results in peripheral and ventral edema. Gross abnormalities of albumin synthesis and portal hypertension, arising as a result of hepatic fibrosis, can lead to increased hydrostatic and oncotic pressure in the intestinal mucosa with a resultant loss of water and proteins into the bowel lumen (diarrhea) and peritoneal cavity (ascites). Horses with significant ascites have a pot-bellied appearance and it may be possible to percuss a fluid thrill across the abdomen.

Tenesmus is thought to be a sign of HE but may also result from constipation.

Steatorrhea with excessive amounts of fat in the feces results from lipid malabsorption secondary to decreased excretion of bile. This is a rare sign in horses as the equine diet is normally low in fat.

Hepatogenic photosensitization (Figs. 2.9 & 2.10)
Horses lacking the normal detoxification capacity as a result of hepatic insufficiency become excessively sensitive to ultraviolet light. Photodynamic agents are derived endogenously as a result of metabolic processes (particularly in the intestine), or from ingested chemicals, including phenothiazine, and some plants, including *Hypericum peroratum* (St John's wort), *Polygonum fagopyrum* (buckwheat) and *Lolium perenne* (perennial ryegrass). Failure to detoxify these photodynamic agents including phylloerythrin (a product of bacterial degradation of the plant pigment chlorophyll) results in accumulation in the circulation. In normal animals any absorbed photodynamic agents are removed from the portal circulation and excreted in bile, precluding the general distribution of the agents to the skin and other organs. Ultraviolet radiation in sunlight causes activation of electrons within the molecules of the photodynamic agent resulting in local free radical formation with subsequent cell membrane damage and

necrosis. Unpigmented areas of skin absorb UV light more efficiently and thus are more severely affected. It is not always only the obvious areas of unpigmented skin which become affected, but the restriction to white skin is almost pathognomonic for photosensitization. The skin first appears erythematous and edematous. Pruritis, pain, vesiculation, ulceration, necrosis and sloughing may occur.

Hemorrhagic diathesis

The liver is also responsible for the synthesis of a wide range of important metabolic proteins including clotting factors, amino acids and other nutrients required for red cell and hemoglobin production. Particularly sensitive to hepatic disease is the synthesis of fibrinogen and the vitamin-K-dependent factors (II, VII, IX, X and protein C), which have short half lives. Vitamin K requires bile acids for proper absorption from the intestinal tract. Hepatic failure then results in a number of related clinical signs, including hemorrhagic diatheses and

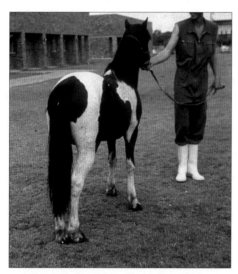

Figure 2.9 Hepatogenic photosensitization. Note that the lesions are limited to the non-pigmented areas of skin.

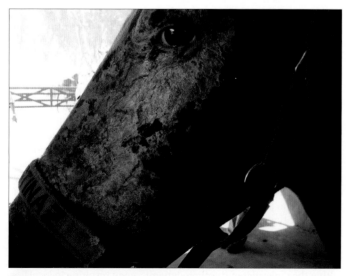

Figure 2.10 Hepatogenic photosensitization as a result of presumed ingestion of a toxic plant. This polo mare was removed from the pasture and stabled and made an uneventful recovery.

anemia. Although overt spontaneous hemorrhage is not a common sign associated with hepatic failure, bleeding into the intestine or into the major conducting airways and prolonged or excessive bleeding from wounds or following venipuncture may be encountered.

Hemolysis

This is rarely seen and the pathophysiology is not exactly known but is thought to be related to increased erythrocyte fragility. When it occurs it is a grave prognostic indicator of severe hepatic failure.

Pruritis and seborrhea

Retention of bile acids and accumulation in the skin may cause pruritis and seborrhea but is rarely reported in horses.

Endotoxemia

Kupfer cells play an important role in removing endotoxin that enters the liver in the portal circulation following intestinal absorption. Therefore decreased function of these cells can result in clinical and laboratory signs of endotoxemia.

Polydipsia, polyuria and the hepatorenal system

Alterations in renal function, serum sodium concentrations, impaired water excretion and urine concentrating ability may accompany severe liver disease.

The heporenal syndrome characterized by acute azotemia and anuria may occur in ponies with hyperlipemia and hepatic lipidosis. The pathogenesis is unclear but may include such factors as reduced effective circulating volume, decreased hepatic inactivation of renin and endotoxemia.

Diagnosis of liver disease

The diagnosis of acute or chronic hepatic failure in the horse is largely based upon the detection of these characteristic, but non-specific, signs and confirmation usually relies heavily upon laboratory studies involving concentrations of hepatic enzymes and plasma proteins. The release of enzymes into the circulating blood from damaged hepatocytes is an index of the extent of the cell damage, although the magnitude of the enzyme concentration increase does not always correlate closely with the degree of hepatic dysfunction.

Liver biopsy, which is a relatively safe and simple procedure, provides definitive histological evidence of the type and extent of the pathological process. As almost all the significant hepatic disorders occurring in the horse are diffuse, biopsy is a most useful aid to their diagnosis. Although chronic hepatic failure may be accompanied by blood clotting disorders the procedure is seldom accompanied by dangerous blood loss. Some of the more common means of assessment of liver pathology are shown in Table 2.3.

Treatment of hepatic insufficiency

The basic goal of therapy is to maintain the animal until the liver regenerates enough to function sufficiently. Thus horses with severe fibrosis often respond poorly as the required regeneration is not possible. In this respect early biopsies are often useful prognostic indicators as therapy may be prolonged in many cases.

- **Sedation.** Horses with HE are often difficult to control and sedation is often required to allow for other treatment, avoid self-inflicted injury and provide safety for the nursing staff. Many tranquilizers are metabolized by the liver and should therefore be used cautiously. Xylazine or detomidine in small doses are safest. Diazepam should be avoided as it enhances the effect of GABA and may exacerbate signs.

- **Fluid therapy.** Fluid deficits and acid–base imbalances should be addressed. Extreme caution should be taken if administering bicarbonate- or lactate-containing fluids as they may result in elevations of blood ammonia levels. Hypokalemia or alkalosis result in increased renal production of ammonia with a corresponding

Table 2.3 Some of the more commonly employed aids to the diagnosis of hepatic disease in the horse

	Relative value of test (and comments)		
	Acute diffuse hepatic failure	Chronic diffuse hepatic failure	Focal hepatic/biliary disease
Ultrasonography	Little value	Useful	Very useful
Liver biopsy	Useful	Very useful	Only if ultrasound guidance available
BSP[1] clearance retention	Should not be used	Useful	Only useful if major obstructive disorder
Bile acids	Little use	Very useful	No value (unless major obstructive disorder)
Aspartate aminotransferase (AST)	Very useful (elevated)	Useful (marginal elevation may be present)	No value (possible increase)
γ-Glutamyl transferase (GGT, γGT)	Very useful (marginal increase initially)	Very useful (significant increase)	No value
Lactate dehydrogenase[2] (LDH$_5$)	Very useful (specialized laboratory)	Very useful (specialized laboratory)	No value
Sorbitol dehydrogenase (SDH)	Very useful (labile enzyme)	Little value	No value

[1]Bromosulphothalein Clearance/Retention Test.
[2]Lactate dehydrogenase isoenzyme-5 (also found in skeletal muscle).

increase in diffusion of ammonia into the CNS, thus treatment with potassium or acidifying fluids may be necessary. As many affected horses are anoretic, continuous infusion of dextrose 5% at a rate of 2 ml/kg/h may be beneficial.

- ***Reducing toxic metabolites.*** Reducing the production or decreasing the absorption of toxic protein metabolites is also an important part of therapy. Methods to reduce production include the oral administration of antibiotics (e.g. neomycin) or lactulose (a syrup containing lactose and other disaccharides). A disadvantage of both is that they may produce diarrhea. Lactulose is also expensive for long-term therapy. Other means of reducing production include alteration of intestinal flora by administration of pro-biotics such as *Lactobacillus acidophilus*. Administration of a low-protein diet (see below) is also advised although this has not consistently reduced signs of HE in humans. Zinc is an important co-factor in many urea cycle enzymes and supplementation may be warranted. Decreasing absorption of toxic metabolites is achieved through the administration of mineral oil or magnesium sulfate.

- ***Dietary management.*** Once horses with hepatic insufficiency become appetent they can be best managed by dietary control. Diets high in carbohydrates, low in protein and rich in BCAAs (branch chain amino acids) should be fed. Oat or other types of grass hay are best. Alfalfa and legumes should be avoided. Grazing should be encouraged. Small feeds several times a day are best because of impaired gluconeogenesis. Vitamin B$_1$, K$_1$ and folic acid should be administered weekly.

- ***Other treatments.*** Anti-inflammatory drugs may be beneficial and include flunixin meglumine, dimethyl sulfoxide and pentoxifylline. Other experimental drugs have been used in human and small animal medicine and may have a future role for management of hepatic insufficiency in horses.

Secondary hepatic failure

Secondary hepatic failure arises in cases of toxemia, septicemia and other apparently unrelated disorders, as a direct result of hepatocyte insult and impairment of one or more of the functions of the organ. **Right-sided heart failure, aflatoxicosis, leukoencephalomalacia (moldy corn poisoning), duodenal ulceration in foals** and several other disorders may progress to hepatic failure. Several **heavy metals** such as **lead, arsenic and mercury** also have hepatic-related effects, although in most of these the hepatic effects are overshadowed by more obvious signs of the poisonings.

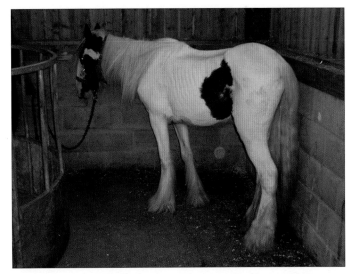

Figure 2.11 Chronic hepatic failure secondary to ragwort (*Senecio jacobea*) poisoning.

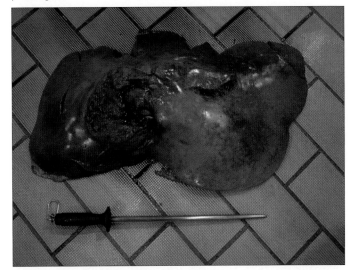

Figure 2.12 Chronic hepatic failure. Liver at post-mortem from horse in Fig. 2.11. Note the small size of the liver typical of ragwort poisoning.

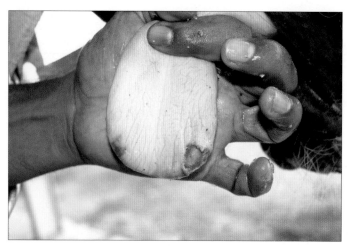

Figure 2.13 Chronic hepatic failure. Tongue ulceration in a horse with chronic liver failure associated with hepatic neoplasia (same horse as Fig. 2.7)

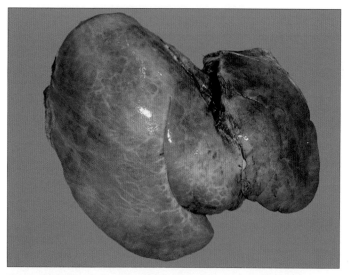

Figure 2.14 Chronic fibrosing hepatitis. Five-month-old male Thoroughbred equine. The horse presented with cholangiohepatitis, bile duct stenosis and pneumonia. The animal became weak, depressed and lethargic, and was euthanized.

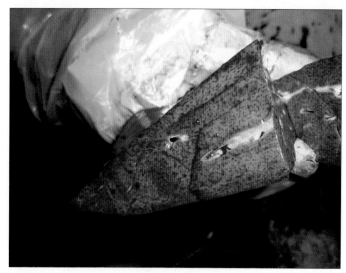

Figure 2.15 Small liver associated with chronic hepatic failure.

Chronic fibrosing hepatitis (Figs. 2.11–2.15)

The differentiation between acute and chronic hepatic failure is often complicated by the fact that the onset of clinical signs in cases of chronic hepatic failure may occur acutely. Hepatoxins are common causes of chronic hepatic failure but essentially any disease entity or intoxication that results in hepatic insufficiency may lead to chronic hepatic failure.

Diagnosis and treatment

- Horses with chronic hepatic failure are frequently hypergamma-globulinemic, but otherwise have similar elevations in hepatic enzymes as horses with acute hepatic failure.
- At post-mortem a small, densely fibrotic liver is usually found. The cut surface is usually dark, dense and fibrous with prominent biliary tracts. The carcass of horses dying from chronic hepatic failure is not often obviously icteric except when secondary bile duct obstruction, either within or outside the liver, has occurred. Generalized edema of the subcutaneous tissues, fluid accumulations in the body cavities and poor body condition may be presented.
- Treatment is largely supportive and similar to that for acute hepatic failure with the prognosis being somewhat more guarded as there is less regenerative capacity.

Non-infectious disorders

Toxic hepatopathy

Toxic insults to the liver are common and may be the result of ingestion of toxic plants, mycotoxins, chemicals or the administration of certain drugs. Other than iron toxicity in foals most result in chronic hepatic failure. Low-level poisoning usually passes unnoticed until ultimately, the damage is sufficient to result in the acute onset of clinical signs which are typical of hepatic failure. Photosensitive dermatosis is often the first reported sign in these cases. It is unusual for the clinical signs to develop slowly but chronic weight loss with ventral edema and soft 'cow-pat' feces may be present in the early stages, and may be indicative of sub-clinical hepatic disease.

Hepatotoxic plants (Figs. 2.16–2.22)

The most common cause is poisoning with plant-derived pyrrolazidine alkaloids, such as are found in *Senecio* spp., *Crotalaria* spp., *Lantana camara*, *Echium plantagineum* (Patterson's curse) and others. Most countries in the world have at least one plant which is capable of inducing chronic liver failure and the local dangerous plants are

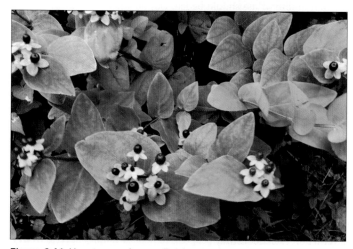

Figure 2.16 *Hypericum perforatum* (St Johns wort).

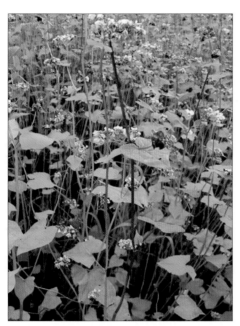

Figure 2.17 Polygonum fagopyrum (buckwheat).

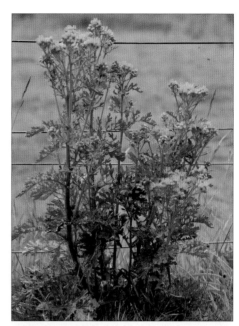

Figure 2.19 Senecio jacobea (ragwort).

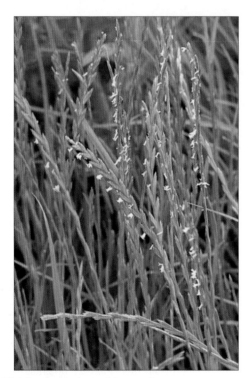

Figure 2.18 Lolium perenne (perennial ryegrass).

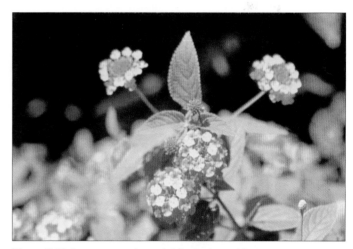

Figure 2.20 Lantana camara (marmalade bush, cherry pie).

are rarely available to horses in sufficient amounts to cause hepatic failure.

Iron-induced hepatic failure in foals has been reported when iron is administered prior to colostrum. Typically 3–5-day-old foals with iron-induced acute liver failure have an acute onset of hepatoencephalopathy (coma, blindness, seizure, etc.) which is almost uniformly fatal.

Mycotoxins (Fig. 2.23)
Mycotoxicosis is uncommon in horses compared to ruminants. The most commonly implicated mycotoxins are aflatoxin and rubratoxin, which may be found in moldy feedstuffs. Generally horses refuse to eat moldy feed and as such avoid exposure. If exposure occurs the extent of hepatic damage depends on the extent and duration of exposure but hepatic failure is uncommon. Fumonisin B1, the mycotoxin of *Fusarium moiliforme*, is associated with contaminated corn and causes leukoencephalomalacia (see p. 427) in horses. The mycotoxin also causes hepatocellular necrosis and periportal fibrosis. However, in these horses signs associated with leukoencephalomalacia predominate and hepatic failure is rare.

usually widely appreciated amongst stock owners. The plants are not usually palatable to grazing horses and ingestion directly from the pasture is not common except where no other food is available. However, the dried or wilted plants appear to be undetectable when they are included in preserved fodder such as hay or silage.

Chemical hepatotoxins
Potential hepatotoxic chemicals include arsenic (pesticide), carbon tetrachloride (fumigant), monensin (ionophore), paraquat (herbicide), and phenol (disinfectant, wood preservative). These and others

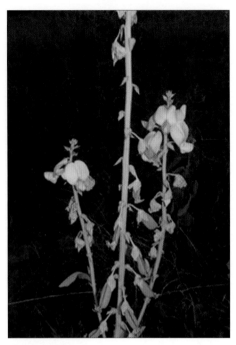

Figure 2.21 Crotalaria crispate.

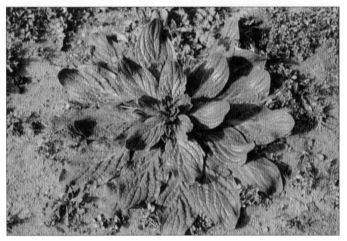

Figure 2.22 *Echium plantagineum* (Patterson's curse).

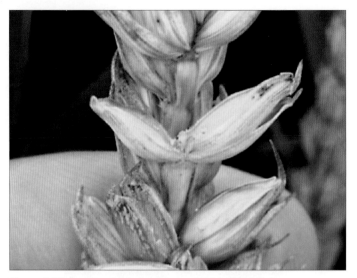

Figure 2.23 *Fusarium* mycotoxin present on moldy wheat.

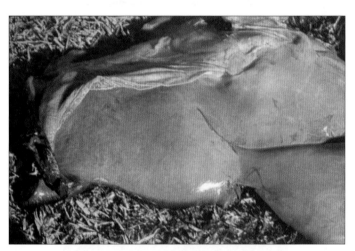

Figure 2.24 Theiler's disease (acute hepatic failure). Generally pale liver with swollen rounded edges.

Diagnosis and treatment

- The diagnosis is often based upon history, clinical signs and laboratory findings of hepatic disease and dysfunction.
- If known ingestion of a toxin occurs administration of activated charcoal or a cathartic may impede absorption. Unfortunately, recognition of ingestion is usually retrospective when clinical signs are noted. This may however allow time for preventative measures to be taken for other horses in an exposed population.
- Treatment is usually supportive but many cases have marked clinical signs and significant hepatic damage when presented.

Theiler's disease (Fig. 2.24)

Theiler's disease (acute hepatic necrosis, serum-associated hepatitis, serum sickness) occurs principally in adult horses. Individuals may be affected but outbreaks involving several horses may also be encountered. Outbreaks of Theiler's disease occur relatively frequently in the autumn months and is most commonly reported in the United States. Many parts of the world have no reported cases. A number of cases have been associated with the prior administration of serum or other biological products and a virus etiology has been suggested in view of some extensive outbreaks amongst horses in close contact. Several other possible causes have been suggested including mycotoxins, alkaloid toxicity and others. To date there has been no single demonstrable etiology.

The clinical signs, which generally have a peracute onset, do not differ significantly from the general signs of acute or chronic hepatic failure. The course of the disease is usually about 5 days with most cases either dying of hepatic failure or gradually recovering over 7–10 days, although commonly recovery may be protracted and incomplete.

Mild forms of the disease are also recognized, presenting with a vague malaise accompanied by elevated serum hepatic enzyme concentrations. Post-mortem examination of affected horses shows the liver to be pale and enlarged with rounded edges. The cut surface shows diffuse mottling giving a characteristic nutmeg-like appearance.

Diagnosis and treatment

- No single laboratory test is diagnostic but a history of recent use of equine-origin biologic with acute onset of clinical signs is highly suggestive. Histopathological findings on a liver biopsy (widespread centrilobular to midzonal hepatocellular necrosis with hemhorrage) although not pathognomonic is also highly suggestive.
- *Differential diagnosis:* Any other cause of acute hepatic failure.
- Treatment is usually general supportive care for hepatic insufficiency.

Liver failure in foals following neonatal isoerythrolysis

Several foals have developed liver failure following a prolonged or refractory course of NI which required two or more transfusions. The etiology of this liver failure is unknown, but may be a result of chronic hypoxia to the liver and/or iron toxicity associated with multiple transfusions or, more likely, a cholangiopathy associated with the hemolysis and bile stasis.

Diagnosis and treatment

- The liver enzymes are all elevated with the GGT elevation most pronounced. Elevations of bile acids and bilirubin are also encountered.
- Ultrasound exam and biopsy of the liver are both abnormal with the ultrasound exam revealing increased echogenicity and irregularity of appearance. The biopsy generally is reported as a hepatopathy with both regeneration and fibrosis.
- There is no proven treatment for this poorly understood liver problem. Certain drugs that may decrease inflammation and/or oxidative injury in the liver and promote bile flow would be recommended. These include pentoxyfilline, S-adenosylmethionine (SAMe) and supplemental vitamin E and selenium.

Bile duct obstruction

In the equine, there are two biliary openings into the duodenum, major and minor biliary papillae. Both drain into the most proximal duodenum in very close proximity.

Foals with gastroduodenal ulcers may develop strictures of the duodenum associated with healing of the duodenal ulcer. If the stricture is at the site of the biliary opening, obstruction of the bile flow will occur. If the stricture is distal to the opening, there will be reflux of ingesta into the bile ducts. The clinical signs are similar with stricture at either site, but the prognosis differs, being grave for strictures at the biliary opening.

There is often a history of a previous illness, e.g., diarrhea, from which the foal seemingly recovered.

Acute bile duct obstruction in adults results in icterus and abdominal pain. It may occur following cholelithiasis or colon displacement. The laboratory abnormalities and clinical signs normally quickly abate following surgical correction of the colon displacement.

Diagnosis

- In foals the history and clinical signs are characteristic of delayed gastric emptying due to gastroduodenal ulceration. Increased levels of bilirubin, GGT and bile acids are usually found. The extent of the elevation of each depends on the degree and duration of obstruction.
- Diagnosis of specific underlying conditions such as colon displacement or cholelithiasis normally allows for a presumptive diagnosis.

Treatment and prognosis

- Treatment of underlying or predisposing conditions is the main goal of therapy followed by metabolic support.

- For foals medical treatment should include intravenously administered H$_2$ blockers in addition to prokinetics such as misoprostil or bethanechol.
- Supportive care such as intravenous fluid administration, regular gastric decompression in foals and parenteral nutrition may be required.
- If the history, clinical signs, endoscopic and radiographic findings suggest chronic obstruction, then medical therapy is unlikely to be curative.

Cholelithiasis (Figs. 2.25–2.29)

Cholelithiasis or the formation of biliary calculi, occasionally results in hepatocellular disease in horses. A **cholelith** is a calculus that forms anywhere along the biliary pathway. A **hepatolith** refers to calculus within the intrahepatic ducts and a **choledocholith** refers to a calculus within the common bile duct. Most hepatic calculi in horses are composed of calcium bilirubinate.

Calculi may be lodged in the common bile duct or the more minor ducts and, in the latter case, there may be almost no helpful

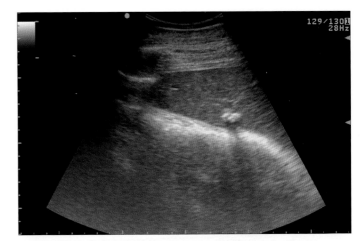

Figure 2.25 This hepatolith was detected ultrasonographically in an otherwise normal horse with no history of hepatic disease. The hepatolith is visualised as a hyperechoic area within the liver, and it casts an acoustic shadow. Measurement of hepatic enzymes was within normal range.

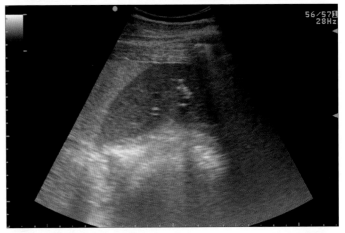

Figure 2.26 This 6-year-old polo mare presented with a history of intermittent colic, weight loss and respiratory disease. She had multiple hepatoliths throughout the liver and ultrasonographically the liver was determined to be of smaller than normal size. She had elevated hepatic enzymes on serum biochemical analysis. The owner decided not to attempt treatment and the mare was taken home where she reportedly died a short time later. No necropsy was performed.

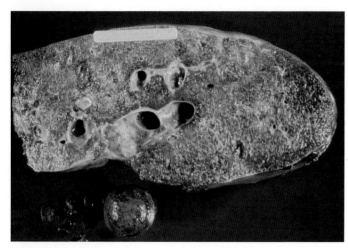

Figure 2.27 Cholelithiasias and cholangiohepatitis. Gross image of the cut surface of the liver from a 12-year-old Stockhorse mare with hepatic failure. Purulent cholangiohepatitis, sabulous cholelithiasis and marked hepatic fibrosis were present.

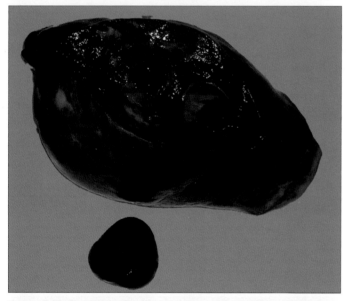

Figure 2.28 Cholelithiasis. This 22-year-old presented with a history of weight loss and anorexia. Due to the presence of this and other intestinal lesions the mare was euthanized.

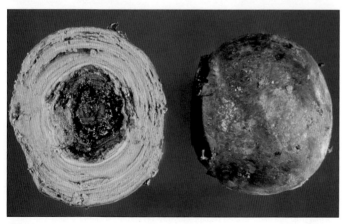

Figure 2.29 Cut surface of choledocholith showing the typical laminated appearance.

pathognomonic clinical signs apart from recurrent colic. Intermittent fever and marked icterus which may vary in severity are sometimes present, particularly when the obstructive lesion is situated in more distal parts of the biliary tract. Complete obstructions of the common bile duct will, of course, result in severe icterus and persistent colic which can become extreme. Biliary calculi, which may also be found incidentally at post-mortem examination, vary in size from 2–12 mm in diameter. Their slow development within the biliary tract is emphasized by their laminated appearance in cross-section.

Diagnosis

- Usually affected animals have a history of previous mild episodes of colic, but it is possible to encounter the disorder without such a history.
- Signs of hepato-encephalopathy are less common than in chronic or acute hepatocellular disorders, particularly with choledocholithiasis (calculi lodged in common bile duct), but dementia and dullness may form part of the clinical syndrome in some cases.
- Laboratory findings suggestive of cholestatic disease include a greatly increased GGT (greater than 15 times normal), increased serum bile acid concentration, hyperbilirubinemia (direct >25% of total) and bilirubinuria.
- Peritoneal fluid is sometimes increased in amount and has an orange-yellow color and may contain a few cells indicative of active inflammation, particularly if bile ducts are disrupted.
- Ultrasonographic examination may be most useful in identifying the dilated bile duct and the choleliths within them. Larger calculi may be more significant and ultrasonography may demonstrate the obstructed bile duct.

Treatment

- If clinical signs of hepatic insufficiency are present supportive care should be given.
- Long-term antimicrobial therapy is usually required to treat secondary hepatitis (see p. 97). Anti-inflammatories are also usually indicated to treat hepatic and biliary inflammation. Dimethylsulfoxide (DMSO) may be beneficial to help dissolve calculi, as it has been shown to be useful for the dissolution of calcium bilirubinate calculi in humans.
- Surgical intervention may be required for occlusion of the bile duct. Unfortunately there is no definitive means by which to assess complete obstruction of the bile duct and thus the decision to intervene surgically is usually made either based on a poor response to medical therapy (persistent fevers and abdominal pain), or markedly severe initial abdominal pain combined with other laboratory or diagnostic indicators of biliary obstruction.
- External massage of the bile duct has been successful at dislodging calculi in the common bile duct (choledocholiths) without choledochotomy. However, if there are multiple calculi throughout the biliary tree, surgical removal is impossible.

Hepatic lipidosis (Figs. 2.30–2.34)

This is one of the commonest forms of acute hepatic failure and is most frequently encountered in overweight ponies in which a dramatic reduction in dietary carbohydrate intake has recently occurred, either as a result of starvation or appetite suppression. Affected ponies (more rarely, horses or donkeys) are often pregnant or lactating. Most cases occur in overweight animals, but body condition may be normal, or even poor. Hyperlipemia has been referred to as an increase in serum triglycerides of less than 500 mg/dl, and hyperlipidemia used to describe increases above 500 mg/dl. However, hyperlipemia is perhaps better described as an increase in serum triglyceride levels without fatty infiltration of the liver or grossly lactesecent blood. Hyperlipidemia refers then to the presence of clinical disease

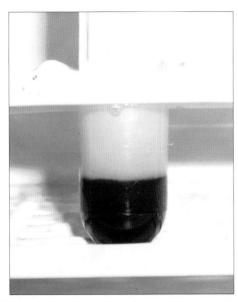

Figure 2.30 Hyperlipidemia. Serum from a horse with hyperlipidemia, note the marked appearance of lipids within the serum.

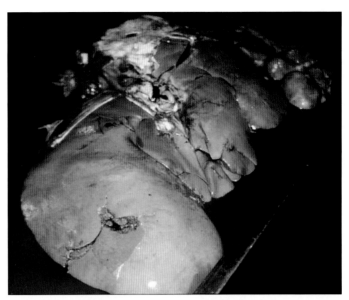

Figure 2.32 Hepatic lipidosis. Enlarged, pale liver associated with fatty infiltration.

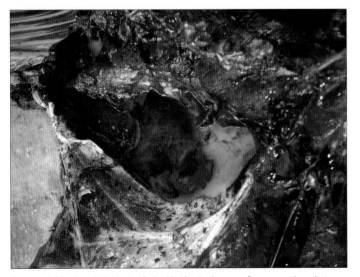

Figure 2.31 Hepatic lipidosis. Marked lipidemic changes of serum evident during necropsy examination of this horse with hyperlipidemia. A 'fatty' film can be seen to have formed.

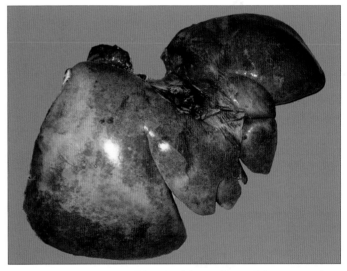

Figure 2.33 Hepatic lipidosis. Enlarged, pale liver with a mottled appearance due to fatty infiltration.

associated with increases in serum triglycerides, including fatty infiltration of the liver and accompanying signs of liver disease.

Affected animals typically show depression and weakness, ataxia, muscle fasciculations, mild colic and dependent edema. Icterus is not usually a prominent sign but individual cases may be obviously icteric. Blood samples are usually noticeably lipidemic and it is often helpful to compare the plasma with that of a normal horse. The extent of the hyperlipidemia is not necessarily proportional to the severity of the clinical syndrome. There may be an intercurrent azotemia and an insulin-resistant hyperglycemia. Secondary laminitis is a common complication. Mortality is usually very high in spite of even the most aggressive treatment and death may be sudden due to hepatic rupture. At post-mortem examination the liver is large, friable, pale-yellow in color and markedly fatty. Pieces of affected liver will float in 10% formal saline.

Primary hepatic lipidosis may also rarely occur due to prolonged administration of high levels of corticosteroids or inappropriately formulated TPN formulations.

Fig. 2.34 outlines the pathogenesis of hepatic lipidosis.

Diagnosis and treatment
- Signalment (miniature equine most commonly) and history of a predisposing disease or event resulting in a period of inappetance. Biochemical findings of elevated plasma triglycerides and liver enzymes. The plasma may be a white color due to the marked elevation in triglycerides (hyperlipidemia).
- Treatment should be directed towards any predisposing disease and nutritional support for the hepatic lipidosis/hyperlipidemia. Parenteral nutrition with amino acids and glucose often combined with insulin can be life-saving in some cases. Crystalloids

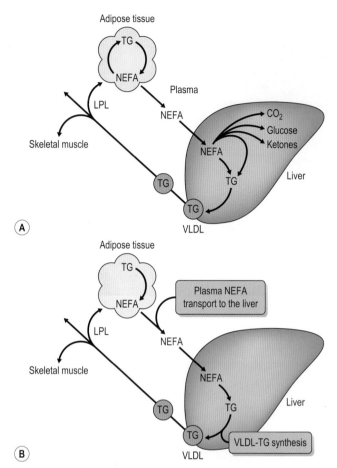

Figure 2.34 Pathogenesis of hepatic lipidosis. (A) demonstrates normal metabolism of non-esterified fatty acids. In cases of abnormal metabolism there is a mobilization of fatty acids usually following a period of inappetance. There follows an abnormal production of very low density lipoprotein (VLDL). TG: Triglycerides; NEFA: Non-esterified fatty acids; LPL: low desity lipoproteins.

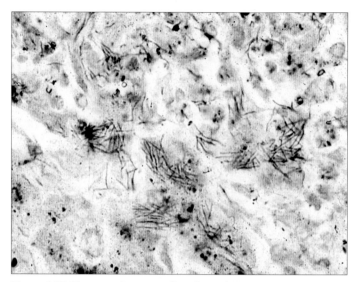

Figure 2.35 Silver stain of a section of liver from a foal with Tyzzer's disease. *Clostridium piliforme* organisms are seen as large rods. Reproduced from McAuliffe SB, Slovis, NM (eds). *Color Atlas of Diseases and Disorders of the Foal* (2008), with permission from Elsevier.

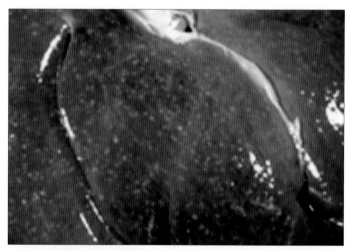

Figure 2.36 Liver of a foal that died of EHV-1 showing focal areas of hepatic necrosis. Reproduced from McAuliffe SB, Slovis, NM (eds). *Color Atlas of Diseases and Disorders of the Foal* (2008), with permission from Elsevier.

should be given intravenously to maintain hydration and prevent azotemia. Multi B vitamins given slowly IV are also recommended.

Infectious disorders

Tyzzer's disease (Fig. 2.35)

Tyzzer's disease is a well-recognized clinical entity caused by *Bacillus pilliformis*. The disease is an acute or peracute, highly fatal, septicemic hepatitis occurring in foals between 1 and 6 weeks of age. Death is often the first sign of the disorder, but cases surviving for over 24 hours are severely depressed, intensely icteric and often show nervous signs attributable to advanced hepatic failure. Although the disease is not considered to be contagious, it may be endemic on some farms, possibly associated with heavier environmental contamination.

Diagnosis and treatment

- A tentative diagnosis is based upon the age of the foal, clinical signs and laboratory findings, which include severe metabolic acidosis, hypoglycemia, and increases in both direct and indirect bilirubin, hepatic enzymes and bile acids in the serum.
- Liver biopsy is rarely performed because the clinical signs and laboratory findings are so characteristic of Tyzzer's disease that a biopsy is not required for a tentative diagnosis and, in fact, due to the frequent occurrence of thrombocytopenia, a biopsy may be

contraindicated. If performed, the large bacteria can be identified in the liver substance on histopathology, and on bacterial culture.
- Although no confirmed cases of Tyzzer's disease have survived, several suspect cases have recovered. Treatment would consist of antibiotics (penicillin +/− aminoglycoside), combined with cardiovascular, nutritional and nursing support.

Equine herpes virus 1 hepatitis (Fig. 2.36)

Mares that become infected with EHV1 late in gestation may deliver a live foal that is jaundiced and weak at birth or the foal may appear normal at birth but develop icterus, vasculitis, respiratory distress, and rarely diarrhea within the first 5 days of life. Due to widespread vaccination of mares this disorder is becoming less common.

Diagnosis

- The diagnosis should be suspected if there is known activity of EHV1 abortion and/or respiratory disease on the farm and a neonatal foal develops the clinical signs listed above.

- Foals with EHV1 are almost always neutropenic and lymphopenic, but this may also be seen with acute bacteremia.
- Buffy coat PCR for EHV-1 could help with an ante-mortem diagnosis.
- Confirmation of the disease occurs at necropsy by finding severe diffuse pneumonia, icterus and hepatic necrosis with viral inclusion bodies.
- On gross examination of the liver, *Actinobacillus*, which is also a common cause of sepsis and acute death in neonatal foals, can cause a similarly abnormal-appearing liver, but usually also has multifocal necrosis of the kidney and absence of diffuse pneumonia.

Treatment
- Treatments are usually unsuccessful if there is multiorgan involvement and severe neutropenia, but some foals do survive.
- Interferon, acyclovir or valacyclovir may be helpful in the treatment, but proper dosages and bioavailability in the foal are not known.
- Affected foals may also be administered granulocyte stimulating factor, but most herpes-1-infected foals seem to have a poor response.
- Antibiotics, oxygen, fluids and supportive care would be indicated.

Infectious necrotic hepatitis

Clostridium novyi type B is the cause of infectious necrotic hepatitis or black disease. It most commonly causes disease in cattle or sheep following migration of *Fasciola hepatitica* through the liver. It has been reported in horses in areas with large populations of sheep but parasitic damage was not apparent in all cases. The onset is acute with rapid progression of clinical signs resulting in death in 2–3 days.

Diagnosis and treatment
- The acute and non-specific nature of the disease make an ante-mortem diagnosis difficult with only mild to moderate elevations in liver enzymes and bilirubin.
- Definitive diagnosis is based on positive staining with fluorescein conjugated antibody specific for the bacteria or isolation at necropsy. The bacteria however are difficult to isolate and require rapid tissue sampling.
- High doses of penicillin and metronidazole are indicated as antibiotics in addition to general supportive care for hepatic insufficiency.

Bacterial cholangiohepatitis (Fig. 2.37)

Primary bacterial cholangiohepatitis has been reported in horses but it is more commonly secondary to biliary stasis, cholelithiasis, chronic active hepatitis, hepatic neoplasia, pancreatitis, enterocolitis, parasitism and intestinal obstruction. It normally results from a reflux of

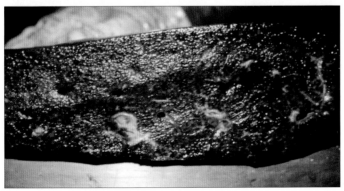

Figure 2.37 Cholangiohepatitis.

enteric organisms and consequently the most commonly isolated organisms are enteric: *Escherichia coli*, *Citrobacter*, *Klebsiella* and *Acinetobacter* spp. Clinical signs include fever, anorexia and icterus.

Diagnosis and treatment
- Laboratory findings may include leukocytosis, hyperfibrinogenemia, increases in SDH, GGT, arginase and direct reacting (conjugated) bilirubin.
- Definitive diagnosis is based on bacterial isolation and histopathological findings from liver biopsy.
- Prolonged courses of antibiotics (4–6 weeks) are normally required in addition to supportive care. Antibiotic selection should be based on susceptibility testing but recommendations for treatment pending culture results are based on the fact that enteric organisms are usually involved and would include trimethoprim-sulfonamide, penicillin and gentimicin, ceftiofur, enrofloxacin and ampicillin.

Liver abscessation/scarring (Figs. 2.38 & 2.39)

Focal, well-circumscribed abscesses in the substance of the liver may be found at post-mortem examination as an incidental finding. While

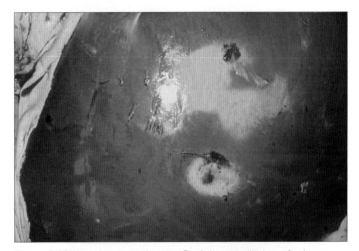

Figure 2.38 Liver abscessation/scarring. Focal abscess in this liver of unknown etiology.

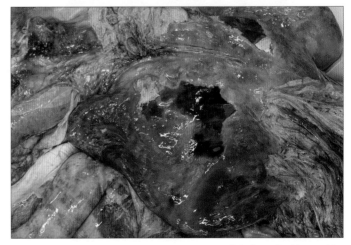

Figure 2.39 Hepatic necrosis. Necropsy appearance of the liver of a 16-year-old Clydesdale mare with clinical signs and blood biochemical abnormalities consistent with hepatic encephalopathy and a marked inflammatory response. The mare was subjected to euthanasia due to deterioration in neurological signs despite treatment. The liver has large areas of infarction and necrosis. The etiology of these changes was not determined.

most are old and no specific organism can be identified, they are usually regarded as the product of septicemic dissemination. Organisms which have been blamed include *Streptococcus equi*, *Staphylococcus aureus*, and *Rhodococcus equi*. Scars or 'milk spots' on the liver capsule are frequently found in normal horses and while the larger of these may reflect normal pigmentary changes in the capsule, others may be scars associated with the hepato-pulmonary migration of *Parascaris equorum*. Even extensive numbers of these lesions appear to cause no detectable harm.

Umbilical vein abscess into the liver
(Fig. 2.40A,B)

Infection of the umbilical structures is common in foals. In many cases, the umbilical vein may be infected and enlarged (>1 cm on ultrasonographic examination) extending from the external umbilical

area into the liver. Affected foals also commonly have failure of passive transfer of immunoglobulins and septicemia and thus often present with non-specific signs or a variety of signs reflecting the different organ systems affected. Enlargement of external umbilical remnants may or may not be present. Liver enzymes are frequently normal.

Diagnosis and treatment

- The diagnosis is based upon signalment and clinical signs, and ultrasound examination of the umbilical structures.
- If the vein is only marginally enlarged, and a positive blood culture is present such that the bacterial pathogen can be identified, then antibiotic therapy may be all that is required.
- If the vein is more enlarged and the abnormality extends into the liver, surgery is recommended. The vein is either removed as far into the liver as possible and the stump cauterized, or the distal part of the vein is removed and the remaining vein (running into the liver) is marsupialized to allow drainage.

Parasitic diseases (Figs. 2.41–2.43)

Parasitic infestation may cause focal hepatic disease but rarely overt hepatic insufficiency. Many parasites migrate through the liver

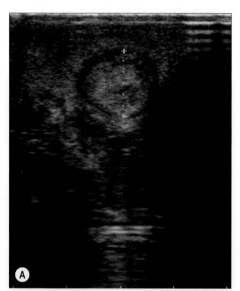

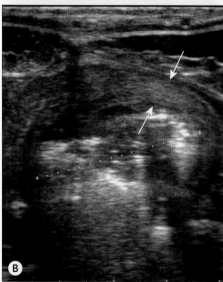

Figure 2.40 Umbilical vein abscess. (A) This ultrasonogram of the umbilical vein obtained just cranial to the umbilicus on the ventral midline shows marked thickening of the walls of the umbilical vein with mixed echogenic contents. (B) Ultrasonogram from the same foal obtained 5 cm caudal to entrance to the liver showing a large abscess of the umbilical vein with contents of mixed echogenicity. Hyperechoic gas reflections can be seen suggesting an anaerobic component to the infection. Note also the thickening of the wall of the vein at this point (between arrows).

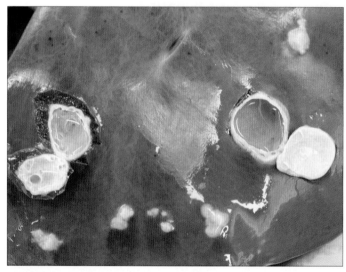

Figure 2.41 Hydatid cysts. Multiple cystic lesions are present which contain proscolices in a clear fluid.

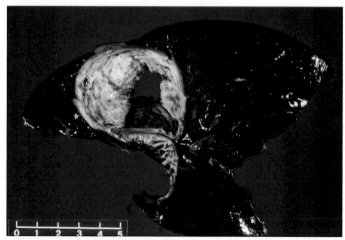

Figure 2.42 Single large hydatid cyst.

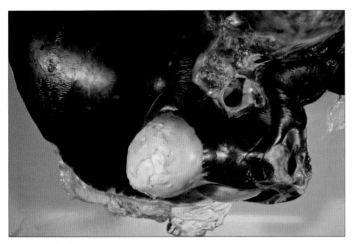

Figure 2.43 Single large intact hydatid cysts.

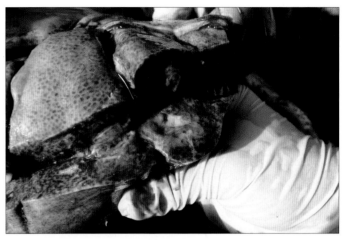

Figure 2.45 Same horse as Fig. 2.44 showing the cut surface of the liver. Focal areas of necrosis were found throughout the liver.

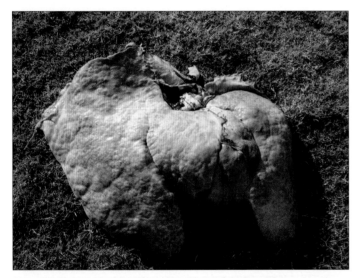

Figure 2.44 Marked enlargement and irregularity of the liver which presented with signs of hepatic insufficiency. Histological examination of the liver confirmed the presence of a cholangiocellular carcinoma. (Same horse as Figs 2.7 & 2.13).

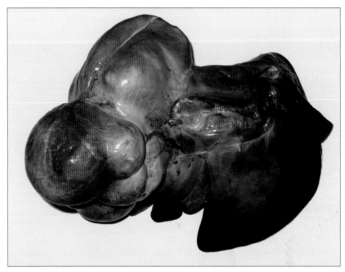

Figure 2.46 Hepatoblastoma. This image is from a 2-hour-old male Thoroughbred foal. Hepatoblastomas can be incidental findings but in this case there were metastatic lesions in all major organs (including brain).

including *Parascaris equorum* and *Strongylus* spp. Considerable numbers of large cysts associated with *Echinococcus granulosis* var. *equinus* may occur in the peritoneal cavity and particularly on the liver capsule. The parasite is a relatively common finding in parts of the world where horses co-exist with infected dogs. Although the appearance may be dramatic they are probably of little clinical significance. The parasite is probably host-specific for the horse and has no known zoonotic importance. Protozoal schizonts may also be rarely encountered.

Infection with the liver fluke is occasionally reported from horses. Prevalences are reported to be highly variable, with some studies reporting less than 1% of horses infected (Bucknell et al. 1995), while others document up to 70% of horses infected on some farms (Fischer and Stoye 1982, Alcaino et al. 1983). As infection is transmitted through snail intermediate hosts, infection rates are believed to be very habitat-dependent. Symptoms caused by *Fasciola hepatica* are unspecific and include ill-thrift and inappetence. Blood work often reveals elevation of the bile duct specific enzyme gamma-glutamyl transferase (GGT) (Campe et al. 2011). Triclabendazole has been reported to be successful for treating *Fasciola hepatica* infection in

horses (Rubilar et al. 1988). Fluke eggs can be detected in fecal samples using a sedimentation technique, but this method is not considered highly sensitive. A serum ELISA test has shown promise for diagnosing *Fasciola* infection in horses (Arias et al. 2012).

Neoplastic disorders

Neoplastic lesions involving the liver substance (Figs. 2.44–2.52, Table 2.4) may be primary or secondary to malignant neoplasia elsewhere. All such disorders of the liver are, fortunately, rare. Cholangiocellular carcinoma is the only primary neoplasm likely to be encountered in the horse and affects older horses exclusively. The

Table 2.4 Neoplasia of the liver and spleen

Liver	Biliary duct carcinoma
	Hepatic adenocarcinoma
	Lymphoma (lymphosarcoma)
Spleen	Lymphoma (lymphosarcoma)
	Hemangiosarcoma

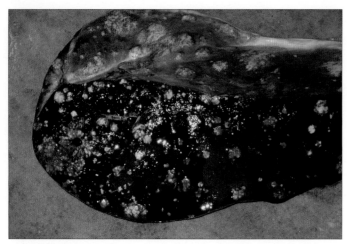

Figure 2.47 Hepatic metastases: necropsy image of multiple and diffuse hepatic metastases of an abdominal carcinoma in a horse which presented for progressive weight loss, inappetence and lethargy. Sonographically, space-occupying lesions in the abdomen and a nodular pattern of the hepatic parenchyma were detected. Peritoneal fluid analysis revealed a modified transudate.

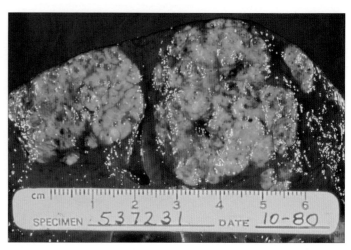

Figure 2.49 Primary hepatic carcinoma.

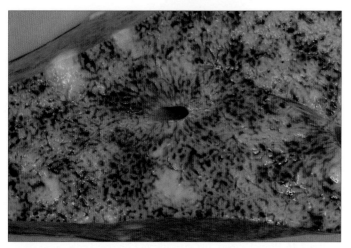

Figure 2.48 Hepatic metastases of colonic adenocarcinoma. Necropsy image of multiple hepatic metastases in a horse which had a primary adenocarcinoma involving the large colon. The horse presented for acute onset of abdominal pain and underwent an exploratory laparotomy, during which neoplastic involvement of the large colon and mesenteric lymph nodes were detected.

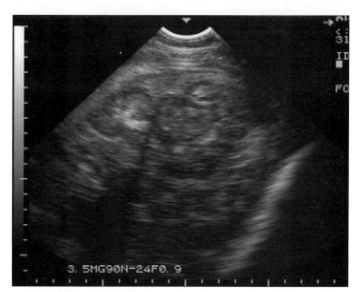

Figure 2.50 Ultrasonographic image of the liver showing discrete masses in a case of multicentric lymphosarcoma.

clinical signs are those associated with biliary obstruction and extensive hepatocellular destruction.

Horses affected by hepatic lymphosarcoma show varying degrees of abdominal distension due to lymphatic and hepatic obstruction with elevation of portal pressure.

The commonest neoplastic changes involving the liver are secondary metastases from malignancies elsewhere. Secondary tumors occurring in the liver substance are usually blood-borne but local transperitoneal metastasis, such as occurs with gastric squamous cell carcinoma, is possible. Secondary tumors of all types are usually multiple, arising from hematogenous spread from a primary lesion elsewhere. Secondary hemangiosarcoma lesions in the liver are soft or spongy, poorly defined and contain dark hemorrhagic amorphous tumor tissue.

Diagnosis
- Definitive diagnosis is usually made based on histopathological examination of a liver biopsy.

- Ultrasonography may show a markedly enlarged liver in cases of primary tumors and more focal lesions in cases of metastatic lesions.
- In cholangiocellular carcinoma the peritoneal fluid is of an orange-red, turbid nature and abnormal cells can be identified easily, although the specific origin of these is almost always impossible to identify in the living horse.
- In cases of hepatic lymphosarcoma, the peritoneal fluid tends to be clear or cloudy but is seldom hemorrhagic. Abnormal lymphocytes can usually be identified in this fluid.

Pancreatic disorders

Pancreatitis
Both acute and chronic pancreatitis have been encountered in the horse. The cause is unknown but theories include grain overload, gastric ulceration, migrating parasites, bacterial and viral infections,

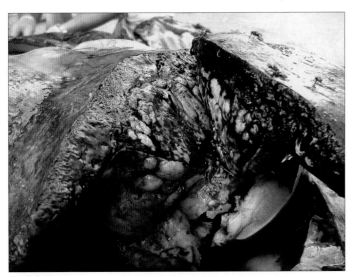

Figure 2.51 Same horse as Fig. 2.50 showing cut surface of liver with multiple neoplastic lesions.

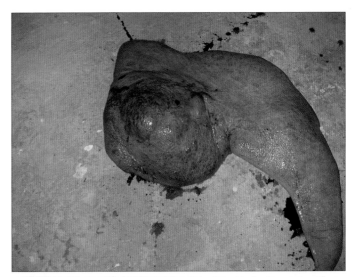

Figure 2.53 Splenic hemangiosarcoma. This mare presented with acute-onset abdominal hemorrhage and died within a short period of time. Post-mortem examination revealed a splenic hemangiosarcoma which had resulted in splenic rupture on the visceral surface (not visible).

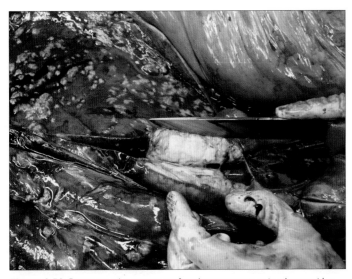

Figure 2.52 Pancreatic adenocarcinoma found at post-mortem in a horse with a history of chronic weight loss.

- Although not pathognomonic, acute pancreatitis cases frequently have voluminous gastric reflux and darkly hemorrhagic, brown-colored, flocculent peritoneal fluid which may be seen to contain large and small globules of free fat.
- At post-mortem examination, the pancreas is diffusely 'mushy' with a dark and often gaseous texture. *Clostridium* spp. bacteria may be identifiable.
- Post-mortem examination of chronic pancreatitis cases shows the pancreas to be severely atrophied.

Treatment
- Medical management of acute pancreatitis is symptomatic with frequent gastric decompression required and administration of large volumes of electrolyte-balanced fluids.
- **Pancreatic neoplasia** (Fig. 2.52) is rarely encountered in the horse. Adenocarcinomas or lymphosarcomas can occur with non-specific signs such as weight loss, diarrhea, icterus and fever.

Splenic disorders (Figs. 2.53–2.60)

Disorders of the spleen are rare but can include neoplasia, splenic hematomas or abscesses and splenomegaly.

Splenic neoplasms

Neoplasia is perhaps the most common splenic abnormality encountered. Splenic neoplasms are frequently as a result of metastasis from other organs. Splenic involvement has been reported in up to 40% of horses with intestinal lymphosarcoma. Primary neoplasia of the spleen is most commonly associated with hemangiosarcoma. Clinical signs include weight loss, anorexia and fever. Splenic rupture may be associated with hemangiosarcomas. There is normally marked splenic enlargement with evident mass(es) bulging from the surface.

Splenic hematoma

Severe trauma associated with caudal rib fractures or falls can result in splenic hematomas or hemoabdomen. Most commonly these incidents are associated with large tears which result in rapid death and the history may simply consist of the animal being found dead in a paddock. In other cases there may be development of a hematoma without splenic rupture. In these cases the hematoma can be detected

immune-mediated damage, vitamin A or E deficiency or vitamin D toxicity. Drugs administered to horses that are known to cause pancreatitis in humans include furosemide, estrogens, tetracycline, corticosteroids and sulfonamides.

Acute pancreatic failure causes a fulminating and rapidly progressive shock and endotoxemia with severe colic, gastric distension and cardiovascular compromise. These signs are also encountered in cases of anterior enteritis and, indeed, the two conditions may be interrelated or co-exist making specific diagnosis even more difficult.

Chronic pancreatic failure results in exocrine pancreatic insufficiency. Affected horses suffer from weight loss and maldigestion but these aspects are masked by the particular characteristics of the horse's digestive tract. Acute or sub-acute episodes accompanied by peritonitis, colic and laminitis may be superimposed upon the chronically failing pancreas.

Diagnosis
- The disorder is rare but may be under-diagnosed as it is most difficult to confirm before death and the signs are not specific.

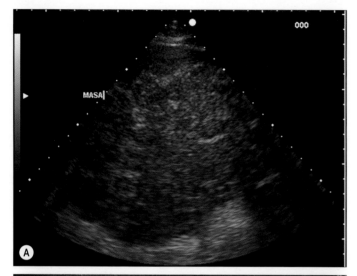

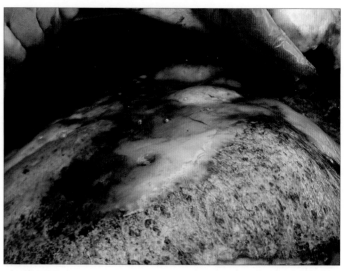

Figure 2.56 Splenic lymphosarcoma (same horse as Fig. 2.54B).

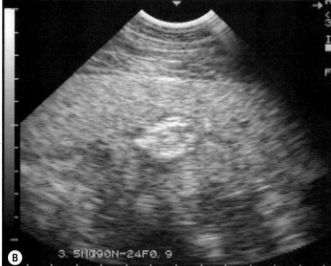

Figure 2.54 Splenic lymphosarcoma ultrasonograms. (A) Sonographically complex mass imaged within the spleen. (B) Hyperechoic nodular mass.

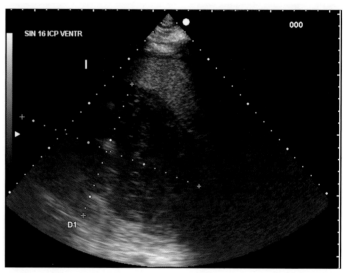

Figure 2.57 Chronic splenic abscess with hemorrhage. Nine-year-old Warmblood gelding, with a history of long-term weight loss and mild colics. The horse was euthanized due to uncertain prognosis. This ultrasound image shows a large hypoechoic mass associated with the spleen.

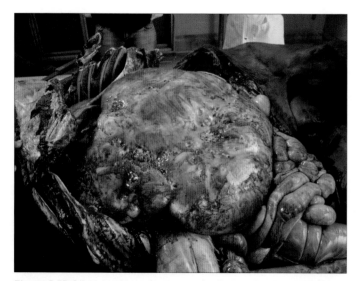

Figure 2.55 Splenic lymphosarcoma as part of multicentric lymphosarcoma.

rectally if the caudal pole or the tail of the spleen is involved or may be imaged ultrasonographically.

Splenic abscess

Splenic abscesses have been reported in horses resulting from extension from local intestinal abscesses, foreign body penetration of the intestine or the abdominal wall or secondary to drainage of a splenic hematoma.

Diagnosis is frequently made by ultrasonography and aspiration. Unfortunately many abscesses are large when diagnosed and therefore difficult to treat.

Splenomegaly

Splenomegaly is a difficult diagnosis in the horse due to the large variation in normal sizes. When pathologic it has been associated with

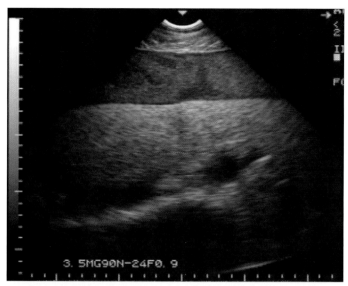

Figure 2.58 This sonogram of the ventral abdomen shows free fluid with the abdomen. In real time this fluid had a 'swirling smoke' pattern consistent with active hemorrhage. An irregular hypoechoic area could be visualized within the splenic parenchyma and the hemorrhage appeared to be originating from that site. The horse was treated symptomatically with blood transfusions and fluid therapy and made an uneventful recovery.

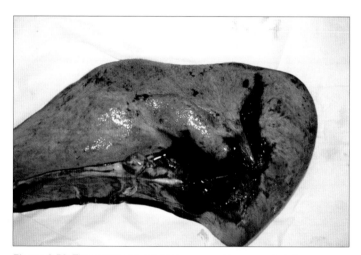

Figure 2.59 This spontaneous splenic tear occurred in a young foal. A splenectomy was performed and the foal made a good recovery.

neoplasia, infarction, extramedullary hematopoiesis or infections such as equine infectious anemia, immune-mediated hemolytic anemias, salmonellosis and piroplasmosis.

Splenic rupture

Ruptures or tears of the spleen may occur secondary to neoplasia or trauma and can also be idiopathic. Depending on the size of the tear clinical signs may vary from depression and weakness to cardiovascular collapse and sudden death.

Treatment depends on the underlying cause. A number of large idiopathic tears in foals have been treated by splenectomy. Smaller tears associated with less severe clinical signs may be treated medically with fluid therapy and blood transfusions (if required).

The prognosis is poor in cases associated with neoplasia. In cases related to trauma, the other injuries sustained are frequently severe and dictate the outcome. Idiopathic cases frequently recover well.

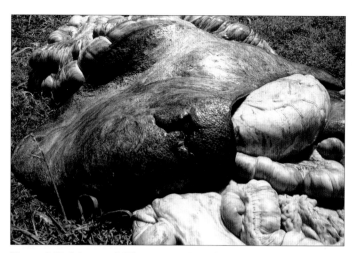

Figure 2.60 Splenomegaly. This was an incidental finding in a horse that was euthanized with a fracture of a thoracic vertebrae. Note also the incidental defect in splenic parenchyma. This defect had smooth edges and the horse had no history of previous trauma prior to the fracture, or clinical signs associated with a splenic tear.

Splenic neoplasia

Splenic hemangiosarcoma can be found as a primary neoplasm. Frequently clinical signs are associated with splenic rupture and acute intra-abdominal hemorrhage.

Splenic lymphosarcoma may occur as a primary or secondary neoplasm. In most instances of splenic lymphosarcoma normal-appearing splenic parenchyma is imaged adjacent to discrete masses with irregular borders and heterogenous echogenicity.

References and further reading

Alcaino, H., Gorman, T., Phillips, J., 1983. Fasciola hepatica infection in thoroughbred race horses in stud farms and hippodromes. Parasitología al Día 7, 37–40.

Arias, M.S., Piñeiro, P., Hillyer, G.V., et al., 2012. Enzyme-linked immunosorbent assays for the detection of equine antibodies specific to a recombinant Fasciola hepatica surface antigen in an endemic area. Parasitol. Res. 110, 1001–1007.

Bucknell, D.G., Gasser, R.B., Beveridge, I., 1995. The prevalence and epidemiology of gastrointestinal parasites of horses in Victoria, Australia. Int. J. Parasitol. 25, 711–724.

Campe, J., Vyt, P., Ducheyne, K., 2011. Fasciolosis in horses on a Belgian stud farm. Vlaams Diergen Tijds 80, 403–406.

Conwell, R.C., Hillyer, M.H., Mair, T.S., et al., 2010. Haemoperitoneum in horses: a retrospective review of 54 cases. Vet Rec 167 (14), 514–518.

Divers, T.J., 1993. Biochemical diagnosis of hepatic disease and dysfunction in the horse. Equine Pract 15, 15.

East, L.M., Savage, C.J., 1998. Abdominal neoplasia (excluding urogenital tract).Vet Clin North Am Equine Pract 14 (3), 475–493.

Fischer, K.L.A., Stoye, M., 1982. Occurrence, significance and control of Fasciola hepatica infections in horses. Zbl Vet Med 37, 268–279.

Mair, T., Divers, T., Ducharme, N., 2002. Manual of Equine Gastroenterology. WB Saunders, Edinburgh, UK.

Mas, A., 2006. Hepatic encephalopathy: from pathophysiology to treatment. Digestion 73 (suppl 1), 86.

McAuliffe, S.B., Slovis, N.M., 2008. Colour Atlas of Diseases and Disorders of the Foal. WB Saunders, PA, USA.

McCornico, R.S., Duckett, W.M., Wood, P.A., 1997. Persistent hyperammonemia in two related Morgan weanlings. J Vet Intern Med 11 (4), 264–266.

Reed, S.M., Bayly, W.M., Sellon, D.C., 2009. Equine Internal Medicine, third ed. WB Saunders, St. Louis, MO, USA.

Reef, V.B., 1998. Equine Diagnostic Ultrasound. WB Saunders, Philadelphia, PA, USA.

Robinson, N.E., Sprayberry, K.A. (Eds.), 2009. Current Therapy in Equine Medicine, sixth ed. WB Saunders, St. Louis, MO, USA.

Rubilar, L., Cabreira, A., Giacaman, L., 1988. Treatment of Fasciola hepatica infection in horses with triclabendazole. Vet. Rec. 123, 320–321.

Southwood, L.L., Schott 2nd., H.C., Henry, C.J., et al., 2000. Disseminated hemangiosarcoma in the horse: 35 cases. J Vet Intern Med 14 (1), 105–109.

Spier, S., Carlson, G.P., Nyland, T.G., et al., 1986. Splenic hematoma and abscess as a cause of chronic weight loss in a horse. J Am Vet Med Assoc 189 (5), 557–559.

Steel, C.M., Lonsdale, R.A., Bolton, J.R., 1998. Successful medical treatment of splenic abscesses in a horse. Aust Vet J 76 (8), 541–542.

Tanimoto, T., Yamasaki, S., Ohtsuki, Y., 1994. Primary splenic lymphoma in a horse. J Vet Med Sci 56 (4), 767–769.

CHAPTER 3

Conditions of the respiratory tract

Congenital/developmental disorders

Wry nose (Fig. 3.1)

Wry nose, or deviated rostral maxilla and associated nasal septal deviation, is a congenital deformity in the horse. The deviation can be very mild to severe. A foal with wry nose will have the upper jaw and nose deviated or turned to one side. A deviated nasal septum is also usually present, which results in obstruction of the airway and difficulty breathing. This is the greatest *functional* concern with wry nose. There will usually be malocclusion (poor alignment) of the teeth, although most foals can still nurse and in most cases are bright and active.

The etiology of maxilla deviations is often unknown. Failure of proper embryologic development of the hard palate and maxilla may be associated with possible genetic defects. Abnormal in utero positioning has also been proposed.

Wry-nosed foals can also have other deformities of the neck and occasionally of the limbs. It is very important to further evaluate the foal for other types of genetic defects.

Diagnosis

- Visual, digital and oral examinations: obvious facial deviations.
- Radiology: helps confirm and further evaluate the degree and severity of the deviation.
- Endoscopic examination: helps assess the deviation and evaluates the soft palate.

Treatment

- Mild cases can potentially survive and live without significant airway problems.
- In more severe cases surgical correction is generally undertaken in multiple stages. This type of reconstructive surgery is expensive and requires significant aftercare. Although the objective of the surgery is usually to make the horse capable of being an athlete, unfortunately, neither the functional nor cosmetic outcome can be guaranteed.

Epiglottic and pharyngeal cysts (Figs. 3.2–3.6)

Epiglottic and pharyngeal cysts are fluid-filled structures that do not communicate with an epithelial surface. These cysts can be found in the subepiglottic tissues, in the dorsal nasopharynx and within the soft palate. In foals these cysts are considered congenital and depending on their location may represent embryonic remnants of the thyroglossal (sub-epiglottic) and craniopharyngeal (pharyngeal) ducts. Thoroughbred and Standardbred foals are most commonly affected. The presence of the cyst at this site may have little effect upon the well-being of the animal and may be detected incidentally at any age during endoscopic examination of the pharynx. The cysts may be relatively small in the early years of life but commonly enlarge slowly with time and therefore a progressively deteriorating respiratory noise

with exercise limitations develops. Horses in which the epiglottis is very prominent and apparently upright, giving the impression of being tightly held by the rostral border of the soft palate, may be so because of an epiglottic cyst under the soft palate. In most such cases, however, no cyst can be identified and radiographic examination will usually confirm or deny their existence. Where no cyst is present the position of the larynx relative to the soft palate is regarded as a normal variant.

Foals with large cysts may present in respiratory distress or be seen to collapse while nursing. Coughing, nasal discharge, nasal milk reflux and aspiration pneumonia are common clinical signs.

Diagnosis and treatment

- **Sub-epiglottic cysts.** Endoscopy is essential for diagnosis. Make sure that swallowing is observed during endoscopy to allow observation of the ventral aspect of the epiglottis and the caudal aspect of the soft palate. Cysts located in the sub-epiglottic tissue may not always be visible while the epiglottis is in its natural position relative to the soft palate, being located under the rostral palatine border. Oroscopic examination may be required for diagnosis.

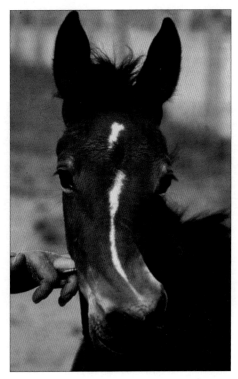

Figure 3.1 Wry nose.

- *Pharyngeal cysts.* These are not directly visible endoscopically, but symmetric or asymmetric dorsal pharyngeal compression, which is not attributable to guttural pouch enlargement, is visible and lateral radiographs of the pharynx confirm their presence.
- Concurrent developmental defects of the epiglottis are sometimes present and these influence the clinical effects and endoscopic and radiographic appearance.
- Repeated dorsal displacement of the soft palate may be present, possibly as a result of inadequate free rostral length or inadequate stiffness of the epiglottis.

- Surgical intervention will be warranted. Surgical resection via a ventral midline laryngotomy works best but with smaller cysts laser ablation may suffice.

Guttural pouch tympany (Figs. 3.7–3.10)

Guttural pouch tympany is a common, possibly developmental, disorder involving usually one (but occasionally both) of the openings (ostia) and/or the pharyngeal component of the auditory tube in the nasopharynx. It is more common in fillies than in colts and Arabians appear to have a breed predilection. The etiology is not exactly known but it appears that the salpingopharyngeal fold (redundant tissue) is excessive, causing the external ostia to act as a one-way valve. This one-way valve action will cause the accumulation of air in the guttural pouch. The affected pouch is distended with air to form a

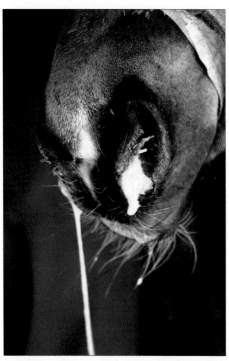

Figure 3.2 Subepiglottic cyst. Nasal regurgitation of milk in a day-old foal with a subepiglottic cyst.

Differential diagnosis:
- Cleft or hypoplastic palate
- Neurologic dysphagia.

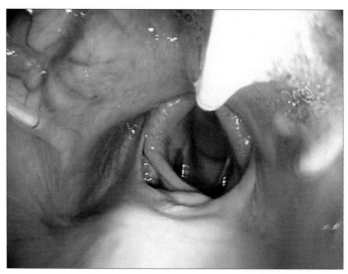

Figure 3.4 Subepiglottic cyst with epiglottic entrapment in a 9 day old foal.

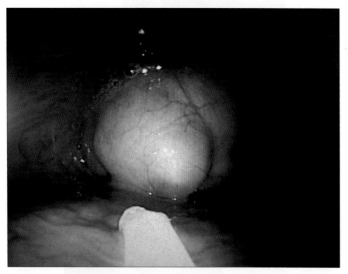

Figure 3.3 Subepiglottic cyst (oral endoscopic view) (same foal as in Fig. 3.2).

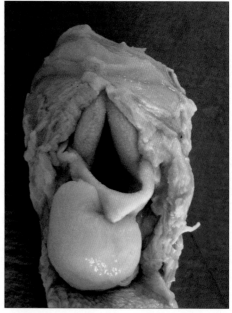

Figure 3.5 Post-mortem image of a subepiglottic cyst. This foal presented with severe aspiration pneumonia related to ineffectual swallowing caused by the cyst.

non-painful, elastic swelling in the parotid region. The swelling is most prominent on the affected side, but can extend across the neck and give the impression of bilateral involvement.

Within the first few weeks of life (but occasionally up to 1 year of age) affected foals develop a prominent, non-painful, non-elastic, tympanitic distension in the parotid region.

Stertorous breathing and possibly dysphagia with nasal regurgitation of food, as a result of dorsal pharyngeal compression or distortion may be evident, particularly if the neck is flexed. Suckling foals may have considerable difficulty feeding from the mare and sometimes adopt bizarre feeding positions in an attempt to limit the pharyngeal distortion and allow normal swallowing.

Diagnosis

- The clinical appearance is typical. Skull radiographs are diagnostic, but endoscopy will confirm involvement of one or both ostia. The free borders of the ostia are often slightly curled in these cases, and noticeably fail to open effectively during the low-pressure (second) phase of swallowing, as the larynx is lowered.
- If in doubt as to the involvement of one or both pouches, air can be released from one pouch by either placing a blunt probe through the ostia on one side or aspirating air percutaneously on one side. If this results in complete resolution of the swelling then only one pouch is affected.

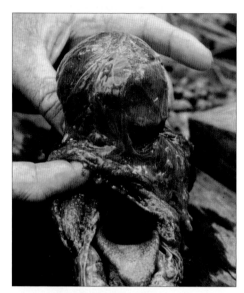

Figure 3.6 Pharyngeal cyst. Post-mortem image.

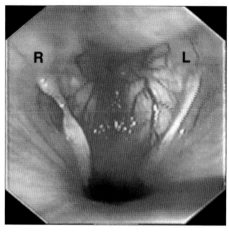

Figure 3.8 Guttural pouch tympany (unilateral) (endoscopic view). Note the curled ostium of right auditive (eustachian) tube. This failed to open effectively during the low-pressure phase of swallowing. Left side normal.

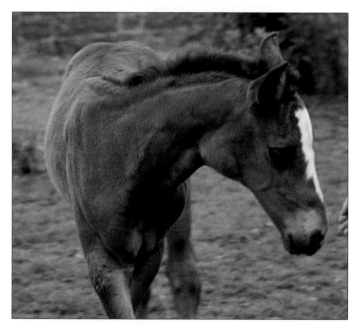

Figure 3.7 Guttural pouch tympany. Typical swelling in throat area. The swelling present is usually bilateral regardless of whether the tympany is unilateral or bilateral. Transcutaneous or endoscopic assisted removal of air from one pouch allows differentiation between unilateral and bilateral conditions as the swelling will persist in bilateral conditions and resolve in unilateral cases.

Differential diagnosis:
- Guttural pouch empyema
- Strangles
- Esophageal cyst
- Branchial cyst
- Salivary mucocele.

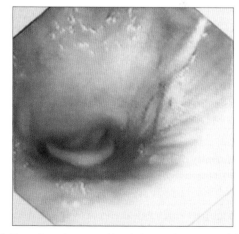

Figure 3.9 Guttural pouch tympany (dorsal pharyngeal compression) (endoscopic view). Collapse of the pharyngeal vault onto larynx causing distortion of arytenoids and occlusion of aditus laryngis.

Differential diagnosis:
- Guttural pouch empyema
- Pharyngeal paralysis (bilateral)
- Hemorrhage in guttural pouch
- Pharyngeal abscess/necrosis
- Dorsal pharyngeal cyst
- Strangles.

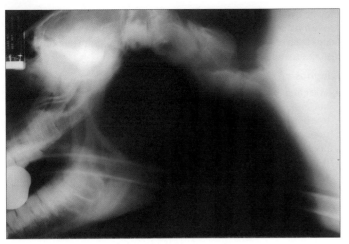

Figure 3.10 Guttural pouch radiograph showing marked distension of the guttural pouch with air.

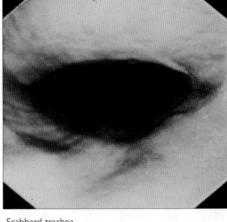

Figure 3.11 Scabbard trachea.

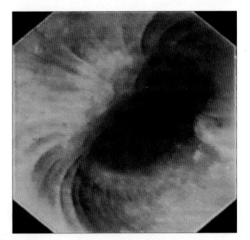

Figure 3.12 Spiral trachea.

Treatment

- For severe cases of pharyngeal collapse the use of a tracheostomy will be warranted.
- For unilateral tympany a fenestration through the median septum is achieved either via endoscopic-guided laser or blunt dissection via a hypovertebrotomy incision which will allow the egress of trapped air from the tympanitic pouch through the normal side.
- With bilateral involvement transendoscopic laser fenestration of the septum or fistulation into the guttural pouch through the pharyngeal recess avoids a surgical incision and the risk of nerve damage.

Tracheal collapse (Figs. 3.11 & 3.12)

Tracheal collapse might be related to abnormal tracheal cartilage matrix and is most often diagnosed in ponies and miniature horses. Limited lengths of the trachea are affected but longer lengths are sometimes involved. The trachea is flattened ventro-dorsally or, more rarely, laterally. The passage of a food bolus through the esophagus can be appreciated during tracheal endoscopy due to the flaccid dorsal ligament which replaces part of the normally solid cartilaginous ring. Some cases are found to have intact tracheal rings with a marked flattening and sharp angles at each side. Typically signs are not noted until the animal is older and is often not noted until adulthood. Severely affected animals will develop a 'honking' inspiratory and expiratory sound. Tracheal stenosis and collapse can also develop dramatic clinical signs, including respiratory stridor, dyspnea and cyanosis. More severe signs are usually associated with concurrent respiratory disease or sudden increased exertional demands.

Spiral deformity of the trachea is a developmental abnormality, also primarily affecting the miniature breeds, in which the tracheal rings take on a spiral contour. This is usually more prominent in the proximal cervical trachea. Animals with spiral deformity of the trachea seldom have any clinical effects, with the defect normally being found incidentally during respiratory tract endoscopy or post-mortem examination.

Diagnosis and treatment

- The diagnosis of tracheal stenosis and collapse is based on signalment, history, clinical signs and endoscopic and radiographic findings.
- No significant treatments plans have been implemented to increase the success of surgical options. The prognosis is usually good for life but poor for athletic functions.

Hypoplasia of the nasal turbinate bones

This is occasionally seen during routine endoscopy and although in some cases it is profound in extent the effect upon the animal is minimal.

Epidermal inclusion cysts (atheroma) (Fig. 3.13)

These are characteristically located in the caudo-dorsal area of the nasal diverticulum (false nostril). These spherical structures are usually unilateral and 2–5 cm in diameter, but in unusual circumstances may be bilateral and much larger. They are only of cosmetic significance. They are occasionally apparent in weanlings but are usually presented in young adults. The cysts are soft, fluctuant and non-painful but may also have a firm texture giving the impression, on palpation, of a solid mass. They may be moveable in the surrounding tissue or relatively fixed, and contain a sterile, gray, creamy, odorless, thick material.

Diagnosis and treatment

- Location and features are usually diagnostic but an aspirate of the cyst material may help differentiate it from a more solid mass.
- Surgical excision is the recommended treatment.

Choanal atresia (Fig. 3.14)

This a rare disorder that is due to a failure of the breakdown of the buconasal membrane. This membrane normally separates the

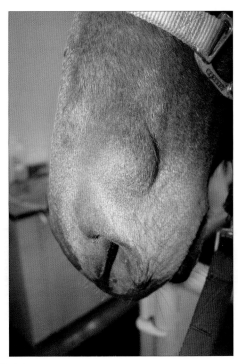

Figure 3.13 Atheroma.

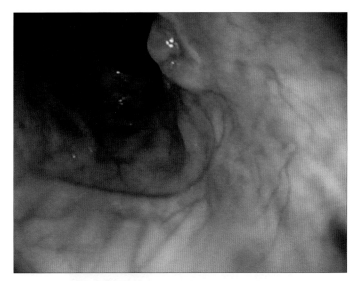

Figure 3.14 Choanal atresia. A 1-year-old Standardbred colt that was presented for exercise intolerance. The yearling was in good general body condition. Endoscopy examination allowed visualization of the ethmoid (top of the picture), but blindly ending middle and ventral meati. There was no communication between the left nasal cavity and the nasopharynx. There were no other congenital or developmental abnormalities.

embryological buccal and nasal cavities and breaks down during later stages of development. There is therefore no communication between the oropharynx and the nasopharynx.

Bilateral atresia results in immediate respiratory distress, cyanosis and decreased/absent airflow from the nares following birth. Unilateral atresia results in a lack of airflow through the affected nasal passage.

Diagnosis and treatment
- Passage of a nasogastric tube will be obstructed at the pharynx. Endoscopic examination will reveal the obstruction in the posterior nares.
- Immediate tracheostomy is warranted during respiratory distress. Surgical intervention has been described with the prognosis for athletic performance being described as poor.

Branchial cysts (Fig. 3.15)
Branchial cysts are uncommon embryonic anomalies of horses. The cysts result from malformation of one of the five branchial arches during embryogenesis. These cysts typically appear as smooth, round, mobile masses and often do not cause any clinical abnormalities, although large cysts may cause discomfort and can disrupt pharyngeal or laryngeal function. Many are not apparent until weaning age with late recognition possibly as a result of delayed secretion of fluid by the epithelial lining.

Diagnosis and treatment
- The clinical appearance of the branchial cysts may be very similar to guttural pouch tympany and enlarged retropharyngeal lymph nodes. Endoscopic examination may reveal collapse of the dorsal pharyngeal wall and compression of the ipsilateral compartment of the guttural pouch.
- Ultrasound examination reveals an anechoic fluid-filled structure with a well-defined hyperechoic capsule. Aspiration of the cysts reveals an amber viscous fluid with a high protein and a low cellularity (lymphocytes and macrophages). Radiographs reveal a large space-occupying soft tissue mass.

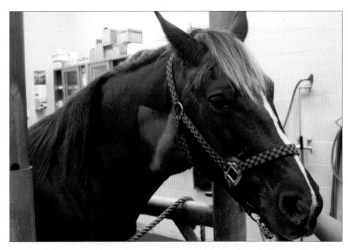

Figure 3.15 Branchial cyst. This aged mare had bilateral branchial cysts which were treated by marsupialization and sclerotherapy. Treatment to resolve the cysts was prolonged, but the mare had no long-term complications.

Differential diagnosis:
- Esophageal cyst/abscess
- Guttural pouch tympany (younger horses)
- Strangles/guttural poch empyema.

- Medical management would consist of marsupialization and iodine sclerotherapy. Surgical excision may be necessary for larger cysts.

Maxillary sinus cysts (Figs. 3.16–3.19)
Congenital disorders of the nasal cavities and paranasal sinuses are very rare. However, unilocular or, more usually multilocular, fluid-filled maxillary cysts may be encountered within the paranasal sinuses in young foals. The caudal compartment of the maxillary sinus is most often affected but the cysts may extend from here into

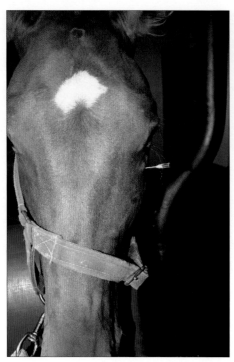

Figure 3.16 Maxillary sinus cyst. This 18-month-old presented for unilateral facial swelling. Radiographs revealed a soft tissue density in the area of the left maxillary sinus. Aspiration of the sinus yielded a serosanguinous fluid. The cyst was removed surgically.

Differential diagnosis:
• Primary/secondary sinusitis
• Sinus mucocele
• Sinus/ethmoid hematoma
• Neoplasia.

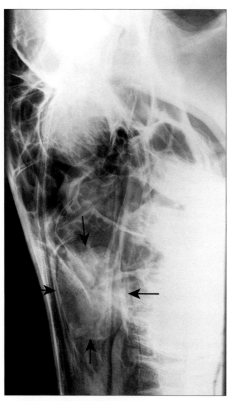

Figure 3.17 Maxillary sinus cyst. Lateral radiograph of the head demonstrating a soft tissue circular-shaped opacity of the maxillary sinus (arrows).

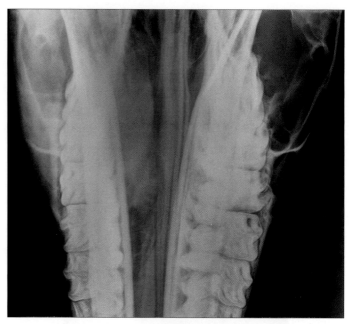

Figure 3.18 Maxillary sinus cyst. Dorso-ventral (slightly obliqued) radiograph demonstrating soft tissue opacity of the maxillary sinus (left side as looking at the image).

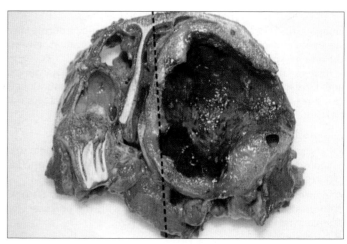

Figure 3.19 Maxillary sinus cyst. Post-mortem. Single fluid-filled cavity with spongy mucosal lining. Severe occlusion of ipsilateral and deviation of nasal septum to occlude contralateral nostril. The mid-line is shown by the dotted line.

the frontal sinus. They are possibly related to the germ buds of the permanent cheek teeth, although most affected foals show no developmental dental defects in later life. Congenital cysts are obvious at birth or develop in the first few weeks of life. Very large cysts have a significant effect upon the nasal cavity and facial appearance. Progressive enlargement results in a worsening obstruction of the nasal cavity and displacement of the nasal septum. Distortion of the maxilla and the nasal cavity, with bony resorption and dental defects, may result.

The clinical effects are largely dependent upon the extent of dental and nasal distortion. Where the erupting premolar teeth are grossly displaced by progressive bone resorption, foals may show difficulty with mastication with food material accumulating in the sides of the mouth. There may also be some loss of solid food from the mouth (quidding) but there is usually no difficulty with suckling, except where the hard palate is also distorted. They often have a marked effect on respiratory function when the distortion of the nasal cavity is sufficient to result in occlusion of both nasal cavities. While most of these cysts have a thick spongy epithelial lining others have a thinner mucosal lining. In both types, incomplete plates of bone are often present. The cyst itself is usually filled with a sterile, turbid, yellowish fluid with little or no odor. In some cases the fluid may be mucohemorrhagic.

Diagnosis and treatment
- Radiographically, fluid-filled structures, with multiple air–fluid interfaces, soft tissue mineralization and gross deviations of the nasal septum are characteristic. Dental distortions and nasal cavity occlusion may be evident endoscopically.
- Frontonasal flap surgery is generally effective. Facial deformity may resolve in young horses following surgery.

Maxillary mucocele
The congenital absence of an effective naso-maxillary opening creates a discrete single-structured secretory cyst within the affected maxillary sinus, and lined by the normal sinus mucous membrane, known as a mucocele. In these cases, the contents of the cyst are thick and mucoid but, in contrast to the sinus cysts and infected sinuses, are usually clear and sterile.

Diagnosis and treatment
- They may be difficult to differentiate from maxillary cysts but, radiographically, gas–fluid interfaces are not usually present.
- Facial deformity is often marked and, as most occur in the rostral maxillary sinus, facial swelling over the third and fourth cheek teeth in foals up to 6 months of age is suggestive of the presence of a mucocele.
- This is a rare condition and as such few treatment options are well described, but surgical creation of an effective naso-maxillary opening is a possibility.

Epiglottic hypoplasia (Fig. 3.20)
The Thoroughbred has been shown to be prone to what is believed to be a developmental epiglottic hypoplasia which may be diagnosed where the epiglottis appears, endoscopically, to be visibly short, or when it appears to be flaccid regardless of the length (which may be normal or, in some cases, greater than normal). Lateral radiographs

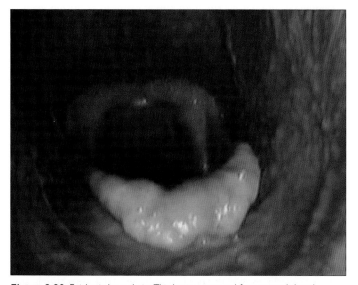

Figure 3.20 Epiglottic hypoplasia. This horse presented for repeated dorsal displacements of the soft palate. Endoscopic examination revealed a shortened epiglottis with thickened edges.

of the pharynx will also identify the shortened epiglottic cartilage which can usually be measured accurately, making allowances for magnification. The normal epiglottic length is 8–9 cm and an abnormal shortening is usually associated with a length of less than 7 cm (some authors say 5.5 cm). These animals appear to be particularly liable to epiglottic entrapment and dorsal displacement of the soft palate (laryngopalatal dislocation). There are few significant primary effects from epiglottic hypoplasia itself, with most of the secondary consequences affecting performance through airway distortions and displacements.

Diagnosis and treatment
- Diagnosis can be challenging and dynamic, endoscopic airway studies performed during treadmill work are often necessary to confirm the effects of the hypoplasia.
- There is no treatment for the hypoplasia itself but measures can be taken to help avoid secondary effects.

Fourth branchial arch defects
This is a rare syndrome of congenital defects resulting from a failure of development of some or all of the derivatives of the fourth branchial arch. Two typical features of fourth branchial arch defects are rostral displacement of the palatopharyngeal arch, which in some cases may only be detected during dynamic studies and defective arytenoid motility.

The condition is important with respect to abnormal respiratory noises and poor exercise tolerance. Most cases are only detected when extra exercise-demands are placed upon them, and they cannot open the *aditus laryngis* to allow an increased air supply. Affected horses show a severe limitation to exercise with harsh rasping inspiratory (and often expiratory) sounds which are localized around the larynx. Other clinical signs include eructation, nasal discharge, coughing and recurrent colic.

Diagnosis and treatment
- Complete evaluation of the extent of defects can only be performed during exploratory surgery or necropsy, but the condition can be suspected on the basis of a combination of palpation, endoscopy and radiology.
- When the upper esophageal sphincter is absent, lateral radiographs reveal a continuous column of air extending from the pharynx into the esophagus.
- There is no effective treatment although laser treatment of rostrally displaced palatopharyngeal arch has been described but affected individuals make poor athletes.

Non-infectious disorders

Foreign bodies (Figs. 3.21 & 3.22)
Foreign bodies may be detected at any site from the nares to the trachea and are often associated with the type of diet the horse is being fed. Thorny twigs, brush bristles and other sharp objects lodging in the pharynx are possibly more common than foreign bodies within the nasal cavity. The presenting clinical signs depend on the site and size of the foreign body.

Clinical signs
- *Nasal cavity*. Those lodged in the nasal cavity result in a unilateral nasal discharge of acute onset, often with small amounts of fresh blood. Affected horses show considerable discomfort, being head-shy and snorting a great deal. Sneezing is unusual in the horse under any circumstances. Untreated cases may result in local abscesses or the development of mineralized concretions within the nasal cavity and a foul-smelling breath from the affected nostril.

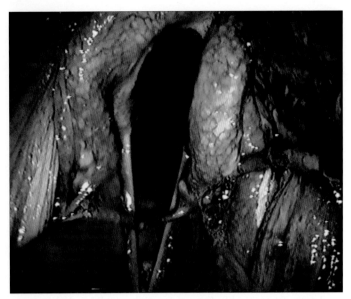

Figure 3.21 Foreign body. This horse was presented for acute-onset coughing and dysphagia. Endoscopic examination revealed a twig in the pharynx. The twig was removed and the horse made an uneventful recovery.

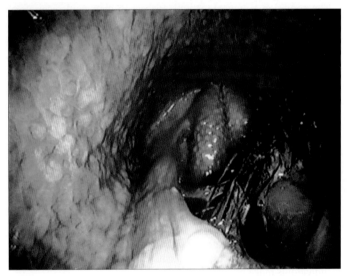

Figure 3.22 Foreign body. This young Warmblood was presented for several days of dysphagia: the wire was a piece of electric fence. It was removed by hand under general anaesthesia and the horse made a good recovery.

- **Pharynx**. Acute-onset dysphagia with complete or partial respiratory obstruction. Large solid objects such as pieces of apple would be expected to have marked effects upon respiration, particularly on inspiration and the effects are consequently dramatic and of peracute onset. In most cases these are transient with the object dislodging spontaneously and resolution is immediate and complete. In some cases, however, the object appears to be firmly lodged and a life-threatening respiratory obstruction may be presented. Horses which habitually chew wooden fences and doors are also liable to pharyngeal obstructions as a result of pieces of wood breaking off. Sharp, small foreign bodies present little immediate threat to life and do not often cause respiratory embarrassment. However, an acute onset of severe and distressing difficulties with swallowing is frequently presented. The affected horse presents with nasal regurgitation of food material and saliva and attempts to drink are accompanied by nasal regurgitation and expressions of pain such

as squealing and arching of the neck. Occasionally unilateral (or in some cases bilateral) epistaxis is present.
- **Trachea**. The inhalation of small grass seeds and particles of dust and grass is common when horses are exercised hard under appropriate conditions. These seldom cause any marked effect and coughing is usually sufficient to dislodge the foreign matter. A residual tracheitis may be present for a day or two thereafter. Plant twigs represent a relatively common tracheal foreign body and are often responsible for an acute onset of a severe and frequently paroxysmal coughing. Tracheal hemorrhage is usual and there is often some inflammation and reflex spasm of the airway.

Diagnosis and treatment

- Endoscopy is usually required for diagnosis even in cases of nasal foreign bodies. In some longstanding cases the foreign body itself may be difficult to identify due to the level of inflammation or secondary infection.
- Removal of the foreign body is the primary goal of treatment followed by treatment of secondary inflammation and infections if present.
- In many instances it may be impossible to remove the foreign body whole without causing further damage and in these cases it may be necessary to break up the foreign body using endoscopic tools.

Facial trauma (Fig. 3.23)

Traumatic lesions involving the facial bones result in variable distortions of the shape of the head, often as a consequence of depression fractures of the facial, frontal, nasal and maxillary bones. Facial trauma may also impair the drainage from the maxillary and/or frontal sinuses. Relatively minor trauma to the facial bones commonly results in damage to, or disruption of, the bony portion of the nasolacrimal duct.

Clinical signs

- Injuries involving the sinuses or the nasal turbinate bones are usually accompanied by slight, moderate or heavy bleeding from the ipsilateral nostril. Even considerable nasal bleeding seldom seems to result in marked distress.
- The immediate consequences of such injuries are related primarily to the bleeding and to any consequent nasal edema and swelling. Sufficient damage to result in an effective occlusion of both nostrils is very rare, even in cases with gross facial damage.
- Damage to the nasolacrimal duct may result in occlusion leading to epiphora.
- Sinus empyema, involving either of the maxillary sinuses and/or the frontal sinuses, represents a serious complication of failure of drainage and infection following traumatic injuries to the face.

Diagnosis and treatment

- The extent of any fractures may be defined by careful lateral and appropriate oblique radiographs. Most fractures are non-displaced and in such cases identification of the fracture site may be difficult if there are no external indicators.
- Evidence of caudal maxillary (and frontal) sinus involvement can be obtained from endoscopic examination of the common drainage pathway of these sinuses in the caudal nasal cavity.
- Treatment depends on the site of the trauma and the involved structures.

Arytenoid chondritis (Figs. 3.24–3.26)

Arytenoid chondritis is abnormal enlargement of the arytenoid cartilages resulting from chronic inflammation. It is seen most commonly in horses working at high speeds and as such Thoroughbreds and Standardbreds are primarily affected. Trauma, inflammation and infection have all been cited as possible causes. Histopathological

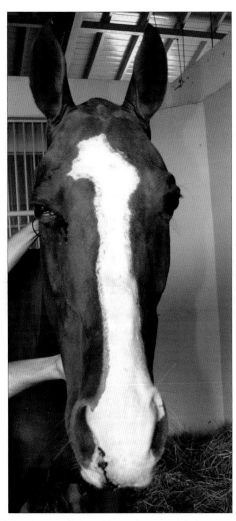

Figure 3.23 Facial trauma. Unilateral hemorrhagic nasal discharge associated with multiple facial fractures sustained during a polo game.

Differential diagnosis:
• Maxillary sinus cyst
• Hemorrhagic diatheses
• Nasal aspergillosis
• Amyloidosis
• Thrombocytopenia
• Guttural pouch mycosis.

findings in most cases are consistent with a chronic inflammatory process. The affected cartilage is thickened and laminated with fibrous connective tissue. The condition is typically unilateral but secondary contact damage ('kissing lesions') between cartilages is common.

A significant loss of effective abduction arises and results in the appearance of a flaccid *aditus laryngis* with collapse of one or both arytenoids into the airway. On some occasions the *aditus laryngis* may be reduced to a mere slit with neither abduction nor adduction present.

Clinical signs
• The onset of signs is usually insidious but in some cases may present acutely with respiratory obstruction.
• Respiratory noise initially during inspiration and later also during expiration.

Diagnosis and treatment
• Endoscopy is normally sufficient for a diagnosis although some cases may mimic laryngeal hemiplegia. Additional findings which

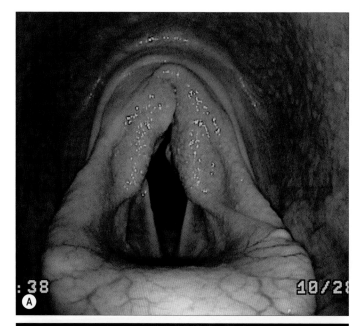

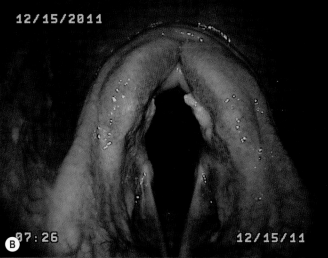

Figure 3.24 Arytenoid chondritis. (A) Enlarged and edematous left arytenoid cartilage. Prominent axial displacement of left arytenoid and impaired abductor function (paralysis) and partial rostral displacement of palatopharyngeal arch which are typical. Narrowing of *rima glottidis*. (B) Bilateral arytenoid chondritis with 'kissing lesions' or areas of ulcerations on the medial aspect of the arytenoids associated with excessive contact between the enlarged arytenoids.

Differential diagnosis:
• Laryngeal hemiplegia (idiopathic and neurological forms)
• Laryngeal neoplasia
• Laryngeal polyps
• Laryngeal granuloma
• Laryngeal cartilage hypertrophic ossification.

are variably present include ulceration, granuloma formation, necrosis and cavitation of the arytenoid cartilage, sinus tracts, deformity of the corniculate process or kissing lesion on the contra-lateral cartilage.
• Medical therapy is normally attempted primarily depending on the level of deformity present. This includes rest, antibiotics and anti-inflammatories. Throat sprays and nebulization are also useful and hyperbaric oxygen therapy has been used in some cases with anec-dotal reports of success.

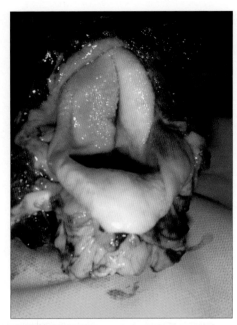

Figure 3.25 Post-mortem image from a horse with arytenoid chondritis showing marked enlargement of the right arytenoid. This horse had been unsuccessfully treated with prolonged courses of antibiotics.

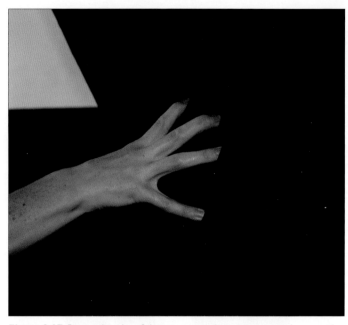

Figure 3.27 Ruptured trachea. Subcutaneous emphysema is commonly seen with tracheal perforations.

Differential diagnosis:
- Clostridial myositis
- Pharyngeal necrosis
- Retro-pharyngeal abscess
- Anthrax.

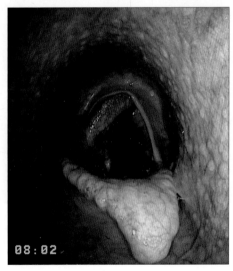

Figure 3.26 Endoscopic view of the larynx following arytenoidectomy of the left arytenoid in a horse with chronic chondritis.

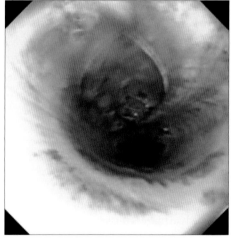

Figure 3.28 Ruptured trachea (endoscopic view).

- In cases in which medical therapy does not give satisfactory results surgical options can be considered. Transendoscopic laser debulking is recommended for horses with granuloma formation. Partial, complete or subtotal arytenoidectomy may be performed depending on the individual case.

Tracheal perforation (Figs. 3.27–3.29)

Blunt trauma to the ventral neck may cause tracheal fracture or avulsion of the tracheo-laryngeal junction. Tracheal perforation with resultant subcutaneous emphysema, secondary to blunt trauma, can also occur. Tracheostomy can also result in secondary subcutaneous emphysema but is usually less extensive than that seen with tracheal perforation. Cases in which the trachea is bilaterally (ventral and dorsal is the most common bilateral lesion) perforated are more likely to develop severe complications.

Clinical signs

- Subcutaneous emphysema which can readily be identified as a non-painful crackling under the skin.
- Stridor may occur but is not consistently present.
- Bilateral hemorrhagic nasal discharge may or may not be present.
- Tachypnea secondary to pneumomediastinum.
- Complicating infection of the original wound or of the emphysematous tissues (particularly where this is due to gas-producing bacteria such as *Clostridium* spp.) results in a similar appearance, but the difference is clinically obvious, with severe inflammation, pain and reluctance to swallow or bend the neck.

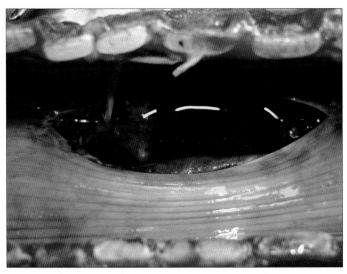

Figure 3.29 Ruptured trachea, post-mortem (same horse as Fig. 3.28).

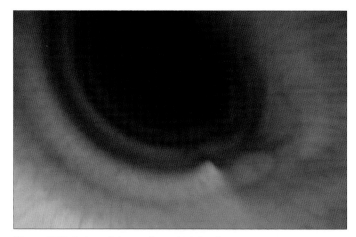

Figure 3.30 Endoscopic image of a tracheal chondroma.

Diagnosis and treatment

- Tracheoscopy is needed for confirmation of the tracheal laceration. Thoracic radiography can aid in the diagnosis of secondary pneumomediastinum
- Small tears may form a fibrin seal rapidly within 24–48 hours. Larger tears should be treated promptly (see below) to avoid infection, obstruction from peritracheal tissue and progression of subcutaneous emphysema to pneumomediastinum with resultant pneumothorax.
- A temporary tracheostomy distal to the site of tracheal perforation may have to be performed in cases where a large tracheal laceration has occurred. This procedure diverts air away from the site of tracheal injury, helping restore airway control by decreasing the subcutaneous emphysema and aiding in the resolution of the injury.

Tracheal chondroma (Figs. 3.30 & 3.31)

The insertion of emergency, or permanent, tracheostomy tubes or traumatic injuries to the trachea are common causes for the development of localized granulation tissue within the trachea. This occurs more particularly when the cartilage rings of the trachea are damaged during the procedure with the resulting tissue being classified as a chondroma, but which may only consist of granulation tissue. The healing of tracheostomy wound sites is often accompanied by distortions of the tracheal rings beneath the mucosa, but it is unlikely that these would be responsible for significant impairment of air flow except where consequent tracheal stenosis or collapse develops, following cartilage damage and/or necrosis.

Diagnosis and treatment

- No signs of damage may be obvious, or there may be a respiratory noise.
- Tracheoscopy is required for diagnosis.
- Intratracheal granulation tissue may respond to laser ablation therapy.

Pneumothorax (Figs. 3.32–3.34)

Pneumothorax is classified as either open or closed. In either case the influx of air into the pleural space causes equilibration of pleural pressure with atmospheric pressure and subsequent lung collapse. An open pneumothorax results from an injury to the thoracic wall leading to an influx of free air into the pleural space. A closed pneumothorax is the leakage of air into the pleural space from a

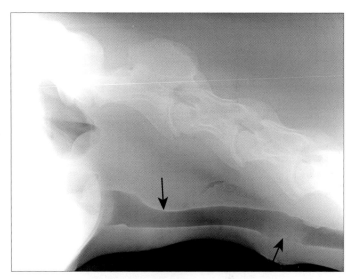

Figure 3.31 Radiograph of tracheal chondroma. This foal had a history of a previous tracheostomy due to *S. equi* infection. Four tracheal rings had been cut to perform the tracheostomy which resulted in a large tracheal chondroma and functional narrowing of the trachea at that point (right arrow). The foal was presented for respiratory difficulty which was in fact due to the continued enlargement of the retropharyngeal lymph nodes which can be seen to be causing compression of the proximal trachea in the radiograph (left arrow).

pulmonary source such as a bronchopleural fistula. A tension pneumothorax occurs when a section of traumatized lung acts like a 'valve' that allows the air to enter but not leave the pleural space. Thoracic drains are a frequent entry point for air into the pleural cavity and horses with thoracic drains in place should be under constant monitoring. Affected horses usually present with exaggerated abdominal lift, elevated respiratory rate and flared nostrils. Bilateral pneumothorax will result in cyanosis and severe dyspnea.

Multiple, smaller bullae in the lungs are a rare complication of longstanding allergic (or other) respiratory diseases which result in loss of pulmonary compliance (elasticity).

Diagnosis and treatment

- Percussion of the chest will establish an abnormal resonance and auscultation will reveal an absence of audible lung sounds over the affected areas.
- Thoracic ultrasonography will reveal horizontal air artifacts in the midthoracic or dorsal regions, thereby not allowing the examiner

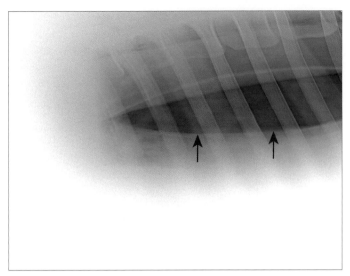

Figure 3.32 Radiograph of pneumothorax. Loss of radiodensity in the dorsocaudal thorax in this horse which had a chest drain in place as part of treatment for a pleuropneumonia. The lung border can be visualized ventrally (arrows).

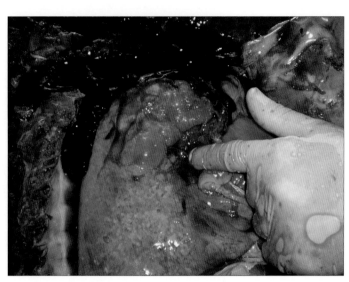

Figure 3.34 Pulmonary emphysema as a complication of longstanding respiratory disease. This can be confused with pneumothorax during ultrasonographic or radiographic examination.

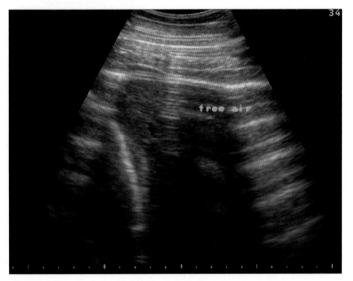

Figure 3.33 This ultrasonogram of the thorax shows an interface between free air and pulmonary air. This is more obvious in real time as the air within the lungs is seen to move cranially and caudally in what is known as the 'curtain sign', whereas the free air does not move.

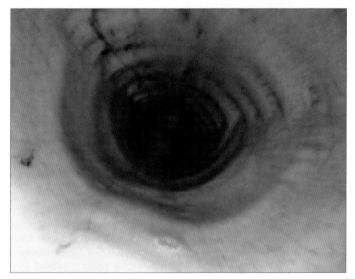

Figure 3.35 EIPH grade 1.

to identify the sliding motion of the visceral pleural against the parietal pleura. Thoracic radiography reveals a horizontal shadow beneath the thoracic transverse processes, which is consistent with a 'line' representing the collapsed lung(s). If radiology and/or ultrasonography are not available, then the clinician can use response to suction via a thoracocentesis as a diagnosis.

- The treatment of choice is *prompt* removal of free air via a thoracocentesis and suction. This procedure rapidly re-expands the lung and relieves the respiratory distress. If an open pneumothorax is diagnosed then surgical closure is indicated.

Exercise-induced pulmonary hemorrhage (EIPH) (Figs. 3.35–3.44)

Horses of all breeds can suffer from pulmonary bleeding during heavy exercise.

Rupture of the alveolar capillaries occurs secondary to exercise-induced increase in transmural pressure. Possible contributors to the pathogenesis include: small airway disease, upper airway obstruction, hemostatic abnormalities, changes in blood viscosity and erythrocyte shape, intrathoracic shear forces associated with gait and bronchial artery angiogenesis. The relationship between exercise-induced pulmonary hemorrhage and chronic airway disorders is reasonably well established, but it is also clear that not all horses affected by one condition will inevitably suffer from the other. Predisposing factors include breed (more common in Thoroughbreds) and age (more common in older horses).

Clinical signs

- Severely affected horses show moderate or severe post-exercise, bilateral epistaxis. In most such horses the bleeding is bright red

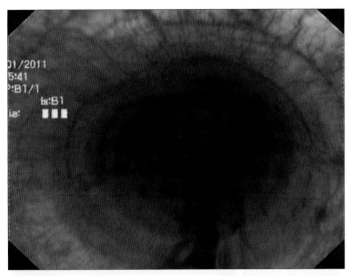

Figure 3.36 EIPH grade 2.

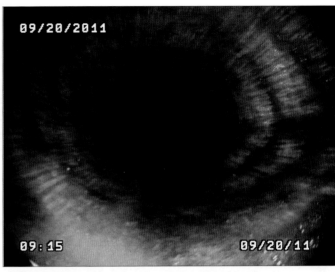

Figure 3.38 EIPH grade 4.

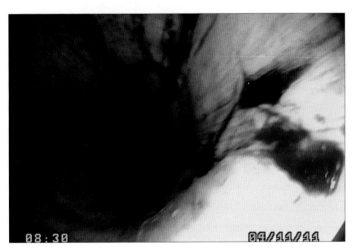

Figure 3.37 EIPH grade 3.

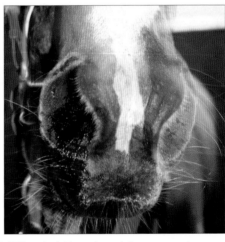

Figure 3.39 EIPH grade 4. Hemorrhage obvious at external nares.

and evident within 30 minutes of exercise. In rare extreme cases, horses may die either during or immediately after racing with extreme arterial-like epistaxis and cyanosis.

- Some affected horses show poor performance throughout the race, while others may 'tail-off' dramatically while others may 'pull-up'. However, poor performance may be attributable to many other causes.
- Milder degrees of exercise-induced pulmonary hemorrhage are commonly detected, endoscopically, in apparently normal racing and other performance horses, without any detectable clinical effect.

Diagnosis

- Tracheobronchoscopy can be used to estimate the severity of EIPH through a grading system (see Table 3.1). However, the relationship between the amount of blood in the large airways and the actual amount of hemorrhage has not been definitively established. This examination is best carried out 30–90 minutes after exercise. If the first examination is negative but there is a high suspicion then the examination can be repeated 1 hour later.

Table 3.1 Grading of EIPH

Grade	Tracheoscopic appearance
Grade 0	No blood detected in the upper or lower airway
Grade 1	Presence of one or more flecks of blood or ≤2 short (<1/4 length of trachea) narrow (<10% of the tracheal surface area) streams of blood in the trachea or main stem bronchi visible from the tracheal bifurcation
Grade 2	One long stream of blood (>half length of the trachea) or >2 short streams occupying less than 1/3 of the tracheal circumference
Grade 3	Multiple, distinct streams of blood covering more than 1/3 of the tracheal circumference. No blood pooling at the thoracic inlet
Grade 4	Multiple coalescing streams of blood covering >90% of the tracheal circumference with pooling of blood at the thoracic inlet

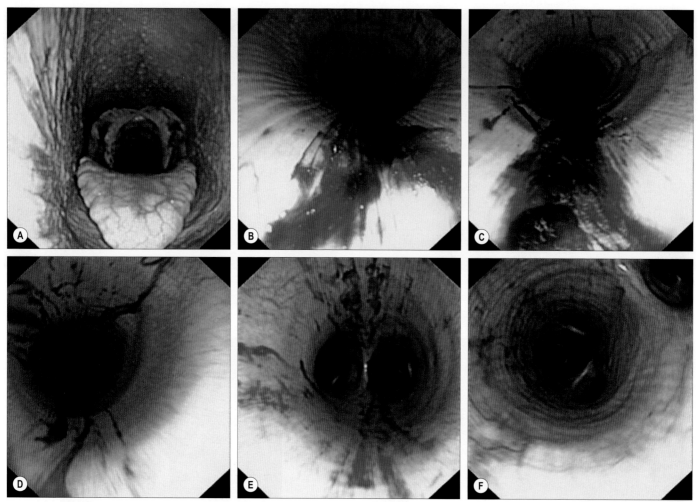

Figure 3.40 EIPH grade 3. Endoscopic view of various areas of respiratory tract showing the different densities of blood: (A) larynx, (B) proximal trachea, (C) mid trachea, (D) distal trachea, (E) tracheal bifurcation and (F) right bronchus.

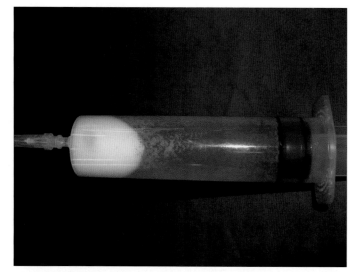

Figure 3.41 EIPH. Mucosanguineous bronchoalveolar lavage fluid.

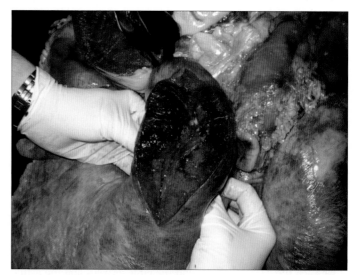

Figure 3.42 EIPH post-mortem. Intrapulmonary blood in dorsal and caudo-dorsal lung regions.

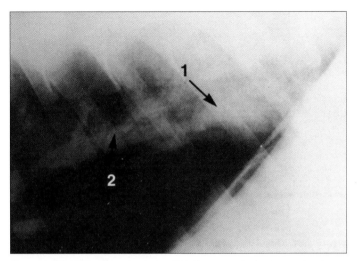

Figure 3.43 EIPH radiograph. Arrow (1) indicates an echodensity associated with the region of intrapulmonary hemorrhage. Arrow (2) shows an echodensity associated with the movement of blood through the bronchial tree.

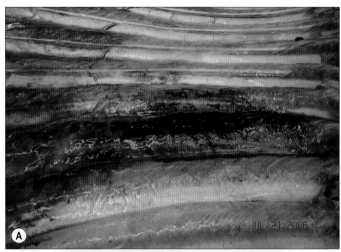

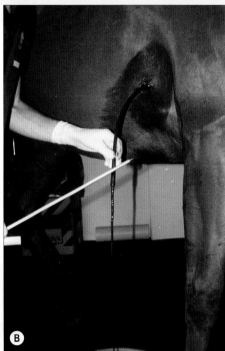

Figure 3.44 Thoracic trauma can also result in hemothorax and in some cases epistaxis. (A) Rib fracture in an adult horse following anesthesia. (B) Hemothorax in an adult horse following thoracic penetration of a tree branch and pulmonary laceration.

- Tracheal aspiration and bronchoalveolar lavage: the presence of red blood cells or hemosiderophages in tracheal fluid or BALF provides evidence of EIPH. Red blood cells are present for at least 1 week after strenuous exercise and up to 21 days in the case of hemosiderophages. These procedures are also useful for the detection of concurrent respiratory tract infections.
- Thoracic radiography may demonstrate the presence of densities in the caudodorsal lung fields but is not indicative of the severity of EIPH. It is most useful for determining the presence or absence of other disease processes that may contribute to the pathophysiology, such as pulmonary abscesses.
- Ultrasonography can also be used with 'comet tail' lesions detected in the caudo-dorsal lung fields associated with areas of hemorrhage.

Treatment and control
- Treatment is aimed at minimizing the effects of recent hemorrhage and eliminating or reducing the severity of subsequent hemorrhage. Difficulties with treatment stem from the fact that the pathogenesis has not been accurately determined and is likely to be multifactorial and different between individual cases.
- The current favored preventative treatment for EIPH is administration of furosemide before intense exercise or racing. It is not permitted in all racing jurisdictions.
- Other considerations are the use of nasal dilator bands and minimization of factors leading to small airway disease, such as the use of non-allergenic bedding.

Prognosis
- The prognosis for horses with clinically significant EIPH is guarded as the condition appears to be progressive with repeated episodes of hemorrhage being common despite treatment and rest. Horses that suffer an episode of EIPH with a concurrent respiratory tract infection appear to have a better prognosis. Many of these cases will not have a repeat episode following treatment of the underlying infection.

Recurrent airway obstruction and inflammatory airway disease (Figs. 3.45–3.49)

Horses and ponies are commonly affected by non-infectious airway diseases such as recurrent airway obstruction (RAO) or inflammatory airway disease (IAD). RAO (also known as heaves) is one of the most common respiratory disorders of the horse in temperate areas of the world, and occurs particularly where horses are stabled for long periods and fed and bedded on preserved cereal and/or grass products. The probable etiology of the disorder is repeated mucosal allergic challenge in the conducting airways. A similar condition is found in some pastured horses and is termed summer pasture-associated obstructive disease. Both conditions are characterized by reversible airway obstruction, with neutrophil accumulation, mucus production and bronchospasm.

IAD is a less well-defined syndrome with different presentations in different groups of horses. The pleasure horse with IAD may have obvious nasal discharge, cough and overheating, whereas the young racehorse may show poor recovery from peak exercise or poor performance. The etiology is believed to be largely the same as RAO with environmental allergens playing a significant role; however, some horses, particularly young racehorses in training, may also have an infectious component to the etiology.

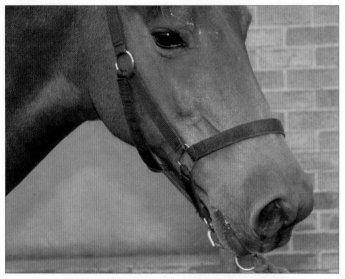

Figure 3.45 Recurrent airway obstruction/small airway disease. Nostril flaring is a typical clinical sign in chronically or severely affected horses. However, nostril flaring associated with respiration can be present in any severe respiratory illness and cannot be used alone to achieve a diagnosis.

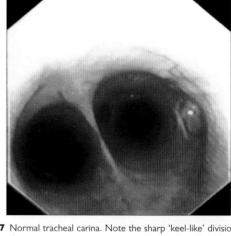

Figure 3.47 Normal tracheal carina. Note the sharp 'keel-like' division at the tracheal bifurcation.

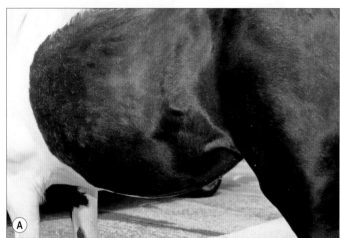

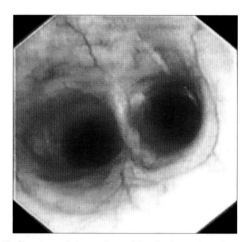

Figure 3.48 Chronic small airway disease (chronic obstructive pulmonary disease (COPD), 'heaves', allergic lung disease) (mild). Note the thickened carina and narrowed bronchial diameter (compare to normal in Fig. 3.47).

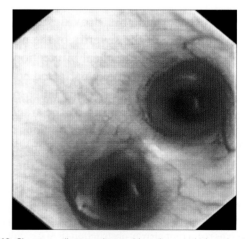

Figure 3.46 'Heave lines' prominent muscular hypertrophy along the caudo-ventral thorax. As the condition progresses these lines become more prominent. (A) Early/mild. (B) Marked.

Figure 3.49 Chronic small airway disease. Note the very thickened carina and marked narrowing of the bronchial diameter (compare to normal in Fig. 3.47).

Clinical signs

- The exercise tolerance of affected horses is frequently adversely affected, with a significant number being presented, initially, for investigation of poor or inadequate athletic performance.
- Cases generally have an abnormally high resting respiratory rate with a variable degree of nostril flare.
- A chronic, harsh, non-productive cough is characteristic.
- Without treatment, the severity of the cough often increases over weeks or months, sometimes with episodes of a more acute syndrome superimposed from time to time.
- Severely affected horses lose weight dramatically and the increased expiratory effort commonly results in marked hypertrophy of the muscles of the caudo-ventral thorax producing the so-called 'heave line'. In the severe cases, an obvious, extra, expiratory 'push' from the abdominal and thoracic muscles is present, possibly with an associated grunt.
- A slight or sometimes more profuse, bilateral, postural, catarrhal nasal discharge is usually present.

Diagnosis

- Clinical signs and history of a seasonal disorder that can be altered by husbandry practices.
- Endoscopic examination of the respiratory tract shows poor mucus clearance from the trachea.
- Broncho-alveolar lavage (BAL) reveals inflammatory cells in proportion to the severity of the underlying disease and this provides an effective quantitative measure of the severity of the underlying pathology. BAL is preferable to transtracheal washing for diagnosing and differentiating RAO from infectious respiratory disease.
- Radiographic examination of the thorax may demonstrate an increase in bronchial and interstitial patterns but this can be difficult to interpret in light of normal changes in bronchial pattern associated with advancing age. Radiography is best used in these cases to differentiate from other, more focal disorders.
- Serum allergen testing and intradermal allergy testing have not proven very useful in identifying specific allergens in the horse's environment.

Treatment

- In horses in which infection is believed or confirmed to be part of the etiology or a complicating secondary factor initial treatment with a course of antibiotics is recommended.
- Environmental management is key to control and treatment of many cases. These changes focus primarily on the reduction of dust in the horse's environment with changes of bedding, soaking of hay or use of hay humidifiers; to all pellet diets in severe cases.
- Pharmacological treatment centers on the use of bronchodilators and corticosteroids. Systemic and/or inhaled drugs are used depending on the severity of clinical signs and cost restrictions. There are a variety of protocols for the administration of these drugs largely dependent on the clinical signs of the individual horse.

Laryngeal hemiplegia (Figs. 3.50–3.56)

The recurrent laryngeal nerve innervates all of the intrinsic muscles of the larynx with the exception of the cricothyroideus. Neuropathy of this nerve results in laryngeal hemiplegia which is defined as a failure of abduction of a structurally normal arytenoid cartilage because of decreased or absent motor fuction in the cricoarytenoideus dorsalis muscle. In most cases no cause for the neuropathy can be found and thus is termed idiopathic. Most frequently, but not exclusively, the left nerve is involved. The paralysis is usually only left-sided, and may be partial (in which there is some abduction movement of the arytenoid) or complete (in which no abduction is visible).

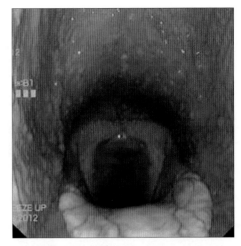

Figure 3.50 Laryngeal hemiplegia grade 1.

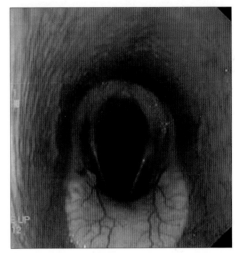

Figure 3.51 Laryngeal hemiplegia grade 2.

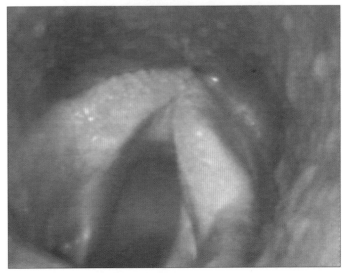

Figure 3.52 Laryngeal hemiplegia grade 3.

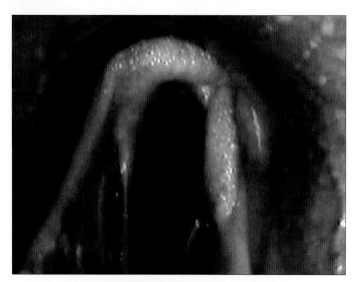

Figure 3.53 Laryngeal hemiplegia grade 4.

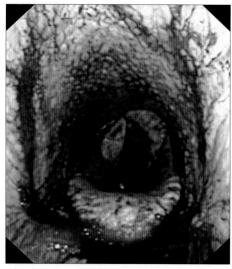

Figure 3.56 Right laryngeal hemiplegia. Note also the blood present in the pharynx associated with an episode of EIPH.

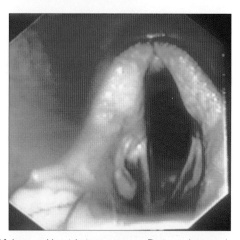

Figure 3.54 Laryngeal hemiplegia post surgery. During real-time endoscopy the left arytenoids is 'fixed' in position and may even appear more abducted than the right side.

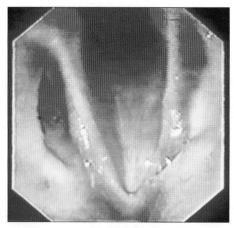

Figure 3.55 Laryngeal hemiplegia post 'hobday' or ventriculectomy surgery. Note thtat the lateral ventricles are no longer present and have been replaced by scar tissue.

Table 3.2 Grading system for recurrent laryngeal hemiplegia

Grade	Anatomy and function
Grade I	Full abduction and adduction of left and right arytenoids cartilages
Grade II	Asynchronous movement such as hesitation, flutters, adductor weakness of the affected arytenoids during inspiration or expiration or both, but full abduction induced by swallowing or nasal occlusion
Grade III	Asynchronous movement of the affected arytenoids during inspiration or expiration or both. Full abduction not induced or maintained by swallowing or nasal occlusion
Grade IV	Significant asymmetry of the larynx at rest and lack of substantial movement of the affected arytenoids

Thoroughbred, Standardbred and Quarter Horse breeds are also affected commonly with a range of mild to severe forms of the disorder with up to 80% of Thoroughbred horses possibly affected to some extent. The majority of these have mild degrees of the condition in which little or no clinical effect is detectable. Most horses with significant laryngeal neuropathy are presented for investigation of inspiratory noises '**roaring**' and/or poor exercise tolerance.

Diagnosis

- The condition may be suspected on the basis of an inspiratory noise but endoscopy is required to confirm the diagnosis. (Table 3.2 outlines a grading system for laryngeal anatomy and function.)
- The 'slap test', which tests the integrity of the thoraco-vagal reflex by observing (or palpating) contralateral laryngeal adduction and abduction in response to a 'slap' applied to the thoracic wall, may also be used to demonstrate the malfunctioning of the affected side. The atrophy of the muscle may be suggested by palpation of the muscular process of the arytenoid on the affected side which becomes characteristically prominent. However, a horse may have normal laryngeal function at rest but still have signs of dysfunction when exercised and atrophy of the *cricoarytenoideus dorsalis* may not be apparent in horses in which the disorder is of recent onset.
- Comparative endoscopic examination of the larynx, at rest and at exercise, is particularly useful in establishing the extent of the dysfunction and to determine whether any prior attempts have been made at surgical relief of the obstruction. Due to possible normal function at rest and abnormal function during exercise traditional methods of detection have consisted of listening for inspiratory

Young horses, between 2 and 6 years of age, and horses over 16 hands in height, are, however, most often affected. Certain breeds, including the Hannovarian, Shire, Irish Draught, Dutch Warmblood and other large breeds, appear to be particularly liable to severe forms of the condition which apparently develop spontaneously. The

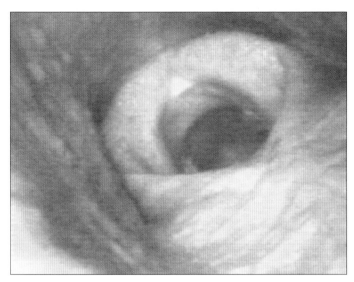

Figure 3.57 Dorsal displacement of soft palate. Epiglottis not visible. This can be seen during endoscopy of normal horses following sedation but is normally easily reversed by stimulating the horse to swallow.

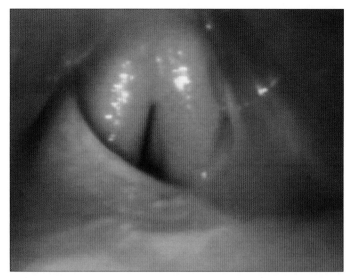

Figure 3.58 Dorsal displacement of the soft palate and laryngeal edema in a young foal with hypoxic ischemic encephalopathy. There was pharyngeal paralysis and severe respiratory disease in this case. The foal was being scoped to aid in the placement of an endotracheal tube prior to commencing assisted ventilation.

noises during exercise in addition to scoping at rest but this may in many instances now be replaced by dynamic endoscopy during exercise in horses which are normal at rest. Right-side and bilateral paralyses are sometimes encountered but the etiology of these are usually better defined.

Treatment

- Surgical correction is required if significant airflow obstruction is present. Laryngoplasty, a prosthetic ligature, is currently widely used to stabilize and abduct the affected arytenoid cartilage. Complications following this procedure include: failure to maintain abduction of the arytenoids cartilage, dysphagia and rarely aspiration pneumonia, chronic infection of the prosthesis, ossification of the cartilage, intraluminal polyps, laryngeal edema and chondritis. Horses which have been subjected to this procedure show a stabilized (immobile) arytenoid on endoscopy.
- Lateral ventriculectomy (Hobday's operation), in which the lateral laryngeal ventricles are surgically ablated, has been used for many years to reduce the respiratory noise. It does not however alleviate the increased impedence to airflow during exercise if used alone. Endoscopic examination will readily detect the absence of one or both laryngeal ventricles.
- Some cases which prove refractory to treatment by the milder surgical interferences are subjected to sub-total arytenoidectomy and the endoscopic appearance of these is very obvious.

Dorsal displacement of the soft palate
(Figs. 3.57 & 3.58)

Abnormal, intermittent or persistent dorsal displacement of the soft palate occurs during exercise (and occasionally at other times) in Thoroughbred and Quarter Horses, in particular. The displacement has a profound effect upon respiratory function, with narrowing of the nasopharynx and consequent air turbulence. The etiology of the disorder is not well understood and many previously proposed causes have been negated. Current theories include dysfunction of the palatal musculature or its innervation, dysfunction of the thyrohyoideus muscle leading to alterations in the positioning of the larynx and hyoid apparatus and alterations in function of laryngeal mucosal receptors. Other possible causes are fatigue, congenital abnormalities of the soft palate, disorders of the epiglottis or pharyngeal discomfort.

The principal clinical signs are respiratory noise with the expiratory noise being very prominent and exercise intolerance. However, up to 30% of affected horses will not have an associated respiratory noise.

Where the dislocation occurs during fast work the performance of the horse may be momentarily affected by a sudden, transient asphyxia. Under these circumstances, the horse shows a characteristic 'gurgling' sound and an abrupt loss of pace.

Diagnosis

- Given the often intermittent nature of the disorder diagnosis in the past has been notoriously difficult. Definitive diagnosis is by recognition of the displacement during endoscopic examination while the horse is exercising at high speed.
- Endoscopic examination following exercise may reveal no abnormalities.
- Endoscopic examination during treadmill work can be used to diagnose the condition but has the obvious disadvantage of the time required to train the horse to a level of fast work on the treadmill. Newer mobile forms of endoscopy are becoming more readily available.

Treatment and prognosis

- Conservative treatment options are often tried initially and include tongue tying for racehorses, use of a figure-eight noseband and nebulization therapy. In addition every attempt should be made to recognize other predisposing factors such as poor conditioning or epiglottic abnormalities.
- Surgical treatments with the greatest popularity are myectomy and staphylectomy.
- The prognosis for all cases should be guarded for athletic function as the results of surgical treatments are frequently unpredictable.

Epiglottic entrapment (Figs. 3.59–3.63)

Epiglottic entrapment occurs when the aryepiglottic fold envelops a portion of or all of the epiglottis. This membrane extends from the lateral aspect of the arytenoids cartilages to the ventrolateral aspect of the epiglottis where it joins with the subepiglottic mucosa and glossoepiglottic fold. In many cases the epiglottic cartilage and soft tissues appear normal. Some cases have epiglottic hypoplasia or concurrent

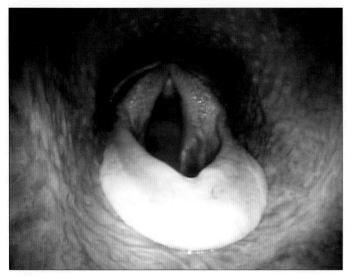

Figure 3.59 Epiglottic entrapment. Crenated border of the epiglottis is not visible.

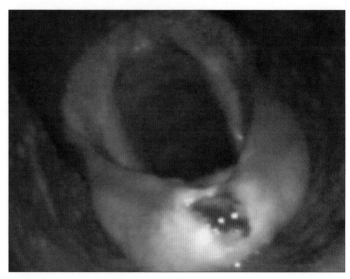

Figure 3.61 Epiglottic entrapment with ulceration. This case was found during routine post-exercise endoscopy. Surgical release of the entrapment was performed.

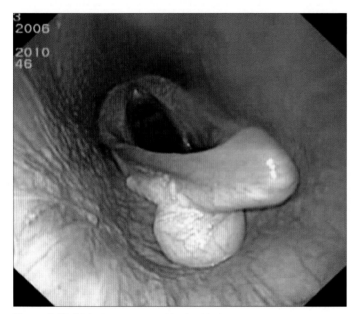

Figure 3.60 Epiglottic entrapment with subepiglottic cyst.

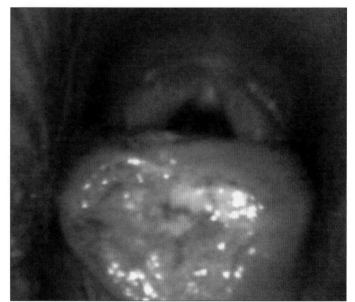

Figure 3.62 This entrapment with severe ulceration was presented for respiratory noise. He was treated with antibiotics and nasal sprays (antibiotics/steroids/DMSO) for 1 month prior to surgical release through a laryngotomy approach.

inflammation of the upper respiratory tract that may contribute to the entrapment. The condition is seen most commonly in Thoroughbred and Standardbred racehorses.

Clinical signs and diagnosis

- Affected horses display abnormal respiratory (inspiratory and occasionally expiratory) noises at exercise. Coughing and a distinct reduction in exercise tolerance are commonly present.
- Diagnosis of this condition is, again, dependent upon endoscopic examination of the pharynx but intermittent or occasional entrapment may not be reliably demonstrated on resting examinations. The extent of the entrapment may vary from minute to minute and some apparently normal horses may be seen to entrap the epiglottis as they swallow. In some mild cases, only the tip of the epiglottis may be entrapped.

- The normal crenated edge and characteristic marginal, radiating blood vessels are lost to view although in many cases the outline shape of the epiglottis is still present. The aryteno-epiglottic folds become abnormally prominent, extending between the base of the arytenoid cartilages and the entrapped epiglottis.
- Extensive, longstanding entrapments often result in ulceration of the overlying mucosa. On rare occasions the mucosa may even become disrupted and the free border of the epiglottis may be seen protruding through the fold.
- Entrapment may be asymmetrical, with only the tip and one lateral border of the epiglottis being lost to view. The caudal margin of the entrapping aryteno-epiglottic fold is, however, always visible. The presence of granulating ulcerations on the surface of the entrapped aryteno-epiglottic fold or on the apex of the epiglottis may support a diagnosis of intermittent entrapment.

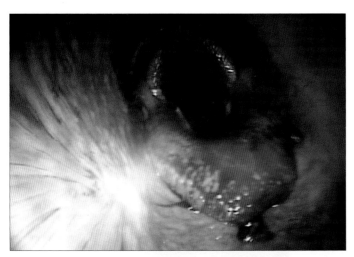

Figure 3.63 Epiglottic liberation post resection of the aryepiglottic fold. (Same horse as in Fig. 3.59).

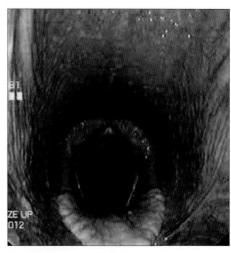

Figure 3.64 Lymphoid hyperplasia grade 1.

- *Differential diagnosis:* in a few cases the disorder also occurs in association with subepiglottic cysts, and particularly with the more flaccid type in which there is an excess of redundant mucosa.

Treatment and prognosis
- In cases of persistent entrapment surgical correction is required. Techniques involve resection or division of the membrane. This can be done by pharyngotomy, laryngotomy or orally under general anesthesia; transendoscopically using a Nd:YAG laser or transnasally/transorally using a hooked bistoury.
- Sequeale of treatments include granuloma formation, chronic cough or low-grade dysphagia.
- The prognosis for horses with concurrent, persistent or frequent, intermittent dorsal displacement of the soft palate, or with obvious deformity of the epiglottis, is much worse as the underlying cause is usually not resolvable.
- Combinations of the various pharyngeal and laryngeal disorders are relatively common in the horse. Thus, horses suffering from hypoplasia of the epiglottis might be affected by any or all of the disorders associated with the positional relationships of the epiglottis.
- Concurrent epiglottic entrapment and dorsal dislocation of the soft palate form a relatively common clinical entity. Similarly, complete dislocation of the palato-pharyngeal articulation results from a simultaneous dorsal displacement of the soft palate and rostral displacement of the palato-pharyngeal arch.
- Horses suffering from a combination of disorders have a poorer prognosis.

Lymphoid hyperplasia (Figs. 3.64–3.67)
Chronic inflammation of the pharynx, termed pharyngeal lymphoid hyperplasia, is a common condition of young horses. The exact etiology is not known but is likely to be multifactorial. Many horses have a history of respiratory disease and husbandry practices (stabling, increased dust, poor ventilation) may exacerbate the condition.

Many horses will show no clinical signs. A mild nasal discharge and submandibular lymphadenopathy may be present. Unless very severe it has not been associated with poor performance.

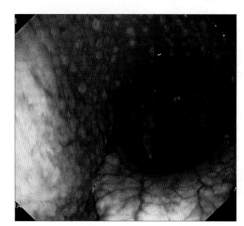

Figure 3.65 Lymphoid hyperplasia grade 2.

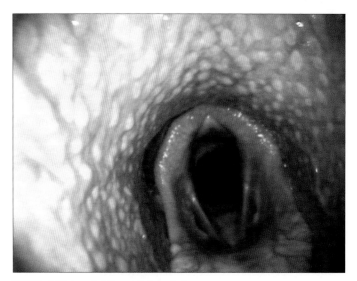

Figure 3.66 Lymphoid hyperplasia grade 3.

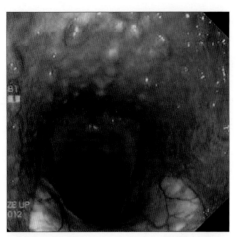

Figure 3.67 Lymphoid hyperplasia grade 4.

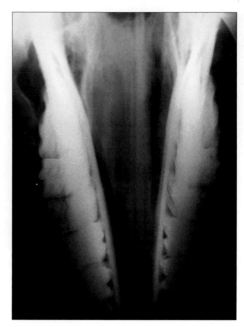

Figure 3.69 Ethmoid hematoma. Dorso-ventral radiograph. Showing soft tissue density of left nasal passage.

Differential diagnosis:
- Nasal polyp
- Neoplasia
- Sinus cyst.

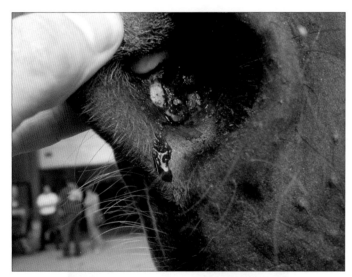

Figure 3.68 Amyloidosis. Minor trauma would result in marked hemorrhage.

Table 3.3	Grading system for pharyngeal lymphoid hyperplasia
Grade	Appearance
Grade I	A small number of inactive white follicles scattered over the dorsal pharyngeal wall. The follicles are small and inactive, a normal finding in horses of all ages
Grade II	Many small, white inactive follicles over the dorsal and lateral walls of the pharynx to the level of the guttural pouch. Numerous follicles that are large, pink and edematous interspersed throughout
Grade III	Many large, pink follicles and some shrunken white follicles are distributed over the dorsal and lateral walls of the pharynx, in some cases extending onto the dorsal surface of the soft palate and into the pharyngeal diverticula
Grade IV	More numerous pink and edematous follicles packed close together covering the entire pharynx, the dorsal surface of the soft palate and epiglottis and the lining of the guttural pouches. Large accumulations appear as polyps

Diagnosis and treatment
- Endoscopy reveals raised hyperemic and edematous follicles distributed throughout the nasopharyngeal walls. A grading system has been proposed for the endoscopic findings (see Table 3.3).
- The ideal treatment remains unclear due to the uncertainty surrounding the etiology. Nebulization or topical administration of anti-inflammatories has anecdotal reports of usefulness.

Amyloidosis (Fig. 3.68)

Amyloid deposition occurs as a result of chronic antigenic stimulation. The nasal cavity is a common site for deposition and may occur alone or in association with cutaneous amyloidosis. A sero-purulent nasal discharge, which may occasionally include flecks of blood or more overt hemorrhage, abnormal respiratory noises, recurrent mild epistaxis from one (or both) nostrils, poor exercise tolerance and weight loss as a result of the primary disease, are associated with the disorder. In such cases lesions are normally concurrently present in other organ systems.

Diagnosis and treatment
- Clinical appearance of raised hemorrhagic nodules in the nasal cavity is suggestive but definitive diagnosis is achieved by biopsy and histological examination.

- Treatment is aimed at any underlying disease. Laser ablation can be used to treat individual nasal deposits.

Ethmoid hematomas (Figs. 3.69–3.71)

Ethmoid hematomas are encapsulated angiomatous masses that develop most commonly from the mucosal lining of the ethmoid conchae and less commonly from the walls of the maxillary and frontal sinus of mature horses, usually over the age of 8–10 years. The etiology of the condition is not known with proposed causes including: chronic infection, repeated episodes of hemorrhage, congenital or neoplastic changes. They have a neoplastic-like appearance but are not recognized pathologically as true neoplastic lesions. They can be

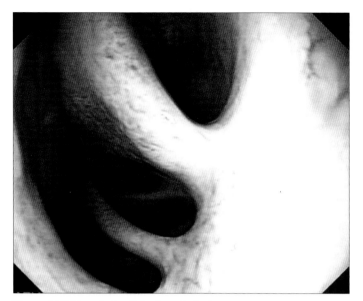

Figure 3.70 Normal ethmoid (endoscopic view).

unilateral or bilateral. All forms of the condition are identical in their gross and histological appearance and their progressive tendency.

As the mass expands the surface mucous membrane ulcerates and a limited loss of blood occurs. This is often combined with an excess of mucus production from the area. This results in an intermittent nasal discharge which can be hemorrhagic, serous or mucopurulent. The nasal discharge may be present for months or years without causing any apparent harmful effect.

As the condition progresses stertorous breathing may be noted due to nasal obstruction. Other signs are facial swelling, exophthalmus malodorous breath, coughing and occasionally the hematoma can be seen to extend from the affected nostril.

Diagnosis

- Clinical signs are suggestive. Endoscopic examination reveals a mass originating in the ethmoid region. It can vary in color from yellow-green or yellow-gray to a red-purple.
- Radiography reveals a space-occupying mass with a soft tissue density and smooth margins. Computed tomography can also be used where available.

Treatment and prognosis

- Treatment options include surgical ablation, laser photoablation, cryogenic ablation, snare excision and injection of formalin or a combination of a number of these methods. The method(s) chosen depends on the size, position and accessibility of the lesion.
- Surgical ablation is most suitable for lesions within the sinus but there is a risk of serious hemorrhage.
- Laser photoablation is most suitable for small (<5 cm) lesions and multiple treatments may be required.
- Cryogenic ablation can be used to augment surgical debulking or for small lesions but care must be taken not to freeze the cribriform plate.
- Intralesional injection of 10% formaldehyde has become increasing popular and is frequently tried as a primary therapy as it has lesser risk of hemorrhage than some other techniques. Repeated treatments are usually required.
- Prognosis following treatment is guarded to good with a recurrence rate of 14–45%.

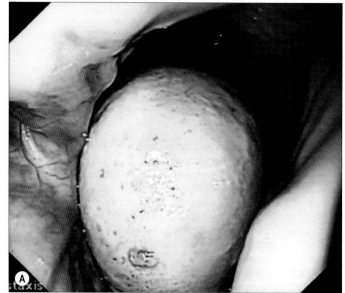

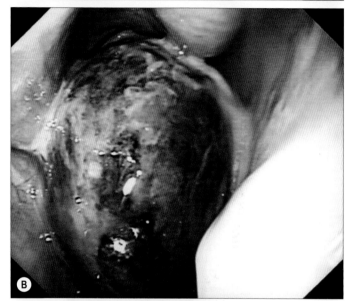

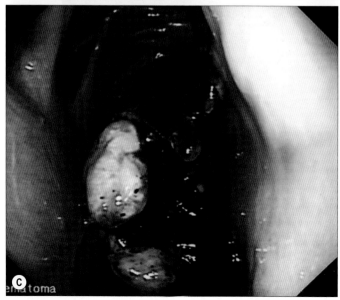

Figure 3.71 (A, B, C) Different examples of the endoscopic appearance of ethmoid hematomas.

Infectious disorders

Nasal discharges (Figs. 3.72–3.83)

Nasal discharges are a common finding in both upper and lower respiratory disease, but can also be seen with some disorders of the gastrointestinal tract and some neurological disorders. The type of nasal discharge and whether it is unilateral or bilateral frequently aids to differentiate the causal conditions.

Viral diseases (Fig. 3.84)

Upper and lower respiratory tract viral infections are some of the commonest infectious disorders encountered in the horse. Respiratory virus infections are a significant cause of acute illness in the horse and frequently predispose to secondary bacterial infections, and to possible subsequent small airway diseases. Whilst single virus infections do certainly occur, complexes of virus and bacterial infections, in which several different pathogenic viruses and bacteria may be identified, are relatively common. In most such cases, a single pathogen may have been responsible for the initial infection but opportunist and commensal potential pathogens become increasingly significant.

Clinical signs

- In general, most of the common respiratory virus infections result in a similar clinical syndrome, with only minor variations associated with particular viruses. Almost all these infections induce some degree of coughing and nasal discharge.
- Most of them initially induce a serous nasal discharge which progresses through catarrhal stages as recovery follows.
- If secondary bacterial infection is present the discharges become progressively more purulent.
- The less-virulent virus diseases are also commonly reported to cause reduction in performance or reduced exercise tolerance without any other overt clinical signs.

Diagnosis

- Diagnosis of a viral infection is frequently made on the basis of clinical signs and hematological findings.
- Definitive diagnosis usually depends on the isolation of virus particles from pharyngeal swabs, and serological tests to confirm the increasing immunological response of the host to a particular virus.

Equine influenza

The equine influenza virus currently consists of one predominantly infectious subtype for horses, H3N8. Within this subtype there are a number of variants. The equine influenza virus is stable antigenically when compared to the human influenza virus with few major antigenic shifts. It has a high morbidity amongst young horses, but has a low mortality in normal healthy horses. The reservoir of equine influenza virus between epizootics is thought to be asymptomatic carriers or other species such as birds which may shed the virus in their feces. The virus has a short survival time in the environment. It is frequently seen in outbreaks of respiratory disease in young racehorses shortly after entering training. Factors such as poor ventilation, inadequate vaccination and rapid transmission of virus from closely stabled adults may play a role in such outbreaks. The incubation period is 1–3 days. Viral infection results in necrosis and desquamation of the respiratory epithelial cells, predisposing to secondary infections. Recovery of the normal epithelial lining can take up to 6 weeks.

Clinical features are pyrexia (103–105°F), serous nasal discharge, anorexia, depression and a dry deep cough. Other signs which can be seen in individual cases are myalgia, myositis and limb edema. Myoglobinuria can occur in some of these cases. Submandibular lymphadenopathy with endoscopic evidence of pharyngitis and tracheitis is frequently present. Exercise exacerbates clinical signs. Secondary bacterial infections are common especially in donkeys and mules. The course of the infection is normally 2–10 days.

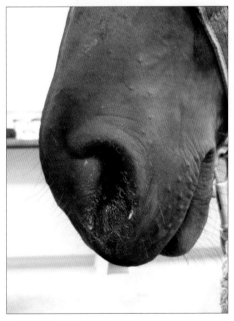

Figure 3.72 Serous nasal discharge.
Differential diagnosis:
- Respiratory tract virus infection (early stage)
- Allergic/irritant rhinitis (e.g. smoke, noxious gas)
- Ethmoid hematoma (chronic, progressive)
- Congestive heart failure.

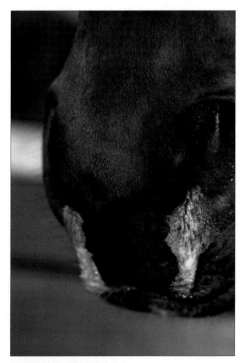

Figure 3.73 Sero-mucoid nasal discharge.
Differential diagnosis:
- Respiratory tract virus infection
- Chronic nasal irritation (smoke, etc.)
- Small airway disease (possibly postural).

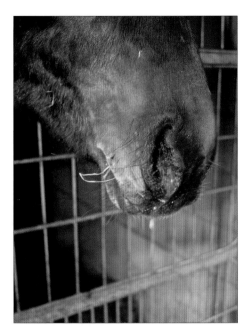

Figure 3.74 Mucopurulent nasal discharge.

Differential diagnosis:
• Secondary bacterial infection following virus infection
• Strangles (*Streptococcus equi*)
• False strangles (*Streptococcus zooepidemicus*).

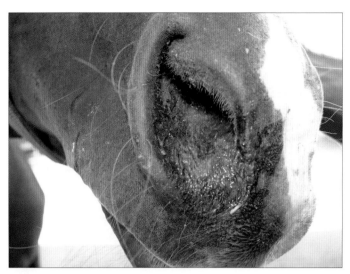

Figure 3.76 Mucohemorrhagic nasal discharge.

Differential diagnosis:
• Respiratory tract infections
• Pleuropneumonia
• Strangles
• Guttural pouch mycosis
• Ethmoid hematoma
• Nasal polyp
• Nasal foreign body
• Rhinal fungal infection.

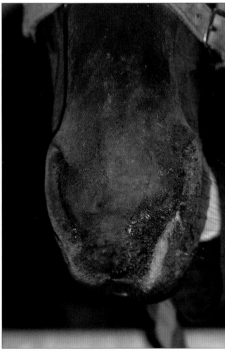

Figure 3.75 Unilateral mucopurulent nasal discharge sinusitis.

Differential diagnosis:
• Maxillary sinusitis
• Guttural pouch empyema
• Maxillary sinus cyst
• Respiratory tract infections.

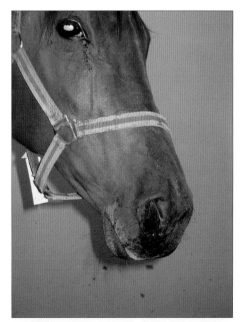

Figure 3.77 Mucohemorrhagic.

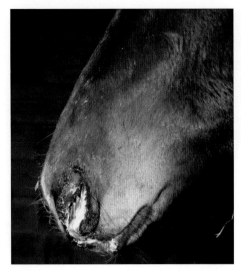

Figure 3.78 Purulent nasal discharge.

Differential diagnosis:
• Bacterial infection
• Bilateral primary sinusitis.

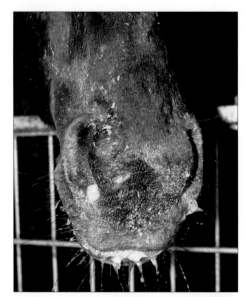

Figure 3.80 Feed contaminated. Yearling with strangles and difficulty swallowing.

Differential diagnosis:
• Choke
• Gastric reflux
• Esophageal stricture
• Neurological dysphagia
• Cleft hard palate (small)
• Cleft soft palate
• Pharyngeal neoplasia (lymphosarcoma, squamous cell carcinoma)
• Esophageal dilatation (megaesophagus)
• Grass sickness
• Pharyngeal foreign body
• Pharyngeal paralysis.

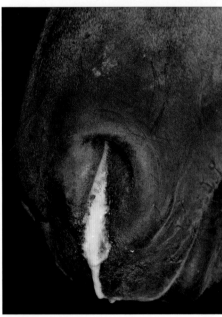

Figure 3.79 Purulent nasal discharge.

Differential diagnosis:
• Strangles (*Streptococcus equi*)
• Pharyngeal/guttural pouch abscess.

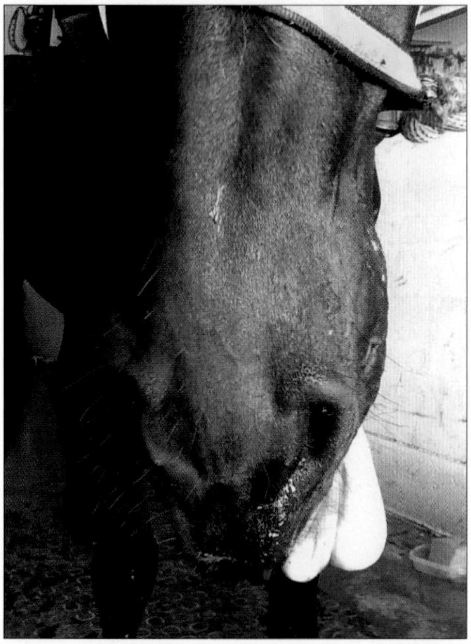

Figure 3.81 Epistaxis unilateral. The identification of the source of epistaxis in the horse is clinically very important. Unilateral hemorrhages may be associated with small venous bleeding within the ipsilateral nasal cavity or from the ipsilateral guttural pouch. Iatrogenic damage from misdirected nasogastric tubes may cause severe hemorrhage within the ipsilateral nostril. Usually this follows introduction of the nasogastric tube into the middle, rather than the ventral, meatus of the nose, and the damage typically involves the ethmoturbinate region.

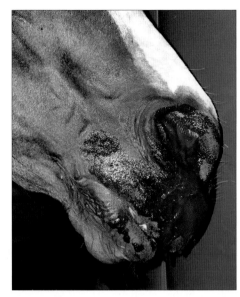

Figure 3.82 Bilateral epistaxis may be a result of simultaneous damage causing bleeding in both nasal cavities, hemorrhage from structures caudal to the nasopharynx, or hemorrhagic disorders, and can be arterial (above) or venous (Fig. 3.83). Heavy (particularly arterial) bleeding from one guttural pouch or from one nasal cavity may also produce bilateral epistaxis.

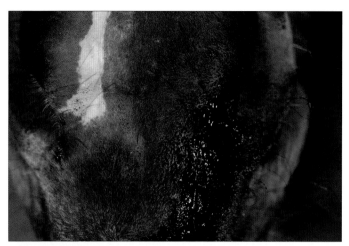

Figure 3.83 Epistaxis (venous).

Differential diagnosis:
- Hemorrhagic diathesis (thrombocytopenia/coumarin/warfarin poisoning)
- Purpura hemorrhagica (immune-mediated vasculitis)
- Guttural pouch mycosis (venous lesion) (usually unilateral)
- Exercise-induced pulmonary hemorrhage (24–48 hours post exercise)
- Disseminated intravascular coagulopathy (DIC).

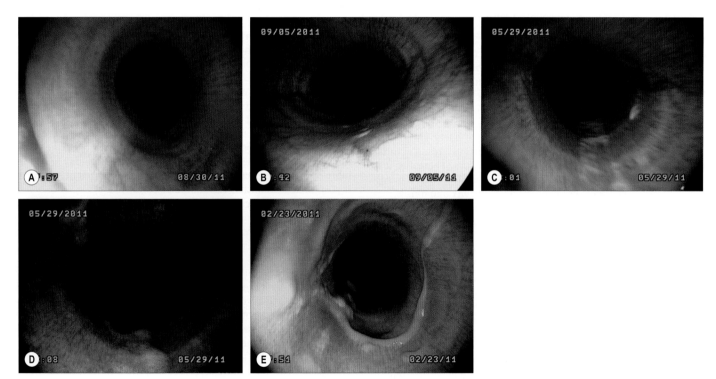

Figure 3.84 Tracheal mucus grading scores. A: Grade 0; B:Grade 1; C:Grade 2; D: Grade 3; E:Garde 4.

Important sequelae are secondary bacterial pneumonia, myocarditis, pericarditis and cardiac arrhythmias.

Diagnosis
- Presumptive diagnosis of a viral respiratory infection is frequently made on the basis of clinical signs and hematological evidence of a lymphopenia followed by a monocytosis.
- Definitive diagnosis involves:
  - Detection of the virus by PCR (most common), or viral culture and isolation (more problematic) from nasopharyngeal swabs.
  - Serological testing. Several methods are available but all involve analyzing acute and convalescent samples.
- There is a proportion of horses however that may not seroconvert following an outbreak.

Treatment and prevention
- Treatment is largely symptomatic with good nursing care an important feature. Judicial use of anti-inflammatories is beneficial and client education to avoid exercise before the respiratory epithelium has adequately recovered.

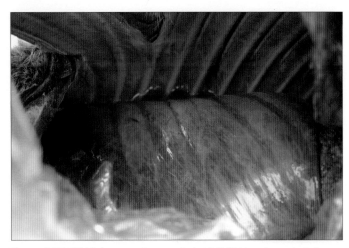

Figure 3.85 EHV. Pulmonary edema in a foal with EHV. Note the marked rib impressions on the lung surface.

- Prevention requires a combination of vaccination and hygienic management practices. The reader is referred to the AAEP (American Association of Equine Practitioners) or OIE (Office for International Epizooties) for current vaccination recommendations for their area. However, it is important to remember that vaccination does not completely eliminate clinical episodes.

Equine herpes virus (Fig. 3.85)

Equine herpes virus type-1 **(EHV-1)** and type-4 **(EHV-4)** are common respiratory pathogens throughout the world. They are also associated with abortions, myeloencephalitis and neonatal deaths. Although both types are universally important EHV-4 has been more frequently associated with respiratory disease alone. Due to widespread vaccination severe epidemics of equine herpes virus infection are now uncommon. The source of infection is recrudescence of latent infection in animals during episodes of stress. Infection occurs as a result of inhalation of the virus or contact with infected tissues. Thereafter it is thought that in the absence of mucosal antibody the virus immediately infects the epithelial lining of the nasopharynx and tonsils.

Clinical signs are usually apparent 1–3 days following infection and respiratory signs can be indistinguishable from influenza infection with a marked rhinopneumonitis and serous ocular and nasal discharges with an obvious diffuse tracheitis. A harsh, non-productive cough during exercise, which is easily induced by tracheal or pharyngeal manipulation, is characteristic. Affected horses do not usually cough while at rest. Pulmonary involvement, which typically affects the most cranial parts of the lung, is audible on auscultation. Once secondary bacterial infection develops the cough may become productive and the nasal discharge is more purulent. Death from a fulminating pneumonitis may occur.

Foals infected in utero are usually stillborn but those born alive are usually weak and die shortly after birth, showing extensive pulmonary, pleural, hepatic and adrenal gland pathology.

More usually, however, the diseases are detected serologically with limited clinical signs occurring simultaneously in a number of in-contact horses and confirmed by virus isolation techniques.

Diagnosis

- PCR performed on nasopharyngeal swabs is currently the most useful method of diagnosis as it is rapid and allows distinction between EHV1 and EHV4.
- Viral isolation from blood samples can also be attempted but is more problematic. There may also be lab variation in the sample requirements. Serological diagnosis is by demonstrating a fourfold rise in antibody titers.

- Post-mortem examination of foals that have died from EHV infection reveals interstitial pneumonia, pleural and peritoneal effusions, hypoplasia of the thymus and spleen and focal necrosis of the liver.

Treatment and prevention

- There is no specific treatment and in most cases the primary concern is to limit spread of infection requiring infected horses to be separated from the rest of the population. In uncomplicated upper respiratory tract infections, rest is generally all that is required. If complicated by secondary bacterial infections antibiotics may be required.
- Prevention is difficult as latent infections and inapparent carriers are common. Herpsevirus can invade the immune system and infect horses that are appropriately vaccinated. The virus is more environmentally stable than influenza virus and can be spread by fomites but is sensitive to many disinfectants.
- Management practices for control and prevention include isolating new horses for 3–4 weeks prior to mixing with resident stock and horses should not be moved for 3 weeks following a clinical episode. Strict hygiene should be maintained in cases of EHV abortion as uterine fluids are highly infectious.
- Current vaccination recommendations can be obtained from the AAEP (American Association of Equine Practitioners) or OIE (Office for International Epizooties) websites.

Other viral infections

There are numerous other virus infections which produce mild or moderate upper respiratory tract infections including **equine arteritis virus**, **equine rhinovirus**, **equine picornavirus** and **equine adenovirus**, but, typically, these are almost asymptomatic, except in immune-suppressed horses such as those affected by combined immune-deficiency syndrome (CID). They may also play a part in mixed infections with other viruses and bacteria.

Hendra virus is a zoonotic morbillivirus that has a fruit bat reservoir and can cause fatal pneumonia and encephalitis in horses and humans. Transmission requires close contact with the bat urine secretions or infected horses. Outbreaks result in high morbidity and mortality rates with associated veterinarian deaths reported in Australia. If suspected local authorities should be contacted.

African horse sickness (Figs. 3.86–3.90) is, possibly, the most serious viral respiratory disorder of the horse. The disease is limited geographically to areas of Africa, the Middle East and Southern Europe and it causes widespread mortality (up to 95% or more) amongst susceptible populations of horses, mules and donkeys. Asymptomatic or mild infections can occur in horses previously infected with a different serotype of the virus, as well as zebras and donkeys. Infected animals or vectors may carry the virus into AHS-free regions. Most countries where the disease is not present have strict regulations regarding its quarantine and control.

African horse sickness results from infection with the African horse sickness virus (AHSV), a member of the genus *Orbivirus* in the family Reoviridae. There are nine serotypes of AHSV. Serotype 9 is widespread in endemic regions, while serotypes 1–8 are found only in limited geographic areas. Serotype 9 has been responsible for the majority of African horse sickness outbreaks outside Africa. Serotype 4 caused one outbreak in Spain and Portugal between 1987 and 1990. African horse sickness is transmitted by nocturnal biting insects of the *Culicoides* group, with *Culicoides imicola* being the most important vector. There is a strong seasonal incidence which closely follows the prevalence of these insects. A variety of clinical syndromes may be encountered, which are dependent upon the susceptibility of the individual horse and the virulence of the strain of virus involved, particularly with respect to its pneumotropism.

Four forms of African horse sickness are described, ranging from a peracute, rapidly progressive, highly fatal form, to a mild, almost

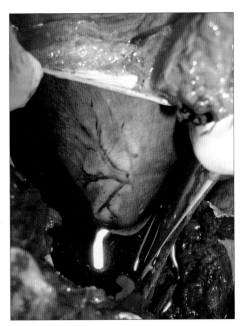

Figure 3.86 African horse sickness. Hydropericardium is a common post-mortem finding.

Differential diagnosis:
- Equine viral arteritis
- Equine infectious anemia
- Hendra virus infection
- Purpura hemorrhagica
- Equine piroplasmosis
- Equine encephalosis
- Toxins, anthrax and other causes of sudden death, as well as diseases that result in severe respiratory distress, should also be considered.

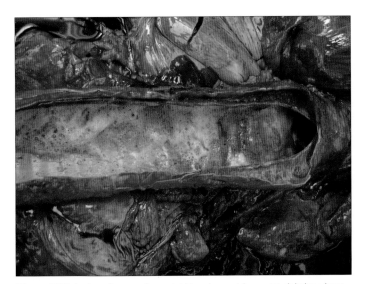

Figure 3.87 In the pulmonary form of African horse sickness, interlobular edema of the lungs and hydrothorax are the characteristic lesions. In the most acute cases, frothy fluid flows from the nostrils and the cut surface of the lungs, which are mottled red, non-collapsed and heavy. In more prolonged cases, there may be extensive interstitial and subpleural edema, and hyperemia may be less apparent. Fluid accumulation can occur in the abdominal and thoracic cavities. Occasionally, extensive fluid accumulation may be noted in the thoracic cavity (hydrothorax), with near normal appearance of the lungs.

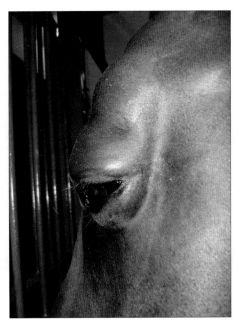

Figure 3.88 Characterisitc supraorbital and eylid edema of subacute African horse sickness.

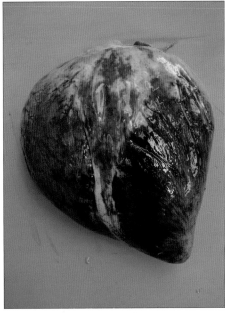

Figure 3.89 The epicardium and endocardium often contain petechial and ecchymotic hemorrhages in acute and subacute forms of African horse sickness.

inapparent respiratory infection. These various syndromes are, however, not well defined and it is not often possible to categorize a specific case into one or other of them. However, all but the mildest types show marked cardiac and respiratory involvement.

In experimental infections, the incubation period can range from 2 to 21 days. In natural infections, the incubation period appears to be approximately 3–5 days for the pulmonary form, 7–14 days for the cardiac form, 5–7 days for the mixed form and 5–14 days for horse sickness fever.

The clinical characteristics of the peracute (pulmonary) syndrome are largely the result of massive, catastrophic pulmonary edema, in which a profuse nasal discharge of yellowish, frothy liquid sometimes blood-tinged is present. Paroxysmal coughing, sweating and a high

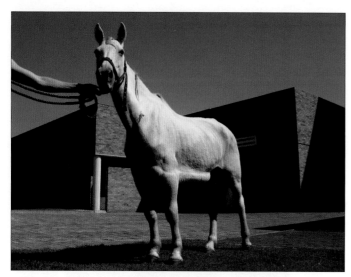

Figure 3.90 African horse sickness. In the cardiac form, ventral edema may be prominent.

fever are prominent features. Death usually occurs between 4 and 24 hours after the onset of clinical signs with high mortality rates (95%). Post-mortem examination confirms the presence of extensive accumulations of froth in the conducting airways and marked pulmonary edema. The lungs exude large volumes of protein-containing fluid, and fail to collapse.

The **subacute** or cardiac form of African horse sickness has a somewhat longer course (5–7 days) and is characterized by swelling (edema) of the head, neck, trunk and limbs. The temporal fossae and eyelids are usually grossly swollen. Prominent chemosis (conjunctival edema) is almost always present in cases which survive beyond 24 hours. Cyanosis, congestion and petechial hemorrhages are usually visible on mucous membranes. Clinically, cardiac tamponade secondary to pericardial effusion may be detectable. Cases which survive for a few days may develop a serious and profound pharyngeal paralysis in which nasal regurgitation of food and water is present. This latter sign may be made even more obvious by the fact that affected horses will often continue to eat and drink, despite apparently severe distress and a high fever. While some cases of the cardiac form of African horse sickness survive, the mortality is nevertheless high (50–90%). Full recovery may, however, take months, or even years in some cases.

A subacute form with myocardial dysfunction, fever and edema of the head and neck can also occur with a lower mortality rate (50%).

The mildest forms of African horse sickness are probably the result of a non-virulent virus attacking a partially immune host or more resistant equidae such as donkeys and zebras. In this form, which is often referred to as **horse sickness fever**, there may be few clinical signs apart from a mild and transient pyrexia, swelling of the eyelids and supraorbital fossae, and occasional, transient dyspnea. Contrary to the more serious types, appetite in these horses is often depressed and the disease closely resembles the respiratory syndromes caused by equine herpes virus, equine influenza virus and equine viral arteritis.

Diagnosis

- African horse sickness should be suspected in animals with typical symptoms of the cardiac, pulmonary or mixed forms of the disease in a suitable geographical area or with history of recent transportation from a suitable geographical area. The supraorbital swellings are particularly characteristic of this disease. The horse sickness form can be difficult to diagnose.
- African horse sickness can be diagnosed by isolating the virus or detecting its nucleic acids or antigens. More than one test should be

used to diagnose an outbreak (particularly the index case) whenever possible.

- Virus isolation is particularly important when outbreaks are seen outside endemic areas. AHSV can be isolated in embryonated eggs, by intracerebral inoculation of newborn mice, or in cell cultures. The isolated virus can be identified by complement fixation or immunofluorescence. The isolate should be serotyped using virus neutralization or other methods.
- AHSV antigens can be detected with enzyme-linked immunosorbent assays (ELISAs). A reverse-transcription polymerase chain reaction (RT-PCR) technique is used to detect viral RNA. A type-specific RTPCR assay can be used for rapid serotyping.
- Serology can also be used to diagnose African horse sickness. Antibodies can be detected within 8–14 days after infection, and may persist for 1–4 years. Available serologic tests include complement fixation, ELISAs, immunoblotting and virus neutralization.
- The indirect ELISA and complement fixation tests are the prescribed tests for international trade. The virus neutralization test is used for serotyping. Immunodiffusion and hemagglutination inhibition tests have also been described. AHSV does not cross-react with other known orbiviruses.

Treatment and control

- AHS is a reportable disease in many jurisdictions with a slaughter control policy.
- In some areas ring vaccination may be used to control outbreaks. An inactivated vaccine is available and is widely used in endemic areas.

Bacterial diseases

Rhodococcus equi *pneumonia* (Figs. 3.91–3.99)

Pneumonia in foals, caused by *Rhodococcus equi* (*R. equi*) is a well-known worldwide problem. Other less common clinical manifestations of *R. equi* infections in foals include ulcerative enterocolitis, colonic/mesenteric lymphadenopathy, immune-mediated synovitis and uveitis, osteomyelitis and septic arthritis.

Inhalation of contaminated dust particles is thought to be an important route for pneumonic infection of foals. Ingestion of the organisms is a significant route of exposure and immunization but may not lead to hematogenous pneumonia unless the foal has multiple exposures to very large numbers of bacteria. It has also recently been demonstrated that infected foals with nasal discharge are a significant form of direct transmission to other in-contact non-infected foals.

Epidemiologic evidence indicates that foals that develop *R. equi* pneumonia are most commonly infected during the first few days of life, but clinical signs do not develop until foals are 30–60 days of age or older.

The most common manifestation of *R. equi* in foals is a suppurative bronchopneumonia with extensive abscessation and suppurative lymphadenitis. The slow spread of the lung infection coupled with the remarkable ability of foals to compensate for the progressive loss of functional lung makes early diagnosis difficult.

Early clinical signs may only include a slight increase in respiratory rate and mild fever. These clinical signs are often missed, allowing the disease to progress.

Therefore, the respiratory signs are often apparently acute in onset. A smaller percentage of these foals may be found dead or more commonly present in acute respiratory distress with high fevers (105–106°F) and no previous history of clinical respiratory disease.

Approximately 50% of *R. equi* pneumonic foals presented to necropsy also had intestinal manifestations characterized by granulomatous or suppurative inflammation of the Peyer's patches and the mesenteric and/or colonic lymph nodes. Interestingly, the majority of

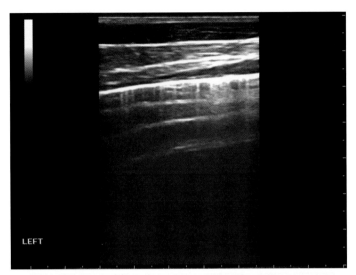

Figure 3.91 *R. equi.* Comet tail artefacts are created by the presence of a small amount of fluid or cellular infiltrate in the pulmonary periphery. The ultrasound beam passes through this area and then encounters air which is highly reflective, creating an air artefact which appears as a comet tail. The finding of comet tails is very non-specific and must be interpreted in conjunction with other findings and considered in relation to the age and use of the animal.

Differential diagnosis for the presence of comet tail artefacts:
- COPD
- EIPH (dorso-caudal lung fields)
- Pulmonary edema
- Acute bronchopneumonia
- Equine influenza
- Scarring from resolving or previous pneumonia.

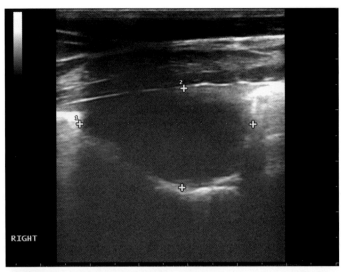

Figure 3.93 *R. equi.* Pulmonary abscesses grade 4.

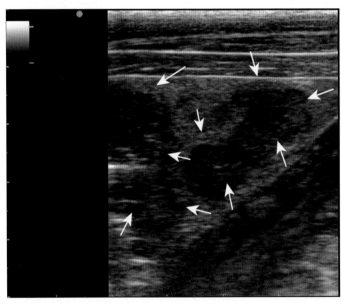

Figure 3.94 *R. equi* grade 10. There is extensive pulmonary consolidation and a cavitated abscess is clearly visible (arrows).

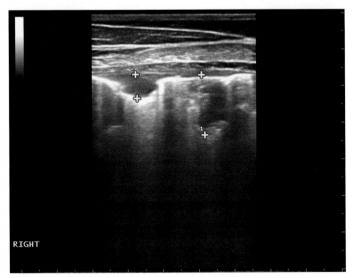

Figure 3.92 *R. equi.* Pulmonary abscesses grade 3. A pulmonary abscess is a cavitated area within the lung parenchyma that lacks the normal pulmonary structures. The cavitated region is normally more anechoic that the adjacent hypoechoic consolidate parenchyma. However, in reality it is frequently difficult to differentiate pulmonary consolidation from pulmonary abscessation.

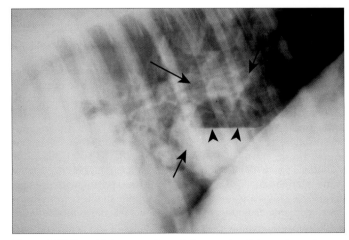

Figure 3.95 *R. equi.* Pulmonary radiograph. Large cavitated abscess (arrows) with evident fluid line (arrowheads).

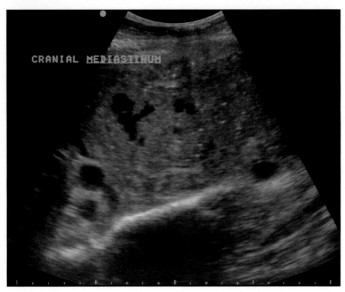

Figure 3.96 *R. equi* mediastinal abscess. Large mediastinal abscess with mixed echogenicity. This abscess in a 6-month-old foal caused dorsal displacement and rotation of the heart in addition to compression of local vessels and lymphatics resulting in a marked pleural effusion. The abscess was surgically reduced and the foal treated with a prolonged course of antibiotics and made a full recovery with no evidence of the abscess at a 6-month follow-up.

the foals with *R. equi* pneumonia do not show clinical signs of the intestinal disease. It has been speculated, however, that foals with subclinical intestinal manifestations may not gain body weight as readily as they should have. In the same study, only 4% of the foals with intestinal *R. equi* lesions did not have pneumonia.

Immune-mediated polysynovitis, particularly the tibiotarsal and stifle joints can be seen in 30% of cases with *R. equi* pneumonia.

Diagnosis

- The insidious course of infection makes early diagnosis difficult. Recognition of foals with *R. equi* pneumonia prior to the development of clinical signs would likely reduce losses and limit costs associated with long-term treatment of affected foals.

- Many diagnostic tests including complete blood cell count, fibrinogen level, thoracic ultrasound, radiographs and serology have all been used to help distinguish R. *equi* pneumonia from that caused by other pathogens.

- However, bacteriologic culture or PCR amplification combined with cytological examination of a tracheobronchial aspirate (TBA) are still the 'gold standards' used to arrive at a definitive diagnosis.

- Serological assays, whether performed on single or paired samples, cannot be used to reliably establish, confirm or exclude a diagnosis of *R. equi* pneumonia in foals. These serological tests are problematic because of the widespread exposure of foals to this organism at a young age which would initiate appropriate antibody production.

- Measurements of white blood cell count (WBC) or fibrinogen concentrations are non-specific indicators of infection or inflammation. On an endemic farm results of a WBC >13 000 cells/μl or noting a foal with a fever would warrant a careful examination by the veterinarian. Foals with a WBC > 14 000 cells/μl with no clinical signs of disease and normal lung sounds should be considered for additional diagnostic tests such as thoracic ultrasonography.

- Ultrasonography may reveal abnormalities of the peripheral pulmonary parenchyma. If these abnormalities are detected then a TBA and/or antibiotic treatment should be initiated. Farms with

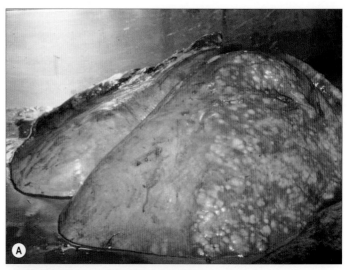

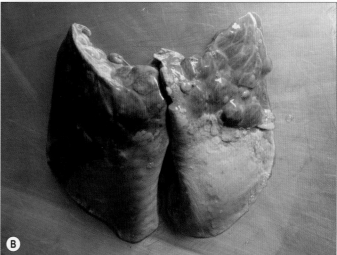

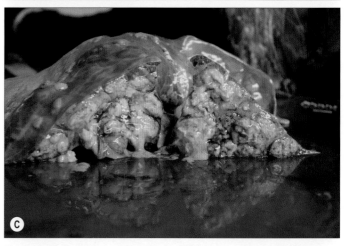

Figure 3.97 *R.equi.* Post-mortem images. (A) Multiple variable-sized abscesses covering half of the lung surface. (B) Large abscess interspaced with areas of consolidation/atelectasis covering the cranial half of both lungs in this foal. (C) Cut surface of the lung (from the same foal as part B) showing the pyogranulomatous content of the abscesses.

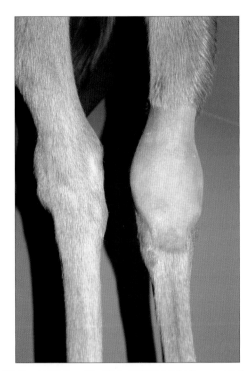

Figure 3.98 *R. equi* polysynovitis. Effusion of the left (right as you look at the image) hock in this foal. Joint fluid analysis was within normal limits. Ultrasonography of the thorax revealed areas of abscessation and culture of a transtracheal aspirate yielded a growth of *R. equi*.

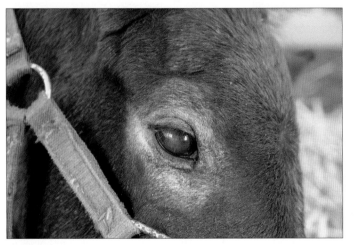

Figure 3.99 *R. equi* uveitis. Differentail diagnosis includes any other possible cause of uveitis (see p. 383) the most important of which in young foals is septicemia.

Table 3.4 Grading system for pulmonary lesions

Grade	Ultrasonographic findings
Grade 0	No evidence of pulmonary consolidation. Pleural irregularities which appear as vertical hyperechoic lines and are described as reverberation artifacts
Grade 1	Less than 1 cm in diameter/depth
Grade 2	Lesions that are 1.0 to 2.0 cm in size
Grade 3	2.0 to 3.0 cm in size
Grade 4	3.0 to 4.0 cm in size
Grade 5	4.0 to 5.0 cm in size
Grade 6	5.0 to 6.0 cm in size
Grade 7	6.0 to 7.0 cm in size
Grade 8	7.0 to 9.0 cm in size. If pleural effusion is present then the lesion is assigned this grade regardless of whether or not you have lesser grades of consolidation or abscessation
Grade 9	9.0 to 11 cm in size
Grade 10	The entire lung lobe is affected

thoracic ultrasonography may be a more sensitive indicator of sub-clinical or early clinical lesions than measurement of WBC.

- The argument exists, however, that many foals are now being diagnosed as *R. equi* positive on the basis of ultrasound findings alone and many cases which may resolve spontaneously are being treated which may lead to antibiotic resistance problems.
- Two grading scales for lesions detected by ultrasonography, ranging from 0 (normal) to 10 (entire lung surface is affected) have been developed to aid in the documentation of lesions, assessment of treatment success and help with the communication and description of pneumonia. Pulmonary lesions are assigned a grade according to the severity. This grading system is outlined in Table 3.4.

Treatment

- Although control trials to evaluate optimal treatment are lacking, the combination of a macrolide (erythromycin, azithromycin or clarithromycin) and rifampin or a macrolide alone in the case of azithromycin are considered standard treatment. Other macrolides have also been examined for treatment of *R. equi* pneumonia. Tulathromycin has not been shown to be effective in clinical trials and gamithromycin which performs well in vitro has not yet had its clinical efficacy or safety established through clinical trials.
- All macrolides may cause hyperthermia and foals should be stabled while on treatment. The cause of the hyperthermia is not exactly known. Other possible adverse effects are antibiotic-induced diarrhea in the foal and colitis in mares which may gain access to the foal's medication, e.g. licking the foal's face following treatments. The incidence of complications appears to be higher with the use of erythromycin than other macrolides.
- Foals that recover from *R. equi* pneumonia and make it to the race track have been shown to perform as well as expected their unaffected peers.

Streptococcus equi *var.* equi *(strangles)*

(Figs. 3.100–3.113)

Streptococcus equi var. *equi* (*S. equi*) is the causative organism of the disease commonly referred to as '**strangles**'. Recent studies indicate that *S. equi* is in fact a clone of the more genetically diverse *Streptococcus zooepidemicus* and reclassification as such has been proposed. Despite marked genetic homology there is no immunological cross-protection. *S. equi* unlike *S. zooepidemicus* is not a normal inhabitant of the equine respiratory tract and does not require prior viral or bacterial infection to produce disease. Based on morphological

endemic *R. equi* that have suffered significant morbidity and/or mortality rates should be monitoring rectal temperatures 2× daily, with febrile foals selected for further testing (thoracic ultrasonography) or treatment. In my experience performing twice-monthly thoracic ultrasonography (starting at 2 weeks of age) has been demonstrated to be very effective for early recognition and reduction of mortality attributed to *R. equi* pneumonia on several endemic farms. The rationale for this early screening is the belief that earlier initiation of specific treatment will not only improve the prognosis for recovery but also reduce the treatment period. Thoracic ultrasonography can also be used to determine when the antibiotic therapy can be discontinued. Additionally, ongoing research suggests that

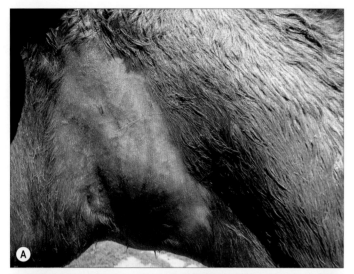

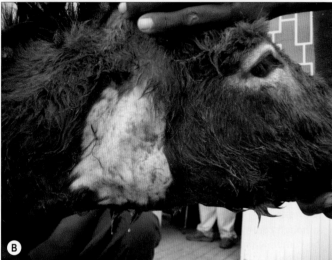

Figure 3.100 (A, B) Strangles; enlargement of retropharyngeal lymph nodes.

Differential diagnosis:
- *Strep. zooepidemicus* infection
- Pharyngeal abscess/emphysema (tracheal rupture)
- Anthrax
- Glanders
- Guttural pouch tympany in foals.

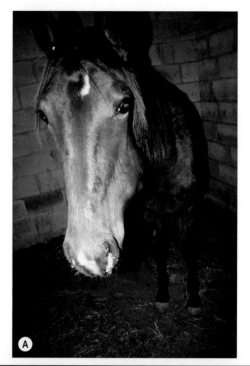

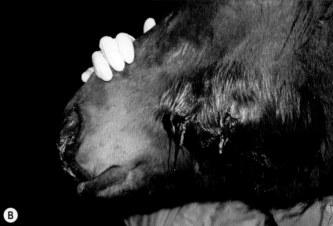

Figure 3.102 (A, B) Strangles abscess on the lateral aspect of the face. Note the concurrent purulent nasal discharge.

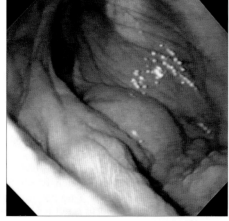

Figure 3.101 Endoscopic image of guttural pouch showing enlarged retropharyngeal lymph node protruding through floor of pouch.

features of bacterial colonies three distinct strains of the organism occur that differ in virulence. The condition may occur in horses of all ages, although those under 5 years of age are probably most susceptible and therefore most frequently affected by serious forms of the disease.

Animals are exposed to *S. equi* from secretions of an affected horse via direct or indirect contact with a sick animal or an asymptomatic carrier. Infected horses shed the organism through the nasal passages so nose-to-nose contact of horses can spread the disease as well as coming in contact with secretions on fomites such as fences, water buckets or troughs, pitch forks, or even a human handler. Horse vans, stalls or public auctions are all possible sources for *S. equi*. Affected animals usually start shedding the organisms several days after onset of fever.

The clinical signs depend largely upon the individual form which the infection takes in a particular animal, and are probably dependent upon the immune status of the host and the virulence of the bacterial strain involved. The initial clinical sign of strangles is a

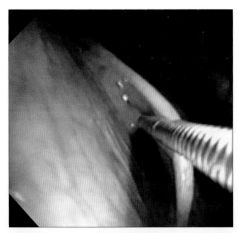

Figure 3.103 Strangles infection with guttural pouch empyema. Endoscopic image of the entrance to the guttural pouch with obvious mucopurulent discharge.

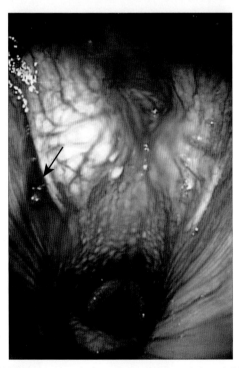

Figure 3.104 Hemopurulent discharge from guttural pouch (arrow) following recent rupture of lymph nodes into the pouch.

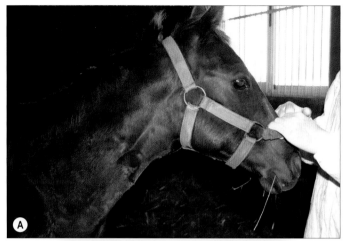

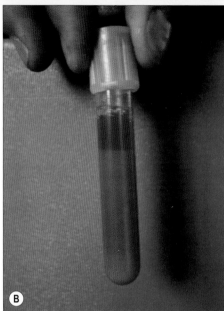

Figure 3.105 (A, B) Guttural pouch empyema. Note enlarged guttural pouches in (A). Ultrasound of the pouches revealed a fluid content and aspiration yielded a mucopurulent content.

fever. Fevers usually occur 3–14 days after exposure. Affected animals may initially have a serous nasal discharge which progresses to mucopurulent and then purulent. The classical form of strangles presents with gross lymphadenopathy and abscessation of the pharyngeal, submaxillary and submandibular lymph nodes. This may be sufficient to result in serious and often life-threatening pharyngeal respiratory obstruction (hence the name 'strangles'). Other lymph nodes of the head such as the parotid and cranial cervical are also commonly involved. Endoscopic examination of the pharynx shows a markedly narrowed pharynx, with dorsal pharyngeal compression. Affected horses frequently hold their necks in extension in an attempt to provide some relief from the pharyngeal pain and respiratory obstruction which may be sufficient to warrant an emergency tracheostomy. The pharyngeal obstruction often causes dysphagia and food material, saliva and purulent exudates from the pharynx may appear at the nose.

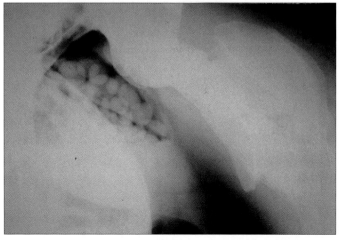

Figure 3.106 Radiographic image of chondroids within the guttural pouch.

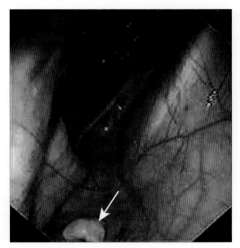

Figure 3.107 Chondroids on the floor of the guttural pouch (arrow).

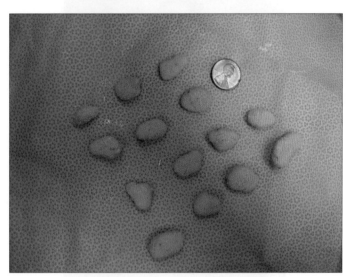

Figure 3.108 Chondroids following removal from guttural pouch.

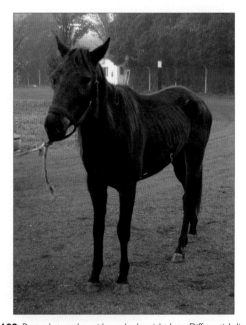

Figure 3.109 Bastard strangles with marked weight loss. Differential diagnosis for weight loss is extensive but a previous history of *S. equi* infection allows inclusion of internal abscessation in the differentials.

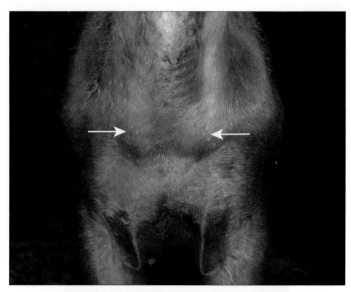

Figure 3.110 Bastard strangles. Enlarged pectoral lymph nodes (arrows).
Differential diagnosis:
• Pigeon fever
• Cutaneous lymphosarcoma.

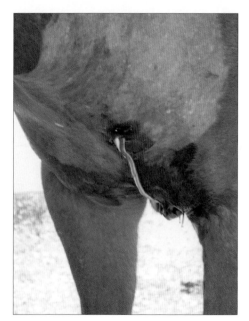

Figure 3.111 Bastard strangles. Pectoral abscess which has been lanced to allow drainage.

The enlarged lymph nodes ultimately burst releasing a creamy-yellow pus, often with some blood. Serum may ooze from the skin before the lymph nodes rupture and drain. While some abscesses burst outwards, others may rupture into the pharynx or guttural pouches, producing a profuse purulent nasal discharge (possibly with some blood). A purulent discharge from the ostia of the auditive tube may reflect the stage of the infection in the pharyngeal lymph nodes, the discharges usually being hemorrhagic immediately after rupture of the abscesses, and purulent thereafter.

Milder forms of strangles in which the extent of pharyngeal lymph node abscess formation is minimal and the systemic effects are much less dramatic are increasingly recognized. Partially immune or mature horses appear more likely to develop the milder forms. In these forms

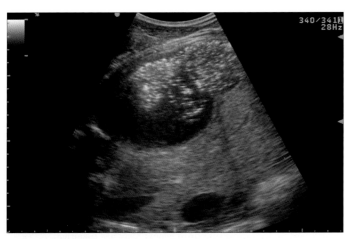

Figure 3.112 Bastard strangles. Ultrasonographic image of large cavitated pulmonary abscess with a thick abscess wall.

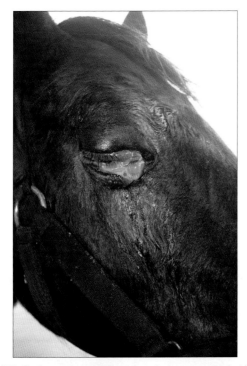

Figure 3.113 Ocular protrusion and conjunctival edema associated with retrobulbar abscessation following *S. equi* infection.

the infection with *Streptococcus equi* closely resembles infection with *Streptococcus zooepidemicus*.

Diagnosis

- A presumptive diagnosis can be based on clinical signs of the characteristic abscesses. The confirming diagnosis via culture can be obtained from a draining abscess, a nasal swab, a pharyngeal wash or a guttural pouch wash.
- A polymerase chain reaction (PCR) can also be used as a diagnostic tool. PCR detects the presence of DNA and does not distinguish between live or dead samples. PCR is considered more sensitive than culture, but may also yield false negatives.

- Serology is available to aid in diagnosis. An ELISA test measures *S. equi* specific M-protein, but does not distinguish between infected and vaccinated animals.
- ***Differential diagnosis: Streptococcus equi* var. *zooepidemicus* lymphadenopathy.** Unlike *Streptococcus equi* var. *equi* this bacterium is considered a secondary pathogen. *Streptococcus equi* var. *zooepidemicus* usually affects horses that have either suffered an upper respiratory infection or are immuno-compromised. It is not considered a primary pathogen like *Streptococcus equi* var. *equi*. Clinical signs are almost identical to *Streptococcus equi* var. *equi*. Cultures are needed to confirm a diagnosis of *Streptococcus equi* var. *zooepidemicus*. Treatment is generally similar to that for *S. equi* with maturation and rupture of abscesses being preferable and antibiotic use reserved for more cases with more severe clinical signs.

Treatment

- Horses with clinically **suspected** *S. equi* should be isolated immediately.
- Most animals affected with *S. equi* do not require treatment or antibiotics, therefore allowing maturation and eventual rupture/ drainage of the abscess.
- Those exhibiting additional clinical signs such as profound fever, depression, anorexia or dyspnea require antibiotic treatment. Penicillin is the antibiotic of choice for strangles. Trimethoprim sulfa has mixed reports on its efficacy against *S. equi*. Rifampin and the macrolides (azithromycin or clarithromycin) have an excellent spectrum of activity against *Streptococcus* infections and can be used in foal cases. Other potential antibiotic choices where owner compliance may be a factor are long-acting tetracyclines and cephalosporins.
- Horses in respiratory distress from abscesses compressing the trachea require a tracheostomy below the affected site.
- Non-steroidal anti-inflammatory medications (phenylbutazone, flunixin meglumine or fetoprofen) may also aid in alleviating fever and improving anorexia.
- Animals affected with guttural pouch empyema should be placed on systemic antibiotics and have their guttural pouches flushed and infused with a pencillin gel.

Sequelae

1) **Abscessation of internal organs**. This is commonly known as 'bastard strangles'; in this form there is 'metastatic' distribution of the organism to lymph nodes and organs other than those of the pharynx and head. While large encapsulated or miliary abscesses may occur in any site, the commonest locations are the lungs, liver, spleen, kidney and brain. Abscesses may also develop in the skin and within synovial structures. Diffuse, multiple-organ abscesses result in a clinical condition which has serious systemic effects upon the horse. These include dramatic weight loss, ventral edema, debilitating and progressive dyspnea and inappetence. A specific diagnosis may be difficult depending on the site of abscessation and differentiation from other causes of chronic debilitation may be difficult. All efforts should be made to achieve a diagnosis as the treatment plans and prognosis may differ significantly. The prognosis is also largely dependent on the site of the internal abscess(es). Cerebral abscesses carry a particularly poor prognosis although there are reports of recovery following surgical removal of the abscesses. Mesenteric abscesses may do surprisingly well with long-term antibiotic therapy.

2) **Purpura hemorrhagica**. This is an aseptic vasculitis (see Chapter 4, p. 177).

3) **Empyema of the guttural pouch** may occur if the retropharyngeal lymph nodes rupture and drain internally into the pouches. The empyema may become inspissated and form chondroids, which are difficult to remove from the pouches. Occasionally, chronic

inflammation of the pouches results in neuropathies related to dysfunction of the glossopharyngeal, vagus, facial and sympathetic nerves which lie within, or adjacent to, the diverticulum. The signs include dysphagia, facial paralysis and Horner's syndrome.

4) Septicemia and development of septic arthritis, pneumonia and/or encephalitis.

5) **Laryngeal hemiplegia** caused by compression of the recurrent laryngeal nerve by enlarged lymph nodes.

6) **Aspiration pneumonia**.

7) **Endocarditis** or **myocarditis**.

8) **Agalactia** in periparturient mares.

9) **Myopathies**. Three different types have been described (see Chapter 8, p 302). One which is characterized by a vasculitis and infarction of skeletal muscle (Infarctive purpura hemorrhagica), a second in which there is significant muscle atrophy and chronic active rhabdomyolysis (Immune-mediated polymyositis) and a third characterized by acute rhabdomyolyis (Acute rhabdomyolysis caused by *S. equi*).

Control of an outbreak

The control measures that are implemented frequently depend on the individual situation, the number of horses involved, the value of the horses and the budget and commitment of the owner. The objectives of control measures are:

• Prevent spread of infection to new or clean areas and control the outbreak within the infected premises. This involves the dedication of 'clean' and 'dirty' areas with infected horses confined to dirty areas and cared for by a dedicated staff. There should be a physical separation between clean and dirty areas and not simply different boxes under the same roof. Strict hygiene measures should be enforced with dedicated feed, water, cleaning utensils and clothing for each area.

• Ensure all horses are free of infection at the end of an outbreak. All recovered cases and in-contacts should be subjected to three consecutive nasopharyngeal swabs (culture) or guttural pouch lavages (culture/PCR) at weekly intervals. Any horse testing positive should be further evaluated and treated accordingly.

• Horses with chondroids may require repeated lavages of the guttural pouches or physical removal of the chondroids. Those without chondroids may be treated with infusion of a penicillin gel into the guttural pouch and should re-test as negative prior to being allowed to re-join the clean group.

Prevention

• To prevent the introduction of *S. equi* into a herd by means of an asymptomatic carrier, all new arrivals should be placed in quarantine and screened for the presence of *S. equi*, ideally with guttural pouch lavages. If positive the horse should be treated (see above) and remain in quarantine until repeat tests are negative.

• Several vaccines are available but none guarantee immunity to infection and there are numerous reports of side effects to live vaccines.

Sinusitis (Figs. 3.114–3.117)

Primary sinusitis with accumulation of exudates within the sinus cavities is a sequela of upper respiratory tract infection. Streptococcal

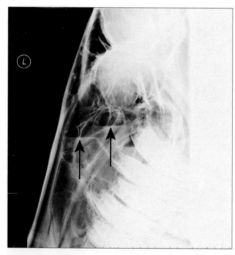

Figure 3.115 Sinusitis. Radiograph showing fluid lines with the maxillary sinus (arrows).

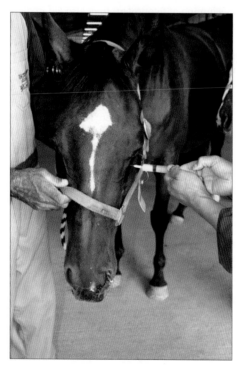

Figure 3.114 Sinusitis facial image. The caudal root of the third cheek tooth (fourth premolar) and the roots of the fourth tooth (first molar) are usually located within the rostral compartment of the maxillary sinus. Infections associated either primarily as a result of bacterial infection extending from the nasal cavity, or secondarily related to disease of the roots of these teeth, usually result in swelling and facial distortion.

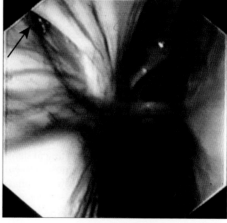

Figure 3.116 Sinusitis. Endoscopy of the maxillary opening demonstrating a mucopurulent discharge (arrow).

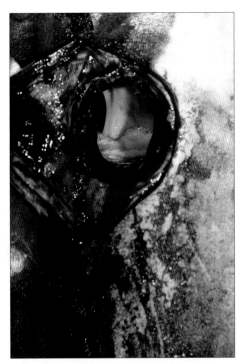

Figure 3.117 Sinus flap showing mucopurulent contents within the maxillary sinus.

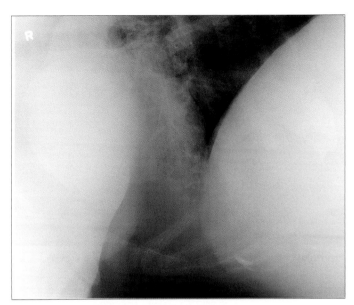

Figure 3.118 Radiographic image of aspiration pneumonia. Note the cranioventral distribution of consolidation.

organisms are most frequently isolated in such cases. Secondary sinusitis occurs most commonly following dental disorders with the first molar being the most commonly involved tooth. It may also occur following traumatic head injuries, development of sinus cysts, with neoplasms or following fungal infection.

Clinical signs depend largely on the initiating cause, which sinus(es) are affected and the chronicity of the condition. It is frequently unilateral with an associated unilateral purulent nasal discharge but can be bilateral. Cases which occur secondary to dental issues or neoplasia may have an associated foul-smelling breath, which is usually restricted to the ipsilateral nostril. Facial swelling and distortion is also frequently found. Other signs that may be seen with less frequency are exophthalmus, dyspnea, epistaxis, epiphora, weight loss and rarely neurological signs secondary to extension of infection through the cribriform plate.

Diagnosis

- History, clinical signs and physical examination (dullness on percussion of the affected sinus and oral examination revealing dental abnormalities) are usually sufficient to make an initial presumptive diagnosis. Further tests are then usually needed to further outline the number of sinuses involved.
- Radiographic examination of the sinus will usually reveal the presence of one or more air–fluid interfaces (fluid level) within the limits of the affected sinus, each associated with separate divisions within the frontal and/or maxillary sinuses. However, where the contents of the sinus have become inspissated, such distinct features may not be visible. Instead, diffuse and irregular opacities within the confines of the sinuses may be detected. The caudal maxillary sinus and the frontal sinus communicate freely and drain by a common ostium into the nasal cavity.
- Endoscopic examination of the caudo-dorsal region of the ipsilateral nasal cavity may reveal fluid and/or purulent discharge descending from the drainage channel created by the converging ventral and dorsal conchae.

- In cases with occluded drainage ostia, particularly where there is an inspissated sinus content, trephination of the affected sinus will allow effective endoscopic examination of the contents and in many cases will establish the etiology. Direct visualization of the tooth roots and the mucosa of the sinus is most useful in this respect.

Treatment and prognosis

- This depends on the inciting cause. Surgical removal of affected teeth, neoplasias or granulomatous tissue and establishment of effective drainage are important.
- Bacterial infections should be treated according to culture and antibiotic sensitivity testing.
- Frequent, repeated flushings of the affected sinus may be required.
- Refractory cases, which generally have poor drainage inhibiting treatment through flushes, may be best treated with facial flap surgery.
- The prognosis is largely dependent on the cause and the bacterial organisms involved. Fungal granulomas and neoplasias generally have a poorer prognosis as does infection with *Pseudomonas* sp. Primary sinusitis generally carries a good prognosis.

Bacterial pneumonia (Figs. 3.118–3.122)

Disorders of the lower respiratory tract are common in horses. The equine lung normally contains small numbers of bacteria that are regarded as transient contaminants that have not yet been removed by clearance mechanisms. However, when pulmonary defense mechanisms are overwhelmed or compromised, bacteria that are normally aspirated from the oropharynx may proliferate and result in pneumonia. Gram-positive organisms such as *Streptococcus* sp. are most frequently involved. These normally invade first, followed by invasion of Gram-negative organisms.

Causative factors in the modification of defense mechanisms include viral infections, transportation, athletic exertion and general anesthesia. Poor management such as overcrowding, poor nutrition and severe weather exposure are also predisposing factors.

In the early stages clinical signs may be inapparent or mild. Fever, depression and inappetence are normally the first signs noted which may coincide with the auscultation of gurgling sounds in the trachea related to mucus accumulation. Nasal discharge is normally

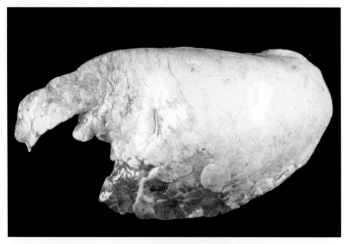

Figure 3.119 Post-mortem image from a horse with aspiration pneumonia.

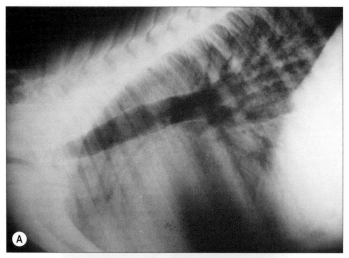

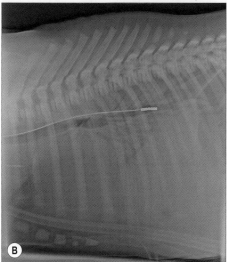

Figure 3.121 Bacterial pneumonia. (A) Diffuse interstitial pattern with coalescing miliary densities with marked airbronchograms.

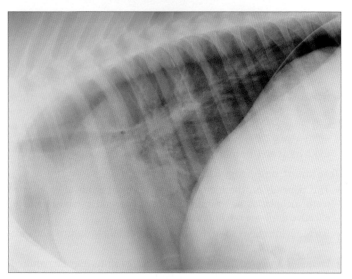

Figure 3.120 Radiograph of the thorax demonstrating an interstitial pattern of pneumonia.

mucopurulent but in some cases may be mucohemorrhagic. Coughing can be easily induced in many cases by manipulation of the trachea.

Diagnosis

- Clinical signs and examination are normally sufficient for a diagnosis but further tests may help to characterize the type and severity of pneumonia and the organisms involved to guide therapy. Auscultation of the thorax reveals harsh sounds dorsally with crackles and wheezes audible ventrally.
- Radiography can be used to determine the type of pneumonic pattern present.
- Ultrasonography can be used to assess the presence of lung consolidation and extension of the infection into the pleural cavity and detect the presence of fluid accumulations within the thorax.
- Clinical pathological findings are suggestive of bacterial infection with leucocytosis, neutrophilia or neutropenia (depending on the organisms involved), hyperfibrinogenemia and hypoalbuminemia as common findings. These are not, however, specific for pneumonia.
- Endoscopy can be used to assess the amount and character of secretions and may help to identify predisposing factors such as

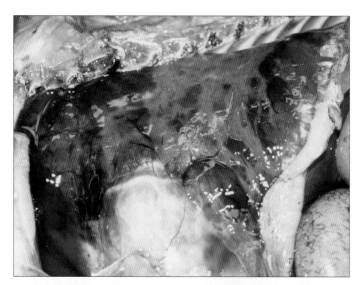

Figure 3.122 Atelectasis post-mortem. This may occur as a post-mortem change or be related to a pathological process. The timing of the post-mortem examination and the history should be taken into account when interpreting such findings.

neuropathies resulting in decreased pharyngeal function or laryngeal abnormalities.

Tracheobronchial aspirates can be used to obtain samples for culture and antibiotic sensitivity testing.

Treatment

- Antibiotic therapy is the cornerstone of treatment and whenever possible it should be aimed at the causative organism as determined by culture results.
- If this is not possible, broad-spectrum antibiotic therapy should be instituted. Common treatments include a combination of penicillin with an aminoglycoside and metronidazole.
- Other frequently used drugs are cephalosporins, trimethoprim-sulfa and tetracyclines.

Pleuritis (Figs. 3.123–3.139)

The other site in which bacterial infection causes severe respiratory disease in the horse is the pleural cavity. The majority of cases arise as an extension of pneumonia or pulmonary abscessation. It can also be seen following thoracic trauma or esophageal penetration. The bacteria involved are similar to those found in cases of bacterial pneumonia and include species that normally reside in the oropharyngeal cavities. Risk factors are the same as those for pneumonia. Fluid accumulates within the pleural cavity as permeability of capillaries increases in association with increased inflammation.

The initial pleural inflammatory response (pleuritis) may be mild and pass unnoticed, but extensive purulent material develops rapidly thereafter and is often complicated by anaerobic infection.

The condition is responsible for the development of intense parietal pain and affected horses are consequently reluctant to move and have a prominent abdominal component to breathing. Pressure applied between the ribs elicits marked pain and an obvious guarding response. Affected horses seldom cough but, when they do, it is soft and obviously painful and there may be an associated grunt, which may also be present at the end of expiration. The elbows are often abducted and there may be considerable sternal (ventral) edema. Horses with extensive, fibrinous, pleural adhesions may show less pain than those in which the inflammatory response is still active and allows movement between the visceral and parietal pleural surfaces.

There is frequently an obvious, foul-smelling, bilateral, purulent nasal discharge which is often flecked with blood or is overtly hemorrhagic. The presence of anaerobic infection within the pleural cavity is accompanied by a severe depression and the nasal discharge becomes particularly foul.

Where the disorder has been present for some weeks a profound non-regenerative iron-deficiency-type anemia will be noticed in most cases.

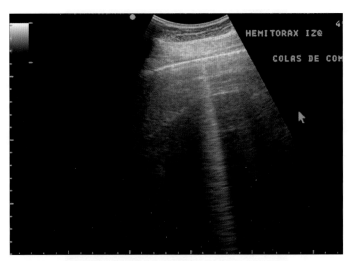

Figure 3.124 Ultrasound comet tails. The most echographic artefacts are comet tails, which are created by the presence of a small amount of fluid or cellular infiltrate in the pulmonary periphery. The ultrasound beam passes through this area and then encounters air which is highly reflective, creating an air artefact which appears as a comet tail. The finding of comet tails is very non-specific and must be interpreted in conjunction with other findings.

Comet tails are found in a large number of pulmonary conditions:
- COPD
- EIPH (dorso-caudal lung fields)
- Pulmonary edema
- Acute bronchopneumonia
- Equine influenza
- Scarring from resolving or previous pneumonia.

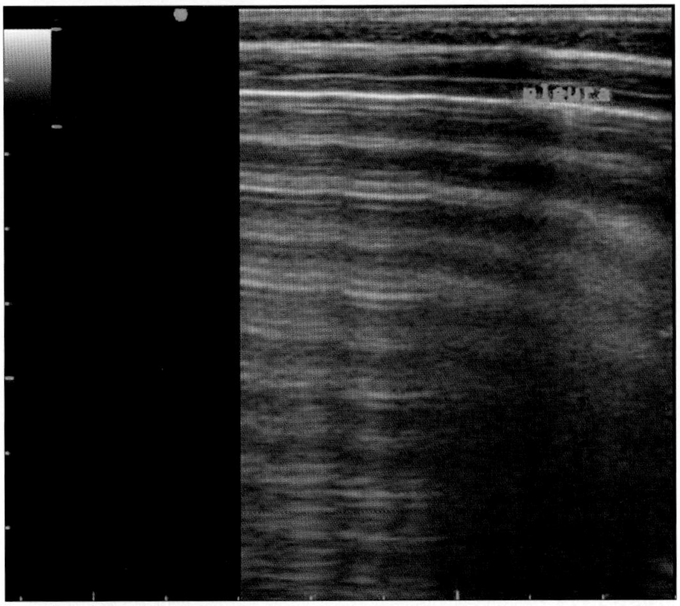

Figure 3.123 Ultrasonographic image of a normal pleura and acoustic echoes.

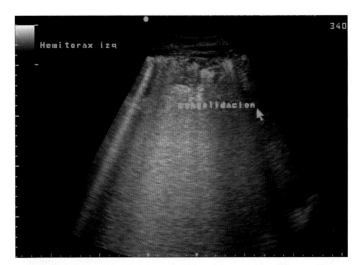

Figure 3.125 Ultrasonogram of the thorax demonstrating pulmonary consolidation. Hypoechoic areas of pulmonary parenchyma that retain the lungs' normal shape are consistent with pulmonary consolidation. These areas are filled with fluid and cellular debris and can have a variety of shapes.

The metabolic effects of the condition are usually serious, with poor, or very poor, oxygenation and progressive sequestration of protein and fluid into the pleural space.

Diagnosis

- Distinguishing a pleuropneumonia from pneumonia on the basis of clinical signs may be difficult and as such a definitive diagnosis usually involves additional imaging modalities with microbiologic and cytologic evaluation of tracheal and pleural fluid aspirates.

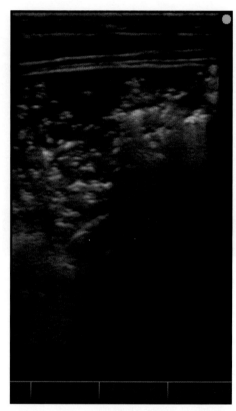

Figure 3.126 Ultrasonogram of thorax demonstrating 'hepatized lung'. A fluid bronchogram is detected when an area of hypoechoic lung parenchyma is seen with fluid-filled bronchial structures. Such areas of lung are called 'hepatized' or 'liver-like' and are associated with more severe pulmonary pathology.

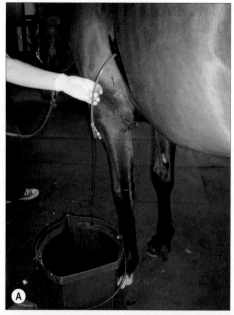

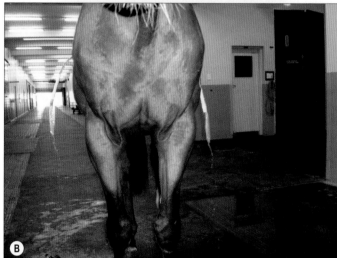

Figure 3.128 (A, B) Pleuritis image of a horse with thoracic drains in place.

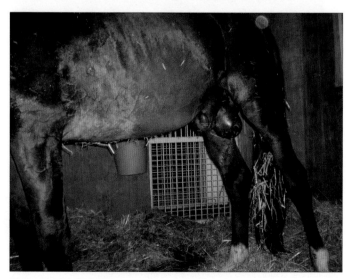

Figure 3.127 Pleuropneumonia results in cachexia with rapid weight loss. Protein loss into the pleural fluid frequently results in ventral edema as in this horse.

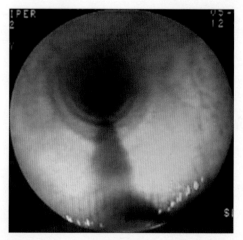

Figure 3.129 Pleuropneumonia endoscopic image showing hemorrhagic exudates in trachea.

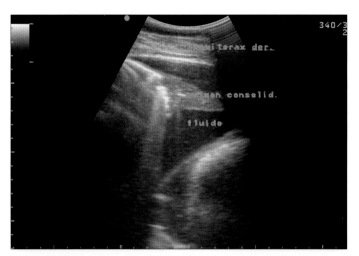

Figure 3.130 Pleuropneumonia. Ultrasonogram showing pleural effusion and consolidation of the ventral lung tip.

Differential diagnosis: most other conditions with significant pleural effusions, such as hydrothorax and neoplasia, have sterile and odor-free pleural aspirates. Very large amounts of fluid which are rapidly replaced in an animal which shows no pleural pain are usually of neoplastic, metabolic or circulatory origin. Pleural effusions may also occur with:
- Thoracic neoplasms
- Thoracic trauma
- Pericariditis
- Peritonitis
- Viral, mycoplasmal and fungal infections
- Congestive heart failure
- Liver disease
- Diaphragmatic hernias
- Hypoproteinemia
- Equine infectious anemia
- Pulmonary granulomata
- Compression of great vessels.

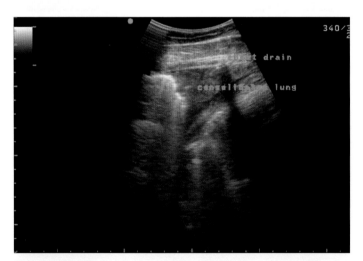

Figure 3.131 Ultrasonographic image of thorax with thoracic drain in place (seen as anechoic shadow). Note the triangular area of pulmonary consolidation.

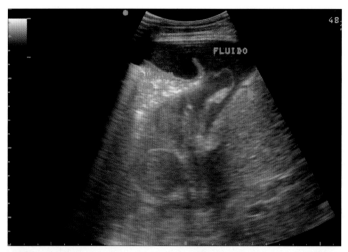

Figure 3.132 Pleuropneumonia pericardial diaphragmatic ligament. This is a membranous structure attached to the diaphragm that is often seen to float in pleural fluid. It should not be confused with fibrin.

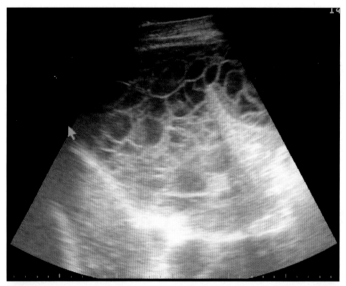

Figure 3.133 Pleuropneumonia. Fibrinous adhesions between lung surface, parietal pleura and diaphragm has resulted in loculation of pleural fluid in this advanced case of pleuropneumonia. Fibrin appears as hypoechoic filamentous strands. The detection of fibrin is associated with a longer treatment period and a poorer prognosis in horses with pleuropneumonia.

- Auscultation may reveal an absence of lung sounds ventrally. Tracheal or bronchial sounds may be heard if lung consolidation is present along with increased radiation of cardiac sounds.
- Palpation may elicit a painful response and percussion reveals decreased resonance ventrally.
- Ultrasonographic examination is the diagnostic aid of choice. It can be used to detect the presence of free or loculated fluid, pleural thickening, pleural, pulmonary or mediastinal abscessation, pulmonary consolidation, fibrinous adhesions and pericarditis. A discrepancy in the height of the fluid levels on the two sides, or differences in the character of the contents, or obvious differences in the ultrasonographic features may indicate a unilateral pleuritis or closure of normal mediastinal fenestrations by fibrin deposition allowing for differing development of the disease process on either side of the thorax.
- Radiographic examination of the chest is a useful adjunct to ultrasonography and will usually identify an obvious horizontal gas–fluid interface which can also be demonstrated by percussion, when the ventral percussible border of the lung will be significantly elevated. However, the purulent material may not always be fluid in consistency and, furthermore, may be loculated into discrete areas making diagnosis more difficult. Some lesions may also be obscured by the cardiac silhouette.

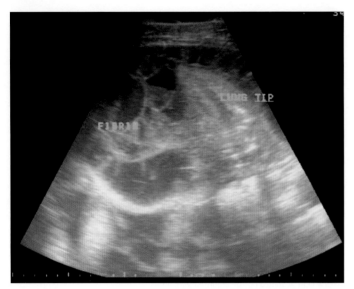

Figure 3.134 (Same horse as Fig. 3.133) This image obtained from the other hemithorax also shows extensive fibrinous adhesions with loculation of pleural fluid.

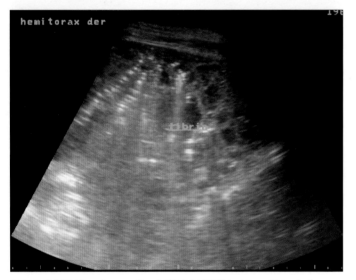

Figure 3.135 (Same horse as Figs. 3.133 & 3.134) This picture obtained a few days later shows a micropolybulbous effusion imaged as pinpoint hyperechoic echoes representing free gas mixed within the pleural fluid. This is highly suggestive of an anaerobic pleuropneumonia or bronchopleural fistula.

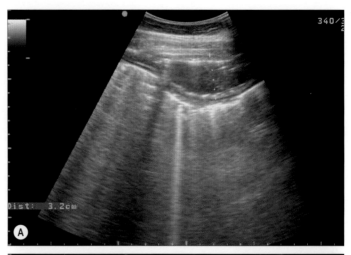

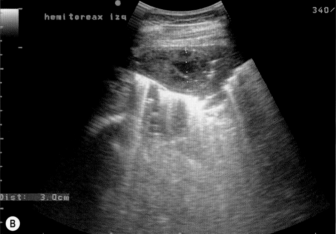

Figure 3.136 (A, B) Pleural abscess. This mare had a penetrating chest injury which resulted in a localized infection and abscess formation. The abscess was drained and flushed in combination with antibiotic therapy. (A) A thick-walled abscess situated between the thoracic wall and lung surface resulting in distortion of the lung surface. (B) Same abscess with a distinct anechoic fluid center and thick fibrous wall.

- Thoracocentesis is indicated to determine the bacteria involved and antibiotic susceptibility. If fluid is present on both sides of the thorax then two separate aspirates should be obtained as the disease process may be somewhat different in the two hemithoraces. Normally the caudal mediastinum is fenestrated in horses but inflammation and the development of fibrin tags may occlude these fenestrations allowing for the differences in the progression of the disease process on either side. Where anaerobic bacteria are present the material obtained by thoracocentesis frequently has a foul odor, which is reflected also in the breath. The fluid will be found to contain a high number of inflammatory cells, most of which will be degenerate, and which form a dense, beige-yellow deposit if the fluid is left to stand for a few minutes.

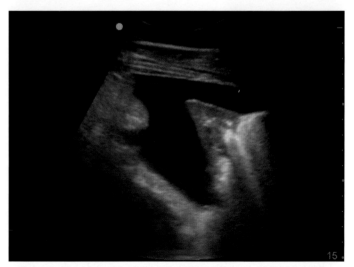

Figure 3.137 Ultrasonographic image of acute pleuropneumonia. Note the hypoechoic fluid with no evidence of fibrin formation. This Thoroughbred returned to racing following treatment including a number of Grade 1 wins.

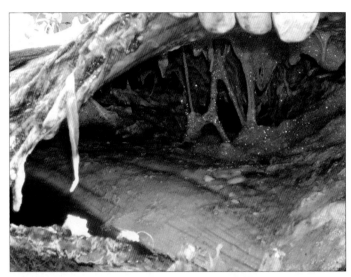

Figure 3.138 Post-mortem findings in cases of infected pleuritis are variable according to the type of bacteria present and the duration of the condition. Longstanding, infective pleuritis cases almost always affect both cavities to about the same extent. Inflammatory debris, fluid in consistency, are reflected in a distinct line of demarcation on the pleural surface, whereas in other cases fibrin will be found over the entire pleural surface. Longstanding inflammation results in the development of extensive (often dense) fibrinous adhesions between the visceral and parietal pleurae.

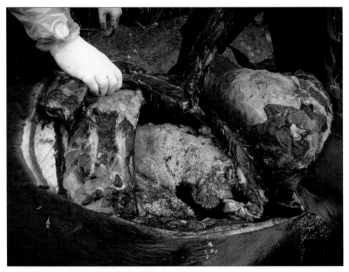

Figure 3.139 Pleuropneumonia post-mortem.

Treatment

The aims of treatment are:

- **Removal of excess pleural fluid**. Pleural fluid is normally removed through the 7th or 8th intercostal space just dorsal to the costo-chondral junction. If small amounts are present drainage with a teat cannula may be sufficient. Placement of an in-dwelling thoracic drain should be considered if:
  - Large amounts of fluid are present
  - The fluid has a pH <7.2 or a nucleated cell count >10 000 cells/μl, and/or protein level >3.5 g/dl
  - Glucose concentration <40 mg/dl or if the horse has responded poorly to prior intermittent drainage.
- **Antibiotic therapy to combat infective processes**. Similar to bacterial pneumonia the ideal antibiotic choice should be based on culture and sensitivity tests. Duration of antibiotic therapy may be

prolonged in many cases and an effort is usually made to change the horse to oral antibiotics as soon as possible based on clinical response.

- **Anti-inflammatory and analgesic therapies**. Pleuritis is a painful condition and efforts should be made to make the horse as comfortable as possible while decreasing the inflammatory response and improving appetite through the judicial use of anti-inflammatories.
- **Supportive care**. This may consist of intravenous fluid therapy, nutritional support and prophylactic treatments for laminitis.

Mycobacterial infection

Although the horse is apparently particularly resistant to infection with *Mycobacteria* spp., pulmonary tuberculosis is recognized in certain parts of the world where the disease associated with this bacterial species in other domestic and wild animals is endemic. Tuberculosis, particularly attributable to *Mycobacterium avium*, in the horse may produce pulmonary or intestinal lesions, and occasionally affects other organs. A chronic, soft cough and weight loss with a bilateral, purulent nasal discharge with some hemorrhage, typical of pulmonary abscess, are the most obvious signs of pulmonary involvement. The pulmonary lesions are characteristically miliary, granulomatous abscesses. Lesions occurring in the intestinal wall are more often single, or few in number and are larger. Intestinal lesions are, in most cases, regarded as the primary lesion resulting from ingestion of the infective organism, from which miliary hematogenous spread occurs to the lungs and other organs.

Glanders

One of the most feared primary contagious bacterial diseases of the horse, donkey and mule is glanders, a disease which has been eradicated from large areas of the world, but which is still endemic in parts of Asia and the Middle East. Glanders has been described for many centuries and its severity and zoonotic nature have resulted in an almost universal fear of the disease. Most countries of the world have strict quarantine measures relating to the control of the infection and these have largely been successful in reducing the incidence and, in many places, completely eradicating it. The ease of worldwide transportation of horses makes its recognition extremely important. The condition is caused by *Burkholderia mallei*. Pulmonary, nasal and cutaneous forms are recognized. All are more or less chronic in their course and characterized by the formation of nodules, ulcers and fibrous scars in the skin and respiratory tract.

Clinical signs

- Acute glanders is rarely encountered in horses but donkeys and mules are often severely affected by this form. There are few pathognomonic features, but most cases have a tenacious, unilateral, hemorrhagic, mucopurulent nasal discharge, and obvious ulceration of the nasal mucosa. The profuse discharge and nasal and laryngeal edema induce severe respiratory obstruction. A marked, non-abscess-forming lymphadenopathy of the glands of the head is a common feature. Death as a result of overwhelming bronchopneumonia, respiratory obstruction and septicemia follows in a few days.
- Horses are more commonly affected by the subacute or chronic pulmonary forms, which have an insidious onset, often lasting several months or even longer. In the early stages there may be few overt pathognomonic features with some cases showing only a mild, tenacious, catarrhal nasal discharge which can easily be mistaken for other respiratory tract infections. Horses with the chronic form of glanders often appear to be remarkably well, and may show a normal enthusiasm for work for extended periods of time. There may be little indication of the potential danger of the nasal discharges, both for the horse itself, and in-contact equidae and humans.

- While, in some cases, the disease may remain in this form for long periods, any superimposed stress (or other disease) will usually result in an immediate development of the subacute form. Coughing, weight loss, intermittent or persistent fever, pneumonia and a high respiratory rate may be present. The chronic form ultimately develops into either the naso-pulmonary form or into '**farcy**' (the cutaneous form). Here, ulcerative nodules, which discharge a brownish, honey-colored pus containing small yellow or brown granules, occur on the nasal, pharyngeal and tracheal mucosae, and along cutaneous lymphatics, particularly over the face, neck and the medial thigh and hock regions. Typically, the nasal lesions heal slowly, leaving a stellate scar. Horses affected with any of the forms of glanders lose weight dramatically, and almost all will finally develop the true pneumonic form which terminates fatally. A few horses recover and return to normal health after a very prolonged convalescence, often lasting some years.

- At post-mortem examination, which is not without major hazard to the operator, characteristic abscesses and lesions in the respiratory tract, lung, spleen and liver will be present. In the chronic form the obvious nasal ulceration takes on a more benign appearance with a 'glassy' hue and is covered with thick, gray, semi-transparent, tenacious mucus.

- In endemic areas the disease may be confused in its early stages with strangles and other lesser respiratory viral infections, but while in a few cases the condition may remain mild for long periods, it seldom if ever resolves.

Diagnosis

- Culture from lesions on blood or meat nutrient agar. Cultures can also be obtained from sputum or urine but blood cultures are frequently negative. PCR tests are available in some laboratories and newer tests can differentiate *B. mallei* from *B. pseudomallei*.

- Serology is rarely useful as high background titers in normal serum complicate interpretation. In addition, serologic reactions to *B. mallei* cannot be differentiated from reactions to *B. pseudomallei* and these tests are not available in all countries. Additionally, positive reactions in agglutination tests develop after 7–10 days.

- Radiography is helpful in the pulmonary form. The lesions may include bilateral bronchopneumonia, miliary nodules, segmental or lobar infiltrates and cavitating lesions.

- ***Differential diagnosis:*** **Melioidosis** is a condition that closely resembles glanders which occurs in the Far East and northern parts of Australia, and is caused by *Burkholderia pseudomallei*. Definitive diagnosis of the disease is usually reliant upon post-mortem examination and bacterial culture. Affected horses develop a fulminating bronchopneumonia, encephalitis and enteritis. While almost every case of melioidosis will be diagnosed in the acute stage, most cases will have been affected previously by an often almost inapparent infection, which may have been present for months before the acute stage develops. The chronic form of the disease affecting the skin and the lungs is probably clinically indistinguishable from glanders.

Treatment

- In many countries glanders is a notifiable disease with a strict slaughter policy due to the implications for human health.

- Glanders can be treated with antibiotics. Few studies have been published on the antibiotic susceptibility of *B. mallei*, but some treatment recommendations are available. Long-term treatment or multiple drugs may be necessary. Abscesses may need to be drained.

- Strict precautions should be taken when handling infected animals and contaminated fomites. Protective clothing including heavy gloves and face shields should be worn when working with infected animals.

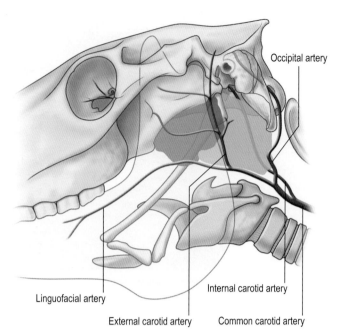

Figure 3.140 Guttural pouch anatomy. The external carotid artery and external maxillary vein course the lateral compartment, along with the pharyngeal branch of the vagus nerve, cranial laryngeal nerve, CNVII (facial) and the mandibular branch of CNV (trigeminal). The internal carotid artery and CNIX and XII can be seen clearly in the medial compartment. CN X (vagus) and CNXI (accessory) and the pharyngeal branch of CN X also course under the medial compartment.

Fungal diseases
Guttural pouch mycosis (see Figs. 3.140–3.146)

Guttural pouch mycosis involves the development of fungal plaques within the mucosa of the walls of the guttural pouches. These are most commonly located on the roof of the medial compartment but can also be seen on the lateral wall of the lateral compartment. They are usually closely associated with underlying vascular structures. Fungal colonization leads to erosion of underlying vascular structures or inflammatory injury to adjacent nerves.

The exact etiology and pathogenesis of the condition is not known. There is no apparent age, sex, breed or geographical predilection.

Clinical signs are generally only noticed when there is vascular or neurological compromise. Epistaxis is the most common sign associated with vascular compromise. A single or repeated mild epistaxis usually involving scanty volumes of dark blood or a somewhat more obvious nasal bleeding is usually reported to precede a severe or extreme bilateral arterial epistaxis which may be precipitated by stress such as transport or restraint.

Neurological signs associated with the condition reflect the affected nerves.

Pharyngeal paralysis is the most frequent neuropathy seen which results in dysphagia and coughing. It likely results from damage to the pharyngeal branches of the vagus and glossopharyngeal nerves. Recovery from pharyngeal paralysis and dysphagia can occur but frequently recovery is incomplete.

Laryngeal hemiplegia (cranial laryngeal nerve) is the next most common but rarely results in signs which can be immediately noticed by the owner. Facial paralysis and Horner's syndrome can also occur (facial nerve).

Diagnosis and treatment

- The condition may be suspected on the basis of the clinical signs but confirmation requires endoscopic identification of a fungal plaque within the guttural pouch.

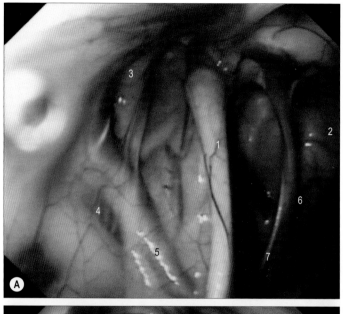

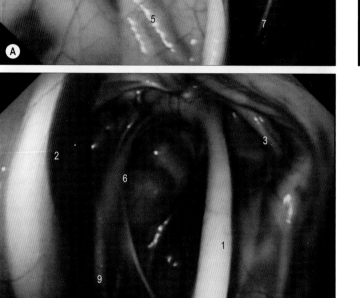

Figure 3.141 (A, B) Different images of normal guttural pouches (endoscopic view). The guttural pouches are reflected around the dorsal border of the stylohyoid bone which divides the pouch into a larger medial and a smaller lateral compartment. 1. Stylohyoid bone; 2. Medial compartment; 3. Lateral compartment; 4. Maxillary vein; 5. External carotid artery; 6. Internal carotid artery; 7. Glossopharyngeal nerves; 8. Hypoglossal nerves; 9. Vagus nerves..

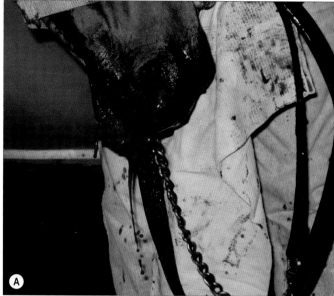

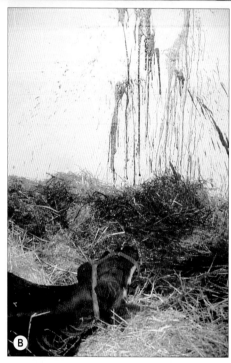

Figure 3.142 Guttural pouch mycosis. (A) Arterial epistaxis. (B) Fatal hemorrhage.

- Endoscopic examination should not be attempted soon after an episode of epistaxis as the plaque may be difficult to visualize if the pouch is full of blood and there is a risk of dislodging a clot to induce another episode of hemorrhage.
- Treatment depends on the stage of the disease. Medical treatment which usually consists of topical and parenteral antimycotic drugs can be attempted if the condition is in the early stages and the clinical signs are not yet marked.
- Frequently a combination of surgical and medical therapy is required with surgery aimed at occlusion of the affected vessels. Supportive care and anti-inflammatories are important in cases demonstrating neurological abnormalities.

Fungal rhinitis (Figs. 3.147 & 3.148)

The nasal cavity of horses may be affected by various fungal infections.

Phycomycosis due to infections by *Pythium insidiosum* or *Entomophthora* coronate (*Conidiobolus coronata*) occurs predominately in the United States of America, occasionally in Australia, and rarely in other warm, wet climatic regions. Infection results in numerous small granulating ulcers or fissures in the rostral part of the nasal cavity. In some cases the size of the lesion and the associated inflammatory response may be sufficient to occlude the affected nostril. Cases are, consequently, presented for the investigation of respiratory stridor, exercise intolerance and/or chronic, unilateral, purulent, nasal

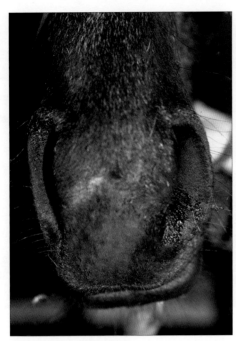

Figure 3.143 Guttural pouch mycosis epistaxis (for differentials see Figs. 3.81–3.83)

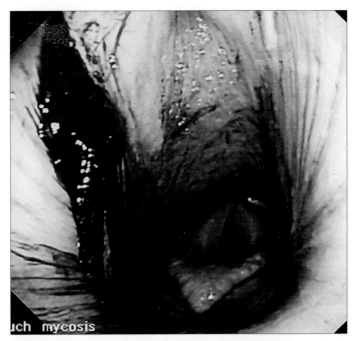

Figure 3.145 Endoscopic view of the pharynx showing hemorrhage from one guttural pouch.

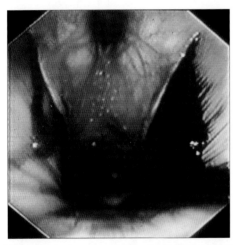

Figure 3.144 Endoscopic view of the pharynx showing hemorrhage from both guttural pouches.

superficial proliferation of fungal mycelium over the surface of the nasal mucosa. Little clinical effect may be present and most such lesions are detected incidentally, although a mild yellowish mucoid nasal discharge may be encountered. The more serious invasive or destructive form occurs on the mucosa of the nasal turbinates and occasionally within the maxillary or frontal sinuses. This form results in extensive destruction of the mucosa and the underlying bone. A surprisingly scanty, foul-smelling, unilateral, purulent nasal discharge, possibly containing some blood, is usually present, reflecting the limited inflammatory response within the nasal mucosa around the active lesion. The erosive lesion is often black or very dark-red in color and a fine white, or gray, mycelium can usually be seen over the surface. Secondary bacterial infection is uncommon. While the larger lesions are pathognomonic for the condition, they may be very small and difficult to appreciate in some cases, and then culture from the nasal discharge or from the surface of the lesions is diagnostic. Topical treatment with enilconazole is generally curative but a treatment course of up to 6 weeks may be required.

Fungal pneumonia
Primary pulmonary pathogens in horses are:

- **Blastomyces dermatitidis** rarely causes respiratory disease in the horse but inhalation of the spores can on occasion result in a pyo-granulomatous pneumonia.
- **Coccidioides immitis**. Inhalation of windborne arthrospores results in pneumonia and pleuritis. Lymphohematogenous dissemination can produce bone, skin and CNS lesions.
- **Cryptococcus neoformans**. Inhalation results in respiratory tract infections with secondary hematogenous spread to the CNS.
- **Histoplasma capulatum**. The horse appears particularly resistant to infection but inhalation can result in respiratory tract infection. However, disease is more commonly seen in the liver, spleen, lymph nodes and bone marrow.

Clinical signs
- Horses with primary fungal pneumonia may have chronic cough, nasal discharge, exercise intolerance, anorexia and weight loss.

discharge which may contain blood. Air flow patterns through the affected nostril may be impaired and where the disease extends into the sinuses these may become dull-sounding on percussion. The lesions are frequently pruritic, resulting in self-trauma. The lesions may be visualized directly or by endoscopy. Surgical excision combined with topical amphotericin B is often successful in the early stages.

Cryptococcosis as a result of infection with *Cryptococcus neoformans* causes granuloma formation and an invasive rhinitis and sinusitis often accompanied by draining tracts through the facial bones. The nasal discharges are usually mucopurulent and sanguineous and have a foul odor which may also be confused with secondary sinusitis. Confirmation of infection is by histology of biopsies, cytology and culture.

Aspergillosis as a result of infection with **Aspergillus** spp. is commonly encountered in most parts of the world and nasal aspergillosis occurs in two main forms. Non-invasive aspergillosis results in a

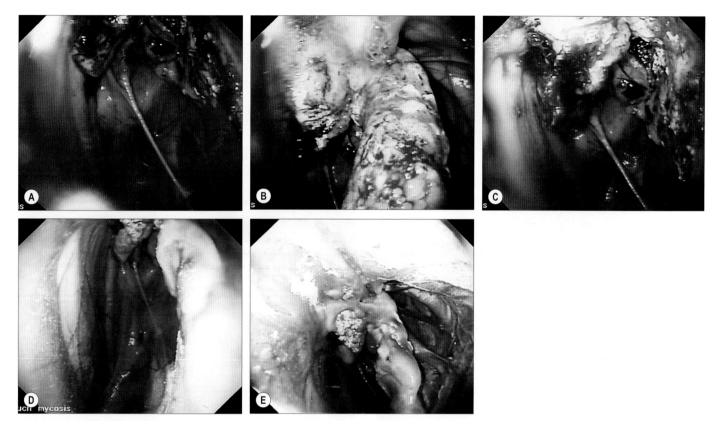

Figure 3.146 Endoscopic images of fungal plaques within the guttural pouch. (A) Extensive lesion along dorsal aspect of medial compartment. (B) Fungal plaque along hyoid bone. (C) Fungal plaque on dorsal wall of medial compartment of pouch. (D, E) Extensive lesion along hyoid bone extending to dorsal wall of medial compartment.

- Tachypnea and respiratory distress are variably present.
- Pleural effusion is found most commonly with coccidiomycosis but has been reported with blastomycosis and cryptococcosis.

Diagnosis

- Radiography and ultrasonography may demonstrate typical pneumonic changes but are not specific for fungal infections.
- Tracheobronchial aspirates may reveal degenerate neutrophils and fungal elements. The difficulty lies in the fact that fungal elements can be obtained from normal horses as the tracheal contaminant.
- Serological detection of an antibody response has been useful with *Coccidiodes* sp., *Cryptococcus* sp. and *Histoplasma* sp.

Treatment

- Long-term administration of antifungal drugs is required for primary fungal infections (10–12 weeks).
- Two classes of antifungal drugs exist:
  - Polyene antibiotics: amphotericin B, nystatin and natamycin.
  - Azoles: miconazole, ketoconazole, itraconazole and fluconazole.
- Drug selection should ideally be based on sensitivity testing.

Secondary opportunistic pathogens in horses
(Figs. 3.149 & 3.150)

***Aspergillus* spp**. These fungi are ubiquitous in the environment. Inhalation of spores is common but disease is rare unless the patient is immuno-compromised. Infection is characterized by hyphal invasion of blood vessels, thrombosis, necrosis and hemorrhagic infarction. Disease is most commonly seen in horses with enterocolitis that have received broad-spectrum antibiotics and anti-inflammatories and that are neutropenic.

***Pneumocystis jiroveci* (formerly *P. carinii*).** Formerly considered a protozoan organism, which has been reclassified as a fungus. The infective stage or source of *P. jiroveci* is unknown but recent investigations suggest that it may be transmitted in water or an airborne route.

P. jiroveci pneumonia is thought to occur primarily in immuno-compromised foals as a complication of some other serious illness such as infectious pneumonia or severe combined immunodeficiency (SCID).

Clinical signs

- Horses with pulmonary aspergillosis may suddenly become febrile and tachypneic with adventitious lung sounds with or without a nasal discharge. Other horses may fail to show signs related to respiratory tract infection and signs related to the primary disorder may predominate.
- In foals with *Pneumocystis jiroveci* dyspnea occurs secondary to the plasmacytic lymphocytic interstitial pneumonia and the flooding of the alveoli with foamy exudate. It is usually an acutely fatal disease.

Diagnosis and treatment

- It is very difficult to obtain a diagnosis ante-mortem. Serological testing to date is not reliable for aspergillosis although a number of experimental assays exist. The use of either a bronchoalveolar lavage or a transtracheal wash has been suggested for identifying *Pneumocystis carinii* intracellularly in macrophages but results may be variable. Confirmation is by identification of the organisms by either silver staining or immunostaining.
- Pulmonary aspergillosis can be treated similar to primary pulmonary fungal infections. Successful treatment with amphotericin B has been reported.
- Prognosis is considered guarded for foals with pneumocystosis but successful treatment has been achieved with the use of either

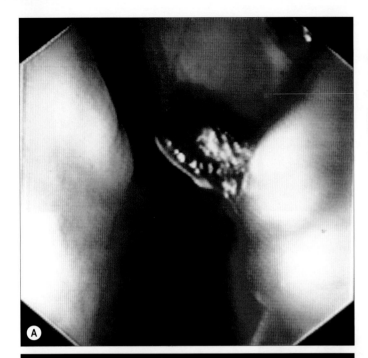

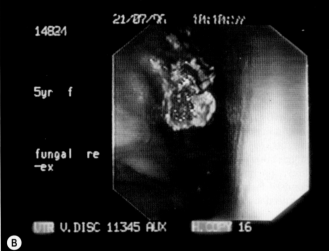

Figure 3.147 Nasal rhinitis. (A) Aspergillosis. (B) Fungal plaque in the nasal cavity.

Differential diagnosis:
- Conidiobolus coronate infection
- Nasal amyloidosis
- Glanders.

potentiated sulfonamides and/or dapsone (3 mg/kg [1.4 mg/lb], PO, q 24 h [dose extrapolated from human data]). Dapsone may be a useful adjunct to traditional treatment for *P. carinii* pneumonia in horses or as a sole medication for horses that cannot tolerate other treatments. Treatment is usually prolonged (45–50 days).

Equine multinodular pulmonary fibrosis
(Figs. 3.151 & 3.152)

Equine multinodular pulmonary fibrosis is a relatively newly recognized and emerging disease of horses. It is regarded as a clinically progressive nodular fibrotic form of inflammatory lung disease that occurs in adult horses with a mean age of 14.5 years. The disorder does not appear to have a sex or breed predilection. It has a characteristic clinical presentation with a history of decreased appetite,

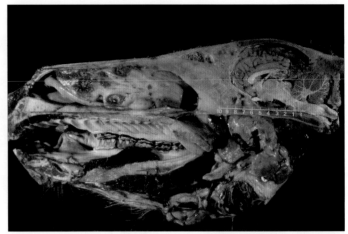

Figure 3.148 Nasal rhinitis. Extensive conidiobolus coronate infection with reactive fibrous tissue resulting in occlusion of the nasal cavity in this horse.

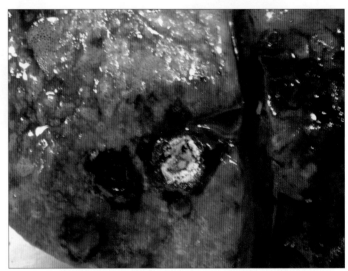

Figure 3.149 Pulmonary aspergillosis. Distinct fungal lesion on the lung surface of a mare that died acutely. She had previously undergone two colic surgeries in the space of 3 days. The pulmonary fungal infection was thought to be secondary to the gastrointestinal problems.

weight loss, cough, tachypnea and respiratory distress. The etiology is not currently understood but it is believed that there may be an association with equine herpesvirus-5 infection. Clinical signs include persistent pyrexia, increased bronchovesicular sounds with wheezes on auscultation and markedly increased respiratory rate and effort.

Diagnosis
- Radiography reveals a diffuse bronchointerstitial pattern with multiple coalescing circular nodules. This appearance may be similar to horses with fungal pneumonia or pulmonary neoplasms.
- Ultrasound examination reveals multiple circular hypoechoic masses involving the periphery of the lung and pulmonary parenchyma. The masses are bilateral and pleural effusion is generally not present.
- Hematology findings of neutrophilic leucocytosis and hyperfibrinogenemia are non-specific.
- BAL and TTW samples reveal neutrophilic and macrophagic inflammation but bacterial culture rarely reveals a growth and virus isolation is also generally unrewarding.

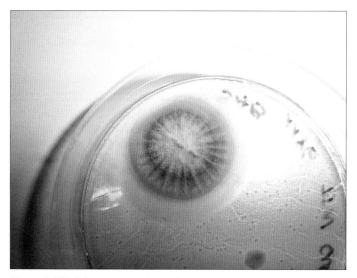

Figure 3.150 Pulmonary aspergillosis culture. Distinct fungal colony of *Aspergillus* sp. from a transtracheal wash sample. The mare in question had initially presented with diarrhea but had subsequently undergone colic surgery. Pulmonary ultrasound changes were noted in association with the onset of fevers. Soon after the TTW sample was obtained the mare started to demonstrate neurological signs and was euthanized. Post-mortem examination revealed a fungal pneumonia and fungal meningoencephalitis.

- Histological examination of biopsy specimens is required for confirmation.

Treatment
- There is a limited number of reported treated cases. In those, a combination of immunosuppressive therapy with dexamethasone (0.4 mg/kg q 24 h) and antiviral therapy with acyclovir (20 mg/kg PO q 8 h) were used.
- The prognosis is considered as poor but in the reported treated cases there was some improvement noted in a number of the horses.

Parasitic diseases
Parascaris equorum
The lifecycle of **Parascaris equorum** in foals involves a period of lung migration. The condition is exclusively found in foals less than 4–6 months old, older horses being solidly immune unless immuno-compromised.

Clinical effects of this migration have not been well defined, though heavily infested young foals may develop a marked productive cough, hyperpnea, loss of weight and very occasionally overt pneumonia.

In many cases, however, the extent of the inflammatory response is marked while few parasites are present.

Diagnosis
- Diagnosis of verminous (ascarid) pneumonia in foals is usually retrospective and speculative where specific treatment results in resolution.
- Endoscopic examination usually shows a profuse mucoid exudate within the trachea, in which the larvae may occasionally be identified.

Dictyocaulus arnfieldi
This **equine lungworm** occurs in most parts of the world but is rarely responsible for disease in horses. It is relatively common in Europe and less so in North America, Africa and Australasia. The primary hosts for the parasite are probably the donkey, mule and the tapir.

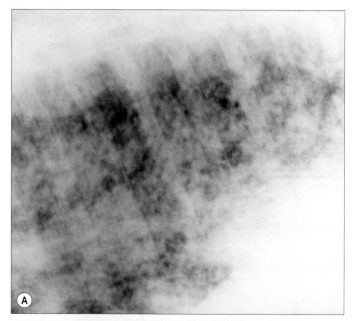
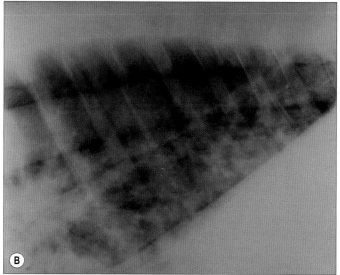

Figure 3.151 (A, B) Multinodular pulmonary fibrosis. The radiographic findings are the most distinctive clinical diagnostic feature. There is a diffuse bronchointerstitial pattern with multiple coalescing circular nodules throughout the lung field.

In primary hosts the parasite causes little or no harmful effect, apart from a mild but persistent, non-progressive cough. Horses grazing the same pasture as donkeys may become infested and this results in a similar clinical syndrome but which is often more severe.

Diagnosis and treatment
- Tracheal aspiration is commonly used to diagnose the disorder when a few parasites, or their eggs or larvae, can be identified in an exudate which contains large numbers of degenerate neutrophils and eosinophils.
- Endoscopic examination may identify the presence of adult or larval forms of the parasite.
- As the horse is not the definitive natural (preferred) host for the parasite, adult, egg-laying worms are less common than in the donkey and consequently examination of feces for larvae is often unrewarding.

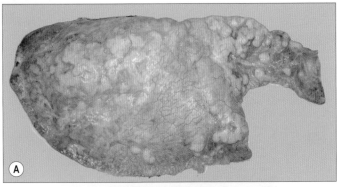

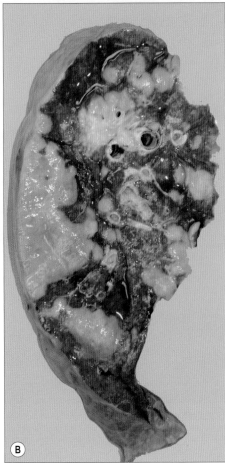

Figure 3.152 (A, B) Multinodular pulmonary fibrosis. This 9-year-old female TB presented with dyspnea, fever and weight loss for approximately a month. The mare had been diagnosed with equine multinodular pulmonary fibrosis via biopsy and was euthanized.

- A specific diagnosis depends upon historical contact with donkeys, identification of the larvae (or eggs) in tracheal aspirations or in feces and a dramatic benefit from specific treatment.
- Moxidectin is 99.9% effective in treating *D. arnfieldi* infections in donkeys. Ivermectin also has good efficacy.

Pulmonary hydatidosis

This represents the intermediate stage of the canine tapeworm, *Echinococcus granulosis* var. *equinum*, and historically has been encountered as an incidental finding during thoracic radiography, when one, or more, radio-dense, cyst like structures may be seen. The presence of a thoracic lesion may be indicative of other (abdominal) lesions and

where these are present in large numbers, particularly on or in the liver, some metabolic effects are to be expected. Large numbers of parasitic cysts may be present without any detectable clinical effect.

Neoplastic disorders

Upper respiratory tract

Perhaps the commonest malignant neoplasm in the airways of the horse is **squamous cell carcinoma**. All forms are rare, but may affect the nasal cavity, sinuses, guttural pouches and pharynx. Occasionally, local invasion occurs and, although they seldom metastasize from these sites, they may have severe local consequences. Primary lesions of **lymphosarcoma** may also be found in the pharynx where, as part of the multicentric form of the disorder, they may cause obvious and debilitating dysphagia with chronic, persistent, nasal regurgitation of food and saliva.

Clinical signs

- The clinical signs associated with neoplasia of the upper airway are frequently non-specific.
- Nasal discharges (often with blood) may be odor-free or, where bone is involved, may have a strong, necrotic odor.
- Airway obstructions are likely where the lesions are present in the nasal cavity, guttural pouches, paranasal sinuses or pharynx.
- Dysphagia may be encountered where lesions interfere with either the physical or neurological function of the pharynx.
- Masses located rostrally in the nasal cavity usually expand outwards producing facial distortions with little encroachment on the nasal cavity itself, whereas lesions occurring more caudally create less facial distortion but more encroachment into the nasal cavity. The latter masses may result in significant and dangerous nasal occlusion when their expansion extends across the nasal septum.

Diagnosis and treatment

- Lateral and ventro-dorsal radiographs may be used to define both their extent and their effect on adjacent bony and soft tissue structures.
- Frequently neoplasia of the upper respiratory tract is advanced when diagnosed, often with extension to regional lymph nodes. This fact combined with surgical difficulties of tumor resection in the area means many of these neoplasms carry a poor prognosis for long-term survival.

Pulmonary neoplasms (Figs. 3.153–3.156)

Primary pulmonary neoplasms are very rare in the horse and, with the possible exception of **lymphosarcoma**, most thoracic neoplasms of the horse are secondary metastatic tumors. Clinical signs attributable to pulmonary lesions are not specific and many cases are largely asymptomatic until they reach an advanced stage.

Gray horses in particular are liable to the development of **melanomas**, which may affect many internal organs, including the lungs.

Malignant tumors (**adenocarcinomata or squamous cell carcinomata**) in any remote organ might be expected to result in secondary masses in the lung. Even secondary lesions will, however, exert a significant effect on pulmonary function, although this may have limited clinical effects upon the horse in the early stages. Poor exercise tolerance, coughing, hemoptysis and a hemorrhagic nasal discharge may be attributable to primary or secondary pulmonary neoplasia but it is surprising how seldom these are presented, even in severe, invasive neoplasia. The difficulties associated with thoracic radiography of the horse, however, mean that many of these cases (particularly where the lesions are very small) may not be detectable before death. At post-mortem examination the lesions of any secondary

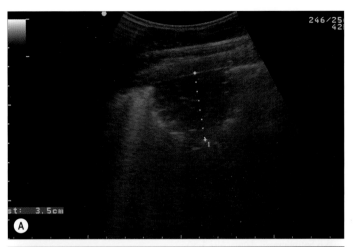

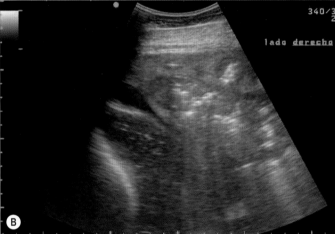

Figure 3.153 Ultrasonographic images of pulmonary neoplasms. (A) A discrete mass is visualised within the pulmonary parenchyma. (B) Multiple masses are visualised within a consolidated lung. These masses were of mixed echogenicity. This horse presented with a recent history of sudden weight loss and intermittent respiratory distress related to exercise. The other lung was normal on ultrasound examination.

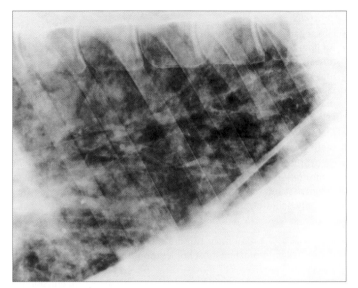

Figure 3.154 Radiograph from a horse with pulmonary adenocarcinoma. Note the diffuse nodules throughout the lung field.

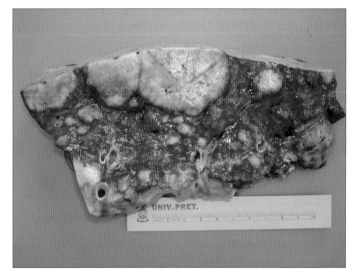

Figure 3.155 Post-mortem pulmonary adenocarcinoma.

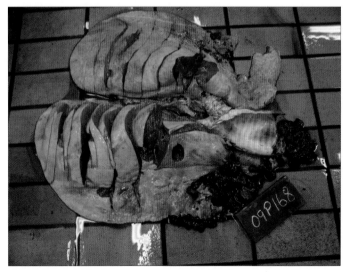

Figure 3.156 Pulmonary metastasis of melanoma. Image courtesy of Irish Equine Centre..

tumor are usually evenly distributed through the lung. Squamous cell carcinomas appear to result in little or no pulmonary interference, in spite of extensive infiltration, and no pleural effusions are usually encountered.

Clinical signs

- Horses with thoracic neoplasia often have a history of sudden-onset dramatic weight loss despite a good appetite, although some may be inappetant.
- Exercise intolerance, intermittent fevers and ventral edema are also frequently seen.
- Many horses will not have clinical signs referable to the respiratory tract, especially those with metastatic lesions where signs related to the primary neoplasm may predominate.
- In others, respiratory signs may include hemorrhagic or mucohemorrhagic nasal discharge, coughing, increased adventitial sounds or decreased adventitial sounds in cases where pleural fluid is present.
- Hypertrophic pulmonary osteoarthropathy characterized by enlargement of joints, bony swelling of distal limbs (especially forelimbs) and generalized stiffness has been reported in cases of granular cell tumors.

Diagnosis

- History and clinical signs may be suggestive in some cases.
- Radiography and ultrasonography may reveal the presence of multifocal interstitial densities (2–3 cm in diameter). Mediastinal masses may be detected in some horses and large amounts of pleural fluid are particularly common with lymphomas. Endoscopy may reveal the presence of bronchial masses in cases of granular cell tumors and bronchogenic carcinomas.
- Pleuroscopy may be indicated in some cases where pleural involvement is suspected.
- Pleural fluid aspirates, trachobronchial aspirates and histological examination of biopsy specimens may aid in the diagnosis, but a negative result does not necessarily rule out neoplasia. Many cases are only definitely diagnosed retrospectively at necropsy.

Treatment

- Most cases of pulmonary tumors have a very poor prognosis; if diagnosed ante-mortem most horses are euthanized to avoid unnecessary suffering.
- Temporary relief can be achieved in horses with pleural effusion by thoracocentesis and short-term therapy with corticosteroids can be considered in pregnant mares to enable delivery of term foals.
- Localized tumors with low metastatic potential such as granular cell tumors can be treated by lung resection.

References and further reading

ACVIM concensus statement: Equine Herpesvirus. www.acvim.org.

ACVIM concensus statement: Rhodococcus equi. www.acvim.org.

Berghaus, L.J., Giguère, S., Sturgill, T.L., et al., 2012. Plasma pharmacokinetics, pulmonary distribution, and in vitro activity of gamithromycin in foals. J Vet Pharmacol Ther 35 (1), 59–66.

Chaffin, M.K., Cohen, N.D., Martens, R.J., et al., 2011. Evaluation of the efficacy of gallium maltolate for chemoprophylaxis against pneumonia caused by *Rhodococcus equi* infection in foals. Am J Vet Res 72 (7), 945–957.

Giguère, S., Cohen, N.D., Chaffin, M.K., et al., 2011. Diagnosis, treatment, control, and prevention of infections caused by *Rhodococcus equi* in foals. J Vet Intern Med 25 (6), 1209–1220.

Khan, I., Wieler, L.H., Melzer, F., et al., 2012. Glanders in animals: A review on epidemiology, clinical presentation, diagnosis and countermeasures. Transbound Emerg Dis 60 (3), 204–221.

McAuliffe, S.B., Slovis, N.M., 2008. Colour Atlas of Diseases and Disorders of the Foal. WB Saunders, Philadelphia, PA, USA.

Mendez, D.H., Judd, J., Speare, R., 2012. Unexpected result of Hendra virus outbreaks for veterinarians, Queensland, Australia. Emerg Infect Dis 18 (1), 83–85.

Reed, S.M., Bayly, W.M., Sellon, D.C., 2009. Equine Internal Medicine, third ed. WB Saunders, St. Louis, MO, USA.

Reuss, S.M., Chaffin, M.K., Cohen, N.D., 2009. Extrapulmonary disorders associated with *Rhodococcus equi* infection in foals: 150 cases (1987–2007). J Am Vet Med Assoc 235 (7), 855–863.

Robinson, N.E., Sprayberry, K.A. (Eds.), 2009. Current Therapy in Equine Medicine, sixth ed. WB Saunders, St. Louis, MO, USA.

Rush, B., Mair, T., 2004. Equine Respiratory Diseases. Blackwell, Oxford, UK.

Tahon, L., Baselgia, S., Gerber, V., et al., 2009 In vitro allergy tests compared to intradermal testing in horses with recurrent airway obstruction. Vet Immunol Immunopathol 127 (1–2), 85–93.

CHAPTER 4

Disorders of the cardiovascular system

CHAPTER CONTENTS

Part 1: The heart and blood vessels

Developmental disorders

Serious and/or complicated congenital defects of the circulation such as **cardiac ectopia** usually result in intrauterine death but some cardiac and vascular anomalies may only become evident after birth, and sometimes much later when the animal starts to work. Defects of structure in the heart usually arise within the first 50 days of gestation, when the rate of development of the heart is maximal.

Persistent neonatal pulmonary hypertension

If the 'normal' anatomical and physiological transitions from fetal to neonatal circulation do not occur, a condition of persistent pulmonary hypertension can arise. This has also been known as 'persistent fetal circulation'.

This condition results in systemic arterial hypoxemia due to increased pulmonary vascular resistance and shunting of pulmonary blood to the systemic circulation. Failure of the pulmonary vascular resistance to lessen post partum despite alveolar expansion and alveolar oxygenation encourages continued variable shunting of blood through the ductus arteriosus and/or foramen ovale with resultant systemic arterial hypoxemia.

A progressive cyanosis is the most prominent clinical feature of this condition with stunting, poor (or extremely poor) exercise tolerance and a secondary polycythemia.

Diagnosis and treatment

- Clinical signs. Auscultation and cardiac echocardiography may demonstrate a PDA or persistent foramen ovale.
- Following O_2 administration, a right foreleg (preductal) PaO_2 will likely show a tension difference/gradient (> 20 mmHg) when compared to a hind limb (postductal) if PDA shunting is substantial. This gradient may not be present, however, if foramen ovale shunting is marked.
- Treatment generally needs to be undertaken at a referral institute and may include mechanical ventilation, decreasing pulmonary hypertension by the use of inhaled nitric oxide or sildenafil.

Congenital cardiac abnormalities

Ninety percent of newborn foals have been reported to have audible murmurs and 96% to have various arrhythmias which normally disappear by 15 minutes post-partum. Hypoxemia and elevated vagal tone likely account for many of these electrical disturbances.

Clinical findings such as widely radiating grade (III/V or greater) murmurs, cyanosis, jugular pulses, peripheral edema, ascites, pleural effusion or syncope, weakness, growth retardation +/− lethargy are suggestive of cardiovascular insufficiency.

Patent ductus arteriosus (PDA) (Fig. 4.1)

The ductus arteriosus in the fetus normally shunts blood from the pulmonary artery to the aorta. It is regarded as physiologically normal for a foal to maintain some shunting of blood in the opposite direction (i.e. from aorta to pulmonary artery) for up to 72 hours after birth. A large persistent PDA typically results in enlargement of the left atrium and ventricle. Over time, if the pulmonary arterial pressure rises substantially, right-sided congestive heart insufficiency/failure may ensue.

The murmur is typically described as a loud, continuous ('machinery') murmur, accompanied by a detectable thrill which is most obvious over the left side at the base of the heart, or slightly above this point. However, by the time many of these foals present the continuous murmur may be absent and replaced by a systolic murmur. This is due to pulmonary hypertension which restricts the flow within the ductus during diastole.

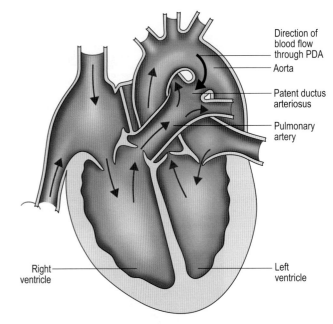

Direction of blood flow through PDA

Aorta

Patent ductus arteriosus

Pulmonary artery

Right ventricle

Left ventricle

Figure 4.1 Schematic representation of a PDA. Reproduced from McAuliffe SB, Slovis NM (eds). *Color Atlas of Diseases and Disorders of the Foal* (2008), with permission from Elsevier.

Clinically, foals with persistent large bore PDAs may have increased peripheral pulse pressure. This increase in pulse pressure is often described as 'bounding' due to the left ventricular increased stroke volume +/− related systolic hypertension and decreased diastolic pressure from the aortic blood pushing into the pulmonary circulation via the PDA. The foal may grow reasonably, but most cases show considerable exercise intolerance and are often noted to be reluctant to play with other foals and lag behind the dam.

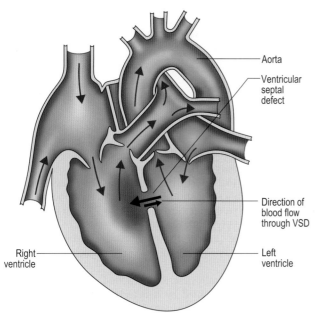

Figure 4.2 Schematic representation of a ventricular septal defect (VSD). Reproduced from McAuliffe SB, Slovis NM (eds). *Color Atlas of Diseases and Disorders of the Foal* (2008), with permission from Elsevier.

Diagnosis and treatment

- Foals in which suspicion that the PDA is functionally patent for greater than 1 week should have further cardiac diagnostic testing with echocardiographic +/− radiographic and blood gas evaluations.
- Since the patency of the PDA is maintained by production of PGE_2 by the ductus arteriosus, prostaglandin suppression through cyclooxygenase inhibitors (i.e. flunixin meglumine, ibuprofen, indometacin, etc.) may elicit closure of the PDA in some cases.

Ventricular septal defect (VSD) (Figs. 4.2–4.5)

Reportedly this is the most frequently occurring congenital cardiac defect in large animals. Foals with VSDs often have readily auscultable murmurs on both sides of the thorax. The majority are situated in the membranous portion of the septum in the left ventricular outflow tract immediately below the right coronary cusp of the aortic valve and the tricuspid valve. Most VSDs are not clinically significant and many are found as incidental findings. In those which are clinically significant there may be a history of lagging behind the dam or disinclination to play with other foals. Young foals with septal defects of clinical significance often show a characteristic exhaustion when suckling and sometimes collapse (faint) during feeding or after only slight exercise. A persistent dyspnea and weakness with an inability or disinclination to stand for reasonable periods of time are often noted.

Diagnosis

- VSDs are usually associated with at least two murmurs. The shunt causes an obvious, loud, pansystolic murmur in the area of the aortic and tricuspid valves. The persistent, undulating, 'machinery type' murmur has a marked precordial vibration (thrill) which radiates widely and is audible on both sides of the chest, but is usually significantly louder on the right. The thrill can often be appreciated merely by palpation of the lower right thoracic wall. This murmur usually becomes more prominent with exercise and rising blood pressure. There is also frequently a second murmur associated with

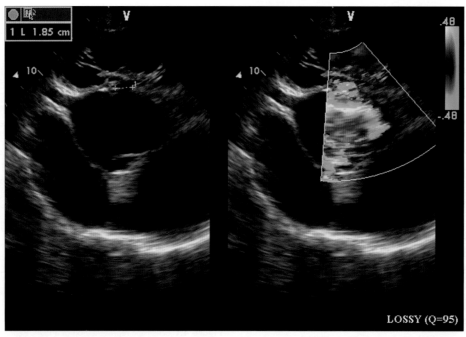

Figure 4.3 VSD muscular. Welsh section A pony 2-year-old at presentation, lethargy and poor exercise tolerance. A VSD was diagnosed on ultrasound; no treatment was given, and there was no follow up.

relative pulmonic stenosis. Although the right ventricular tract is normal there is an increased volume of blood leaving the right ventricle which results in a loud holosystolic crescendo–decrescendo murmur over the pulmonic valve in the left third intercostal space. This murmur is usually at least one grade lower than the VSD murmur.

- Peripheral signs of circulatory status and electrocardiographs are usually normal.
- Ultrasound studies including Doppler are the best diagnostic tools as they not only determine the presence and size of the defect and the shunt velocity but can also be helpful to assess the hemodynamic burden.
- Major septal defects, which shunt significant volumes of blood into the relatively lower-pressured right side, result in gross right-sided enlargement and this may be detected on percussion or, more precisely, by radiographic and ultrasonographic examination of the chest.

Treatment and prognosis

- Membranous defects that are smaller than 25 mm and demonstrate a shunt velocity of greater than 4 m/s may be exercise-tolerant.
- In smaller breeds of horses and ponies it is also useful to compare the size of the VSD with the diameter of the aortic root. Those which are less than one third of the aortic root carry a better prognosis.
- Muscular ventricular septal defects, defects with aortic insufficiency, or other anomalies are likely to be intolerant of strenuous exercise.
- Foals with membranous VSD larger than 35 mm in diameter or muscular VSDs tend to have decreased life expectancy. VSD may also be a component of complex cardiac anomalies carrying a poor prognosis.

- Treatment of significant defects is generally impractical and owners should be advised against using the horse for athletic purposes or breeding.

Atrial septal defect (ASD) (Fig. 4.6)

Atrial septal defects are uncommon in the equine neonate. Most are a component of complex congenital cardiac anomalies.

Three types of ASD are most described: ostium primum, ostium secundum and sinus venosus; however, a fourth, 'unroofed coronary sinus' which is a coronary sinus septal defect occurs less commonly.

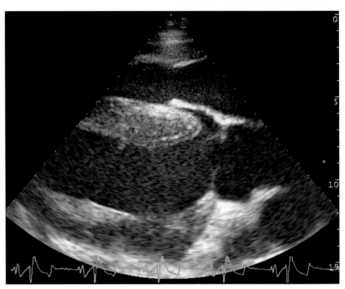

Figure 4.5 Echogram of subaortic VSD. Right parasternal long-axis echocardiogram optimized for the left ventricular outflow tract from a 10-year-old Welsh Mountain pony gelding without exercise intolerance. A paramembranous VSD is present, adjacent to the right coronary cusp of the aorta and the septal leaflet of the tricuspid valve. The small size (<0.25 of the aorta diameter) of the defect and the high peak shunt velocity across the defect (> 4.8 m/s) are consistent with a restrictive VSD that is not hemodynamically important.

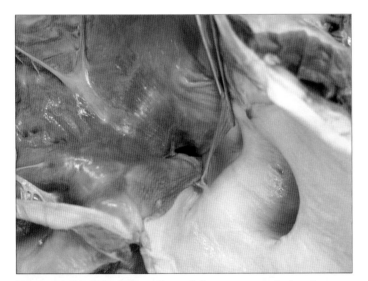

Figure 4.4 PM of VSD (VSD membranous). Post-mortem examination of a restrictive ventricular septal defect viewed from the left side, in a horse subjected to euthanasia for a non-responsive periocular tumor. The VSD measured approximately 1 cm in diameter in the perimembranous region of the ventricular septum immediately cranial to the septal leaflet of the tricuspid valve and adjacent to the right coronary leaflet aortic valve. Ante-mortem the VSD was associated with a grade 4/6 pansystolic murmur over the right heart apex and a grade 2/6 holosystolic murmur over the left heart base. The size of the VSD and velocity of shunt blood across the defect as detected by spectral Doppler ante-mortem (>5 m/s) supported the characterization of the defect as a restrictive VSD.

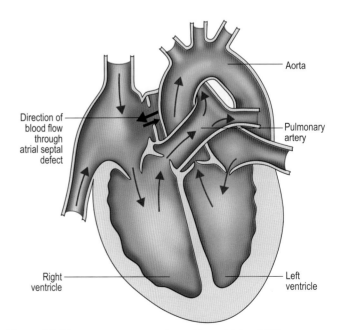

Figure 4.6 Schematic representation of an atrial septal defect (ASD). Reproduced from McAuliffe SB, Slovis NM (eds). *Color Atlas of Diseases and Disorders of the Foal* (2008), with permission from Elsevier.

Diagnosis and treatment

- Most cases are obvious in the first few weeks of life with a pronounced heart base murmur and are frequently exercise-intolerant at presentation.
- Clinical signs of right-sided volume overload predominate (jugular pulsation, ascites, pleural effusion, peripheral venous distension and edema) and supraventricular arrhythmias (especially atrial fibrillation) are not uncommon due to right atrial enlargement.
- Definitive diagnosis is made with echocardiography. Color flow Doppler may be required to differentiate a residual, non-functional foramen ovale from a true ASD.
- No treatment is usually undertaken as the prognosis is poor.

Tetralogy of Fallot (Figs. 4.7 & 4.8)

Pulmonary valve stenosis, ventricular septal defect, overriding aorta and right ventricular hypertrophy make up this complex cardiac defect. If a patent ductus arteriosus also is present, then pentalogy of Fallot is present. Right-to-left shunting results in cyanosis and lethargy.

Many of the affected foals are born dead or die shortly after birth, having shown marked respiratory distress, polypnea and cyanosis. The foals may appear to faint spontaneously and collapse at the slightest exertion. Exercise intolerance, difficulty nursing and dyspnea are frequently encountered. Frequently foals are presented for suspected respiratory disease and when questioned the owners frequently reveal a history consist with congenital cardiac abnormality.

Diagnosis and treatment

- Clinical signs are diagnostic. A loud grade 4/6 to 6/6 pansystolic murmur, with palpable thrill over the left heart base, with point of maximal intensity (PMI) over the pulmonary valve area. The defect may also be audible on the right side but is usually less intense on this side.
- Radiographic examination of the thorax will usually identify the grossly enlarged right ventricle and a very prominent ascending aorta.
- There is no treatment and the prognosis is grave.

Tricuspid atresia

Tricuspid atresia is a rare defect in foals that often accompanies complex cardiac anomalies. Persistent foramen ovale, ventricular septal defect, ventricular dilation and mitral dysplasia have been reported with this defect.

Diagnosis and treatment

- Two-dimensional echocardiography demonstrates echo banding in the tricuspid valve region, fallout of the aortic root, enlarged left ventricle, small right ventricle, and variable atrial enlargement and mitral excursion variations.
- Contrast echocardiographic techniques confirm intracardiac shunting of blood from right to left atrial chambers then to left ventricle if shunting is suspected.
- There is no treatment available for this condition.

Great vessel transposition (Fig. 4.9)

This condition consists of the aorta exiting the right ventricle and the pulmonary artery exiting the left ventricle. Foals born with this anomaly may survive for several days postpartum but are markedly cyanotic and frequently recumbent.

Auscultation often reveals a louder right-sided systolic murmur compatible with VSD as well as the continuous, crescendo–decrescendo 'machinery'-type left heart base murmur of the PDA.

Diagnosis and treatment

- Echocardiography demonstrates a characteristic 'twin pipe' appearance as the two outflow tracts exit the ventricles in near parallel instead of their normal twisted configuration.
- There is no treatment available for this condition.

Truncus arteriosus (Fig. 4.10)

Incomplete or failed septation of the embryonic truncus arteriosus leads to a common 'trunk' through which the aorta and pulmonary artery flow. A ventricular septal defect is also usually evident. This leads to mixing of oxygenated and non-oxygenated blood, variable cyanosis and often pulmonary vascular overload. Decreased PaO_2, right heart insufficiency and pulmonary edema often ensue. Since pulmonary vascular resistance is lower than systemic vascular tone, blood is preferentially pushed into the pulmonary vascular system driving pulmonary vascular overload with resultant clinical signs.

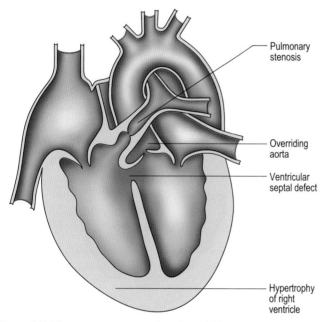

Figure 4.7 Schematic representation of tetralogy of Fallot. Reproduced from McAuliffe SB, Slovis NM (eds). *Color Atlas of Diseases and Disorders of the Foal* (2008), with permission from Elsevier.

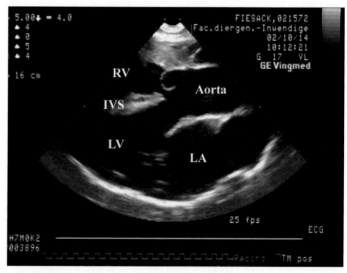

Figure 4.8 Echocardiogram demonstrating an overriding aorta as part of tetralogy of Fallot.

Clinical signs

- Exercise intolerance.
- Stunted growth.
- Dyspnea or syncope may be noted.
- Grade 4/6 to 6/6 crescendo–decrescendo cardiac murmur with palpable thrill over left heart base.

Treatment

- None is usually undertaken and the prognosis is regarded as poor although there have been a number of suspected cases that have survived for a number of years.
- Surgical repair is the treatment of choice in human infants with this condition.

Non-infectious disorders

Dysrhythmias: atrial fibrillation (Fig. 4.11)

Atrial fibrillation is the most common atrial arrthymia associated with poor performance and exercise intolerance. It may be found as an incidental finding in some horses or can occur in horses with concurrent EIPH, congestive heart failure, respiratory distress, pulmonary hemorrhage, ataxia or collapse and myopathy.

It may be paroxysmal or sustained. The paroxysmal form is often associated with a single episode of poor performance and normally disappears spontaneously within 24–48 hours. Hypokalemia and other electrolyte abnormalities, which are frequently seen in horses with diarrhea or following furosemide therapy, predispose

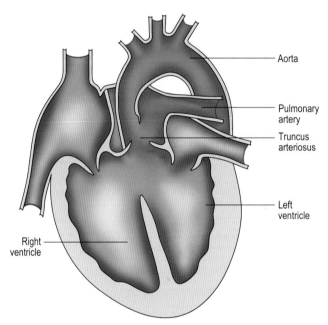

Figure 4.9 Great vessel transposition. Reproduced from McAuliffe SB, Slovis NM (eds). *Color Atlas of Diseases and Disorders of the Foal* (2008), with permission from Elsevier.

Figure 4.10 Truncus arteriosus. Reproduced from McAuliffe SB, Slovis NM (eds). *Color Atlas of Diseases and Disorders of the Foal* (2008), with permission from Elsevier.

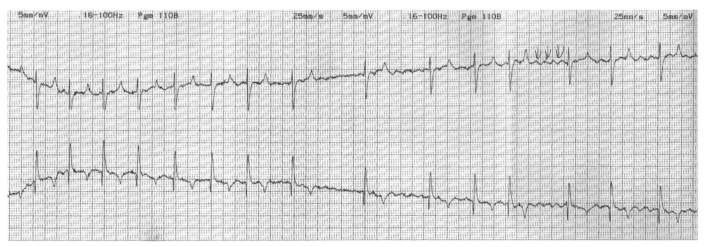

Figure 4.11 Atrial fibrillation. Classic electrocardiogram of atrial fibrillation revealing no definitive P waves, F waves (flutter) of the atria and normal-appearing QRS complexes arising at irregular intervals.

the equid to paroxysmal atrial fibrillation as can excessive resting vagal tone.

Sustained atrial fibrillation is less common but easier to diagnose. Some of these horses may have no other evidence of heart disease.

Diagnosis and treatment

- On auscultation it is classically described as an 'irregularly irregular' rhythm.
- Atrial fibrillation is easily identified on an ECG strip as multiple rapid atrial 'f' waves preceding regular QRS complexes. In horses with sustained atrial fibrillation an echocardiogram should be performed to determine whether there is any underlying cardiac disease.
- Laboratory studies for determination of electrolyte abnormalities may be useful for horses with paroxysmal atrial fibrillation.
- Therapy with β-blockers, class 1A antiarrhythmics (quinidine, procainamide, etc.), class 1C (flecainide, etc.), class III medications (amiodarone, etc.) and electroconversion should only be reserved for intractable or persistent atrial fibrillation (greater than 48 hours duration) without spontaneous conversion to normal rhythm or with clinical signs of exercise intolerance, lethargy, etc.

Prognosis

Negative prognostic factors include:

- Congestive heart failure (CHF)
- Consistently elevated resting heart rate (>60 beats/min)
- Dilated cardiomyopathy
- Valvular regurgitation with cardiomegaly
- Prolonged history of sustained atrial fibrillation (>6 weeks)
- Prior episodes of atrial fibrillation
- Unresponsive to therapy.

Premature atrial beats (PAB) (Fig. 4.12)

Premature atrial depolarizations arise within atrial foci not often associated with the SA node. Therefore, atrial p waves of often variable morphology occur earlier than expected in the ECG recording. Most have a normal QRS that follows. Infrequent premature atrial beats can be found in apparently normal horses. PABs are more likely to be clinically significant if:

- They are frequent at rest
- They are associated with atrial tachycardia

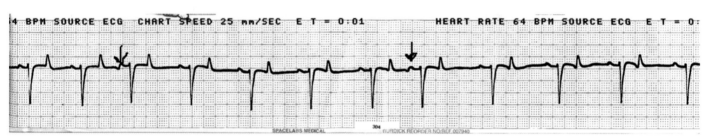

Figure 4.12 Premature atrial beats (arrows) in a 3-week-old foal. The foal had been bitten 3 days previously by a Western Diamond Back Rattlesnake. The foal had disseminated intravascular coagulation (DIC) and had to be hospitalized for 2 weeks; 6 weeks after initial presentation the arrhythmia resolved. Reproduced from McAuliffe SB, Slovis NM (eds). *Color Atlas of Diseases and Disorders of the Foal* (2008), with permission from Elsevier.

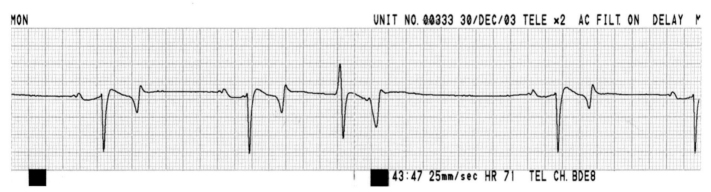

Figure 4.13 Ventricular premature contractions (VPC). Characteristic 'bizarre' QRS complex with lack of preceding 'P' wave.

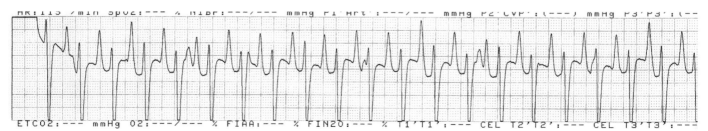

Figure 4.14 Ventricular tachycardia.

- They are related to poor performance
- They precipitate paroxysmal atrial flutter or fibrillation
- They develop along with other signs of cardiac disease.

Diagnosis and treatment

- Auscultation reveals a regular sinus rhythm that is interrupted by an obviously premature beat. Confirmation is by electrocardiogram (ECG). Documentation during exercise may be required to demonstrate a relationship with poor performance.
- Therapy is not often recommended unless atrial tachycardia arises. Atrial tachycardia is defined as more than four consecutive premature atrial beats. Transient atrial tachycardia can occur in structurally normal hearts during exercise, catecholamine release, hypoxia, hypovolemia, electrolyte alterations and caffeine therapy due to increased automaticity or triggered activity.
- Quinidine or procainamide can be considered but are impractical for long-term use. Digoxin is an alternative therapy but its effectiveness in such cases has not been evaluated in large studies.
- Other considerations of therapy are maintenance of normal serum potassium levels and treatment of any underlying cardiac disease such as myocarditis.

Ventricular premature contractions (VPC)
(Figs. 4.13 & 4.14)

These premature contractions arise within the myocardium of the ventricles. Reportedly, premature ventricular contractions can transiently occur in approximately 14% of clinically normal horses during a 24-hour monitoring period. Isolated or rare VPCs can also be observed occasionally in normal individuals immediately post-exercise. Premature ventricular contractions that occur during exercise or are occurring frequently (> 7 VPCs per minute) are abnormal. These VPCs can be caused by hypoxia, hypokalemia, hypomagnesemia, hypercalcemia, elevated catacholamines, adrenergic medications, endotoxemia/sepsis, and primary cardiac disease (myocardial, pericardial or contusive cardiac insults).

Diagnosis

- Early beats can be heard via auscultation and pulse deficits are common.
- ECG findings reveal lack of p waves preceding wide and/or tall ('bizarre') QRS complexes. If the QRS complex morphology varies, these VPCs are considered polymorphic and are assumed to arise from multiple/variable foci within the ventricles indicative of more diffuse myocardial disease.
- A pronounced jugular pulse with the VPC may be observed due to atrioventricular asynchrony (cannon A wave) and the follow-up beat after a VPC may be stronger due to the increased left ventricular filling that occurs with a compensatory pause following the VPC. This is known as extrasystolic potentiation leading to greater intensity of this beat.
- A physical examination, complete blood count, serum chemistry, blood gas (arterial +/− venous), echocardiogram and ECG evaluations should be considered to define the inciting cause(s).
- Evaluation of electrolyte abnormalities, as well as measurement of ionized calcium and magnesium, is recommended. Hypokalemia and hypomagnesemia are frequent causes of VPCs and electrolyte derangements may affect the usefulness of specific antidysrhythmic agents such as lidocaine.
- Measurement of cardiac Troponin 1 and other cardiac enzymes can be used to document underlying cardiac disease; 95% of normal healthy foals in one study had cardiac Troponin 1 values <0.49 ng/ml. Values ≥1 ng/ml are highly suggestive of myocardial disease/inflammation.

Treatment

- The majority of horses with VPCs will have spontaneous resolution of the arrhythmia after 4–8 weeks of rest.
- Patients with abnormal VPCs should be closely monitored such that **ventricular tachycardia (VT)** does not arise, i.e. heart rate >100–120 beats per minute with the rhythm being initiated from below the bundle of His (ventricular origin). Although potassium imbalance (both hypo- and hyperkalemia), other electrolyte disorders (hypomagnesemia), toxicants, vitamin E/selenium deficiency and stimulants can lead to VT, primary myocardial disease is most associated with ventricular tachycardia.
- Therapy should be directed at the inciting cause with primary myocardial disease a likely complicating issue. Class I anti-arrhythmic medications (lidocaine, procainamide, quinidine, propafenone) are often effective in VT patients with clinical signs of cardiac insufficiency while at rest, if multimorphic VT is noted, R waves are superimposed onto T waves on ECG, or if the heart rate is excessive for the age group patient.
- Although not as rapidly acting as lidocaine, magnesium sulfate (2–4 mg/kg q 2 minutes) can be useful to control ventricular tachycardia with a total dose not to exceed 50 mg/kg.
- The use of corticosteroids may be indicated if primary cardiac disease is deemed to be the inciting cause.

Acquired valvular heart disease

Valvular pathology is probably the most common cause of significant murmurs in the horse. These are sometimes accompanied by physiological disturbances of blood flow and exert consequent effects on the well-being and exercise capacity of the horse. In particular, defects of the mitral valve appear somewhat more likely to result in clinically significant murmurs. Mild, chronic, progressive valvular disease resulting in systolic murmurs form the commonest group of acquired disorders of the equine heart. The murmurs are usually of low intensity, and the sounds remain localized over the affected valve. Serious valvular dysfunction results in poor exercise tolerance and prolonged recovery after exercise. There is usually a high resting heart rate which shows a poor recovery rate to normal resting levels following even limited exercise but some cases affected by apparently severe murmurs show no detectable clinical effect on either performance or well-being. Causes of valvular regurgitation are listed in Table 4.1. Further discussion of more common causes is given below.

Clinical signs

- **_Mitral regurgitation_**. The murmur of mitral insufficiency is holo- or pan-systolic, typically band-shaped and is loudest over the fifth

Table 4.1 Causes of valvular regurgitation

Mitral insufficiency	Aortic insufficiency	Tricuspid insufficiency
Degenerative thickening	Degenerative thickening	Degenerative thickening
Idiopathic disease	Idiopathic disease	Idiopathic disease
Prolapse of the valve	Prolapse of the valve	Prolapse of the valve
Ruptured chordae tendinae	Congenital valvular disease	Congenital valvular disease
Bacterial endocarditis	VSD	Bacterial endocarditis
Non-infective valvulitis	Non-infective valvulitis	Pulmonary hypertension
Primary or ischemic myocardial disease	Ruptured aortic sinus aneurysm	Myocardial disease
Congenital malformation of the valve		Ruptured chordae tendinae
		Chronic tachycardia

intercostal space, radiating caudo-dorsally if it is severe. It may be an incidental finding or horses may show signs of poor performance or clinical signs of heart failure. The tolerance is often largely dependent on the type of work the horse is doing, with horses in vigorous training showing an expected poorer tolerance for the condition. In some horses the condition may be complicated by atrial fibrillation which further compromises cardiac function. Depending on the cause other clinical signs may be present such as fever, weight loss or polyarthritis which can occur in cases of bacterial endocarditis.

- **Aortic regurgitation**. The murmur of aortic insufficiency is typically pan, holo or early diastolic decrescendo and has its point of maximal intensity over the aortic valve in the left fifth intercostal space and radiates variable distances ventrally. It may be musical or have a 'creaking' quality in some horses. In most horses, aortic regurgitation (AR) is an incidental finding and commonly occurs as a result of valvular degeneration in horses greater than 10 years of age. The existing murmur can vary greatly in intensity and is not indicative of the prognosis. Although degenerative valvular changes are generally regarded as being slowly progressive, studies have indicated that horses with AR have a shorter survival time and are more prone to developing congestive heart failure or sudden death. The quality of the arterial pulses is a good indicator of the severity of the AR as bounding pulses are associated with volume overload and moderate to severe AR with a poorer prognosis.
- **Tricuspid regurgitation**. A soft, grade 2–3 pansystolic murmur with the point of maximal intensity on the right side of the tricuspid valve is most commonly found incidentally. Endocarditis less commonly affects the tricuspid valve and thus associated signs are not frequently seen. The prognosis for horses with TR is generally good.

Diagnosis

History and clinical findings may allow for a provisional diagnosis but definitive diagnosis and assessment of cardiac function requires thorough echocardiographic examination.

Ruptured chordae tendinae (Figs. 4.15 & 4.16)

Loud, widely radiating murmurs with an abrupt onset and a marked thrill develop in cases where there is rupture of one or more of the *chordae tendinae* (tendinous strands running from the papillary muscles to the free borders of the atrio-ventricular valves). The mitral valve is most often affected. This elicits a pronounced mitral valve insufficiency +/– cardiac insufficiency (edema, atrial enlargement, arrhythmias) and in some cases collapse and death.

Clinical signs, diagnosis and treatment

- Horses which are seen alive show an abrupt onset of severe respiratory distress and pulmonary edema, which is often audible and may be evident as a blood-stained, frothy, bilateral nasal discharge and cyanosis.
- Echocardiography is diagnostic.
- Treatment is supportive and dictated by the cardiovascular state although the prognosis is frequently poor.

Endocarditis (Figs. 4.17–4.24)

Bacterial endocarditis can affect the endocardium and/or one or more valve components. It occurs sporadically and can be seen in horses of all ages. The aortic and mitral valves are most commonly affected with mural lesions less common. Although they do occur on the valves of the right side, the effects of emboli are likely to be less obvious, possibly even passing unnoticed. Bacterial invasion and colonization secondary to a bacteremia is the most likely pathogenic mechanism but pre-existing valvular disease or endocardial changes as a result of jet lesions may predispose to the condition. Microthrombi production during severe illness, i.e. sepsis, etc., can also lead to turbulent or

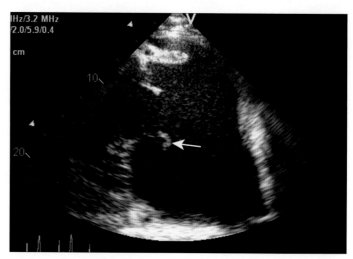

Figure 4.15 Ruptured chordae tendinae. Echocardiogram obtained from the left side showing a long-axis view of the mitral valve. Note that the ruptured chordae (arrow) can be appear to "flap" with movements of the valve.

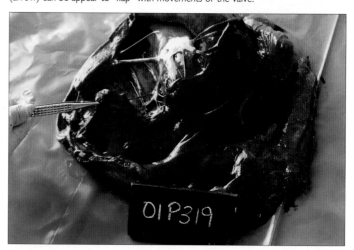

Figure 4.16 Post-mortem image revealing a ruptured chordae tendinae from a horse that was found dead. Image courtesy of the Irish Equine Centre.

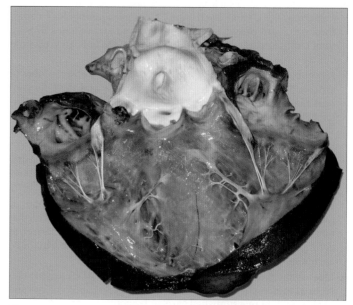

Figure 4.17 Endocarditis. This 1-year-old TB had a history of prior illness and subsequent poor growth. Valvular insufficiency was suspected on the basis of an auscultable murmur and echocardiography confirmed the presence of a vegetative endocarditis associated with valvular insufficiency.

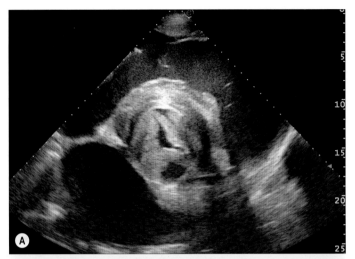

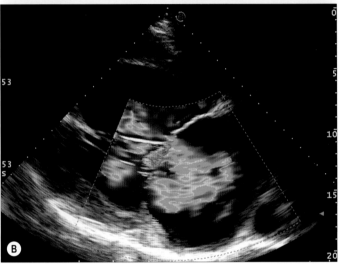

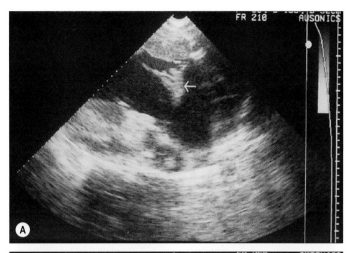

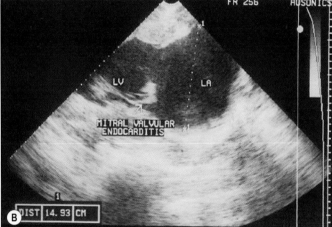

Figure 4.20 Echocardiogram of the mitral valve showing marked thickening and shortening of the valve associated with endocarditis.

Figure 4.18 (A, B) Echocardiograms obtained from a Thoroughbred broodmare with endocarditis involving the aortic and mitral valves. The clinical findings at presentation were weight loss, lethargy, tachycardia, pyrexia, increased jugular pulses and grade 4/6 pansystolic and holodiastolic murmurs, loudest on the left side. Marked vegetative lesions involving all leaflets of the aortic (A) and mitral valves and valvular insufficiency were evident during B-mode and color flow Doppler imaging (B). Moderate mature neutrophilia, marked hyperfibrinogenemia and hyperglobulinemia were present, consistent with a marked inflammatory process. The horse was subjected to euthanasia without treatment and post-mortem examinations confirmed the ante-mortem diagnosis of endocarditis. No bacteria were cultured from blood or valvular tissue.

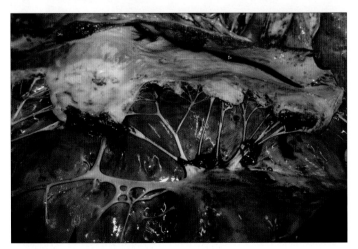

Figure 4.19 Endocarditis with thickening of the mitral valve.

traumatic endocardial damage which allows adhesion by transient bacteremic organisms and subsequent infective endocarditis. The organism involved is largely dependent on the origin of the bacteremia (gastrointestinal, respiratory, skin, oral cavity, surgical wound or intravenous catheter). *Streptococcus* sp., *Actinobacillus* sp., *Pasteurella* sp. and *Staphylococcus aureus* are most frequently isolated although many other bacteria and even fungi have been reported. Thrombophlebitis and catheter sepsis have been associated with the development of endocarditis in the horse.

Valvular inflammation results in ulceration and inflammation of the valve leaflets and although affected valves may not appear to be grossly thickened, there are serious consequences in relation to valve movement and the development of valvular endocarditis lesions which act as a focus for the accumulation of fibrin; extensive blood clots are commonly present attached to the damaged valves. Organization of the fibrinous accumulations (with the enclosed bacteria) produces friable **vegetative lesions**, from which infective emboli may be disseminated into the circulation. These have, therefore, considerable potential as sources of emboli, of both infective and non-infective types. Progressive organization of the inflammatory foci in the valve leaflets has profound effects on valve closure and the site and type of the lesion may be of great importance. Smooth, longstanding and well-organized thickening of the valve cusps typical of chronic valvular endocarditis is somewhat less likely to result in serious embolism than the more irregular, friable lesions associated with acute bacterial endocarditis.

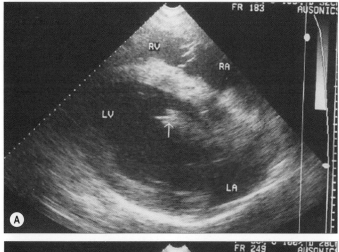

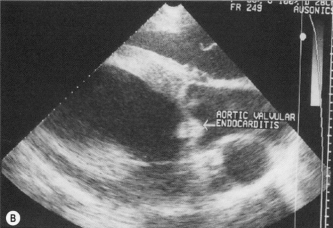

Figure 4.21 Echocardiogram demonstrating an endocarditis lesion of the aortic valve (same mare as Fig. 4.20). She presented with a history of bilateral shifting hindlimb lameness with variable swelling of the hindlimbs and intermittent fevers. Both mitral and aortic valves were incompetent.

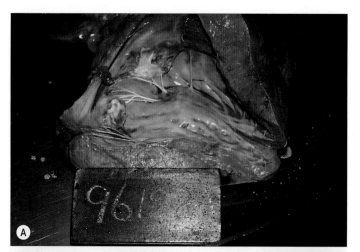

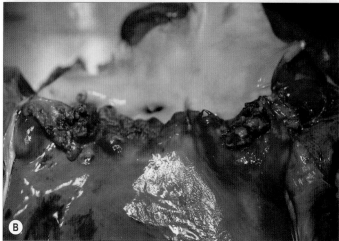

Figure 4.23 (A, B) Necropsy images from horses with vegetative endocarditis. Note the marked thickening and shortening of valves with vegetative lesions of the valve cusps. Image courtesy of Irish Equine Centre.

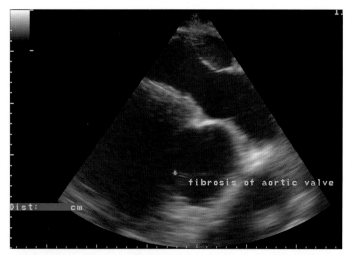

Figure 4.22 Long-axis view of the aortic valve showing thickening of the left coronary cusp of the valve. This thickening often appears as an echogenic thickening parallel to the free edge of the valve leaflets and corresponds to parallel fibrous band lesions which are frequently noted at necropsy.

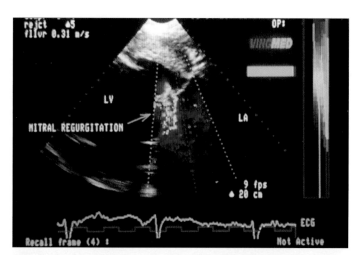

Figure 4.24 Mitral valve incompetence (color flow Doppler, ultrasound). Blood flow coded red, flowing from left ventricle (LV) to right atrium (LA) during systole. The signal has aliased, as shown by the central core change from blue through to red (i.e. traveling so fast that signal received as if traveling in the opposite direction).

Clinical signs

- Most horses with bacterial endocarditis present with intermittent pyrexia, weight loss, depression, malaise, intermittent lameness and clinical indications of cardiac insufficiency attributable to the chamber/side of heart affected.
- A predisposing condition or concurrent infection or the history of such may be present but many horses present with no other obvious signs of disease and no history of a prior disorder.
- Valvular lesions often incite regurgitant murmurs best heard over the valve involved. Therefore, atrioventricular valve endocarditis results in a systolic murmur whereas aortic or pulmonic valve endocarditis results in a diastolic murmur. Mural endocarditis and small vascular lesions may not produce heart murmurs, especially if the right side of the heart is affected. The quality or intensity of the murmur may change during subsequent examinations and arrythmias may also be present.
- Right-sided vegetative lesions that dislodge may create embolic pneumonia or focal pulmonary abscesses, whereas left heart vegetations can dislodge to spread septic emboli to other organ systems with swelling of joints and tendon sheaths commonly seen.

Diagnosis and treatment

- Diagnostics include serial blood culture during or just after febrile episodes, CBC, chemistry, echocardiography and thoracic radiography.
- Complete blood counts frequently demonstrate a moderate to marked neutrophilic leukocytosis and hyperfibrinogenemia.
- Treatment is initially broad-spectrum antimicrobials with long-term (4–8 weeks) antimicrobial selection based on blood culture results. Bacteremia is considered continuous but the number of bacteria at any given time may fluctuate.

Prognosis

Prognosis for left-sided vegetative valvular endocarditis is often poor. Right-sided lesions may have a slightly better prognosis (guarded). The guarded to poor prognosis is based on the facts that a bacteriological cure is difficult to obtain and progressive valvular damage may occur as the vegetation heals and results in valvular scarring. In horses which appear to have been treated successfully periodic follow-up checks are therefore important.

Pericarditis (Figs. 4.25–4.30)

Pericardial inflammation and/or infection is uncommon in the horse. It may, however, when it occurs lead to life-threatening cardiovascular compromise and is most commonly associated with pericardial effusion and fibrinous pericarditis. Viral and bacterial infections are most commonly implicated but primary pneumonia, pulmonary abscesses, trauma and neoplasia-associated cases have been reported. Not all cases of pericarditis are septic but given the consequences should be regarded as such until proven otherwise. Additionally, although sepsis is by far the most common cause of pericardial inflammation, culture from the fluid (or even from the pericardium at post-mortem

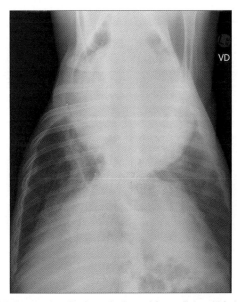

Figure 4.25 A ventrodorsal radiograph obtained from a 7-day-old foal with pericarditis that presented with a 2 day history of lethargy, inappetance and increased respiratory effort. There is a globoid enlargement of the cardiac silhouette due to marked pericardial effusion and scalloped lung margins asscociated with pleural effusion, most evident in teh right hemithorax. Concurrent septic conditions present in the foal were polyarthritis and omphalophlebitis, consistent with disseminated bacterial infection.

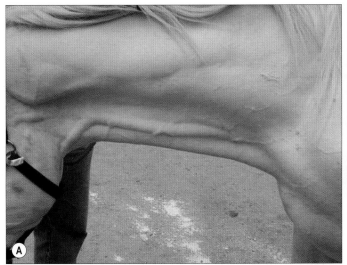

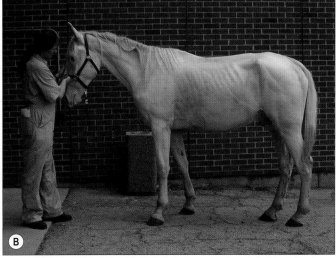

Figure 4.26 (A, B) Jugular distension in a 16-year-old Thoroughbred gelding. The horse presented for weight loss and the signs of generalized venous congestion. Jugular pulses, ventral edema and cardiac cachexia were identified. Echocardiography confirmed the right-sided congestive heart failure was secondary to severe restrictive pericarditis. Euthanasia was recommended and the necropsy image is shown in Fig. 4.29.

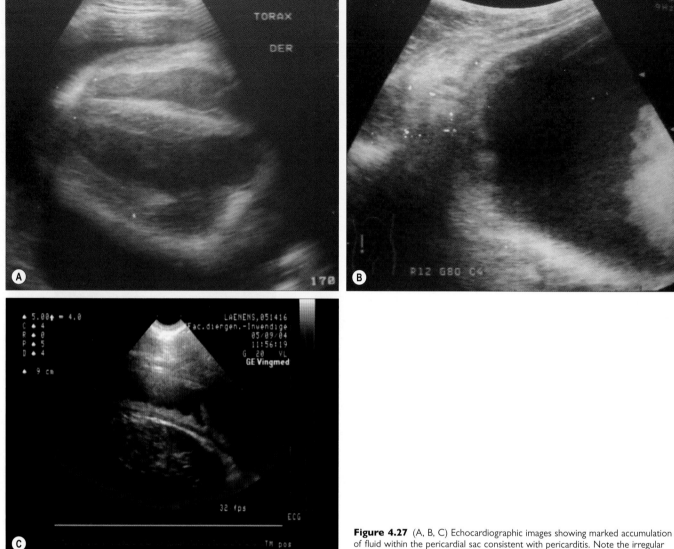

Figure 4.27 (A, B, C) Echocardiographic images showing marked accumulation of fluid within the pericardial sac consistent with pericarditis. Note the irregular surface of the myocardium consistent with fibrin deposition (C).

examination) is frequently unrewarding. The pathogenesis of non-infective pericarditis is unknown.

The clinical signs associated with the disorder vary according to the extent and nature of the exudate within the pericardial sac. Where the disease is secondary to respiratory tract disease, the respiratory signs may be prominent and the presence of concurrent pericarditis might easily be overlooked. Affected horses typically are pyrexic, partially to completely anorexic, lethargic and may be reluctant to move.

Extensive pericardial effusions result in diminished or muffled heart sounds and evidence of cardiac tamponade (compression of venous return to the heart due to increased volume of fluid in the pericardium). The signs of tamponade are those of right-sided cardiac failure, including prominent jugular distension and pulsation, tachycardia, poor pulse pressure (hypotension) and ventral edema. In some cases the apex beat of the heart may not easily be palpable, but a number of other conditions, including obesity and pleural effusions, may also produce the same result. A pericardial 'rub' is often present during auscultation of the ventrolateral thorax. Other clinical signs may be related to the underlying cause, e.g. infection or neoplasia.

Diagnosis

- Clinical signs may be suggestive but echocardiography is fundamentally diagnostic where the thickened pericardium and the presence of variable amounts and consistency of effusion will usually be obvious.

- Pericardiocentesis with fluid analysis and culture may be required to identify the causal agent and its susceptibility profile. *Streptococcus* spp., *Actinobacillus equuli*, *Pseudomonas aeruginosa* and *Pasteurella* sp. have all been reported. Pericardiocentesis may be performed between the fourth, fifth or sixth left intercostal space midway between the shoulder level and the sternum. This technique is relatively easy and safe. Simultaneous ultrasound may provide accurate guidance for the aspiration needle. Normal pericardial fluid is limited in volume and contains few cells and low protein levels, whereas in most cases of pericarditis, whether septic or not, both cell and protein content increase markedly.

- The electrocardiogram of horses affected with pericarditis shows a characteristically diminished QRS voltage and/or repeated

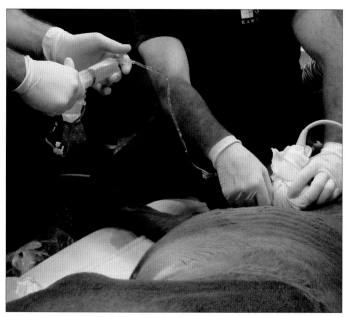

Figure 4.28 Pericardial drainage in a foal with pericarditis. This septic foal was noted to have marked accumulation of fluid within the pericardial sac on routine thoracic ultrasound. He was treated by drainage and lavage of the pericardial sac in addition to systemic antibiotics and made a full recovery.

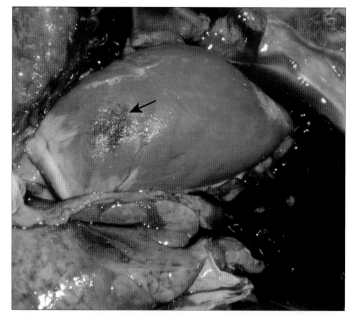

Figure 4.30 Pericardial accumulation of blood. Pericardial and myocardial laceration (arrow) caused by a severely displaced fractured rib resulted in pericardial accumulation of blood and death of this foal.

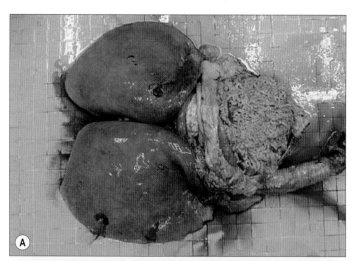

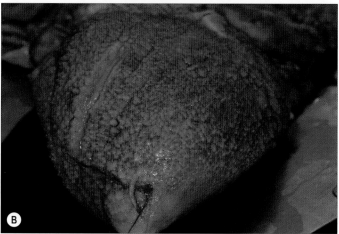

Figure 4.29 (A, B) Post-mortem images. (A) Heart and lungs showing marked fibrin deposition on the myocardium following opening of the pericardium. (B) Fibrinous pericarditis.

variations in QRS amplitude, which may be attributable to the movement of the heart within the distended pericardial sac.

- Thoracic radiography may also be used to demonstrate an enlarged, rounded cardiac silhouette but is limited by any concurrent pleural fluid and the technical problems of thoracic radiography in all but the smaller horses.
- CBC results are variable with the majority of horses demonstrating a moderate to marked neutrophilic leukocytosis with elevated fibrinogen. Animals suffering from pericardial tamponade will frequently present with azotemia due to decreased cardiac output and subsequent reduced renal output. Central venous pressure (if routinely monitored) greater than 10–12 mmHg is suggestive of cardiac tamponade and should prompt further diagnostics/therapy.
- Post-mortem examination reveals a markedly thickened pericardial sac and the presence of exudate which may be purulent or partially organized and, in longstanding cases, fibrinous. There is commonly some intercurrent valvular endocarditis.

Treatment and prognosis

- Therapy is aimed at the inciting cause with broad-spectrum antibiotics and anti-inflammatory medications initially; specific culture results may dictate longer-term treatment.
- Pericardiocentesis is indicated in all cases of septic effusion and cases of cardiac tamponade. Electrocardiographic monitoring during the drainage procedure allows recognition of arrthymias.
- Pericardial lavage can be performed in cases of septic pericarditis. It should be repeated daily until the accumulation of fluid declines (<1 L in 12 hours for an adult), clinical signs have improved and the cytological characteristics of the fluid indicate the presence of less inflammatory cells.
- Surgery is rarely required but could be considered in cases of constrictive pericarditis that are non-responsive to other therapies.
- Traditionally the prognosis for horses affected by pericarditis has been poor, however, there have been recent reports of successful outcomes.

Myocardial disease (Figs. 4.31–4.32)

This may arise directly from intercurrent endocarditis or pericarditis. In many cases of myocarditis there is a detectable dysrhythmia with supraventricular or ventricular extrasystoles or atrial fibrillation. Many cases in which myocardial inflammation is suspected have no overt clinical evidence, and it is likely that many viral diseases (including equine herpes virus, equine influenza virus, African horse sickness, etc.) may be associated with some pathological inflammation. The significance of the myocarditis may be overshadowed by the more obvious clinical features but its importance should not be overlooked. Myocardial injury can also occur idiopathically or as a result of a diet

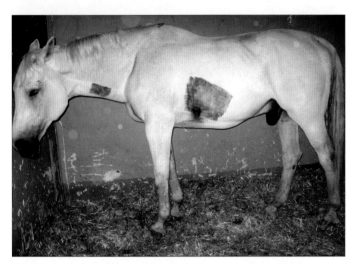

Figure 4.31 This gelding was presented with signs of congestive right-sided heart failure. On presentation, he had exercise intolerance, jugular distension and atrial fibrillation. The atrial fibrillation was pathological and attributed to cardiomyopathy.

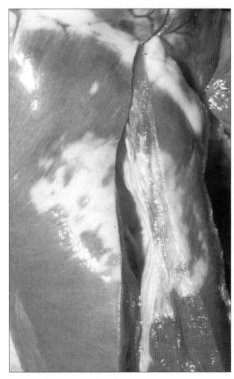

Figure 4.32 Myocardial fibrosis (infarct).

deficient in selenium and vitamin E, toxins (ionophore antibiotics, poisonous plants), ischemia, hypoxia, systemic bacterial infections, parasite migration, heavy metals, trauma, persistent tachyarrhythmias, metabolic disease or other nutritional deficiencies. Extension of and infiltration with local neoplasias or rarely amyloidosis is another possible cause.

The level of compromise of cardiac function varies greatly from horse to horse from no detectable clinical signs to weakness, staggering and occasionally collapse and death.

With progressive cardiac enlargement there are further changes in physiologic function and the pathological processes involved in producing progressive clinical signs are as follows:

- Reduced myocardial contractility and ventricular ejection function
- Diastolic dysfunction with impaired ventricular filling
- Mitral or tricuspid valve incompetency as a result of cardiac dilation or papillary muscle dysfunction
- The development of arrhythmias.

Clinical signs frequently are not noted for some time after the initial myocardial injury and in many such cases the disease process has continued to progress unnoticed, complicating identification of the initiating cause and in many cases complicating treatment and diminishing the prognosis. Horses suffering from the acute stages of myocardial degeneration often have intercurrent skeletal (and possibly smooth) muscle involvement and may be presented with all the clinical features of colic.

Diagnosis

- Resting clinical examination may be normal in many of these horses. Post-exercise clinical examination may reveal an abnormally and persistently high heart rate. Others may have audible irregularities and murmurs.
- Creatine kinase (CK) and lactate dehydrogenase (LDH) isoenzyme studies on horses suspected of having acute myocardial pathology may be helpful in supporting a diagnosis. Serum Troponin I measurement is a more specific indicator of myocardial injury.
- The relative size of the heart can be assessed radiographically. Findings may include upward displacement of the trachea and/or obvious enlargement. Physiological cardiac hypertrophy is common in fit performance horses but this should not affect the relative position of the trachea in the chest.
- Ultrasonographic assessment using M-mode may be used effectively to identify the thinner-than-normal atrial and ventricular walls, a loss of compliance (contractility) and a gross distension of the cardiac chambers.
- Post-mortem examination may show generalized myocardial pallor, gross distension or focal areas of fibrosis within the myocardium.

Treatment and prognosis

- Treatment is primarily supportive with both treatment and prognosis being determined by the severity of the myocardial injury and the hemodynamic consequences.
- All affected horses should be stall-rested until myocardial function, ECG, cardiac isoenzymes and serum troponin I levels return to normal. This may take several weeks.
- Antiarrhythmic therapy may be required in some cases but in many the arrhythmias return after removal of therapy.
- ACE inhibitors such as enalapril or ramipril may reduce myocardial remodeling and unload the ventricle.
- Once CHF has developed, digoxin and furosemide can be used as part of therapy but digoxin should not be used where monensin

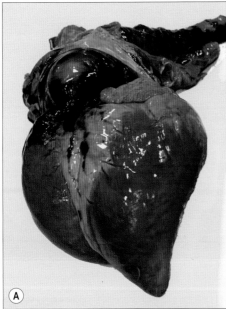

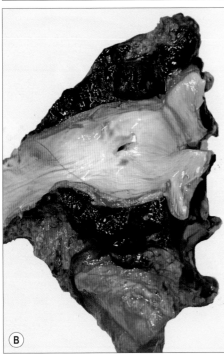

Figure 4.33 (A, B) Aortic rupture. These images are from a 1-year-old TB colt that was found dead in the paddock. The lesion was regarded to be the cause of death.

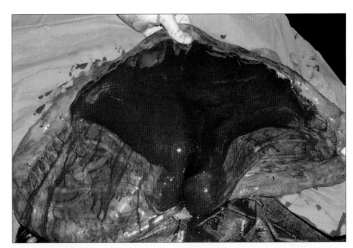

Figure 4.34 Mesenteric hematoma following rupture of mesenteric vessel. Note that the bleeding is confined only to the mesentery.

Rupture of major vessels

A dramatic cardiac failure is induced by **rupture of the cardiac annulus**. This highly fatal disorder results in gross distortion of the valvular integrity. While some cases may be seen alive, in extremis, with very high heart rates and severe congestive heart failure with extreme cyanosis and prominent, pulsating and engorged jugular veins, most cases are found dead.

Aorta (Fig. 4.33). Rupture of the aorta at its base (or the pulmonary artery) is a rare but important clinical syndrome in stallions in particular. Sudden death is usual, although some survive long enough to allow the identification of extensive hemothorax or pulmonary bleeding. Rupture of the aorta into the right atrium (aorto-atrial fistula) results in a catastrophic cardiac failure although death is often delayed for some hours and minor fistulation resulting in lesser degrees of arterial shunting may be present. The pressure gradient is such that the condition does not remain static and progression is to be expected. Cardio-aortic (dissecting) aneurysm results in aortic bleeding into the atrial and ventricular septal muscle and again a catastrophic loss of myocardial function with gross electrical abnormalities results in rapid death.

Middle uterine artery. Rupture of the middle uterine or the ovarian artery occurs in the brood mare as a complication of foaling (see p. 457). Death occurring less than 24 hours after parturition is more usual than sudden collapse immediately after delivery. Rupture of the middle uterine artery within the broad ligament may result in the development of a large hematoma which may be sufficiently extensive to result in colic and clinically significant blood loss, without any overt signs of bleeding. Rectal examination will usually identify the lesion as a large discrete fluid-filled mass lying cranial to the pelvic brim on one or other side.

Mesenteric vessels (Fig. 4.34). Ruptures of mesenteric vessels, resulting in large hematomas within the mesenteric confine, are also encountered and may be the result of parasitic damage. This is a possible cause of colic. Obvious anemia is unusual but a blood-stained peritoneal fluid and extreme pain usually encourage exploratory laparotomy, during which the hematoma is obvious.

Umbilical artery. Rupture of the umbilical artery occurs in neonatal foals subjected to excessive cord tension at delivery. Although the outward extent of hemorrhage may be relatively minor, it is often sufficient to result in death, particularly as a significant volume of the foal's blood is usually left in the placenta. Overt hemoperitoneum may

toxicosis is suspected. Digoxin and monensin have an additive effect causing calcium to flood into the myocardial cell increasing myocardial cell injury and death.

- If immune-mediated disease or non-infective processes are thought to be involved in the etiology, corticosteroid therapy may be beneficial.
- Horses already in CHF when presented have a poorer prognosis but there have been cases that have recovered and returned to previous function.

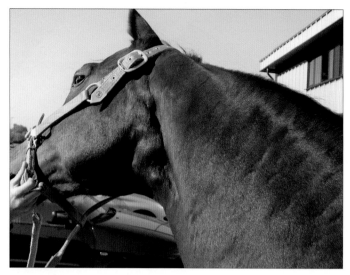

Figure 4.35 Arteriovenous fistula. Swelling in the throat latch area would become more pronounced with jugular occlusion.

Differential diagnosis:
• Congestive heart failure
• Anterior thoracic mass
• Jugular thrombosis.

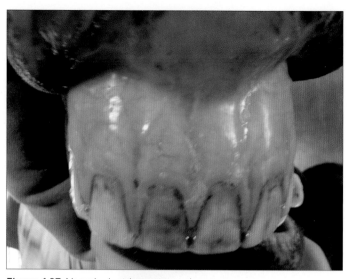

Figure 4.37 Normal pale pink mucous membranes.

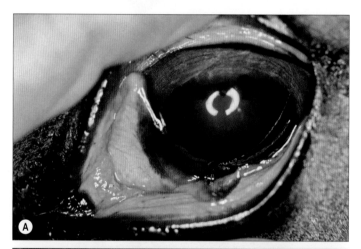

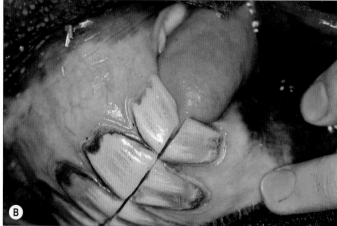

Figure 4.38 Mild anemia in a horse with multiple myeloma.

Differential diagnosis:
• Blood loss
• Hemolytic diseases (usually rapidly progressive)
• Bone marrow suppression, e.g. chronic infection, iron deficiency, neoplasia (usually slowly progressive)
• Deficiency disorders
• Clotting disorders
• Malabsorbtion syndromes
• Lymphosarcoma
• Equine infectious anemia.

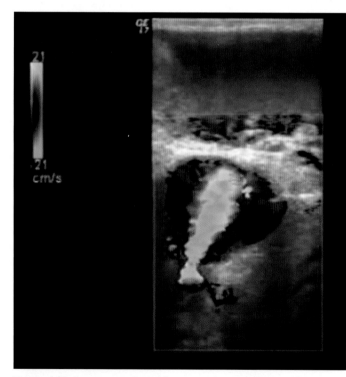

Figure 4.36 Arteriovenous fistula. Ultrasonographic image of the carotid artery showing admixing of blood as noted by the yellow and green coloration.

be present and detectable by abdominal paracentesis but in some cases there is none detectable and in these the hemorrhage is usually confined within the falciform and round ligaments.

Arteriovenous fistula (Figs. 4.35 & 4.36)

Peripheral arterial aneurysms or shunts (arteriovenous fistula) may be either congenital or acquired as a result of local trauma (often venepuncture). The congenital shunts occur almost anywhere including the distal limbs, and particularly at the hock. They are usually incidental findings, having little or no pathological significance. Only lesions associated with the more superficial vessels are likely to be detectable. Large lesions involving major vessels may result in disorders of cardiac flow and, ultimately, congestive heart failure. A fistula between the carotid artery and the jugular vein in the mid-cervical region is probably the commonest iatrogenic form of the disorder, and follows misdirected intravenous injections (of irritant drugs, in particular). The proximity of the carotid artery to the medial wall of the jugular vein makes inadvertent intracarotid injection relatively easy. The high-pressure differential between the two vessels ensures that once a small fistula has been created it is likely to enlarge progressively and result in gross enlargement of the jugular vein(s).

Diagnosis

- A diagnosis can be confirmed from the clinical appearance of a large pulsating jugular vein (often with fremitus at the site) and the presence of arterial (or nearly arterial) blood within the vein.
- The ipsilateral distal arteries (including the easily palpable posterior facial and facial arteries) have a very poor pulse pressure when compared to the normal side.

Treatment

Depending on the location and consequences of the fistula, some may be treated surgically but many are left untreated.

Mucous membranes (Figs. 4.37–4.46)

The mucous membranes are a significant and important indicator of the circulatory status of the horse and may, furthermore, show significant changes in color and appearance in many other disease conditions.

Vasculitis (Figs. 4.47–4.53)

Vasculitis (inflammation of the blood vessels) can occur as a primary disorder but is more commonly found secondary to immune-mediated, infectious, toxic or neoplastic disorders.

Clinical signs depend on the type of vessel affected and the severity of the inflammatory response. Increased vascular permeability results in edema and hemorrhage, as fluid and cellular components of blood leak into the extravascular space. Most equine vasculitis syndromes have the characteristics of a well-demarcated area of cutaneous edema. The ventral body and distal limbs are affected most frequently and in many cases the edematous area is hot and painful. Extensive serum exudation from the inflamed and edematous skin lesions is a common sign and may ultimately result in extensive sloughing. Petechial hemorrhages may be visible in the skin (although this is usually difficult to identify) and in the mucous membranes of the mouth, eyes and vulva. More extensive, ecchymotic hemorrhages may also occur in any mucous membranes. Affected horses are often stiff and reluctant to move, giving the impression of laminitis, and may show marked respiratory distress due to obstructive edema of the upper respiratory tract. Anemia and spontaneous nasal bleeding (in spite of normal clotting profiles and normal platelet counts) are also encountered in some cases. A wide variety of apparently unrelated clinical signs including colic, weight loss, azotemia, lameness, dyspnea and ataxia may be encountered and are probably the result of multiple/secondary organ involvement.

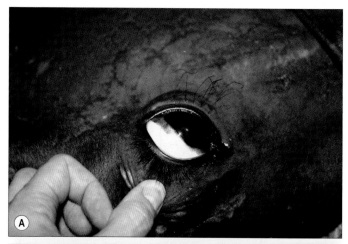

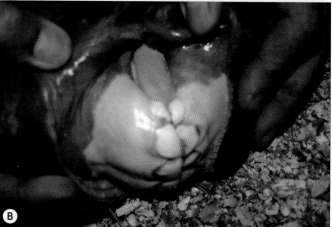

Figure 4.39 Severe anemia. This mare when examined had a HCT of 7%. She had previously been in a barn fire and had extensive burns of all limbs. On examination she had a large intra-abdominal hematoma of unknown origin.

Differential diagnosis:
- Blood loss (hemorrhage or hemolysis which may or may not be obvious)
- Severe bone marrow depression.

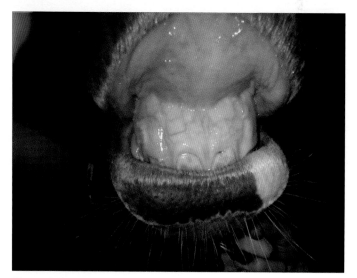

Figure 4.40 Oral mucous membranes with both mild anemia and icterus.

Differential diagnosis:
- Neonatal isoerythrolysis
- Babesiosis
- Equine infectious anemia (adult horses).

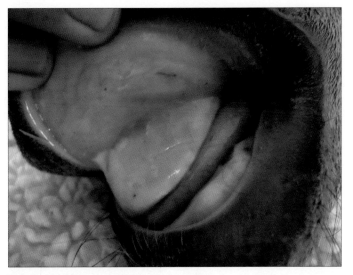

Figure 4.41 Pale and cyanotic mucous membranes.

Differential diagnosis:
- Circulatory compromise/congestive heart failure
- Respiratory obstructions/failure
- Hemorrhage.

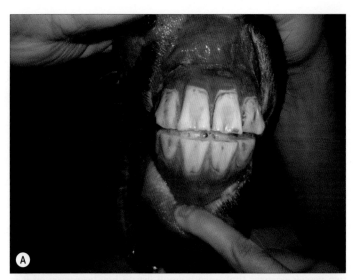

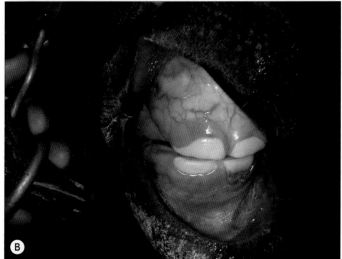

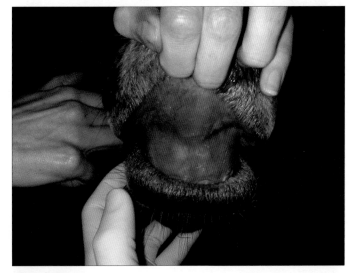

Figure 4.43 Congestion and cyanosis.

Differential diagnosis:
- Circulatory compromise
- Respiratory failure
- Severe endotoxemia.

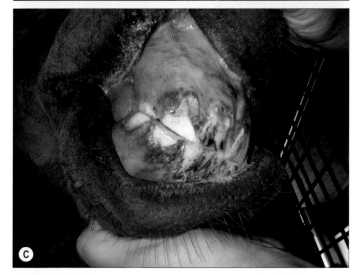

Figure 4.42 Congested mucous membranes. Congestion of the mucous membranes may appear as diffuse congestion or may present as an area of congestion bordering the teeth (known as a 'toxic line').

Differential diagnosis:
- Endotoxemia
- Circulatory obstructions
- Congestive heart failure
- African horse sickness
- Acute renal failure.

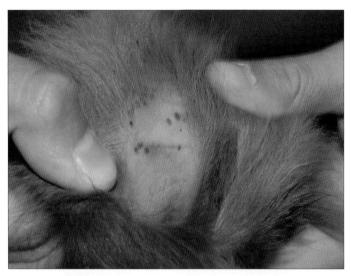

Figure 4.44 Petechiation.

Differential diagnosis:
• Hemorrhagic diatheses
• Thrombocytopenic purpura
• Purpura haemorrhagica
• Septicemia
• Toxemia
• Vasculitis (systemic lupus erythematosus-like syndrome of horses)
• African horse sickness
• Viral arteritis
• Equine infectious anemia.

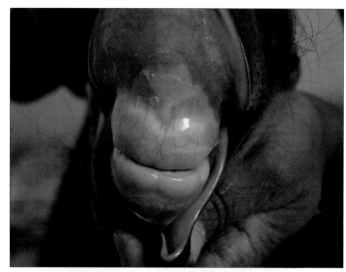

Figure 4.46 Severe icterus.

Differential diagnosis:
• Neonatal isoerythrolysis
• Severe hemorrhage or hemolysis
• Hepatic insufficiency
• Biliary obstruction.

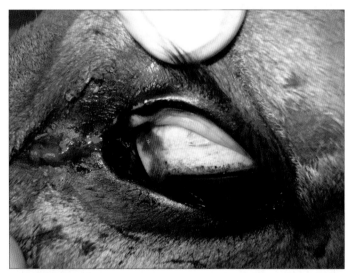

Figure 4.45 Ecchymotic hemorrhages.

Differential diagnosis:
• Vasculitis (immune-mediated and infectious)
• Toxemia
• Hemorrhagic diatheses
• Immune-mediated thrombocytopenia
• Systemic lupus erythematosus-like syndrome.

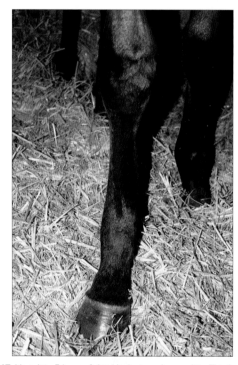

Figure 4.47 Vasculitis. Edema of distal limbs in early vasculitis. This foal had an immune-mediated vasculitis with a recent history of respiratory tract infection. He was treated with corticosteroids and made an uneventful recovery.

Infectious diseases associated with vasculitis are equine infectious anemia (EIA), equine viral arteritis (EVA) and equine granulocytic ehrlichiosis.

Most other non-infectious causes of vasculitis in the horse are thought to be immune-mediated. Perhaps the best recognized **immune-mediated vasculitis** is **purpura hemorrhagica** which, in the horse, in spite of its name, is a non-thrombocytopenic purpura (i.e. platelet numbers are generally normal). It is most often encountered in young horses, some weeks after recovery from an upper respiratory tract virus or bacterial infection (in particular, equine influenza virus and/or *Streptococcus equi*). Some non-infectious causes have been identified, including the administration of drugs and vaccines. In addition to the typical signs of vasculitis these horses are often markedly febrile. The factors that determine which individuals develop hypersensitivity vasculitis remain unclear. Genetic predisposition, altered immunoregulatory mechanisms, and amount, size and

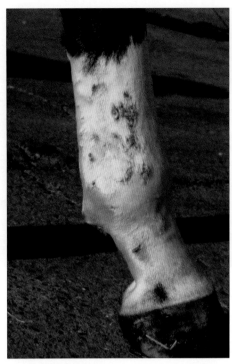

Figure 4.48 Vasculitis. Note the distinct areas of serum exudation in this case.

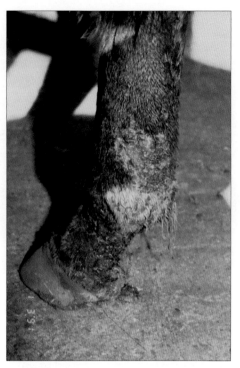

Figure 4.50 Severe vasculitis in this case has resulted in local edema, serum exudation and skin sloughing.

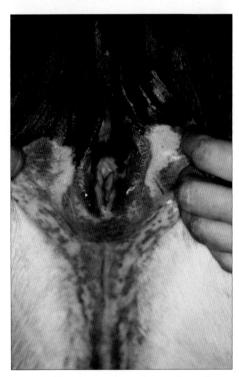

Figure 4.49 Vasculitis. Note the extensive ecchymotic hemorrhages visible on the mucous membranes of the vulva and surrounding skin.

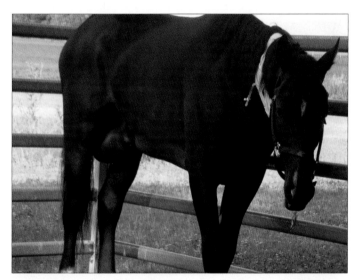

Figure 4.51 Vasculitis. Marked edema of ventral abdomen, scrotum and limbs in this horse which developed widespread vasculitis secondary to septicemia.

Treatment

- **Provide supportive therapy.** This includes hydrotherapy and limb wraps to limit edema formation. Nutritional and fluid support as many animals will be markedly depressed and disinclined to eat or drink. A tracheostomy may be required in cases of edema of the upper respiratory tract.

- **Remove the antigenic stimulant if possible.** No treatment effectively eliminates the viruses of EIA or EVA from the body. The course of equine ehrlichiosis may be shortened by the administration of oxytetracycline. Where the cause is not clearly known and is suspected to be immune-mediated, any drugs being administered at the time of presentation should be stopped. A search for underlying

type of complement components in circulating immune complexes may also possibly be important in relative risk of developing vasculitis. Purpura hemorrhagica following *S. equi* infection is the result of deposition of circulating immune complexes to IgA and *S. equi* subsp. *equi* M protein in small subcutaneous vessels.

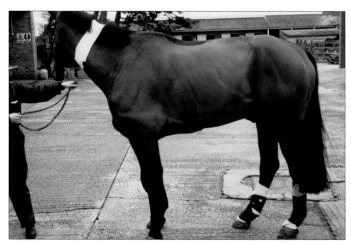

Figure 4.52 Purpura hemorrhagica. Sharply demarcated edema of the fore-limb at the level of elbow.

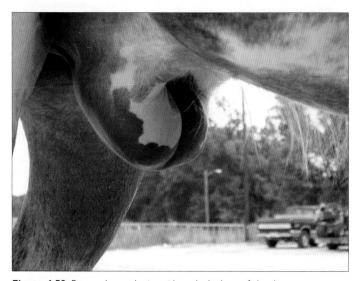

Figure 4.53 Purpura hemorrhagica with marked edema of sheath.

Differential diagnosis:
- Equine viral arteritis
- Protein losing condition
- Congestive heart failure.

infection or neoplasia should be undertaken. Many cases of purpura hemorrhagica following *S. equi* infection occur after the infection has resolved but if a *Strep.* sp. infection is suspected of having been involved penicillin should be administered as unrecognized ongoing sepsis and antigen production will prolong the ongoing vasculitis.

- ***Reduce vessel wall inflammation.*** NSAIDs can be used to decrease vascular inflammation and provide analgesia. Some cases may require or warrant corticosteroid administration (see below).
- ***Normalize the immune response.*** Clinical experience suggests that corticosteroid therapy is useful in horses with idiopathic vasculitis syndromes. The decision on whether or not to administer corticosteroids will in many cases depend on the severity of the case. Mild cases may resolve wihout immunosuppressive therapy but more severe life-threatening cases are candidates for immediate aggressive corticosteroid therapy. Dexamethasone is generally given as first choice (0.05–0.2 mg/kg q 12–24 h IV or IM). Prednisolone can also be used orally at 0.5–1 mg/kg, but anecdotally it is not as successful possibly due to poor oral absorption. Once edema and

hemorrhages start to resolve the dose can be reduced by 10–15% every 1–2 days. Relapses are common and may require the dose to be temporarily increased. Horses with purpura hemorrhagica frequently require therapy for 4–6 weeks.

Prognosis

- The prognosis depends on the initiating disease process. Cases related to EVA and equine ehrlichiosis carry a good prognosis. Horses with EIA are infected persistently and may have relapses. Horses with idiopathic syndrome have an unpredictable response to therapy and as a result an unpredictable prognosis.
- Many horses with purpura hemorrhagica recover but require aggressive prolonged therapy and many may have numerous sequelae such as laminitis, cellulitis, skin sloughing and thrombophlebitis.

Infectious disorders

Viral diseases

Equine viral arteritis (see also Chapter 12, pp. 474, 490 and 511) This virus is probably distributed worldwide, though little serological evidence of it has been found in Britain or Japan. While, in some parts of the world, this produces a severe and highly fatal disease, milder or completely inapparent infections, which are only detectable serologically, are more common. The clinical signs are the result of a panvasculitis and are similar, in most mild cases, to those caused by equine herpes and equine influenza viruses and to some extent those of the milder forms of African horse sickness. Affected horses show typical signs of upper respiratory tract virus infection with pyrexia, cough, palpebral edema, chemosis (conjunctival edema) and conjunctivitis with lacrimation. The significant specific clinical signs are related to the panvasculitis and the consequent increased vascular permeability of small arteries and capillaries which results in blood-stained tears. There is commonly a prominent edema of the limbs, head and neck in a very similar way to African horse sickness. The ventral abdomen and the genitalia of stallions are often edematous. The severe forms of the disease present with many of the typical clinical signs of purpura haemorrhagica, but are usually also febrile and show lacrimation, chemosis (edema of the conjunctiva), swelling of the eyelids, diarrhea and weakness. Petechial hemorrhages are commonly encountered in the mucous membranes. Cutaneous edema and urticaria-like plaques are less common in viral arteritis than in purpura haemorrhagica. Abortion is a particularly common and serious effect of the virus. Secondary pleural and peritoneal effusions are present in the severe forms. Many infections are entirely subclinical without any overt clinical signs, only being detectable serologically. The similarity of this disease to several other conditions in which upper respiratory tract infections and/or vasculitis are present makes its diagnosis particularly important.

Diagnosis and treatment

- Antibodies to EAV can be demonstrated by complement fixation and virus neutralization tests. Semen samples with sperm-rich fraction should be collected for virus isolation of suspected infected stallions.
- EAV can be isolated from both fetus and placenta by virus isolation, especially from placenta, fetal spleen, lung and kidney and fetal/placental fluids.
- Supportive care is the most important element of therapy. For prevention see Chapter 12, p. 474.

Equine infectious anemia (EIA)

This is a retroviral disease transmitted by blood-feeding arthropods, which occurs worldwide, but which has been effectively controlled in some areas. The acute syndrome is usually associated with the first episode of infection and is clinically similar to that caused by equine viral arteritis with transient petechial hemorrhages, thrombocytopenia and fever. Recurring cycles of fever and progressive anemia, ventral and dependent edema, icterus and weight loss are typical of the subacute or chronic form of the disease. The severity of the anemia increases with each succeeding viremic, febrile episode and while successive episodes are usually milder, the disease progresses inexorably. Consequent severe, prolonged anemia results in organ failure which, along with the anemia, may be detected at post-mortem examination. The clinical signs usually become less severe with time but any stress may result in the development of an acute or peracute episode. There is a population of horses in which clinical signs are inapparent and these represent a carrier state which is a severe threat to unaffected horses.

Diagnosis and management

- The agar gel immunodiffusion test (Coggin's test) is extremely sensitive and very easily performed, and has been largely responsible for the control and eradication of the disease over large areas of the world. False-negatives can occur early in the course of the disease. False-positives can occur in foals following passive transfer of antibodies from the dam. Additionally there is a small percentage of chronically infected horses that may test negative. In these instances repeat testing at a 30-day interval is recommended.
- An enzyme-linked immunosorbent assay test is also available and while more rapid is not as sensitive for chronically infected horses.
- There is no treatment that results in viral clearance and animals, once infected, appear to remain viremic for the rest of their lives.
- In most jurisdictions horses that are found to be positive for EIA must be reported to government authorities.

African horse sickness

African horse sickness (see p. 132) is also characterized by an extensive and diffuse vasculitis with petechiation and protein loss into tissues and organs. The clinical signs of the disease can be attributed almost completely to the development of an extensive and severe vasculitis in the lungs and other major organs.

Thrombophlebitis (Figs. 4.54–4.61)

This is a common complication of catheter placement. Thrombosis without inflammation results in a hardened, 'cord-like' vein. This arises as a result of the thrombogenic nature of the catheter or in most instances as a result of a hypercoagulable state (activation of clotting system in septicemia, disseminated intravascular coagulation, toxemia or as a result of dehydration). Thrombophlebitis results when there is concurrent infection or inflammation. This can arise as a result of poor technique during catheter placement, secondary to septicemia or from irritant drugs, e.g. oxytetracycline.

Thrombosis (or other occlusion) of arteries has catastrophic effects upon the distal tissues, particularly where the collateral circulation is inadequate to maintain oxygenation. Thus occlusion of a digital artery in the limb by a neuroma may result in gangrene and sloughing of the foot. Occlusion of a major mesenteric artery may cause extensive and catastrophic ischemia, whereas occlusion of a minor mesenteric vessel has less local effect. Occlusion of major veins, whether through thrombosis or obstruction, results in increased venous pressure on the capillary bed it serves. This causes edema and ischemia which result in further damage and progressive deterioration. Common sequelae of thrombosis are generalized venous engorgement and coagulation and gross edema, venous distension and/or necrosis of the tissues in the distal capillary beds.

Clinical signs

The rate of development of vascular occlusion and arterial damage has a profound effect upon the extent of signs. Thus, slowly

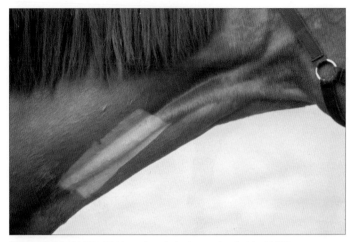

Figure 4.54 Phlebitis. Thickened corded vein associated with phlebitis.

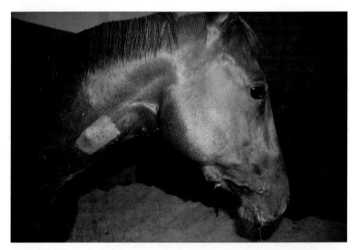

Figure 4.55 Jugular thrombophlebitis. Note that the thrombophlebitis appears to be more localized in this case with a distinct swelling in the mid-jugular area corresponding to the location of previous catheter placement.

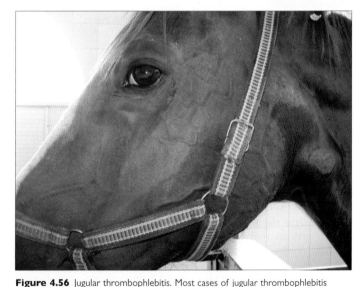

Figure 4.56 Jugular thrombophlebitis. Most cases of jugular thrombophlebitis arise secondary to the injection of irritant drugs or the placement of intravenous catheters. The subsequent inflammation can move proximally and distally within the vein to result in large areas of venous occlusion with thrombus formation. This mare had an intravenous catheter placed distally but developed a large thrombus through most of the length of the jugular vein which can be seen here at the angle of the jaw. The subsequent venous occlusion has resulted in distension of the veins of the face.

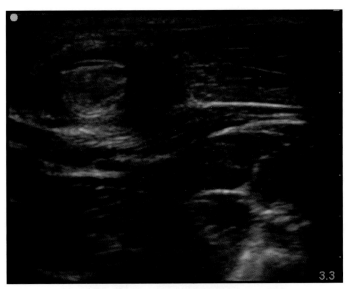

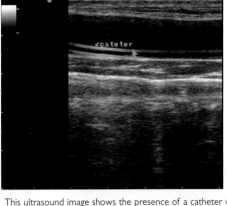

Figure 4.59 This ultrasound image shows the presence of a catheter within the jugular vein. The catheter is imaged as a hyperechoic linear structure within the vein. The development of venous thrombi can be more sensitively detected by ultrasound than by external changes such as heat or swelling.

Figure 4.57 Thrombophlebitis. This ultrasound image of the jugular vein shows the presence of a large thrombus.

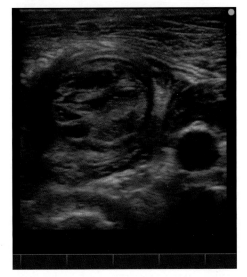

Figure 4.58 This ultrasound image is of a septic thrombus within the jugular vein. Note the septate appearance which is characteristic of a septic thrombus.

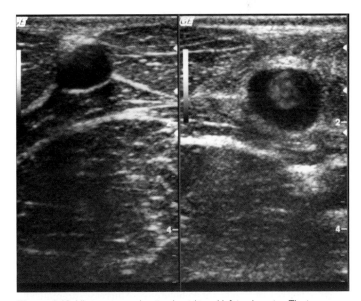

Figure 4.60 Ultrasonogram showing the right and left jugular veins. The image on the right shows a thrombus resulting in partial occlusion of the vein. Note also the distension of the vessel which results from thrombus formation.

progressive occlusion of one (or even both) jugular vein is usually adequately compensated by collateral circulation. In these cases swelling of extremities is less evident, although it is usually possible to identify distension of the superficial veins distal to the lesion.

Rapidly developing, complete venous occlusion induces severe edema, which in the case of the jugular vein is exacerbated by the tendency for the affected horse to hang its head down.

- **Thrombosis.** The clinical signs of thrombosis are dependent largely on the vessel affected. Thus thrombosis of mesenteric vessels would commonly result in signs of colic, thrombosis of limb vessels would result in lameness and thrombosis of both jugular veins would result in marked edema of the proximal neck and head.
- **Thrombophlebitis.** Heat, pain and swelling are the most common signs when there is a septic thrombophlebitis.

- Consequent Horner's syndrome and other circulatory effects such as facial swelling and congestion of facial vessels may be present.

Diagnosis and treatment

- Clinical examination and history. Ultrasonographic examination should be employed to assess the extent of venous occlusion and to determine whether there is an infection present. Cavitations of the thrombus or identification of fluid pockets is suggestive of a septic process.
- If a septic thrombophlebitis is present broad-spectrum antibiotics should be administered in addition to anti-inflammatories.
- Topical therapy such as hot compresses, ichthammol or DMSO may help to reduce inflammation. Drainage of focal abscesses may be required. In rare cases surgical resection of the vein may be required.

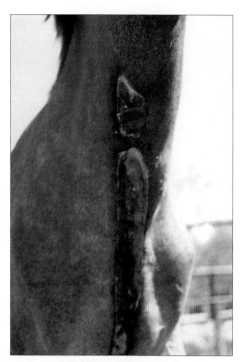

Figure 4.61 Necrosing phlebitis caused by perivascular injection of an irritant drug. The resultant slough included jugular vein, carotid artery and vago-sympathetic trunk. Right-side Horner's syndrome and laryngeal paralysis were present.

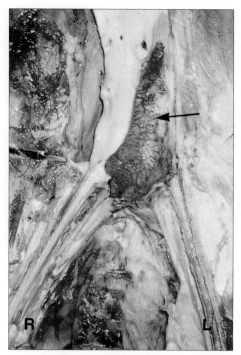

Figure 4.62 Aorto-iliac thrombosis (arteriosclerosis). Note the dense nature of tissue narrowing the aortic diameter (arrow). Marked asymmetry of occlusive lesion resulting in a more severe left iliac occlusion than right.

Prognosis

Many cases of venous thrombosis resolve spontaneously over months or years with some effective cannulation of major and lesser vessels. Potential sequelae of thrombophlebitis of the jugular vein include:

- Unilateral vascular occlusion: limiting venous access.
- Bilateral jugular occlusion: results in impaired venous return from the head and upper neck. Such cases present with edema of the head and dyspnea as a consequence of laryngeal compression. Emergency tracheostomy may be required.
- Thromboemboli to distant organs such as heart, lung, kidney or other vascular beds occur rarely but the consequences can be grave. The risk of significant embolic disease increases dramatically where the site is infected due to an increased tendency for disruption of the thrombus.
- Septicemia or bacteremia could also occur.
- Ipsilateral laryngeal paralysis.

Aorto-iliac thrombosis (Fig. 4.62)

This thrombosis involving the distal aorta, its quadrification and the major hind limb arteries is an important clinical disorder of unknown etiology. Historically related to parasite migration it is now thought unlikely that this is the only cause. Affected horses show intermittent lameness which is characteristically brought on or aggravated by exercise. The extent of the clinical signs is largely dependent upon the speed of onset and the ultimate extent of the occlusion. True saddle thrombus occurring at the bifurcation of the aorta as a result of a massive, peracute occluding embolus, and resulting in complete occlusion of the iliac arteries, is very rare in the horse. Affected animals have cold hind limbs and rapidly developing, complete hind-quarter paralysis. The slowly developing diffuse thickening of the distal aorta, the aortic quadrification and the iliac vessels,

characterized by narrowing of the arterial lumen is much more common. The extent of the thrombosis and narrowing is variable, often with one hind leg being more severely affected than the other. Bilateral cases in which there is little apparent difference between the hind legs are, however, encountered. The affected limb is relatively cool and sweating is very limited. Very poor subcutaneous venous definition will invariably be present in the affected limb(s). A weak, or even absent, arterial pulse in the arteries of the distal limb may help to define the position and severity of the obstruction. Differences in peripheral pulse quality between the two hind limbs is usually strongly indicative of an occlusive lesion in the more proximal arteries although this may, of course, in some very rare cases, be due to other obstructive conditions. All of the typical signs are consistent with the reduced blood supply, which may be adequate when there is little or no demand upon circulatory efficiency. Immediately following exercise, affected horses commonly exhibit clinical signs of colic, often lying down, flank watching and stamping their feet. There may be muscle wasting over the hind-quarters although this is uncommon.

Diagnosis

- Clinical signs are suggestive in many cases.
- A definitive diagnosis may be achieved with careful rectal and ultrasonographic assessment of the pelvic arteries. Not all the branches of all the arteries will be affected equally, some may be partially occluded, others may have no occlusion, while others may be totally obstructed. Occlusive lesions which extend down to the major muscle branches of the hind limbs are relatively frequent.
- At post-mortem examination the extent and the chronic, atherosclerotic nature of the lesion, can be appreciated.

Treatment

- Treatment aims at improving collateral circulation and preventing additional thrombus formation.

sinuatrial or interventricular node, may induce serious irregularities of electrical activity and consequent arrhythmia, including atrial fibrillation and ventricular ectopic contractions, and may be responsible for sudden and unexpected deaths.

Diagnosis is, in most cases, made at necropsy.

Part 2: The blood, lymphatic vessels and lymph nodes

Disorders of the blood and blood-forming organs produce a limited number of clinically detectable signs, prominent amongst which are anemia, bleeding and icterus (and their associated implications). A wide variety of clinical disorders may ultimately present with apparently similar clinical features identified primarily by changes in the mucous membranes. Accurate and careful clinical assessment will usually enable the clinician to establish a tentative diagnosis which may then be confirmed with the aid of appropriate laboratory investigations. The responses of the equine erythron to decreasing numbers is notoriously slow and unspectacular and even longstanding cases of anemia may show only mild changes in circulating cell morphology and numbers. Nucleated red cells are very rarely encountered in peripheral blood and reticulocytes probably do not appear at all. The responses of the red and white cell series to disease processes are useful aids to the diagnosis of many diseases, but the changes are fickle and they should not be given undue significance without supporting clinical evidence.

Developmental disorders

Congenital abnormalities of the blood and lymphatic system of the horse are, in general, very rare conditions.

Coagulation defects (Figs. 4.64 & 4.65)

Several congenital clotting defects in horses have been reported. However, all of these are very rare. They include:

- Protein C deficiency: protein C is a vitamin-K-dependent molecule which is a natural hemostatic inhibitor.
- Prekallikrein deficiency has been reported in Belgians and miniatures. Prekallikrein is needed for the activation of the intrinsic coagulation cascade. It is one of several contact activation factors that interact with the negative charged surfaces (e.g. collagen) in the subendothelial matrix.
- Von Willebrand's disease has been reported in Thoroughbreds and Quarterhorses. Laboratory clotting times are normal. This disease results in failure of platelet aggregation and activation resulted in increased tendency to bleed.
- Hemophilia A (inherited factor VIII deficiency) is the most common clotting deficiency encountered and has been reported in a number of breeds. This is the most common disorder and is encountered in Thoroughbred, Standardbred and Arabian foals, and may be sex-linked to the male and genetically carried by apparently normal females. Most of these conditions are certainly hereditary and laboratory evaluation will enable a definitive diagnosis to be made of the specific factor deficit.

Clinical signs

Clinical signs are attributable to a bleeding diathesis characterized by large-vessel hemorrhage, usually including spontaneous hemorrhages into the subcutis, multiple hematoma formation and a progressive (regenerative) anemia which ultimately becomes nonregenerative. Hemarthrosis (bleeding into joints) is also a common

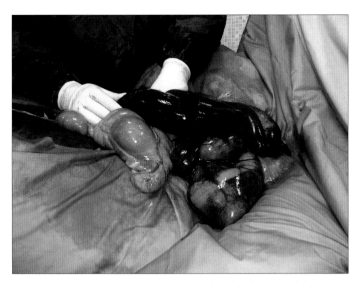
Figure 4.63 Verminous arteritis has resulted in thrombus formation of this mesenteric vessel with secondary bowel ischemia.

- There are no controlled studies of treatment but a variety of anticoagulants, anthelmintics, anti-inflammatories and controlled exercise programs have been used.
- Early recognition and therapy are essential.

Parasitic diseases (Fig. 4.63)

Lesions arising in the wall of the major arteries form an important group of disorders. Although now less commonly seen in the developed world due to the extensive use of anthelmintics, they are still important in developing countries and may become more common as resistance to currently available anthelmintics increases. Lesions occurring in the arteries are frequently attributable to the migratory habits of *Strongylus vulgaris*. Damage to the *tunica intima* of the cranial mesenteric artery and/or the aorta leads to damage which may either result in narrowing of the arterial lumen or to a localized (but often severe and extensive) arteritis surrounding variable numbers of larvae. Destruction or disruption of the muscular layer of the arteries allows the development of a localized enlargement or ballooning (aneurysm) of the arterial wall. The most dramatic form of verminous arteritis results in rupture of the affected vessel and catastrophic blood loss, but such a scenario is rare. Much more commonly, the localized inflammatory response results in embolic occlusion of larger or smaller mesenteric arteries and this results in focal areas of ischemia of the jejunum, colon or cecum. The clinical consequences of this occlusion are heavily dependent upon the extent and efficiency of collateral circulation and upon the amount of devitalized intestine.

Neoplastic disorders

Primary neoplastic disorders of the heart are very uncommon, but secondary lesions may develop in the myocardium, epicardium, endocardium or within the pericardial sac. The commonest lesions are those of lymphosarcoma, hemangiosarcoma and melanoma (predominantly in gray horses). Lesions occurring in and around the heart valves produce valvular distortions and murmurs are audible. Ultrasonographic examination will detect the thickened and distorted valve and incompetent valve closure but will not usually identify the type of lesion present. Masses within the myocardium, such as melanoma and lymphosarcoma, may be asymptomatic but, particularly where these are located in the interventricular septum or at either the finding and consequently both joint swelling and lameness are presented. Aspiration of blood-stained synovial fluid from more than one joint of a young foal is highly suggestive of a coagulation disorder, particularly when other evidence also exists. Colic as a result of intra-abdominal bleeding, epistaxis, hemoptysis, depression and dyspnea are less common signs. Prolonged bleeding after minor trauma or routine procedures, e.g. passage of a nasogastric tube, can result in severe and prolonged hemorrhage. Other signs include petechial hemorrhages, melena, anemia or frank blood in the urine.

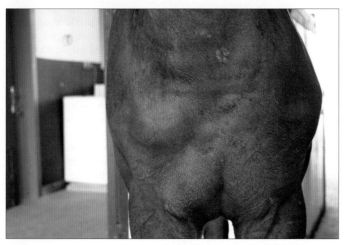

Figure 4.64 Inherited defects: hematoma formation.

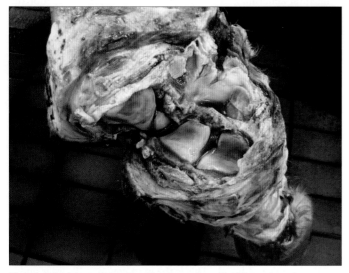

Figure 4.65 Inherited disorders: blood-stained joint fluid (hemarthrosis).

Diagnosis

A series of laboratory tests can be used to establish a diagnosis of a clotting disorder and to distinguish between the various disorders (see Table 4.2). These tests are:

- Bleeding time (BT). The time taken for a small cutaneous or gingival pinprick to stop bleeding. Normal time is 3–4 minutes
- First stage prothrombin time (PT)
- Activated partial thromboplastin time (APPT)
- Clotting time (CT). This is an in vitro test and is the time taken for a blood sample to clot in a glass tube at 37°C. Normal values are between 4.5 and 7 minutes
- Factor VIII determination. In humans with hemophilia A, the severity of the disorder varies inversely with this value
- Von Willebrand's disease is diagnosed on the basis of measurement of plasma concentrations of VWF: Ag.

Treatment and prognosis

- Emergency treatment is often undertaken in a hemorrhaging foal prior to diagnosis. Such treatments can include plasma or whole blood administration. However, catheter placement in these foals can in itself result in severe hemorrhage.
- There is no effective long-term treatment for these disorders and euthanasia is frequently recommended. Carrier females should be removed from the breeding population.

Thrombocytopenia

There are three main types of thrombocytopenia:

1) **Reduced platelet production** may result from bone marrow aplasia, suppression or marrow infiltration due to neoplasia or severe inflammation
2) **Increased platelet consumption** such as disseminated intravascular coagulation (DIC)
3) **Increased platelet destruction** such as immune-mediated thrombocytopenia (IMTP). IMTP is either primary (idiopathic or autoimmune) or secondary, induced by drug administration, infection or neoplasia.

Disseminated intravascular coagulopathy (Figs. 4.66–4.69)

DIC is a systemic thrombohemorrhagic disorder. Activation of coagulation, inhibition of fibrinolysis and consumption of coagulation inhibitors and platelets lead to a hypercoagulant state with subsequent thrombus formation in small and large vessels resulting in ischemia in the major organs and body tissues. Many disease conditions including acute gastrointestinal diseases, endotoxemia, shock, septicemia, hemorrhage and protein-losing enteropathy have been implicated as causes of this condition. It is not however limited to the above conditions. In the pathogenesis of DIC, two proteolytic enzymes, thrombin and plastin, are activated and circulate systemically; it is the relative balance between the two that determines whether a given horse develops a thrombotic or bleeding tendency. Thrombin activation leads to increased fibrin formation with which an activated coagulation state results in fibrin deposition in the microvasculature.

Table 4.2 Diagnostic features of the more common congenital clotting disorders

	Deficit	BT (min)	CT (min)	PT (s)	APTT (s)
Hemophilia A	Factor VIII	>20	Prolonged	Normal	Prolonged
Von Willebrand's disease	vWF	Normal	Normal	Normal	Normal
Reference value		2–4	4–7	9–12	47–73

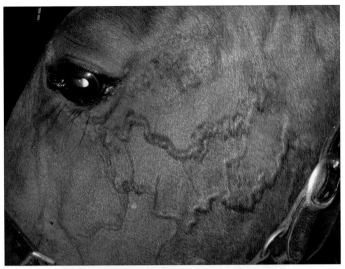

Figure 4.66 DIC. Note the marked venous distension in this mare with DIC secondary to intestinal salmonellosis. The mare in this image died a few moments after this photograph was taken and DIC was confirmed at necropsy.

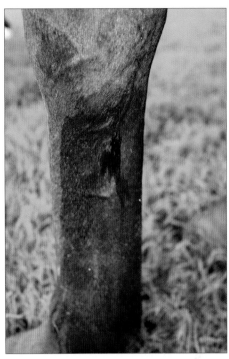

Figure 4.68 DIC. Delayed clotting time in a horse with DIC following a nerve block.

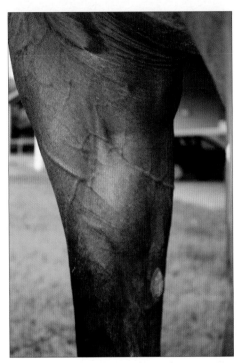

Figure 4.67 DIC. Hematoma formation at site of venepuncture.

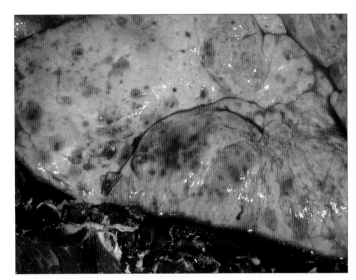

Figure 4.69 DIC. Hemorrhages throughout the lungs of a horse that died with DIC.

These microthrombi lead to tissue ischemia and organ dysfunction. This is usually first clinically obvious at sites where venepuncture has been carried out. Jugular thrombosis in response to venepuncture is a common manifestation of the early stages of the condition.

Concurrently anticoagulation mechanisms are suppressed and inhibitory proteins of the coagulation cascade are defective with resultant impairment of fibrinolysis despite high levels of plasmin. Consumption of coagulation factors and platelets may then result in excessive bleeding, especially in advanced or more severe cases. Bleeding from even minor surgical wounds and venepuncture sites and spontaneous hematoma formation indicate the onset of the advanced hemorrhagic stages. Petechiation and ecchymotic hemorrhages on

mucosa, inner pinna, retina (in foals), melena and epistaxis form the overt clinical signs of the condition. Damage to the kidney or other internal organs may ensue from the development of thrombi, ischemia and bleeding within the capillary beds, resulting in further damage and further collagen exposure.

It is also important to remember that subclinical hyperactivation of coagulation without clinical signs of DIC is common in horses with colic, especially those that have undergone surgical procedures.

Diagnosis

The condition in many cases can be suspected on the basis of clinical signs but this would obviously preclude subclinical cases. A 'definitive' diagnosis depends on the alteration of three of the following six values:

- aPTT. This is considered to be the most sensitive parameter and is increased in DIC
- PT. Prolongation of PT times are normally seen
- Fibrinogen concentration. Frequently within normal limits
- Antithrombin concentration. The activity of antithrombin is usually severely decreased
- D-dimer concentration. Typically there are marked elevations
- Platelet count. Thrombocytopenia is rare except in the most severe cases.

Treatment

- Early recognition, especially of the subclinical stages, is important as early intervention is associated with much improved success rates of therapy and an improved prognosis.
- The first aim of therapy is to remove the inciting cause and therefore appropriate treatment of the primary disorder is paramount.
- Other recommendations are the administration of fresh frozen plasma and heparin. The ideal amount of plasma to be administered is unknown but is thought to be between 5–10 L per 500 kg, with many clinicians choosing an intermediate dose of 7 L per 500 kg. However, because of the potential of plasma to actually promote coagulation, concurrent heparin administration is recommended as it potentiates the inhibitory action of antithrombin and inhibits formation of new thrombi. It does not have any effect on thrombi that have already formed. Low-molecular-weight heparin is preferred as it has the advantage of neither decreasing hematocrit nor increasing aPTT. It is used at a dose of 50–1 000 anti-FXa IU/kg q 24 h.

Immune-mediated thrombocytopenia (IMTP)

IMTP is, again, most often associated with other pre-existing infections (such as upper respiratory tract infections), or other serious intercurrent diseases such as lymphosarcoma or chronic infectious processes. In many cases, however, no other condition can be identified at the time of presentation.

Clinical signs

- The onset of the clinical syndrome is characteristically insidious and the signs of hemorrhagic diatheses are often the most obvious presenting features. Thus, mild or occasionally more severe, spontaneous intermittent or persistent, unilateral or bilateral epistaxis is a common finding and occurs when the platelet count falls sufficiently.
- As one of the primary functions of the platelets is the maintenance of the vascular endothelial integrity, dramatic reductions in their numbers result in the development of petechial or larger, ecchymotic hemorrhages, which are most prominent on the more stressed mucous membranes of the nasal cavity, pharynx and vulva.
- Hyphema (bleeding into the anterior chamber of the eye) and micro-hematuria are commonly encountered but may easily be overlooked.
- There are usually few other signs of overt illness, but spontaneous and/or trauma-induced hematomas and prolonged bleeding from injection sites or minor cuts may be encountered. Chronic (persistent) bleeding commonly occurs into the lumen of the intestine and results in significant, detectable blood and blood products in the feces.

Diagnosis

- The response to corticosteroid therapy is highly supportive of the diagnosis but the specific detection of antiplatelet antibodies is definitive. However, the latter tests are insensitive and are, at present, poorly defined for the horse.

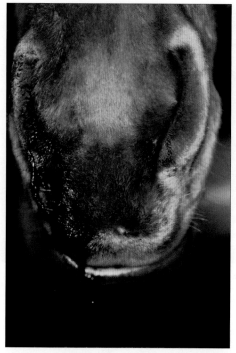

Figure 4.70 Thrombocytopenia in this horse has resulted in spontaneous epistaxis.

- The absence of hot, painful, skin swellings helps to differentiate the disorder from purpura hemorrhagica and the absence of febrile response and other systemic signs of illness preclude infectious causes of anemia.

Idiopathic thrombocytopenia (Fig. 4.70)

Idiopathic thrombocytopenia in which no underlying explanation (either immunological or infectious or iatrogenic) can be found, also occurs in horses. The disorder presents in the same way and the clinical course follows the same pattern as the autoimmune disorder but fails to show any response to therapy. Bone marrow examination is a useful, underutilized, means of assessing the response to all of these conditions.

Clinical signs

- Thrombocytopenia results in hemorrhagic diathesis when platelet counts fall below 30×10^9/L characterized by ecchymotic and petechial hemorrhages.
- Other clinical signs include epistaxis, hematuria or spontaneous hemorrhages.
- Clinical signs related to an underlying disorder may be predominant in cases of DIC or immune-mediated thrombocytopenia, thus aiding differentiation from these disorders.

Diagnosis

- Thrombocytopenia ($<100 \times 10^9$/L) should be confirmed. Pseudo-thrombocytopenia is frequently seen as a result of platelet interaction with ethylenediaminetetraacetic acid (EDTA) anticoagulant. This should be suspected when platelet clumping is reported on the blood smear and a second sample in 3.8% sodium citrate anticoagulant should be analyzed for comparison.
- When abnormal PT, APTT and fibrin degradation products (FDP) accompany thrombocytopenia, DIC should be suspected.
- When a normal PT, APTT, plasma fibrinogen and FDP accompany thrombocytopenia, bone marrow disease or IMTP should be suspected.

- Direct immunofluorescence and flow cytometry can be used to identify surface-associated Ig molecules in IMTP.
- Alloimmune thrombocytopenia should be suspected in thrombocytopenic foals in which sepsis has been ruled out and platelet antibody tests are positive.

Treatment
No treatment exists for bone marrow hypoplasia. Treatment for IMTP should include:

- Whole blood or platelet rich transfusions are indicated in life-threatening cases
- Withdrawal of any medication and adjustment of antibiotic therapy (if it is required) to molecularly dissimilar agents
- Identify and treat any possible underlying diseases.
- Dexamethasone (0.05–0.1 mg/kg IV q 12–24 h) should be administered with the dose decreased to 0.01 mg/kg when the platelet count is $>10 \times 10^9$/L. The platelet count should be normal for at least 5 days prior to withdrawal of steroid therapy
- Corticosteroid refractory immune-mediated thrombocytopenia may be treated with azathioprine (0.5–3 mg/kg PO q 24 h) or vincristine (0.014 mg/kg IV q 10 days).

Hemolytic anemia (Fig. 4.71)
Hemolytic anemia, which can be intravascular or extravascular, results from accelerated removal of red cells from the circulation. Intravascular hemolysis is classically associated with icterus and hemoglobinuria and is usually acute in onset. Extravascular hemolysis is associated with icterus without hemoglobinuria.

Intravascular hemolysis
Oxidative damage to red cells can occur from exposure to wilted red maple leaves, phenothiazines or onions. This oxidative damage results in Heinz body formation, increased fragility of red cells and changes in cell permeability with subsequent intravascular hemolysis along with increased removal by mononuclear phagocytic cells in the spleen and liver. Oxidative changes also result in methemoglobin formation with resultant decreased oxygen-carrying capacity.

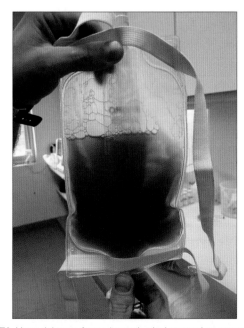

Figure 4.71 Hemoglobinuria from a horse that had received an excessively rapid administration of DMSO solution intravenously.

Red maple leave toxicity is the most common type of oxidative damage and is frequently seen in the eastern United States. Combined hemolytic anemia and tissue hypoxia as a result of methemoglobin formation result in clinical signs of fever, tachycardia, tachypnea, icterus and hemoglobinuria.

Diagnosis
- A combination of clinical signs and history of exposure to an oxidative agent is usually sufficient for a presumptive diagnosis but supportive clinical laboratory data of oxidative damage are easily obtained.
- Hematological abnormalities seen include: anemia, increased mean corpuscular hemoglobin (MCH), increased mean corpuscular hemoglobin concentration (MCHC), free plasma hemoglobin, anisocytosis, poikilocytosis, eccentrocytes, lysed erythrocytes, agglutination, Heinz bodies and neutrophilia.
- Serum chemistry findings include: increased direct and indirect bilirubin, serum creatinine and serum urea nitrogen levels; reduced RBC glutathione levels, increased AST, SDH, CK and GGT activities. Additional changes which may be found are metabolic acidosis, hypercalcemia and hyperglycemia.
- Urinalysis typically reveals hemoglobinuria, methemoglobinuria, proteinuria, bilirubinuria and urobilinogenuria.
- ***Differential diagnosis:*** familial methemoglobemia or nitrate toxicity.

Treatment and prognosis
- The aims of therapy are to provide supportive care, reduce the fragility of red cells, maximize tissue oxygenation and maintain renal perfusion. This may include oxygen therapy for patients with hypoxia and severe tachypnea. Removal of the horse from the source of the oxidative damage is important, and administration of activated charcoal (8–24 mg/kg up to 2.2 kg via nasogastric tube) may help reduce further absorption. Fluid therapy helps to maintain renal perfusion and diuretics in those patients with acute renal failure. Whole blood transfusions may be required in severe cases. Dexamethasone (0.05–0.1 mg/kg IV q 12–24 h) may help to stabilize cell membranes. Ascorbic acid and vitamin E administration may also be beneficial for improving cell membrane stability.
- Methylene blue has been historically used to treat methemoglobinemia but there is little evidence to support its use.
- The prognosis is guarded for horses with severe hemolysis due to the high incidence of sequelae such as renal failure, cerebral hypoxia, laminitis, bowel hypoxia and DIC. Red maple leaf toxicosis has a mortality rate of up to 60%.

Other causes of intravascular hemolysis
- Microangiopathic hemolysis can occur following vessel thrombosis and is a potential sequel to chronic DIC.
- Liver failure can result in hemolysis with the proposed pathogenesis being changes in RBC lipoprotein as a result of increased bile acids.
- Snake bite envenomation can result in hemolysis in addition to altered coagulation.
- Bacterial exotoxins may result in hemolysis and are most commonly seen in septicemic neonates.
- *Leptospira* spp. infections although rare may also result in hemolysis.
- Heavy metal intoxication.
- Intravenous administration of hypotonic fluids, poorly diluted DMSO or excessively rapid administration of appropriately diluted DMSO can all result in intravascular hemolysis.

Extravascular hemolysis

Immune-mediated hemolytic anemia

In contrast to the hemolytic disease of newborn foals, immune-mediated, **(autoimmune) hemolytic anemia** in adult horses is rare. The condition may be primary, in which antibody is produced directly against the animal's own erythrocytes, or secondary when antibody is produced against other antigens which become adherent to erythrocytes. The former state is particularly rare, while the latter is somewhat more common and is associated with underlying disease with an infectious agent (notably equine infectious anemia, *Babesia* organisms and *Anaplasma* phagocytophilia), neoplasia, or following drug administration. Some infectious agents have been thought to be responsible for changes in epitopes of the red cell membrane, while others are thought to result in neoantigens adherent to erythrocytes that contribute to enhanced removal by immune mechanisms. Most often the progression of this disease is slow and insidious, with a longstanding, chronic anemia. Pallor, weakness and poor exercise tolerance are the major presenting clinical features. Icterus and hemoglobinuria are rarely present, presumably as the destruction of red cells takes place within the reticuloendothelial organs and is therefore extravascular. However, in some cases a combination of extravascular and intravascular hemolysis is possible, especially when IgM antibodies or complement are involved.

Diagnosis

- History and clinical signs are suggestive but may be overshadowed by other signs associated with the primary disorder.
- Autoagglutination suggests surface-bound antibody. If erythrocytes agglutinate after dilution of the sample 1:1 with saline, they can be considered positive for surface-bound antibody.
- When autoagglutination is absent direct or indirect Coombs test can be used. The direct test is more sensitive but it is important to realize that false-negatives may be obtained if an incomplete set of reagents is used, if the test is not performed at both 40°C and 37°C, or if severe hemolysis has already resulted in the removal of the majority of antibody-coated RBCs from the circulation.
- Newer methods of diagnosis include direct immunoflorescence assay with class-specific antibodies to equine IgG, IgM and IgA.

Treatment

- Any current drug administration should be stopped. If drug therapy is required for an underlying infection a different class of antimicrobials should be chosen. Penicillins and cephalosporins are most commonly associated with IMHA.
- Other possible causative underlying infections should be ruled out.
- Immunosuppressive therapy is required in most horses with dexamethasone (0.05–0.2 mg/kg IV q 24 h) being most commonly used. Patients should be monitored for response by frequent monitoring of packed cell volume (PCV). If a rapid response reflected by stabilization of PCV is not seen then the dose may be increased. It may take a full week of therapy to observe the full effect in terms of a rise in PCV but once stabilized at 20% the steroid therapy should be tapered.
- Azathioprine and cyclophosphamide have been used to manage rare refractory cases.

Anemia as a result of nutritional deficiencies

Nutritional deficiencies of protein, iron, folate, vitamin B$_{12}$, copper and cobalt have all been implicated in chronic progressive anemia in foals and adult horses. In both adults and foals normal dietary components are usually sufficient in all these respects but dietary deficiency or failure of absorption and chronic infections may affect the availability of one or more of them. Anemia associated with acute, massive blood loss in the absence of overt bleeding from wounds etc. is usually the result of internal bleeding which in the foal may be from gastric ulceration, or from the rupture of one or more of the major blood vessels. Significant blood loss may arise in young foals from premature rupture of the umbilical cord. Bleeding into the internal cavities renders most of the iron temporarily unavailable to the animal, although a significant proportion of the red cells may be re-introduced into the circulation via the lymphatic vessels.

Chronic infection (and other persistent immune stimulant conditions including neoplasia) is one of the commonest causes of **non-regenerative anemia** in both foals and adult horses. Pleuritis, pneumonia, chronic internal abscesses and neoplasia are potentially responsible for the development of a typical **iron-deficiency anemia** which arises from a lack of available iron, although total body-iron is usually normal. Affected horses show a profound progressive microcytic, hypochromic anemia with little or no bone marrow response. Deficiencies of other nutrients are supposedly responsible for the development of clinically important anemia but it is unlikely that, in the absence of underlying disease, horses ingesting a normal diet will be found to be deficient in any of the more significant nutrients.

Polycythemia

Polycythemia is an increase in red blood cell mass. Relative polycythemia results from plasma volume reduction such as occurs in dehydration, endotoxemia or splenic contraction. Absolute polycythemia is an increase in red cell mass without a change in plasma volume. Primary absolute polycytemia is when red cell mass increases without a concurrent increase in erythropoietin concentration. Secondary absolute polycythemia is an increase in red cell mass in response to increased erythropoietin. Examples of causes are congenital heart defects which result in right-to-left shunting and hypoxia. Most other documented cases have occurred as a result of some form of hepatic disease, such as hepatic neoplasia, chronic active hepatitis and obstructive cholelithiasis.

Clinical signs include lethargy, weight loss and mucosal hyperemia. These signs are non-specific and in more severe cases (PCV >60%) other signs such as abnormal mentation, tachycardia and tachypnea as a result of increased blood viscosity and impaired oxygen delivery may be noted.

Diagnosis

- Diagnosis is based on measurement of persistently increased PCV, hemoglobin concentration and RBC count in the presence of normal plasma volume.
- Diagnosis of the causative disorder in secondary absolute polycythemia may be more challenging and the diagnostic plan should include blood gas determination, cardiopulmonary examination, complete blood chemistry and bone marrow assessment.
- Measurement of erythropoietin requires biopsy and is not routinely performed.

Treatment

- Phlebotomy is indicated if the PCV remains consistently above 50%; 10–20 ml/kg of blood is removed and replaced by an equal volume of polyionic fluid. This procedure can be repeated as often as required. Hydroxyurea has been used in humans and dogs but its efficacy in horses is not proven.
- Many underlying conditions which result in polycythemia carry a poor prognosis.

Ulcerative lymphangitis (Figs. 4.72–4.75)

Ulcerative lymphangitis is a bacterial infection of the cutaneous lymphatic vessels, most commonly involving the hind limbs, and usually associated with *Corynebacterium pseudotuberculosis*. Other organisms including *Streptococcus equi*, *Rhodococcus equi* and *Pasteurella hemolytica* have been isolated from some cases. Bacterial contamination of superficial wounds usually precedes the development of skin nodules

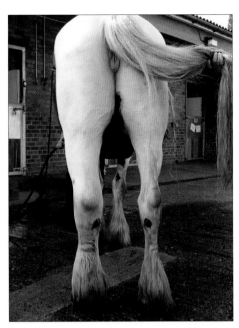

Figure 4.72 Typical appearance of acute lymphangitis with marked swelling and edema of the affected limb compared to the non-affected limb.

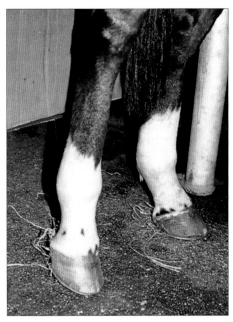

Figure 4.74 Sporadic lymphangitis ('Monday-morning leg'). Edematous swelling (pits on pressure) resolved easily following short walking exercise. Recurred regularly while horse was stabled.

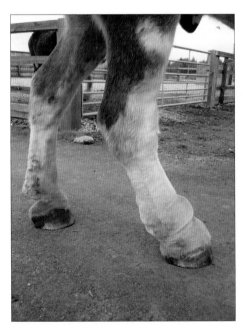

Figure 4.73 Chronic lymphangitis. The swelling in this case is more localized but again note the marked difference between the affected and normal limb.

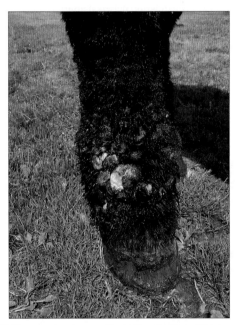

Figure 4.75 Ulcerative lymphangitis. Corded lymphatic vessels and purulent discharge from ulcerated sites. Chronic thickening and exudate over distal parts of limb.

Differential diagnosis:
- Exuberant granulation tissue
- Botryomycosis
- Glanders (farcy).

along the course of the lymphatic vessels which ulcerate and drain onto the skin surface. Where the condition is longstanding and, more particularly where it is due to *Corynebacterium pseudotuberculosis*, there is usually a massive and extensive fibrosis and local and distal edema. A very similar appearance is presented in cases of sporotrichosis, due to infection with the fungus *Sporothrix schenkii*, farcy (glanders) due to *Pseudomonas mallei* and pythiosis, which also appear to track along lymphatic vessels in skin and subcutis and which present with chronic, discharging, ulcerated, dermal nodules.

Horses which are stabled for long periods of time, and in particular those which are immobile during such confinement, either due to

voluntary or enforced immobility, are often found to have swollen ('filled') distal limbs. The hind legs are often particularly affected and the swelling may be considerable in some cases. The condition, known as **sporadic lymphangitis** or '**Monday-morning leg**', can readily be differentiated from the more sinister causes of distal limb edema by the fact that rapid resolution usually follows even short exercise, and no underlying disease process is present. As its colloquial name implies, it is commonly seen on a Monday morning after a rested weekend in a stable.

Diagnosis, treatment and prognosis

- The clinical appearance is diagnostic but culture where possible will allow identification of the causative organism.
- Antibiotic therapy is essential and ideally should be guided by culture and sensitivity testing. However, it is usually necessary to institute therapy before culture results are available, in which case broad-spectrum antibiotics should be used.
- Non-steroidal anti-inflammatories should be used and some clinicians like to add a diuretic if the lymphatic inflammation has resulted in marked edema of the limb.
- Adjunct therapies include controlled exercise such as hand-walking or turnout in a controlled area combined with hydrotherapy.
- The prognosis is largely dependent on the causative organism and the chronicity of the condition when presented for treatment. Longer-standing cases that already have marked ulcerative lesions when presented have a poorer prognosis.

Protozoal diseases

Protozoal infections in the horse form an important group of diseases in various parts of the world. In general, they require the presence of suitable vectors for transmission between animals and most are therefore species-specific and seasonally and geographically restricted.

Potomac horse fever

Potomac horse fever is a seasonal disease due to *Ehrlichia risticii* and which is geographically restricted to limited areas of North America. The disease has some enigmatic features relating to its transmission and epidemiology and appears to occur in a number of different circumstances affecting horses in different ways. A short disease course lasting from 1–3 days with soft ('cow-pat') or diarrheic feces due to an acute typhlocolitis, accompanied by fever, general malaise and anorexia are seen in the milder forms of the infection. Colic and profuse watery diarrhea may be seen in more severe cases and endotoxemia and laminitis are common sequelae from which horses seldom recover. While the diagnosis cannot be confirmed from the clinical features alone even the laboratory tests are difficult and sometimes misleading (see Chapter 1, p. 69).

Piroplasmosis (Figs. 4.76–4.78)

Equine babesiosis (piroplasmosis) is an acute or chronic disease caused by either *Babesia caballi* or *Theileria equi* (or both), and is transmitted by ticks. *Babesia caballi* is transmitted transovarially from one generation of tick to the next. *Theileria equi* is transmitted horizontally by species of *Dermacentor*, *Hyalomma* and *Rhipicephalus*. While *Babesia caballi* causes a milder (and often inapparent) disease and has an almost world-wide distribution where vectors exist, the smaller *Theileria equi* causes a more recognizable and serious disease and is more restricted geographically.

The clinical effects of either infection are largely similar, varying only in degree, and are dependent upon the degree of immunity of the host. In endemic areas most horses are symptomless carriers in a preimmune state, and overt infection may only emerge when the balance between the host and the parasite is altered, especially if the host-immunity is allowed to wane or is reduced by stress, such as that associated with racing, transportation or pregnancy. The clinical signs of acute babesiosis include fever, depression and icterus, which is rendered more prominent by the intercurrent anemia. Moderate supraorbital edema is a common sign and terminally, this extends to

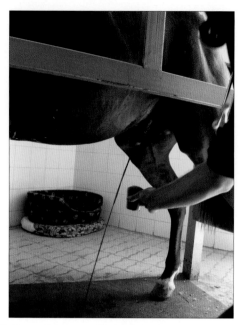

Figure 4.76 Hematuria in horse with piroplasmosis.

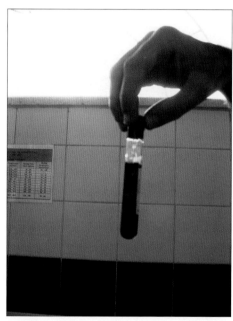

Figure 4.77 Hemolysis secondary to piroplasmosis.

peripheral and dependent edema of the limbs and ventral abdomen. Infected red cells are removed by the spleen which is often grossly enlarged and this can be recognized during rectal examination.

Fetal foals may be infected with *Babesia equi* and are sometimes born with a severe, often overwhelming, parasitemia. They are febrile and icteric from birth and mortality is particularly high. In endemic areas **neonatal babesiosis** may be confused with neonatal isoerythrolysis syndrome and Tyzzer's disease.

Diagnosis

- Observation of parasitized RBC with Giemsa-stained blood smears.
- Serology (complement fixation, indirect fluorescent antibody test, polymerase chain reaction) is regarded as the most definitive means

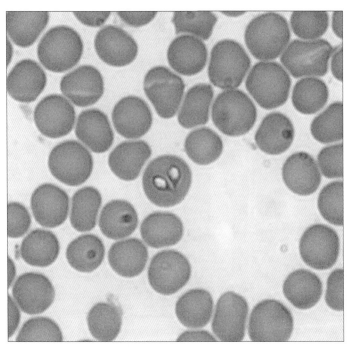

Figure 4.78 Peripheral blood smear showing the presence of the typical 'tear-drop' shaped *Babesia caballi*.

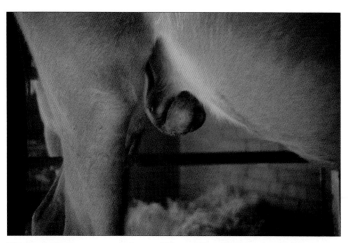

Figure 4.79 Trypanosomal infection. Edema of the sheath in a horse with dourine.

of diagnosis but antibodies will not be produced for a minimum of 14 days post infection and as such paired samples are normally required and in many instances therapy has to be instituted on the basis of clinical signs and relevant history before the diagnosis can be confirmed.

- Post-mortem examination of horses with overt piroplasmosis reveals a grossly enlarged spleen and a pale flabby heart. Most major organs are pale, degenerate and/or icteric. Obvious edema of the renal capsule is usually present.

Treatment

- Imidocarb dipropionate is the most effective means of treatment.
- Clearance of *B. caballi* is achieved by the administration of two doses at 2.2 mg/kg im at an interval of 24 hours. It should be administered deep intramuscular and can be associated with severe muscle soreness and local abscessation. Some clinicians recommend splitting the dose and injecting mixed with procaine penicillin into the pectoral muscles.
- *T. equi* is more difficult to treat and parasite clearance requires 4–6 doses at 4 mg/kg at 72-hour intervals. Some clinicians will decide to administer a lower dose and allow the horse to develop immunity to the parasite, especially if in an endemic area. Parasite clearance becomes of greater concern in competition horses required to test negative for international travel.
- Imidocarb is an anticholinesterase and treated horses should be carefully monitored for associated side effects such as colic and hypersalivation. Donkeys are particularly sensitive to imidocarb and should not receive the higher dose.

Equine ehrlichiosis

Equine ehrlichiosis is caused by the rickettsial organism *A. phagocytophilia*. This organism is also the cause of tickborne fever in ruminants and human granulocytic ehrlichiosis. The disease is most commonly reported in California but can be seen in other areas. Clinical signs include fever, depression, ventral edema, reluctance to move and ataxia.

Diagnosis and treatment

- Clinical signs are suggestive but are normally combined with hematological findings of granulocytopenia, anemia and thrombocytopenia. Serology can be used to demonstrate a fourfold rise in antibody titers.
- ***Differential diagnosis:*** purpura, EVA and encephalitis.
- Supportive care includes NSAIDs, IV fluids and efforts to control the limb edema (hydrotherapy and limb wraps). Intravenous oxytetracycline (7 mg/kg diluted in 0.5–1 L of saline IV q 24 h for 5 days) is effective in clearance of the organism. Clinical improvement in response to oxytetracycline therapy is usually rapid and is used by many clinicians to retrospectively confirm the diagnosis while awaiting serology results.

Trypanosomal infections (Figs. 4.79 & 4.80)

Trypanosomal infections of the horse present different clinical signs depending on the infective organism. With the exception of ***Trypanosoma equiperdum*** which is transmitted venereally and causes **dourine**, the other organisms require specific vectors for transmission and are therefore geographically restricted to areas where these occur. Infection with ***Trypanosoma brucei***, which is transmitted by tsetse flies (*Glossina* spp.), is restricted to areas of north and central Africa and causes the disease known as **nagana**. Recurrent pyrexic episodes of variable severity are accompanied by anorexia, dramatic weight-loss and progressive hind-quarter weakness with ataxia. The superficial lymph nodes are enlarged and may be visible from a distance. Ventral edema, particularly of the prepuce, scrotum and lower limbs, anemia with tachycardia, and dyspnea are typical signs of the disease but these closely resemble the signs of babesiosis. Conjunctivitis, epiphora and photophobia are sometimes present. The diagnosis may be confirmed from peripheral (capillary) blood smears when the parasites can be readily identified. In many cases, however, the extent of parasitemia is low in circulating blood and thick smears, serological methods or cerebrospinal fluid examination are then helpful.

Surra

Surra is a trypanosomal infection due to ***Trypanosoma evansi*** and is particularly important in India, but has been found in other parts of the world. It is transmitted by biting flies (and possibly other insects) and occasionally by injudicious re-use of needles and syringes. The signs are indistinguishable from nagana.

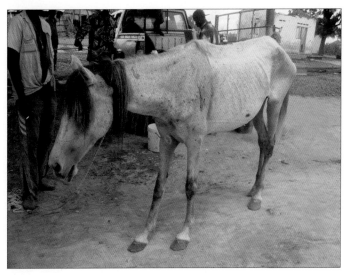

Figure 4.80 Chronic wasting and poor body condition in a horse with dourine.

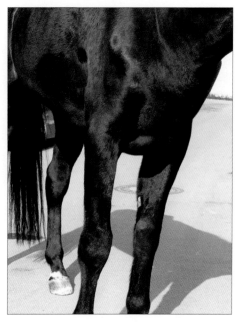

Figure 4.82 Ventral thoracic edema in a horse with a mediastinal lymphosarcoma.

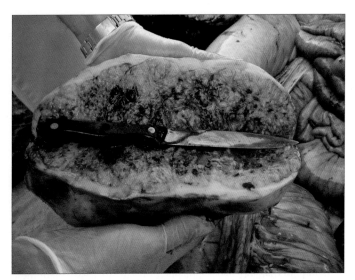

Figure 4.81 Multicentric lymphosarcoma. Enlarged mesenteric lymph node from mare with multicentric lymphosarcoma (same mare as Figs. 1.251 and 2.56).

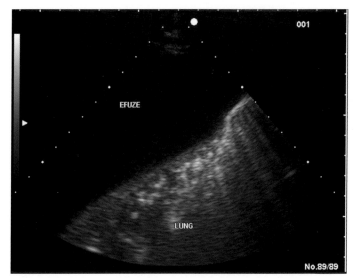

Figure 4.83 Ultrasonographic image of the thorax from the (same horse as Fig. 4.82) showing an accumulation of thoracic fluid and pulmonary consolidation.

Neoplastic disorders

Lymphoma (Figs. 4.81–4.86)

Lymphoma is the term to denote malignant transformation of lymphoid cells. Lymphosarcoma is the malignant transformation of lymphoid cells into solid tumors.

Lymphoma in its various forms is probably the commonest internal neoplasm in the horse and is certainly the most frequent tumor of the hemopoietic system. It is probably the most common neoplastic cause of death in the horse. While most lymphocytic cells occur in the lymph nodes, spleen, intestinal walls, bone marrow and pharynx, they are also present in lesser numbers in almost all tissues. Therefore, tumors involving lymphocytes are possible in almost all sites including the skin and the central nervous system. Four more-or-less distinct equine lymphosarcoma syndromes are recognized. These are:

- The multicentric form (50%)
- The alimentary form (19%)
- The mediastinal form (6%)
- The extranodal form (25%).

With the exception of the cutaneous (extranodal) form, metastasis of the primary tumors is particularly common and consequently, multiple organ involvement is frequent. Where secondary (metastatic) tumors are present clinical signs may be attributable to (multi-) organ failure and are very variable. Horses of all sexes, ages and breeds are liable to the condition and, while most cases are to be found in middle-aged horses (4–15 years of age), younger and older horses are by no means precluded. The general signs of lymphosarcoma of all the forms are similar, with depression, progressive weight loss, peripheral and dependent edema, diarrhea (particularly in the diffuse intestinal form) and intermittent, recurrent, pyrexic episodes

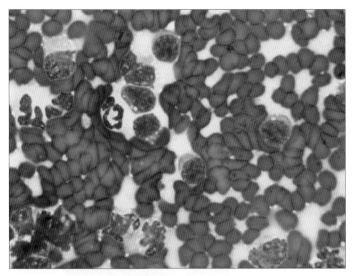

Figure 4.84 Cytological examination of the fluid obtained from the thorax in the horse in Fig. 4.83 revealed an abundance of lymphocytes.

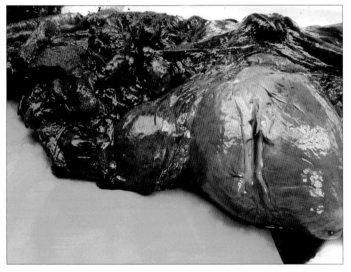

Figure 4.85 Necropsy image of horse in Fig. 4.83 showing a neoplastic mass at the heart base.

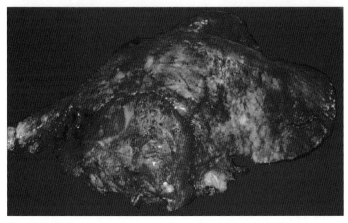

Figure 4.86 Necropsy image showing the presence of a mediastinal neoplasm (lyphosarcoma) wrapped around the heart.

at variable intervals. Secondary effects, including immune-mediated hemolytic anemia and thrombocytopenia, are sometimes the first and most obvious clinical manifestations.

Interference with vascular or lymphatic circulation by enlarged lymph nodes in the abdomen or thorax results in localized edema and accumulations of fluid within the body cavities. This fluid often contains cells of diagnostic value. Hypoalbuminemia, hyperfibrinogenemia and gammopathies are good supportive laboratory findings in all forms of the disease. Plasma calcium concentrations are often, but not always, significantly elevated. In some cases of lymphosarcoma, the hematological and biochemical findings may be disappointing in relation to the severity of the underlying pathology. With the exception of the extranodal form where horses have been reported to survive for several years following diagnosis, the rate of progression is usually rapid, with significant deterioration apparent within 2–4 months, at most.

Generalized (multicentric) lymphosarcoma

The most frequently affected tissues are lymph nodes, liver, spleen, intestine, kidney and lung. The clinical signs are very variable and depend heavily upon the organ(s) most affected. Obvious peripheral lymphadenopathy is usually presented in these cases. Physical enlargement of lymph nodes induces secondary respiratory signs, dysphagia and exophthalmos. Signs attributable to organ dysfunction such as icterus, colic, weight loss and anemia are common. This is the most common form to be associated with circulating neoplastic lymphocytes. The course of the disease is usually rapid once clinical signs become evident.

Alimentary (intestinal) lymphosarcoma

This form occurs in two well-recognized ways.

Diffuse intestinal lymphosarcoma. This is the most common of the alimentary types and is more prevalent in younger horses than the focal form. Horses affected have a grossly impaired intestinal absorptive capacity, which is caused by diffuse intestinal infiltration by abnormal blast cells. Weight loss, peripheral and dependent edema, lethargy and ascites are common signs. Recurrent pyrexia is a frequent finding and, in the later stages when the cells invade and affect the water-absorptive capacity of the cecum and colon, diarrhea is often present. Metastases are slow to develop but grossly enlarged mesenteric lymph nodes at the root of the mesentery are often palpable per rectum. Abdominal fluid frequently contains cells of diagnostic value and rectal biopsy may occasionally be diagnostic and is easy to obtain. A definitive diagnosis is often, however, only possible from biopsy specimens obtained from the intestine at laparotomy.

Focal intestinal lymphosarcoma. The general signs of lymphosarcoma are also present in this form. Post-prandial abdominal pain, as a result of non-strangulating (sometimes partial or intermittent) small intestinal obstruction, is a presenting sign and, with weight loss, is often the first overt clinical evidence of the disease. Rectal palpation frequently identifies significant mesenteric lymph node enlargement at the root of the mesentery and sometimes the intestinal mass(es) may be appreciated. Rectal biopsy is not often of diagnostic value but significant blast cells may be found in peritoneal fluid. Laparotomy is often the best method for making the diagnosis.

Mediastinal lymphosarcoma

The progression of this form is usually particularly rapid. Clinical signs of thoracic involvement are attributable to circulatory effects of masses within the mediastinum and include coughing, dyspnea or tachypnea, and exercise intolerance. There is usually some obstruction of one or both jugular veins, and the thoracic lymphatic ducts are frequently obstructed. Consequent edema of, at first, one forelimb and then both with jugular engorgement and edema of the head and neck are typical. Owners might report the forequarters to be 'good' and the hindquarters to be 'poorly developed or wasted'. Massive pleural effusion of clear or hemorrhagic fluid which is replaced almost as fast as it is withdrawn is characteristic. It is not unusual to remove up to 35 liters of the fluid from the chest only to have to repeat the procedure within 12–24 hours. The fluid contains cells of diagnostic value in almost all cases. Although the site of the most obvious lesions is in the cranial parts of the thorax, the disorder seldom involves the thymus except in very young horses. Extensive tumor masses in the mediastinum and its associated lymph nodes may be found at post-mortem examination. In some cases the malignancy extends to the dorsal thoracic and abdominal lymph nodes and hind limb edema, ascites and diarrhea may then be present.

Extranodal lymphosarcoma

The most common sites of extranodal tumor development are the skin, upper respiratory tract, eyes and central nervous system. Lesions may occur only in the skin (cutaneous form) or can occur concurrently with lesions at other sites.

Multiple cutaneous nodules, which may be firm or fluctuant, or may resemble edematous plaques, which may ulcerate, can be found all over the body. Similar lesions are found in the pharynx and nasal cavity where they may induce dysphagia and respiratory obstructions respectively. This is the only form of lymphosarcoma which may take a protracted course and metastases seem particularly slow to develop.

Secondary lymphosarcomatous tumors may develop in almost any organ including the liver, spleen, kidney and heart.

Diagnosis and treatment

- The diagnosis of lymphosarcoma, and related lymphoproliferative and myeloproliferative disorders, often presents the clinician with considerable difficulties in that many of the signs are non-specific and, as the disorder carries a hopeless prognosis, ante-mortem confirmation is very desirable.
- Suitable biopsy specimens from affected tissues (including tissue aspirates from lymph nodes, cutaneous masses, pleural, pericardial or abdominal fluids) is the only satisfactory and definitive way of confirming the diagnosis at present.
- Treatment is rarely attempted due to the poor prognosis, expense and possible toxicity of chemotherapy agents. However immuno-suppressive glucocorticoid therapy may be palliative for steroid-responsive tumors and also aid in diminishing immune-mediated sequelae. There have been a few reports of specific anti-neoplastic agents in the treatment of lymphoma in the horse.

Myeloid leukemias

Myeloproliferative disorders are characterized by medullary and extramedullary proliferation of bone marrow constituents. Classification schemes are based on the degree of differentiation of the trans-formed cell line, e.g. acute myeloid leukemia involves myeloblast cells whereas chronic myeloid leukemia involves neutrophils and late pre-cursor cells. Reports of myeloproliferative disorders of horses are rare but those available show no breed, sex or age predilection. Clinical signs have included weight loss, ventral edema, depression and enlarged lymph nodes.

Diagnosis and treatment

- All reported cases have had anemia and thrombocytopenia with circulating neoplastic cells.
- Bone marrow examination confirms the diagnosis.
- Treatment is rarely attempted but specific agents such as cytosine arabinoside have been used.

Lymphangioma (Figs. 4.87 & 4.88)

Lymphangiomas are rarely encountered neoplasms of lymphatic vessels. Most reported cases have been in young horses with a predilection for the medial thigh and prepuce. Characteristically there is sponge-like edema of the affected tissue.

Diagnosis is possible based on biopsy ante-mortem.

There have been no successful reports of treatment. Treatment in humans involves resection of the affected tissue but location and large affected areas have precluded treatment in cases reported to date.

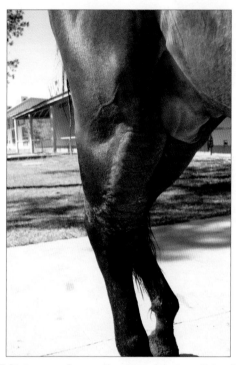

Figure 4.87 Distinct area of sponge-like edema of the inner thigh and prepuce in an 18-month-old TB colt. The edema had been present for a number of months and was unresponsive to therapy.

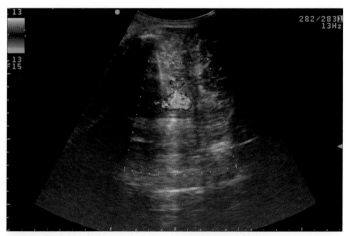

Figure 4.88 Ultrasonographic image of the medial thigh area of the colt in Fig. 4.87. Note the extensive edema and area of arteriovenous fistulation close to the bone.

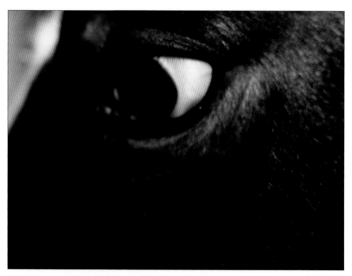

Figure 4.89 Marked anemia associated with a plasma cell tumor.

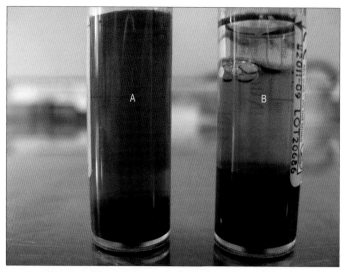

Figure 4.90 Blood from the horse in Fig. 4.89 (A). Note the low packed cell volume when compared to a normal horse (B).

Plasma cell myeloma (Figs. 4.89 & 4.90)

Plasma cell (multiple) myeloma has been reported in horses between 3 months and 22 years of age. It induces similar clinical signs to lymphoma with signs related to the site of tumor invasion and expansion.

Diagnosis and treatment

- In all reported cases there has been a detectable monoclonal gammopathy.
- In most cases due to the poor prognosis, treatment is not attempted but there are a number of reports of prolonging survival times up to 1 year after diagnosis with the use of chemotherapeutic agents.

Hemangiosarcoma

Primary hemangiosarcomas occurring in the walls of blood vessels within muscles and elsewhere are very inclined to metastasize to remote sites and lesions may therefore occur in any or all of the major organ systems, including the lung, myocardium and heart valves and liver. Chronic and persistent blood loss and impaired circulation within body cavities results in massive accumulations of blood-stained fluid and/or hematuria and melena. Ultimately, such blood loss commonly results in the development of disseminated intravascular coagulopathy and chronic, blood-loss anemia. Other clinical signs depend on the primary and secondary tumor sites but signs can be very variable and non-specific.

Further reading

Bonagura, J.D., 1985. Veterinary Clinics of North America: Equine Practice. Symposium on Cardiology, Volume 1, Issue 2. WB Saunders, St Louis, MI, USA.

Marr, C.M., Bowen, M., 2010. Cardiology of the Horse, second ed. WB Saunders, Oxford, UK.

McAuliffe, S.B., Slovis, N.M., 2008. Colour Atlas of Diseases and Disorders of the Foal. WB Saunders, Philadelphia, PA, USA.

Messer, N.T., 1995. Veterinary Clinics of North America: Equine Practice. Clinical Pathology, Volume 11, Issue 3. WB Saunders, St Louis, MI, USA.

Reed, S.M., Bayly, W.M., Sellon, D.C., 2009. Equine Internal Medicine, third ed. WB Saunders, St Louis, MI, USA.

Robinson, N.E., Sprayberry, K.A., (eds.), 2009. Current Therapy in Equine Medicine, sixth ed. WB Saunders, St Louis, MI, USA.

Rose, R.J., Hodgson, D.R., 1999. Manual of Equine Practice. WB Saunders, St Louis, MI, USA.

CHAPTER 5

Urinary tract disorders

While the incidence of clinically significant disorders of the urinary tract of the horse is less than in many other species, pathological changes are quite frequently recognized at post-mortem examination and it is possible that subclinical urinary tract disease passes largely unnoticed. Foals are markedly more prone to renal disease than adult horses, and this may be associated with the neonatal maladjustment syndrome and septicemic disorders. Normal horse urine has a markedly cloudy appearance, particularly towards the end of the flow, due to the very high calcium carbonate content, and is frequently mucoid or viscid in consistency.

As with some other organ systems, damage to the urinary tract organs may be reflected clinically in a limited number of ways. Thus the clinical appearance of different disorders may be similar and the specific identification of a given problem may be difficult. The general signs of urinary tract disease are associated with variations in the volume of urine produced and abnormalities of micturition including abnormal frequency of urination, or dysuria (difficulty or pain during or after micturition).

Furthermore, the kidney itself has a very large functional reserve and damage may only become clinically obvious when over 70% of the available tissue is non-functional. The implications of this fact for diagnosis and therapy of renal disease are particularly important as the opportunity for therapeutic measures has often been lost before clinical disease is recognized.

Separation of renal disorders into infectious and non-infectious is not always clear-cut as there is frequently an overlap or combination of conditions contributing to renal failure and thus the clinical signs seen.

Diagnosis of urinary tract disorders usually involves obtaining a good history and physical examination coupled with diagnostic imaging and supportive clinical pathology.

Developmental disorders

Congenital or hereditary disorders of the kidneys and ureters are particularly unusual in the horse. Unilateral disorders are likely to be incidental findings at post-mortem examination, whereas bilateral disorders are likely to result in recognizable, if non-specific, clinical signs or the early demise of the foal, possibly even intrauterine death.

Renal agenesis, hypoplasia and dysplasia
(Figs. 5.1 & 5.2)

Renal agenesis is the complete absence of renal tissue. It may be unilateral or bilateral. Unilateral is reported more frequently but this simply may be a reflection of the fact that bilateral agenesis is incompatible with life. Other congenital abnormalities such as atresia ani may occur simultaneously. Unilateral disorders are frequently

identified incidentally in otherwise healthy horses or may be identified during reproductive examinations or when renal disease is present in the remaining kidney. There is no confirmation of a hereditary basis but this may simply be due to a lack of data and repeat matings of the same sire and dam should be discouraged.

Renal hypoplasia is defined as a kidney 50% smaller than normal or total renal mass decreased by more than one third. If the condition is unilateral there is commonly hypertrophy of the contralateral kidney and normal renal function. As such the hypoplasia may go undiagnosed. Hypoplasia may occur bilaterally, resulting in renal failure, or can occur with renal dysplasia. In many cases the diagnosis is made post-mortem but may be suspected ante-mortem on the basis of ultrasound examinations or computed tomography.

Renal dysplasia is defined as disorganized development of renal tissue. The proposed mechanisms are anomalous differentiation, fetal viral infection, teratogens or intrauterine ureteral obstruction. Renal

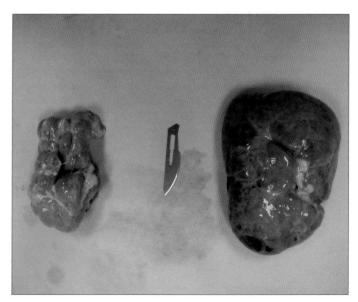

Figure 5.1 Renal hypoplasia and dysplasia. Right and left kidneys from a 3-month-old foal. The left kidney is notably small and misshapen. The right kidney although of normal size is misshapen. Histopathological examination revealed dysplastic changes in both kidneys. This foal surprisingly was not in renal failure but was noticeably smaller than his herd mates. The hypoplasia of the left kidney was suspected on the basis of ultrasound examination. Reproduced from McAuliffe SB, Slovis NM (eds). *Color Atlas of Diseases and Disorders of the Foal* (2008), with permission from Elsevier.

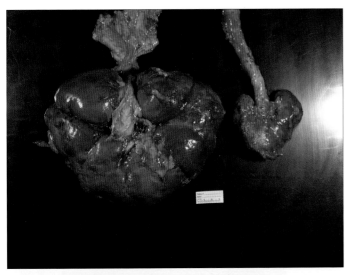

Figure 5.2 Renal hypoplasia (unilateral).

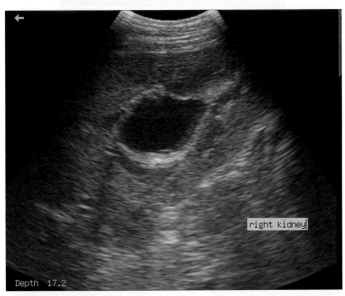

Figure 5.3 Single renal cyst found incidentally during abdominal ultrasound examination in a foal with diarrhea.

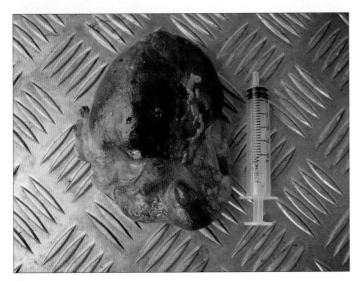

Figure 5.4 Renal cyst.

dysplasia may occur unilaterally and not be associated with renal failure or may occur bilaterally or in association with renal hypoplasia where it leads to chronic renal failure at a young age. This condition may be somewhat more difficult to diagnose ante-mortem as the kidneys may be of normal size and function tests are non-specific for cause.

Treatment
There is no specific treatment for any of the above conditions.

Renal cysts (Figs. 5.3–5.6)
Polycystic kidney disease and glomerulocystic disease
Polycystic kidney disease (PKD) is a disorder in which multiple variable-sized cysts are found throughout the cortex and medulla. In PKD cysts may also be found in the bile ducts and pancreas. In comparison glomerulocystic disease consists of microscopic cysts limited to Bowman's spaces. Both conditions have been described in foals. PKD has been described in a number of adult horses presented for renal failure.

Diagnosis, treatment and prognosis
- Both conditions can be diagnosed with reasonable certainty based on ultrasonographic findings.
- There is no available treatment and prognosis depends on the size and number of cysts present and existing renal dysfunction at presentation.

Hereditary nephropathies
There are few reports of nephropathies in horses other than nephrogenic diabetes insipidus (see below) but as these disorders may not result in renal failure it is likely that they are perhaps under-recognized in the horse.

Vascular anomalies
Renal arteriovenous malformations or intrarenal vascular anomalies are rare and may be silent for many years when present. Common clinical signs include hematuria and flank pain.

Anomalies of the vascular supply to the kidneys are also rare and have been associated with hematuria, hemoglobinuria, partial urethral obstruction or hydronephrosis.

Diagnosis and treatment
- Cystoscopy is used to determine if the condition is unilateral or bilateral, by visualization of hematuria from one or both ureteral orifices. Ultrasonographic examination and contrast radiographic studies are also used for diagnosis.
- If the urinary tract bleeding is minor then conservative treatment consisting of close observation and repeated examinations may be all that is required.
- If the bleeding has resulted in anemia or there is danger of exsanguinations then unilateral nephrectomy may be considered.

Pendulent kidney
A pendulous kidney is an extremely mobile kidney attached to the dorsal body wall by a thin band of tissue. The condition is rare and is generally thought to be congenital although it is possible that perirenal trauma, hydronephrosis or extreme weight loss could result in a similar condition.

Diagnosis and treatment
- Diagnosis is usually made by rectal examination and no treatment is normally required unless displacement or rotation leads to ureteral obstruction.

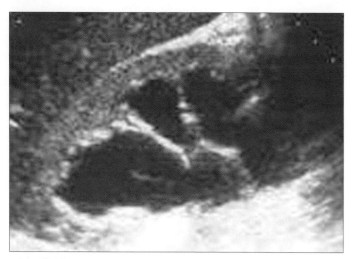

Figure 5.5 Polycystic kidney disease. Incidental ultrasound finding in adult horse.

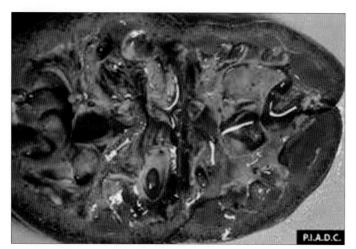

Figure 5.6 Polycystic kidney disease.

Rectourethral and rectovaginal fistulae
(Figs. 5.7 & 5.8)

These are rare anomalies that are associated with failure of separation of the urorectal folds. These conditions are frequently associated with atresia ani or other congenital conditions such as agenesis of the coccygeal vertebrae and tail, scoliosis, microphthalmia and severe angular limb deformities.

Diagnosis and treatment

- Diagnosis is visually obvious in many cases with passage of feces from the vagina or urethra but in some cases contrast radiographic studies may be required.
- Several foals have had surgical correction of fistulae and accompanying atresia ani. However, the decision for surgery should be based on the number of accompanying congenital defects and several surgical procedures may be required.
- There is some evidence to suggest that the condition is hereditary and as such if affected animals are surgically corrected they should not be used for future breeding.

Ectopic ureter (Fig. 5.9)

In individuals with ectopic ureters, one or both ureteral ostia empties into the bladder or urethra at some point distal to the functional sphincter. In some animals, the aberrant ureters may open into the uterine lumen or vaginal tract.

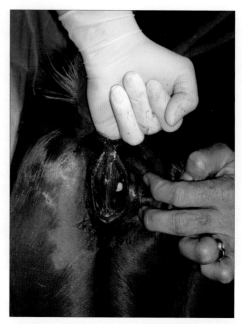

Figure 5.7 Rectovaginal fistulae in a day-old foal that had presented with atresia ani.

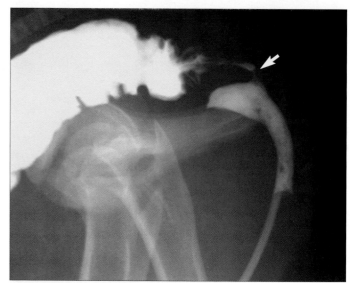

Figure 5.8 Rectourethral fistulae. A positive contrast urethrogram in a 3-day-old burro that had atresia ani and intermittent passage of fecal material from the urethra. A catheter passed via the urethra and contrast agent injected into the catheter resulted in accumulation of a large amount of contrast agent in the rectum and a lesser amount in the intrapelvic portion of the urethra. A small amount of contrast agent is visible in the urethrorectal fistula (arrow). (Reproduced from Reed SM, Bayly WM, Sellon DC (eds). Equine Internal Medicine, 2nd edition (2004) with permission from Elsevier.)

Diagnosis and treatment

- The diagnosis may be suspected on the basis of clinical signs such as urine dribbling but definitive diagnosis requires endoscopy or cystography.
- This malformation can only be corrected by means of reconstructive surgery or, if the condition is unilateral, nephrectomy. Reconstructive surgery is rarely successful as it is technically difficult to perform and post-surgical complications such as renal infections are common.

- Nephrectomy is also a difficult surgical procedure but the success rate is higher with this approach.

Patent urachus (Fig. 5.10)

The persistent dribbling of urine from the umbilicus in a neonatal foal should alert the clinician to the possibility of a patent urachus. Foals may be born with the urachus normally closed but then be observed dribbling urine from the external umbilical remnant on the first or second day of postpartum life. This may occur in foals that are constipated or have meconium impaction and strain to defecate; the intra-abdominal pressure created by abdominal press can lead to re-opening of the urachal lumen and the exit of urine via the urachal remnant. Re-opening of the urachus may also occur as a result of infection and is also frequently seen in foals that are largely recumbent for other reasons, e.g. septicemia. Where the urachus fails to close adequately at birth, the patent structure provides a portal for the entry of bacteria, and local abscess, particularly of the umbilical vessels, or even septicemia may result. Ascending infections from the urachus into the bladder (and thence to the ureters and kidneys) and from the umbilical vessels into the general circulation have particularly serious systemic consequences.

Diagnosis and treatment

- The observation of urine dribbling from the umbilical stump of a young foal is the basis for making a diagnosis of patent urachus,

although sonographic imaging may be used to confirm the patent status of the structure internally and assess associated structures.

- Currently many practitioners recommend treatment consisting of 5–7 days of antimicrobial support and keeping the foal's ventral abdomen clean and dry, with twice to four-times-daily dipping of the external umbilical stump with a 1:4 chlorhexidine:water or dilute iodophore solution.
- Topical applications of silver nitrate are no longer routinely recommended.
- In cases of foals which are largely recumbent it may be useful to catheterize the bladder, thus removing the physical pressure of bladder distension which may contribute to maintaining a patent urachus.

Uroperitoneum (Figs. 5.11–5.18)

Uroperitoneum, or urine in the peritoneal cavity, is a common problem of neonatal foals. It is a sign of rupture of some portion of the urinary tract. The urinary bladder is the most common site of rupture, but renal, urachal, ureteral and urethral ruptures or injuries also occur and result in leakage of urine into the peritoneal cavity.

Uroperitoneum arising from bladder rupture may occur from disruption of the urinary tract during parturition or as a result of a congenital abnormality. Bladder rupture can also result from septic foci and consequent necrosis and when caused by sepsis may be seen

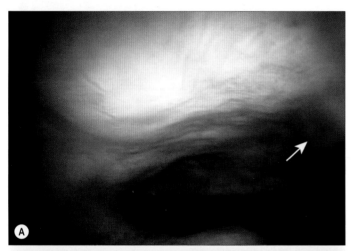
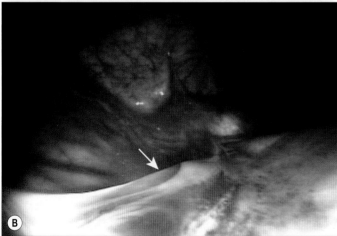

Figure 5.9 Ectopic ureter in an 8 month old filly. (A) Cystoscopic examination demonstrated a normal ureteral opening in the right dorsal wall of the bladder (arrow), but left ureteral opening was absent. (B) Vaginoscopic examination revealed the left ureter opening into the ventral vagina, where urine could be clearly seen coming from the opening (arrow).

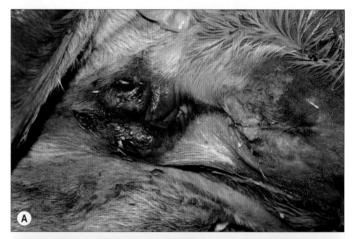
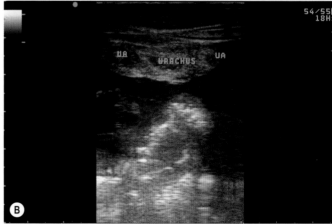

Figure 5.10 Patent urachus. (A) This image is from a foal whose umbilicus closed normally following birth but who later developed diarrhea and septicemia at which time the urachus re-opened. (B) Ultrasound image of a patent urachus; the urachus which in this image contains hypoechoic fluid is readily apparent between the two umbilical arteries. This image also shows the presence of free abdominal fluid which in this case was urine.

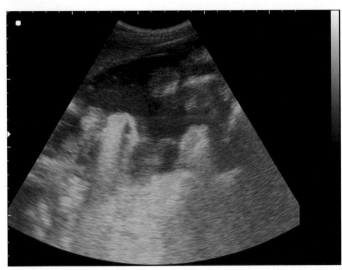

Figure 5.11 Ultrasonographic image obtained from the ventral abdomen in a 3-day-old foal, demonstrating large amounts of anechoic free fluid with loops of small intestine floating in the fluid. Abdominocentesis and comparison of creatinine levels in abdominal fluid and blood confirmed a uroperitoneum in this case.

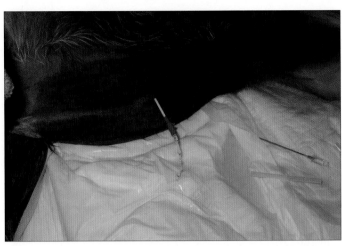

Figure 5.13 Uroperitoneum. If large amounts of fluid are present it is best to drain the abdomen prior to surgery; this decreases abdominal pressure which adversely affects respiration and prevents the absorption of additional potassium from the urine within the abdomen. Hyperkalemia can have profound cardiac effects and for that reason uroabdomen is generally considered more of a medical than surgical emergency.

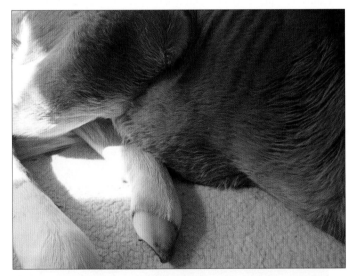

Figure 5.12 Uroperitoneum. The increased abdominal pressure associated with large accumulations of fluid (urine) in the abdomen can result in fluid accumulation in the scrotum or subcutaneously around the umbilicus.

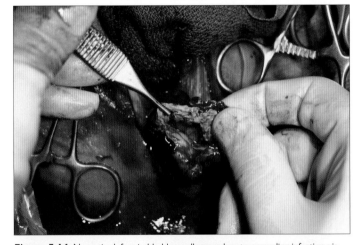

Figure 5.14 Necrotic defect in bladder wall secondary to ascending infection via the umbilicus resulted in uroperitoneum.

in older foals. Males appear to be affected more frequently but the incidence in the sick or hospitalized is approximately equal between the sexes. Clinical signs of uroperitoneum characteristically develop between 1–3 days after birth, the foal having been normal up to this point. In some cases however the reduced or absent urinary output may have been recognized from an early age. Foals which have septic necrosis of the urachus or bladder may develop signs much later.

Clinical signs

- The earliest sign is usually frequent stranguria and repeated posturing to urinate. Sick foals, especially those that are recumbent, may not show these signs and stranguria is frequently confused with tenesmus.
- Affected foals show progressive abdominal distension and depression with a palpable fluid thrill may be detected across the abdominal cavity.

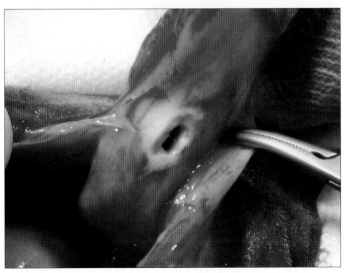

Figure 5.15 Urachal tear which resulted in uroperitoneum.

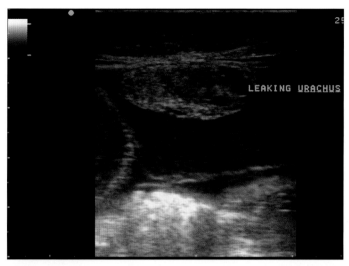

Figure 5.16 Ultrasonographic image of umbilical remnants. This image shows a large amount of free hypoechoic fluid within the abdomen. A tear in the urachus could be visualized in real time.

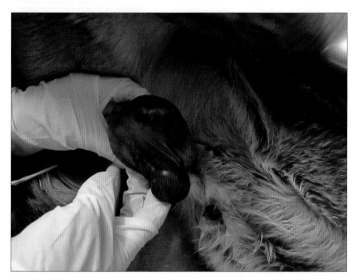

Figure 5.17 Urethral tear. Four-day-old foal with a tear in the urethra resulting in urine accumulation in the prepuce and scrotum. In most of these cases the swelling will be more obvious on one side indicating the location of the lesion. The subcutaneous accumulation of urine in these cases can result in scrotal rupture and/or local necrosis of tissue.

- The foal may still continue to void urine through the urethra and as such the observation of the passage of urine does not preclude a diagnosis of ruptured bladder.
- As the condition progresses these foals develop **hyponatremia, hypochloremia, hyperkalemia and azotemia.** Depending on the timing of presentation, the metabolic derangements that develop can result in other signs: hyponatremia can result in neurologic disturbances including convulsions; progressive hyperkalemia results in cardiac dysrhythmias.
- Uroperitoneum may also be caused by disruption of the urethra, urachus or ureters (rarely). In cases of urethral leakage in colts subcutaneous accumulation of urine in the scrotal area is frequently seen. Depending on the site of injury this may occur alone or in combination with uroperitoneum. Uroperitoneum associated with urachal disruption may also be accompanied by subcutaneous leakage of urine in the umbilical area.

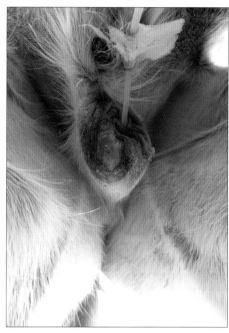

Figure 5.18 The same foal as Fig. 5.17, 4 days after the placement of the urinary catheter. An area of necrotic skin is apparent; this section was resected and the foal made an uneventful recovery.

- Progressive accumulation of fluid which may be accompanied by persistent straining will force significant amounts of urine down the inguinal canals and result in swelling of the scrotum and prepuce.

Diagnosis

- Transabdominal ultrasound is very useful in examination of foals with suspected uroperitoneum, and quickly reveals anechoic-to-hypoechoic fluid free in the peritoneal cavity, with bowel loops and other viscera floating on and in the fluid. The rent in the bladder, whether congenital or acquired, is nearly always located in the dorsal wall but is generally difficult to visualize.
- A fluid sample may be obtained via abdominocentesis and assayed for creatinine concentration. If the creatinine concentration in the peritoneal fluid is twice or higher than the serum concentration, a diagnosis of uroperitoneum may be rendered. However, it is important to note that serum electrolyte and creatinine concentrations may be normal in the early stages of the disorder and should not be used as a means of ruling out the condition.

Treatment

- In most instances slow drainage of the abdomen is initiated. Removal of urine from the abdomen helps to prevent worsening of the metabolic condition. In cases of severe abdominal distension resulting in respiratory compromise, abdominal drainage is a must.
- Uroperitoneum is a metabolic rather than a surgical emergency and surgery should be delayed to allow for correction of electrolyte abnormalities. Correction of hyperkalemia to a serum concentration <6 Eq/L is the most important consideration prior to general anesthesia. Administration of 1–3 L of 0.9% NaCl/5% glucose solution can be used to treat the hyperkalemia.
- In foals for which surgery is not an option or in foals with urethral or urachal tears, placement of an indwelling urinary catheter in combination with an indwelling peritoneal drain may facilitate sufficient removal of urine to permit healing.
- Placement of a urinary catheter for a couple of days post surgery to maintain an empty bladder is not usually required but should be

used in foals where bladder rupture was deemed to be secondary to sepsis with necrosis of the bladder wall. Balloon-tipped Foley catheters with 10–30 ml of sterile saline solution in the balloon to keep it in a dependent position in the bladder lumen work well, but rigorous monitoring and nursing care, including the administration of broad-spectrum antimicrobials, is necessary.

Prognosis

- In foals, the prognosis for full recovery, barring complications, is very good.
- Uroperitoneum may recur after surgery in an occasional foal as a result of ongoing leakage or further necrosis. When this occurs and the volume of fluid in the abdominal cavity is small, it can be managed conservatively by the placement of an indwelling catheter for 3–5 days. A second celiotomy may be required in some cases.

Non-infectious disorders

Bladder rupture (Fig. 5.19)

Bladder rupture has been recognized in adult horses as an accident of parturition or in horses which are repeatedly catheterized, particularly where there is an intercurrent cystitis. More unusually, the bladder may rupture as a result of severe and total urethral obstruction such as might occur with urethral calculi, which is effectively restricted to the male. The speed with which abdominal accumulation of urine occurs depends upon the extent of and reasons for the rupture. Progressive azotemia and hyperkalemia are common sequels to any disruption of the urinary tract within the abdomen. However, it appears that peritonitis is not a common feature, the peritoneum appears to tolerate the presence of urine fairly well, unless there are bacteria present. The possible exception to this is mares that have suffered a ruptured bladder as a result of parturition trauma as in many cases they have also endured bruising or damage to the gastrointestinal tract resulting in translocation of bacteria through the bowel wall.

Diagnosis and treatment

- The presence of free urine in the abdominal cavity (sometimes with blood-staining and inflammatory cells) may be detected by paracentesis. Cystoscopy and/or ultrasound examination of the bladder may help to identify the site of rupture and the size of the lesion which will influence the treatment.
- Instillation of dye such as methylene blue into the bladder which can then be recovered from the abdomen may help to identify small defects.
- Depending on the cause and extent of damage surgical repair can be attempted. Medical management would involve placement of a urinary catheter in conjunction with an abdominal drain. This is only likely to work in cases where the defect is very small.

Polyuria/polydipsia (Fig. 5.20)
Diabetes insipidus

Diabetes insipidus (DI) of central origin arises from failure of the pars distalis of the pituitary gland to produce anti-diuretic hormone (ADH). This occurs secondary to viral encephalitis or to compression of the pituitary gland as part of the Cushing's disease syndrome.

Nephrogenic diabetes insipidus occurs as a result of failure of tubular response to ADH. In can be inherited as a nephropathy or can occur secondary to bacterial infection, drug therapy, obstruction of the urinary tract or neoplasia.

Cushing's disease

This is accompanied by a loss of diurnal rhythm of cortisol which results in a persistent increase in plasma cortisol concentration which in turn results in increased glomerular filtration rate. Concurrent hyperglycemia also induces polyuria.

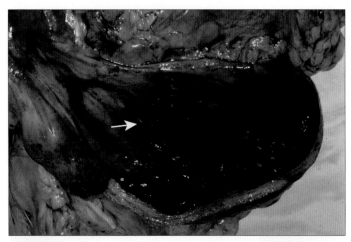

Figure 5.19 Bladder perforation in an adult following dystocia (arrow).

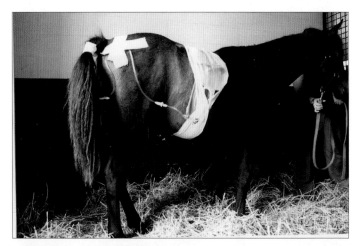

Figure 5.20 Polyuria/polydipsia (PU/PD). This yearling Morgan filly presented with a history of polydipsia. Measurement of water intake and urine output confirmed PU/PD. Necropsy indicated the presence of a meningoencephalitis.

Sepsis and endotoxemia

Prostaglandin E_2 production in response to endotoxemia results in vasodilation of renal blood vessels and decreases sensitivity of collecting tubules to ADH. Combined these effects can result in increased urine production in the face of dehydration.

Diabetes mellitus

Destruction of pancreatic islet cells resulting in hyperglycemia and resultant dieresis is rare in horses but can be found occasionally as a sequel to parasitic migration.

Iatrogenic causes of polyuria

These include administration of large volumes of intravenous fluids and exogenous administration of corticosteroids.

Psychogenic polydipsia

Psychogenic polydipsia is perhaps the most common cause of polyuria/polydipsia (PU/PD) in young adult horses. It is regarded as a vice associated with boredom in stabled horses. Dietary factors such as a high intake of dry matter or compulsive salt consumption may also contribute. These horses are normally in good body condition with no evidence of renal failure. Horses with a recent onset may concentrate their urine in response to the water deprivation test whereas longer-standing cases may have washout of renal medullary electrolytes resulting in an inability to concentrate urine in response to this test.

These horses will have a positive response to the modified water deprivation test although a number of days may be required for normal urinary concentrations to be reached.

Diagnosis and differentiation

- A good history is imperative to determining if the primary problem is polydipsia or polyuria. While they occur together one is usually a physiological response to the other. Therefore a horse for example with psychogenic polydipsia will as a result have polyuria. While similarly, a horse with polyuria due to renal failure will have a physiological polydipsia as a result.
- A good history should also rule in or out behavioral factors, drug administration, concurrent disease that is already being treated or clinical signs consistent with other disorders such as renal failure or Cushing's.
- In many cases it may be necessary to measure water intake and urine output over a 24-hour period. A complete blood count and serum biochemistry profile should be performed in addition to urinalysis.
- *Water deprivation test.* If the horse shows no clinical or laboratory features of renal failure, endotoxemia, sepsis or Cushing's disease then a water deprivation test can be performed to assess the ability of the renal tubules to respond to ADH. The horse is weighed and a urine sample obtained for determination of specific gravity (SG). The horse is then confined without access to water and urine samples collected every 2 hours. The test ends when the urine has a specific gravity (SG) of 1.025 or the horse has lost 5% of its body weight, whichever comes first. If the horse responds by producing urine with a SG >1,025 then he can be diagnosed as a psychogenic water drinker; if he fails to concentrate the urine, then a modified water deprivation test should be performed.
- *Modified water deprivation test.* Water access is restricted to 40 ml/kg/day for up to 4 days. This will result in concentration of urine in horses with psychogenic polydipsia that have washout of renal medullary electrolytes. The horse should still be weighed daily and the test ended if the horse has lost 10% of its body weight and SG is still <1.025 as these cases may have diabetes insipidus.
- *Desmopressin response test.* Administration of 20 µg of desmopressin acetate (DDAVP) allows differentiation between central and nephrogenic diabetes insipidus. If the urine concentrates in response to the DDAVP then the diabetes insipidus is central, if not it is nephrogenic.

Treatment

- Many cases of PU/PD respond to treatment for the underlying condition, e.g. Cushing's, renal failure, endotoxemia, etc.
- Psychogenic polydipsia can be controlled by alterations in management to allow for less boredom and control of water intake.
- *Diabetes insipidus* (DI) may be somewhat more difficult to treat and there are few reports of long-term therapy. Central DI can be treated with intraocular desmopressin but cost of treatment may be prohibitively expensive in some cases. It should be borne in mind however that most cases of post-encephalitis DI in humans are transient and production of ADH may return to normal.
- There is no treatment for nephrogenic DI but the animal may be able to lead a relatively normal life. However, due to the uncertain heritability of the condition the animal should not be used for breeding purposes.

Displacements of the urinary bladder
(Figs. 5.21–5.23)

These are effectively limited to the female. The most common of these disorders is **bladder eversion**, where the bladder is everted through the urethra and the mucosal surface is then visible at the vulva. The vesico-ureteral openings, from which urine will be seen to issue in

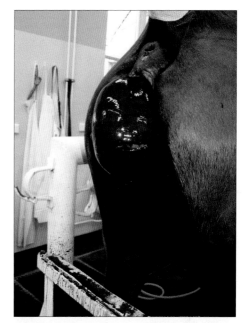

Figure 5.21 Urinary bladder prolapse which occurred during a dystocia. A fetotomy was performed and the bladder was replaced. The bladder ruptured during replacement, was sutured and re-replaced. The mare died 48 hours later due to peritonitis and toxemia. The exposed serosal surface of bladder was reddened in this case due to trauma associated with transportation.

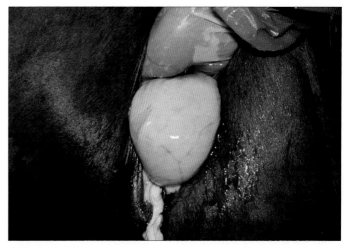

Figure 5.22 Bladder prolapse. This prolapse also occurred during a dystocia delivery.

pulses every few minutes, may be readily visible on the dorsal surface. **Urinary bladder prolapse** usually occurs through a tear in the vaginal wall at parturition and in these cases the smooth reddish serosal surface is visible. This is distinctly different from the mucosal surface visible in bladder eversion. In contrast to the free issue of urine in the everted bladder, in these cases, the bladder is unable to empty due to the kinking of the urethra and, consequently, the organ may become grossly distended and may ultimately rupture. Both of these conditions are most often associated with, and accompanied by, tenesmus (excessive involuntary straining) such as might occur during or after normal or assisted parturition, dystocia, colic due to small colon obstructions, rectal prolapse and vaginitis, or perineal lacerations occurring during foaling.

It is unusual for neurological disorders of the bladder or cystic calculi to result in displacements of this type. Mares affected with either condition will also strain incessantly as a result of the

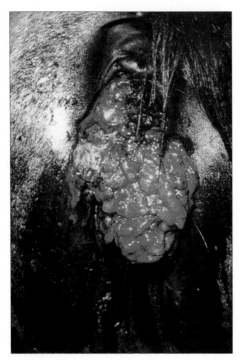

Figure 5.23 Bladder eversion.

Differential diagnosis:
• Bladder eversion
• Impending parturition (amnion/chorioallantois)
• Prolapse of intestinal loop.

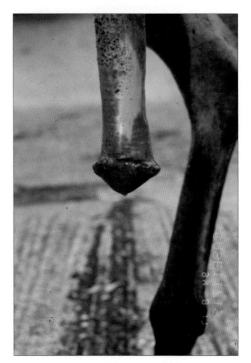

Figure 5.24 Bladder dysfunction. Penile prolapse and constant dribbling of urine were present in this gelding with paralytic bladder syndrome.

Differential diagnosis (urine dribbling with penile protrusion):
• Sorghum poisoning
• Polyneuritis
• Spinal or sacral trauma.

displacements, thereby making matters considerably worse, and possibly inducing secondary rectal prolapse and gross perineal edema. Persistent tenesmus of this type is exhausting and affected mares become very tired after a relatively short period.

Diagnosis and treatment
• The diagnosis is usually obvious upon clinical examination.
• ***Bladder prolapse***. The exposed surface of the bladder should be cleaned gently and replaced to the abdominal cavity through the vaginal laceration. In most cases a caudal epidural and aspiration of the bladder contents is required. If possible the vaginal laceration should be repaired immediately. In cases where the severity of trauma does not permit immediate repair, a caslick should be performed to minimize bacterial aspiration and in some cases placement of a urinary catheter may be required.
• ***Bladder eversion***. The exposed mucosal surface should be thoroughly cleaned and examined for defects. Application of sugar solutions may be required to help decrease edema of the exposed surface. Once cleaned and lubricated the bladder should be gently replaced through the urethra. In some cases a small incision in the urethral sphincter may be required to facilitate replacement. This incision should be repaired immediately if required. Placement of a urinary catheter should be performed to lavage the lumen and ensure complete repositioning.
• Broad-spectrum antibiotics and anti-inflammatories should be applied in both cases.

Urinary incontinence and bladder dysfunction
(Fig. 5.24–5.28)
Bladder dysfunction in horses essentially falls into three groups:

• **Upper motor neuron (UMN) or reflex bladder** (also known as spastic or autonomic bladder). These cases are characterized by increased urethral resistance despite the presence of a full

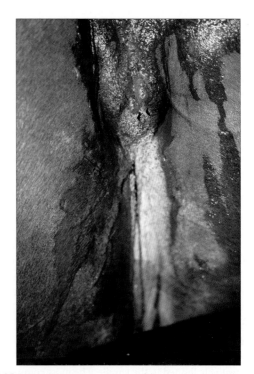

Figure 5.25 Urinary incontinence in a mare following a dystocia delivery. Urinary scalding of perineum and extensive crystalline deposits on the caudo-medial thigh due to evaporation of the urine being dribbled out continuously.

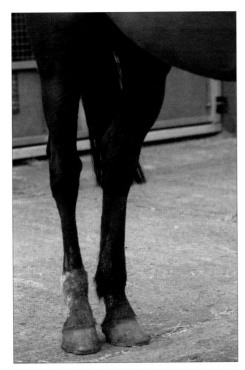

Figure 5.26 Urinary scalding of the hind legs due to urinary incontinence.

Differential diagnosis (urine dribbling without penile protrusion):
- Cystic calculus
- Cystitis
- Urethral calculus
- Penile or preputial neoplasia
- Sorghum poisoning
- Cauda equina neuritis
- Spinal or sacral trauma
- Equine herpes virus-1 neurological syndrome
- Urethritis.

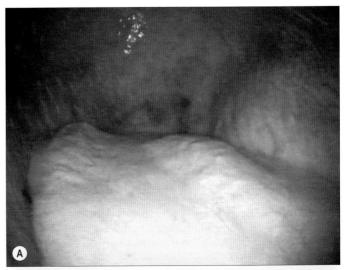

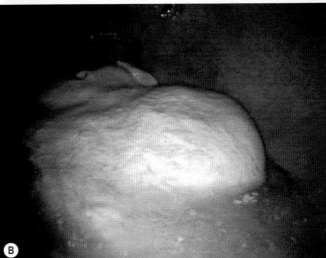

Figure 5.28 (A, B) Cystoscopic images from a mare with sabulous urolithiasis. The mare had accompanying neurological examination findings of cauda equina syndrome, including urinary incontinence. The urolithiasis was treated by bladder lavage, dietary manipulation to increase urinary acidification and orally administered trimethoprim-sulfonamide. Sabulous urolithiasis re-occurred and neurological findings worsened, including development of hindlimb ataxia and paresis, and the mare was subjected to euthanasia.

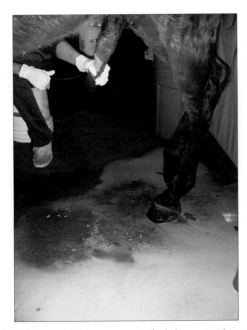

Figure 5.27 Sabulous cystitis. Large amounts of sabulous material were obtained from this gelding upon catheterization of the bladder. This horse had a long history of urinary incontinence. He was thought to have commenced as a LMN/paralytic bladder but had secondary myogenic dysfunction.

bladder making catheterization difficult. It is normally seen in association with deep and/or broad spinal cord lesions. Such lesions are normally accompanied by other more obvious and significant clinical signs such as inability to stand.

- **Lower motor neuron (LMN) or paralytic bladder.** This may be encountered in several neurological disorders including **cauda equina neuritis**, **equine herpes virus-1 neurological syndrome**, sorghum or Sudan grass poisoning and other traumatic, inflammatory or neoplastic conditions affecting the spinal cord or peripheral nerves in the sacral and caudal lumbar regions. It may also follow a difficult parturition or caudal epidural anesthesia. In most of these circumstances bladder dysfunction is not the only sign which is present and any or all of the following may be seen concurrently: loss of anal sphincter tone, tail paralysis, perineal hypalgesia or analgesia, hindlimb weakness or muscular atrophy of the hip or hindlimb.

- **Myogenic or non-neurogenic bladder.** This is normally seen in geldings and frequently lacks an identifiable cause at the time of diagnosis. It usually develops slowly in association with accumulation of sabulous material, which in time leads to increased detrusor muscle stretching and dysfunction. These cases unlike those of UMN or LMN origin occur without other neurological signs.

Other non-neurogenic causes of bladder dysfunction include hypoestrogenism and chronic cystitis.

Bladder dysfunction is normally recognized when some degree of urinary incontinence is present. In the male intermittent, or continuous, dribbling of small volumes of normal urine results in urine-scalding of the hind limbs and extensive preputial inflammation and excoriation. In mares, exercise, coughing or vocalization may result in spurting of urine from the urethra and persistent dribbling of urine results in perineal excoriation and crystallization of urine in the hair of the caudo-medial thigh and tail. The development of sabulous urolithiasis, made up of a homogeneous sludge of calcium carbonate and cellular and mucoid debris in the bladder, carries a poor prognosis as this is usually secondary to serious and longstanding bladder paralysis.

Diagnosis
- Rectal examination reveals a large distended bladder, which in LMN lesions can be easily voided by placing pressure on the bladder per rectum; in UMN lesions, voiding is difficult due to the increased tone in the urethra.
- Catheterization of affected horses results in a relatively clear initial flow of urine but there is usually a very dense sediment in the dependent part of the bladder.
- Endoscopic examination of the bladder is usually required to identify the presence of extensive sabulous urolithiasis.
- Cystometry, which involves the inflation of the bladder with volumes of sterile water, saline or carbon dioxide, can be used to determine the intravesicular pressure at which micturition occurs. The contraction threshold is the pressure which reflects detrusor muscle contraction. In normal horses this threshold is about 90+/−20 cmH$_2$O. The higher the pressure the better the prognosis is but there are few available reports to date in clinical cases.

Treatment
- Without other serious problems horses with UMN bladder may recover spontaneously with time.
- Cases of LMN or myogenic bladder dysfunction are frequently not recognized until the atonia is irreversible. If a particular cause can be identified, e.g. equine protozoal myeloencephalopathy, it should be treated. Otherwise, the basic aim of therapy is to avoid retention of urine leading to secondary complications such as accumulation of sabulous material and cystitis. This can be achieved by intermittent or permanent catheterization. However, while facilitating drainage secondary cystitis is a common problem associated with catheterization.
- Bethanechol chloride is a parasympathomimetic agent with a selective effect on the smooth muscle of the bladder wall. However, it has no effect when the bladder is completely atonic or areflexic. If cystometry indicates that some contractions are possible then bethanechol may be useful.

Obstructive disorders of the urinary tract

While the prevalence of obstructive disorders of the urinary tract of the horse is low, they form an important group of conditions with potentially serious consequences. Most urinary tract obstructions can be attributed to one or other form of urolithiasis and this can occur at any site in the urinary tract. Other causes of urinary tract obstruction are neoplasia, displacement and trauma. The clinical signs seen

depend on the site and degree of obstruction with incomplete obstructions frequently resulting in mild abdominal pain, incontinence and dysuria. Complete obstruction results in severe pain which subsides following bladder or urethral rupture to be replaced by depression and progressive metabolic derangements.

The pathogenesis of urinary calculi is uncertain, but it is likely that some underlying metabolic or inflammatory process precedes their development. Any condition that results in retention of urine or incomplete urine voiding increases the chance of nucleation and crystal growth. Similarly any nidus of cellular debris or a foreign body will predispose to calculus formation. There are two commonly encountered types of calculus, one composed largely of calcium carbonate and the other composed largely of calcium phosphate, often with various additional inorganic components including magnesium, phosphate, ammonium and/or oxalate ions.

Urethral calculi (Figs. 5.29–5.31)

Urethral calculi are the preserve of the male horse, as the long narrow urethra is far more likely to become obstructed by relatively small

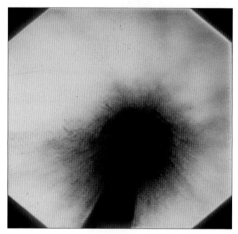

Figure 5.29 Endoscopic image of the urethra showing a blood trail. This could be found with a urethral or cystic calculus.

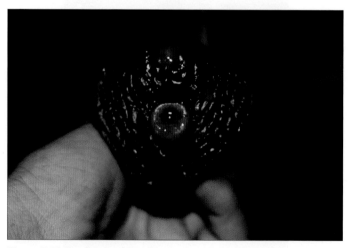

Figure 5.30 Blood staining of urethra due to persistent bleeding from the urethra and frequent attempts at urination.

Differential diagnosis:
- Urethral calculus
- Neoplasia of urinary tract, kidneys, penis or prepuce
- Hemorrhagic disorders of urinary tract
- Cystitis
- Accessory gland inflammation (bulbo-urethral glands).

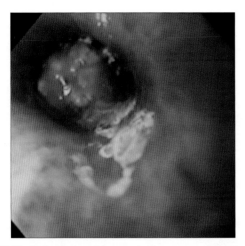

Figure 5.31 Urethral endoscopy demonstrating the presence of a urethral calculus.

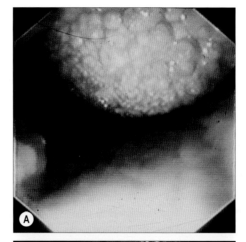

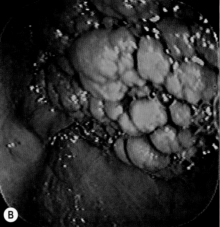

Figure 5.32 (A, B) Cystoscopy demonstrating the presence of a large cystic calculus.

calculi than the short widely dilatable urethra of the mare. They can form at sites of previous damage or strictures or arise as a result of cystoliths passing down the urethra which may lodge either in the pelvic segment of the urethra, near the ischial arch, or in a more distal portion of the urethra (often in the penile urethra). Urethral calculi lodging at the urethral process should not be confused with concretions of smegma in the urethral fossa, which can sometimes become large and very firm. Careful examination will easily define the difference between these two conditions.

Clinical signs and diagnosis

- The penis is often protruded for prolonged periods while the horse maintains a posture of urination.
- Small amounts of blood may be seen at the end of the urethra.
- Rectal examination reveals a very large, extremely tense bladder which is obviously different from the flaccid distension encountered in the paralytic bladder syndromes.
- Eventually bladder rupture and uro-peritoneum will inevitably arise.
- The condition can be suspected on the basis of the above clinical signs and failure to pass a urinary catheter beyond the site of obstruction.
- Rectal, ultrasonographic and particularly endoscopic examination may identify the site and character of the obstruction.
- The successful passage of a urethral calculus is almost always accompanied by urethral ulceration which may be obvious endoscopically.

Treatment and prognosis

- Treatment depends on location. Calculi lodged at the ischial arch can be removed through a perineal urethrotomy which is normally left to heal by second intention.
- Calculi which are palpable in the distal urethra can be removed in some cases following sedation and transurethral crushing of the calculus.
- Unpalpable calculi may be removed endoscopically or in some cases require urethrotomy.
- All cases should be given a guarded prognosis; even when removal of the calculus is successful, there is a high incidence of complications such as stricture formation, reoccurrence, and secondary upper urinary tract disorders, such as pyelonephritis.

Cystic calculi (Figs. 5.32–5.34)

Cystic calculi are the commonest clinically significant form of urolithiasis in the horse. Males are far more frequently affected clinically than females, but large and/or numerous calculi may also be present in mares. Persistent dribbling of bloody urine results in the scalding of the hind legs of geldings and in perineal excoriation and crystalline deposition in mares. Most cystic calculi are rough-surfaced, moderately friable, yellowish and spiky and these result in significant bladder inflammation. These calculi are predominantly composed of calcium carbonate.

Urine passed by horses affected with this type of stone immediately following exercise is characteristically intensely hemorrhagic and this is almost pathognomonic of cystic calculus.

The smoother (often multiple) type of calculi is very hard, white or yellow in color, composed predominantly of calcium phosphate and causes less local bladder inflammation.

Diagnosis and treatment

- Cystic calculi are almost always very readily appreciated during rectal examination, though in some cases with bladder distension it may be necessary to empty the bladder to allow for easier palpation of the calculus. In some cases multiple calculi can, during rectal examination, be felt to be rubbing against each other, like a bag of stones.
- Cystoscopy can not only be used for diagnosis but also allows for determination of the extent of bladder inflammation and the number and type of the calculi present.
- The size of the calculus, sex of the horse and surgeon's preference often determine the type of treatment.

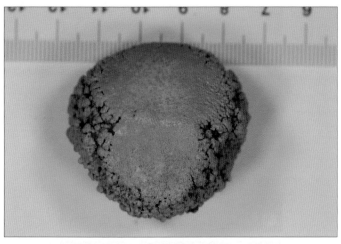

Figure 5.33 Cystic calculus. Facets indicating the presence of at least two more calculi.

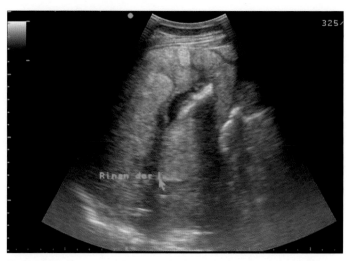

Figure 5.35 Ultrasonographic image of right kidney. Note the acoustic shadows (arrow) cast by the presence of renal calculi; also note the dense hyperechoic cortex in this end-stage kidney.

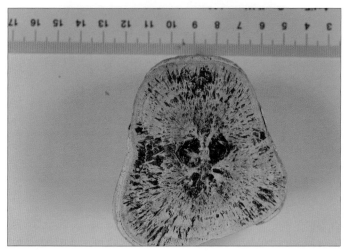

Figure 5.34 Cystic calculus cut surface showing typical laminated appearance.

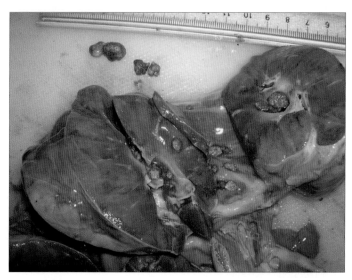

Figure 5.36 Renal calculi. Numerous small calculi and single larger calculus in renal pelvis (same horse as Fig. 5.35).

- Laparocystotomy through a midline or paramedian incision is the preferred approach in males, especially those with large calculi. Smaller calculi can be removed through perineal urethrotomy. Calculi in mares are nearly always removed through the urethra with a lithotrite being used to crush larger calculi prior to removal.
- Complications such as recurrence are common and recommendations to help prevent recurrence include post-operative antibiotics, urinary acidifiers (not well proven) and dietary modifications to decrease calcium excretion and promote diuresis.

Nephrolithiasis (Figs. 5.35–5.39)

Renal calculi, which are often multiple and which may be present in both kidneys, develop within the renal pelvis or the kidney substance where they may be smooth or they may conform to the shape of the renal pelvis at that site. They are often asymptomatic, being incidental findings at post-mortem examination. However, a significant proportion of cases affected by unilateral or bilateral renal calculi have other, concurrent, urinary tract disease such as pyelonephritis, renal hypoplasia or neoplasia. Sometimes vague back pain, hematuria, which can be traced endoscopically to one ureter, or even failure to perform up to

expectation may be associated with the stones but, unless they are extensive and bilateral, signs of renal failure will not usually be present.

Ureteral calculi are particularly rare and may have serious consequences with ascending infection into an inflamed and compromised ureter resulting in pyelonephritis and renal failure ultimately affecting both kidneys.

Diagnosis

- The diagnosis of calculi in the renal substance, renal pelvis or ureter is generally confirmed by percutaneous or transrectal ultrasonographic examination. The detection of a calculus in one kidney may be a strong indication that the contralateral kidney is also affected. It is important to remember that calculi measuring less than 1 cm may not be diagnosed in this manner.
- The loss of patency of one or both ureters may be detected by endoscopic examination of the vesico-ureteral openings when the normal pulsatile urine release, which usually occurs at about one to two pulses per minute, may be lacking.
- Complete ureteral obstruction results in a unilateral hydronephrosis which may be detectable during a thorough rectal examination but seldom causes any detectable signs of renal failure.

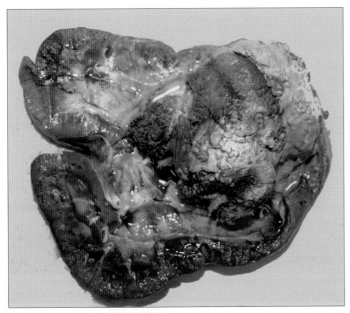

Figure 5.37 Single large renal calculus. This 11-year-old female Thoroughbred equine died following colic surgery. The renal calculus seen was an incidental finding at necropsy.

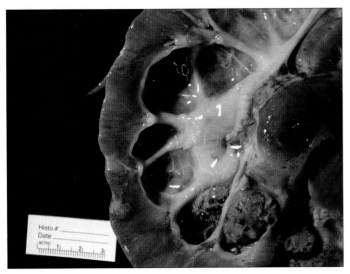

Figure 5.38 Renal calculi and hydronephrosis.

Treatment

- Many horses with renal or ureteral calculi are in chronic renal failure at the time of presentation and thus poor candidates for therapy.
- In cases of unilateral renal calculi nephrectomy would be the treatment of choice.
- Other therapies that have been attempted with variable success have included: nephrotomy, vestibulourethral passage of a basket stone dislodger, percutaneous nephrostomy and electrohydraulic lithotripsy.
- Extracorporeal shock wave lithotripsy is being increasingly used in other species.

Acute renal failure (Figs. 5.40–5.44)

Acute renal failure (ARF) is the clinical syndrome associated with an abrupt reduction in glomerular filtration rate (GFR). Continued

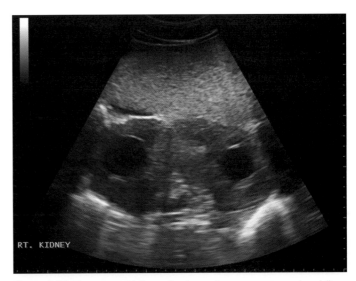

Figure 5.39 Ultrasonographic image showing cystic appearance to renal medulla (same horse as Fig. 5.38).

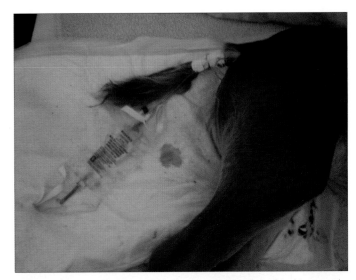

Figure 5.40 Acute renal failure. Lack of urine production (anuria) in this neonatal foal.

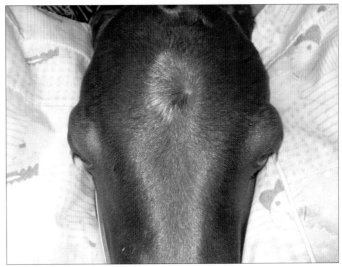

Figure 5.41 Acute renal failure. Periorbital edema. With failure of urine production fluid administration results in edema in many organs and tissues. Periorbital, limb and pulmonary edema are frequently seen.

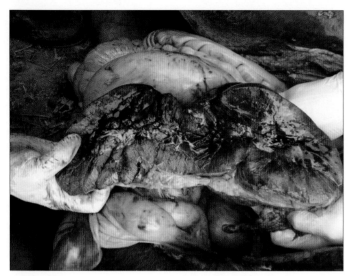

Figure 5.42 Acute renal failure. Amorphous appearance of kidney with extensive hemorrhage and loss of architecture due to severe myoglobinuria over a 3-day period.

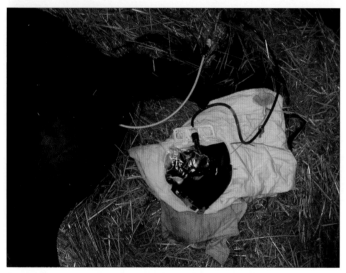

Figure 5.43 Acute renal failure secondary to myoglobinuria.

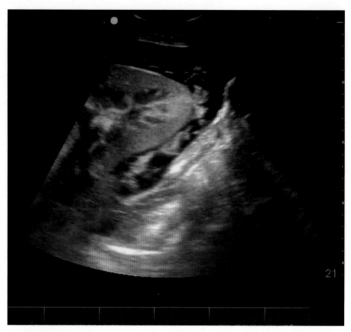

Figure 5.44 Ultrasonographic image of the right kidney from a mare with diarrhea and endotoxemia with acute renal failure. Note: Marked perirenal edema.

reduction in GFR is associated with decreased ability of the kidneys to excrete nitrogenous wastes resulting in azotemia along with disturbances in fluid, electrolyte and acid–base balances. Causes of acute renal failure have been classified into three groups, prerenal, renal or post-renal.

1) **Prerenal** renal failure (most common) is associated with decreased renal perfusion which in turn can be a result of decreased cardiac output or increased renal vascular resistance. Decreased cardiac output is commonly associated with conditions such as diarrhea, endotoxemia, acute blood loss, shock or prolonged intense exercise.
2) **Renal** causes of ARF include ischemic or toxic damage to tubules, tubular obstruction, tubulointerstitial inflammation or glomerulonephritis. It should be noted though that prerenal causes and ischemic tubular necrosis are really a continuum, when decreased renal blood flow persists long enough or is severe enough to result in tubular cell death. Intrinsic renal disease may be further

classified according to the primary area of the kidney affected: tubules, interstitium, glomeruli or vessels. Acute tubular necrosis (ATN) is the form most frequently recognized in horses being associated with ischemia and administration of nephrotoxic drugs the most important of which are aminoglycosides and NSAIDs. Less common causes are exposure to heavy metals (mercury), vitamin D or K_3 or endogenous pigments (myoglobin or hemoglobin).

3) **Post-renal** or obstructive renal failure can occur following disease of the renal pelvis, ureters, bladder or urethra. Other than ruptured bladder syndrome in foals post-renal renal failure is relatively uncommon.

Many plants, including the oak (*Quercus ruber*) and its acorns, are liable to induce tubular degenerations within the kidney when ingested in quantity. Almost all these poisonings result in clinical signs which are associated with acute renal failure and reflect a dramatic and extensive renal damage involving more than 75% of the renal tissue. Pathologically the condition is recognized by acute tubular necrosis which results in oliguria (or anuria) and terminally a severe intravascular hemolytic crisis is encountered. In terminal cases, limited, or sometimes excessive, amounts of urine are passed containing obvious red-brown pigment which is identifiable as hemoglobin but which closely resembles myoglobin.

Clinical signs
- In most horses with prerenal renal failure the most common clinical signs are referable to the disorder which resulted in a decrease in cardiac output such as acute colitis or sepsis.
- Other clinical signs of acute renal failure are vague and often limited to depression and anorexia. Dysuria, laminitis, peripheral/dependent edema, colic and diarrhea may be present.
- Urine production in horses with ARF is variable. Oliguria is common but polyuria is also common, especially with exposure to nephrotoxins and in the recovery phase. Anuria is rare and is more commonly seen in foals than adults.
- Oliguria in the face of fluid administration is a sign that significant renal damage is present.

Diagnosis

- The presence of azotemia suggests renal compromise but does not indicate a cause, therefore initial diagnostics are based on determining if a prerenal, renal or post-renal cause is present.
- Rectal examination may, in some cases, detect the presence of an enlarged, edematous and often painful kidney. A soft, amorphous kidney may also be identified and this finding reflects a dramatic loss of renal architecture. The latter state is most often encountered after severe hemodynamic or hypovolemic/shock syndromes, complicated by profound, acute, renal failure.
- Post-renal causes, although uncommon, are frequently suspected on the basis of clinical signs and history.
- Measurement of specific gravity in the azotemic horse is commonly used to determine the presence of prerenal ARF. In these cases the value is greater than 1.025 and frequently as high as 1.055.
- In practice the diagnosis is often retrospective based on the response to fluid therapy. In prerenal ARF, volume repletion should restore renal function with a decrease in the value of azotemia of 50% or more during the first 24 hours of therapy.
- Determination of the subtypes of intrinsic renal failure depends on the analysis of urine and urine sediment.

Chronic renal failure (Figs. 5.45–5.50)

This is recognized most commonly in adult horses and can be the result of glomerular or tubular disease (or both). It is an uncommon disorder but this may be in part due to the large functional reserve of the kidney, requiring more than two thirds of the nephrons to be non-functional before clinical signs are seen.

Many of the causes of chronic renal failure are also causes of acute renal failure with the extent and timescale of injury determining the speed of onset of clinical signs.

Glomerular injury may be immune-mediated or initiated by ischemic, toxic or infectious events, which usually also result in tubulo-interstitial damage.

Other causes of tubulointerstitial disease are neprotoxic compounds, aminoglycoside antibiotics, NSAIDs, vitamins D and K_3, acorns and heavy metals. Obstructive disorders resulting in pyelonephritis, hydronephrosis and other inflammatory renal disease ultimately progress to chronic renal failure, which represents the end stage of all these disorders.

Less common causes of CRF are amyloidosis, renal neoplasia and possibly oxalate poisoning (experimental studies have failed to produce renal failure as a result of oxalate ingestion).

Clinical signs

- Clinical signs of chronic renal failure in horses under 4–5 years of age are more likely to be the result of congenital abnormalities than acquired renal disease.
- Horses affected by chronic renal failure have pronounced weight loss and inappetence, which has no other obvious cause.

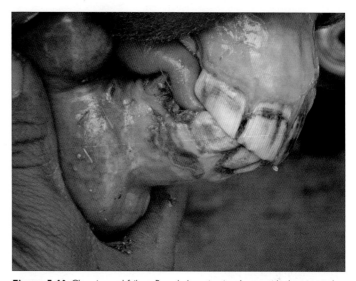

Figure 5.46 Chronic renal failure. Buccal ulceration in a horse with chronic renal failure.

Differential diagnosis:
- Physical trauma
- Plant fibers, awns
- Chemical burn.

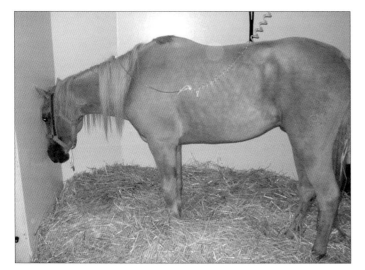

Figure 5.45 Chronic renal failure. Depression and neurological signs in a horse with marked electrolyte abnormalities due to chronic renal failure.

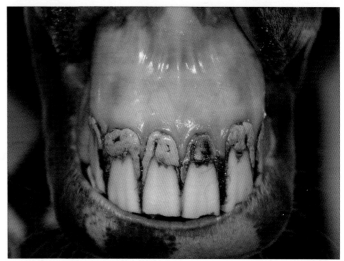

Figure 5.47 Increased tartar in a horse with chronic renal failure.

Differential diagnosis:
- Incidental finding in a normal horse
- Equine motor neuron disease (EMND). In these cases the tartar is normally black in colour.

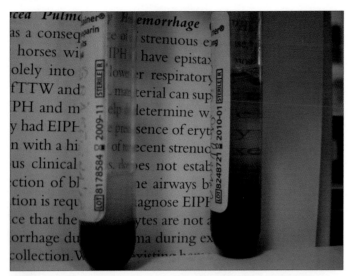

Figure 5.48 Hyperlipidemia in chronic renal failure. The exact etiology of the hyperlipidemia is unknown.

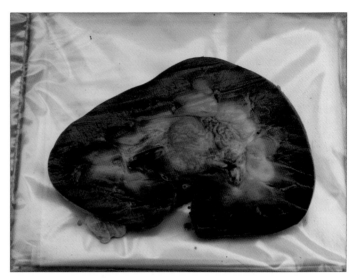

Figure 5.50 Small shrunken kidneys from a horse with chronic renal failure.

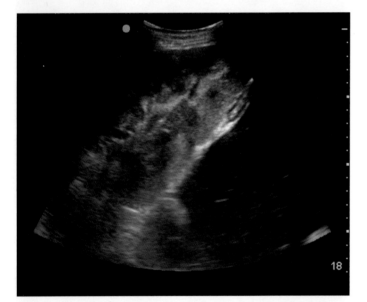

Figure 5.49 Ultrasonographic image of chronic renal failure. Small irregular kidney in an old horse with end-stage kidney disease (ESKD). Horses with ESKD often have small, dense kidneys that are more echogenic than normal due to sclerosis and possible tissue mineralization.

- Polyuria, polydipsia, laminitis and intermittent pyrexia are typically vague but important signs of the condition.
- Oral ulceration, which initially affects the tip of the tongue, 'furring' of the tongue, excessive dental tartar, hypertension and the development of ventral edema consequent upon loss of protein in the urine and severe hypoproteinemia are some of the signs which may be present.

Diagnosis
- Rectal and ultrasonographic examination will usually identify dense, small kidneys which are seldom painful. Less commonly, the kidneys and ureters may be enlarged and painful, if obstructions by uroliths, infection or neoplasia are present.
- The ratio of blood urea nitrogen (BUN) to serum creatinine concentration (BUN:Cr conc) is typically >10:1 in horses with CRF compared to horses with acute renal failure or prerenal azotemia is often less than 10:1. While this is useful it should be noted that

BUN is influenced by dietary protein and as such cannot always distinguish between acute and chronic renal failure.
- Other than elevations in BUN and creatinine other abnormalities found on laboratory analysis include anemia, hypoalbuminemia, hyponatremia, hyperkalemia, hypochloremia, hypercalcemia, hypophosphatemia and metabolic acidosis.
- Some horses with CRF develop hypercholesterolemia and hyperlipidemia.
- Ultrasonography can be used to determine the size of the kidneys in addition to assessing the presence or abscence of uroliths or cysts. Urine produced by horses with chronic renal failure is persistently isosthenuric (with a specific gravity between 1.008 and 1.014), and the urine is usually clear and watery, containing little or none of the cloudy, mucilaginous character encountered in the normal horse.
- Renal biopsy can also be used to detect renal disease but frequently lesions found are consistent with ESKD and reveal little if any information regarding the inciting cause.
- At post-mortem examination the kidneys are small, dense and fibrotic with a narrow cortex.

Treatment
- CRF is progressive and irreversible, meaning that the long-term prognosis is grave. It is also difficult to predict initially which patients will progress more slowly than others. Recent history and early response to management strategies for maintaining weight can be useful indicators. Animals that continue to eat well and maintain their body weight have the best short-term prognosis.
- The aims of therapy are to avoid complicating conditions (e.g. dehydration and continued use of nephrotoxic drugs), and provide a palatable diet to encourage appetite and help maintain body condition. Close monitoring of dietary protein is essential as decreasing protein can help alleviate clinical signs but because of protein-losing nephropathy the level has to be sufficient to match needs and losses.

Vascular disorders

The only vascular disorder of consequence in the urinary tract of horses is **rupture of a renal artery** which is usually due to verminous arteritis, possibly as a result of migrating *Strongyle* larvae. Clinically affected horses show moderate, persistent colic over a course of several days, and most often have free blood in the peritoneal cavity which can be detected by abdominocentesis. Hemorrhage may however be more restricted in some cases with retroperitoneal bleeding which may remain localized or extend into the diaphragm and sublumbar muscles. Where this is present some horses show a synchronous diaphragmatic flutter. In some cases the extent of blood loss may therefore be limited and the signs of the disorder are restricted to mild or recurrent colic and progressive anemia. Jaundice may be present where the capacity of the liver to excrete hemoglobin by-products is exceeded. In this event there will be an elevation of the total and the unconjugated bilirubin.

Urinary tract infection (Figs. 5.51 & 5.52)

Urinary tract infections are uncommon in horses compared with other species. When they do occur, ascending infections are most common with the exception of septic nephritis most commonly associated with bacterial septicemia in foals. The urinary bladder is strongly resistant to infection in normal horses as a result of both the repeated flow of urine through the organ, which tends to dilute and flush out any residual bacteria, and the natural mucosal/epithelial resistance to the ingress of bacteria. Other factors tending to inhibit bacterial proliferation in the bladder include local secretory immunoglobulins and the varying pH of the urine. Thus any condition which causes turbulent or irregular flow of urine may predispose to the development of a UTI.

Cystitis (Figs. 5.53–5.55)

Cystitis is uncommon as a primary disease, most cases being secondarily associated with urolithiasis, bladder paralysis, anatomical

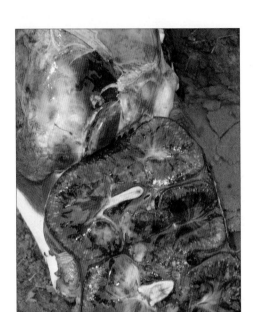

Figure 5.51 Nephritis. Miliary abscesses present in the kidneys of this septicemic foal.

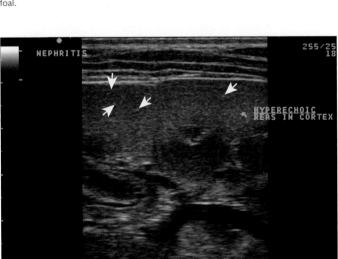

Figure 5.52 Nephritis. This foal presented with septicemia and diarrhea. Serum creatinine concentrations began to rise during hospitalization and urine analysis showed increased white cells and the presence of bacteria. Multiple hyperechoic areas throughout the cortex could be visualized on echographic examination of the kidneys. The foal was treated with antibiotics and the echographic changes resolved as the foal's clinical condition improved.

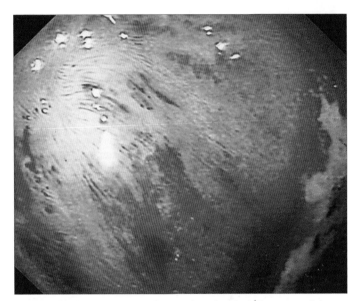

Figure 5.53 Cystoscopic image of cystitis showed marked inflammation of the mucosal surface.

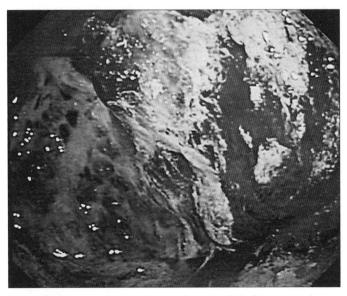

Figure 5.54 Cystoscopic image of cystitis showed marked inflammation and thickening of mucosa.

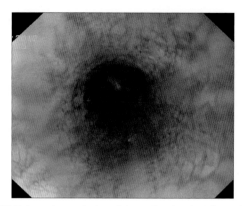

Figure 5.55 Endoscopic examination of the urethra showing inflammation and prominence of the vasculature, a typical appearance in horses with cystitis.

defects, catheterization and vestibular and vaginal infections in the mare. The shorter female urethra possibly accounts for the relatively higher incidence of cystitis, when compared to the male horse. The clinical signs are the result of an intercurrent urethritis and frequent painful attempts at urination with prolonged straining, and small, dribbling amounts of urine passed frequently.

Diagnosis

- Ultrasonographic and cystoscopic examinations may be used effectively to identify mucosal damage and the extent of bladder wall thickening.
- While in some cases the urine may look normal, sediment analysis may reveal blood, presence of bacteria (in some cases) and increased white cell counts (>10 leukocytes per high-power field).
- A definitive diagnosis requires quantitative culture results; >10 000 colony-forming units (CFU) per milliliter in a urine sample collected by midstream catch or catheterization. If not to be cultured immediately the sample should be refrigerated as bacterial numbers may increase in samples stored at room temperature.

Treatment and prognosis

- Aims of therapy are correction of any predisposing problems if possible (e.g. urolithiasis) and administration of systemic antibiotics.
- Antibiotic selection is best based on culture and sensitivity results. If not available factors to be borne in mind are: most UTIs are caused by Gram-negative bacteria, minimal treatment time is 1 week and often 4–6 weeks of therapy are required for horses with recurrent infections so ease of administration and cost are important considerations. Drug metabolism should also be borne in mind as many drugs are almost completely metabolized before reaching the urinary tract.
- Relapses are common as bacteria remain dormant in the bladder wall.

Pyelonephritis (Figs. 5.56–5.59)

Ascending or hematogenous bacterial infection may result in a severe obstructive inflammation of the ureters with consequent hydronephrosis and pyelonephritis. Ascending infections usually develop from bladder infection and/or stasis while hematogenous infection usually extends directly down the ureters from the kidney and renal pelvis. In foals, infection may also arise from urachal infection and ascend via the bladder into the ureters and the renal pelvis. While the majority of cases arise from ascending infection, in adult horses descending infection from pyelonephritis (usually a consequence of *Corynebacterium* spp.) is occasionally responsible for the development of cystitis. Pyelonephritis on its own may be unilateral or bilateral, although the latter is more common. Chronic pyrexia, weight loss and malaise are

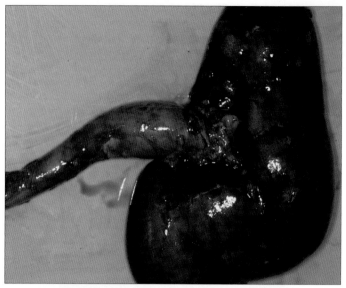

Figure 5.56 Renal and ureteral enlargement associated with pyelonephritis.

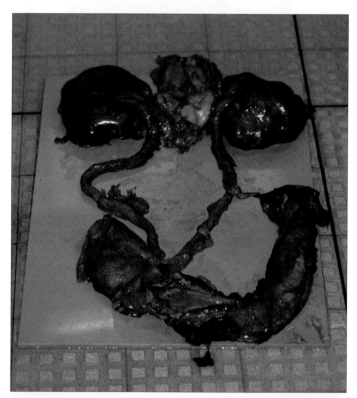

Figure 5.57 Pyelonephritis and cystitis. Enlarged kidneys and ureters with thickening of bladder wall associated with cystitis. These findings are consistent with an ascending infection.

the usual vague clinical signs. The bladder is invariably additionally affected and cystitis is a common complication.

Diagnosis and treatment

- Alterations in urine character and appearance are commonly present but in unilateral cases the urine may be apparently normal and biochemical parameters of renal function may also be totally normal.
- Percutaneous or transrectal ultrasonography is a most useful aid to the diagnosis of pyelonephritis.

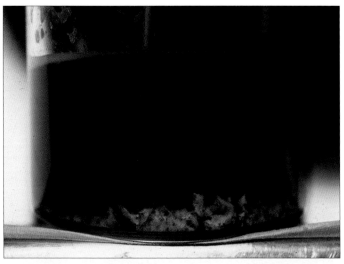

Figure 5.58 Pyelonephritis. Urine sample from a horse with pyelonephritis. There is obvious hematuria and cellular precipitate.

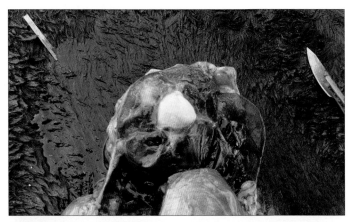

Figure 5.59 Renal abscess. This abscess was found in a foal that died suddenly but was not believed to be related to the cause of death.

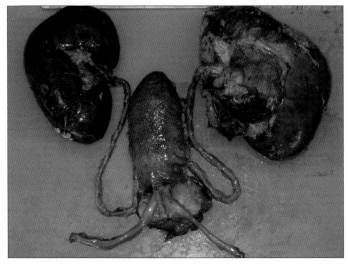

Figure 5.60 Renal lymphoma. This horse had multicentric lymphoma.

- Cystoscopic examination can help differentiate infection in one or both kidneys and/or ureters.
- Examination per rectum reveals a grossly thickened and tortuous ureter on the affected side(s), although in longstanding cases the kidney may be small and dense consistent with ESKD.
- At post-mortem examination the extent of the infective process may be appreciated. It is usual for the renal pelvis to be markedly affected.
- Long-term antibiotic therapy is usually required and should be based on culture and sensitivity testing. In selected cases of unilateral disease a nephrectomy may be performed (unilateral urolithiasis, poor response to antibiotics, abnormal structures and normal laboratory results for renal function indicating the remaining kidney is disease-free).

Neoplastic disorders

Primary neoplastic disorders in the urinary tract are extremely rare, accounting for fewer than 1% of equine tumors. They include adenomata, renal cell carcinomata and nephroblastomata.

Renal neoplasia (Figs. 5.60–5.63)

Renal adenomata are small well-circumscribed lesions in the renal cortex that are usually found incidentally at necropsy. Nephroblastoma is an embryonal tumor that arises in primitive nephrogenic tissue or in foci of dysplastic renal tissue.

Renal cell carcinoma is the most common renal tumor. It is frequently large and unilateral. Secondary neoplastic lesions arising from metastatic spread are encountered, with lymphosarcoma and hemangiosarcoma being the most frequent, although melanomas and adenocarcinomas can also be encountered.

Clinical signs of renal tumors may be diverse and non-specific including weight loss, colic, depression and poor performance. Other more specific signs include hematuria.

Diagnosis and treatment

- Rectal palpation to detect the presence of a mass in the area of either kidney.
- Determination of the presence of hematuria and cystoscopy to determine if it is unilateral or bilateral.
- Ultrasonographic examination revealing the presence of a tissue mass destroying the normal architecture of the kidney is highly suggestive of renal neoplasia.
- Cytological examination of peritoneal fluid and urine for the detection of neoplastic cells.
- Biopsy of the tissue mass may be indicated but it should be borne in mind that many of these neoplasms are well vascularized or rapid growth may have led to the development of arteriovenous fistulae and as such there is a higher risk of fatal hemorrhage associated with the procedure.
- Nephrectomy of the affected kidney is the treatment of choice but is not always possible due to the large size and adhesions to surrounding organs in many cases. Renal cell carcinoma is also frequently associated with early metastasis to local organs.

Bladder neoplasia

Squamous cell carcinoma is the most frequently reported bladder neoplasm of the horse but lymphosarcoma, leiomyosarcoma, transitional cell carcinoma and fibromatous polyps have also been reported. Hematuria is the most common clinical sign.

Diagnosis and treatment

- Palpation or ultrasonographic determination of a bladder mass. Cytoscopic examination and urine cytological examination. Biopsy.

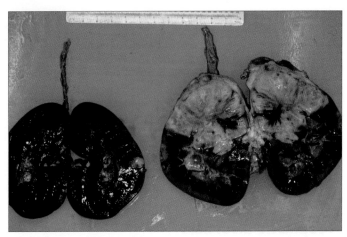

Figure 5.61 Renal lymphoma. Cut surface of kidneys (same horse as Fig. 5.60).

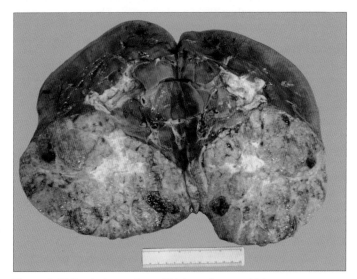

Figure 5.62 Renal adenocarcinoma. This image from an adult horse was an incidental finding at necropsy.

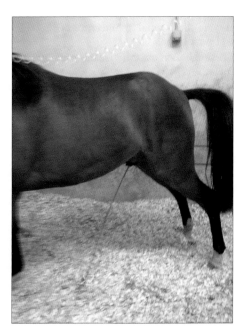

Figure 5.63 Hematuria is a frequent finding in horses with renal neoplasia.

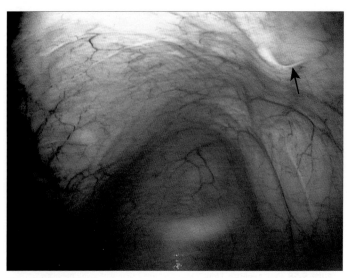

Figure 5.64 Normal opening of ureter in dorsolateral bladder wall (arrow). Cystoscopic examination of the openings in cases of hematuria may assist in determining the source of the hematuria.

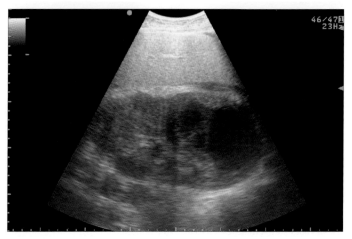

Figure 5.65 Renal hemangiosarcoma. Transabdominal ultrasonographic image of the left kidney from a one year old TB that presented with a history of shock and collapse. A hemabdomen was presented associated with a splenic tear but abnormal fluid filled masses were found in multiple abdominal organs and were later confirmed to be hemangiosarcomas. This image demonstrates an enlarge kidney with poor differentiation between cortex and medulla and a large fanechoic fluid filled posterior pole.

- Partial bladder resection of intravesicular instillation of 5-fluorouracil but there are no reports of successful outcomes to date which are most likely related to the extent of bladder involvement at the time of diagnosis.

References and further reading

Brown, C.M., Parks, A.H., Mullaney, T.P., et al., 1988. Bilateral renal dysplasia and hypoplasia in a foal with an imperforate anus. Vet Rec 122 (4), 91–92.

Fischer Jr., A.T., Spier, S., Carlson, G.P., Hackett, R.P., 1985. Neoplasia of the equine urinary bladder as a cause of hematuria. J Am Vet Med Assoc 186 (12), 1294–1296.

Hurcombe, S.D., Slovis, N.M., Kohn, C.W., Oglesbee, M., 2008. Poorly differentiated leiomyosarcoma of the urogenital tract in a horse. J Am Vet Med Assoc 233 (12), 1908–1912.

Jaeger, E.D., Keersmaecker, S.D., Hannes, C., 2000. Cystic urolithiasis in horses. Equine Vet Educ 12, 20–23.

Kranenburg, L.C., Thelen, M.H., Westermann, C.M., et al., 2010. Use of desmopressin eye drops in the treatment of equine congenital central diabetes insipidus. Vet Rec 167 (20), 790–791.

LeRoy, B., Woolums, A., Wass, J., et al., 2011. The relationship between serum calcium concentration and outcome in horses with renal failure presented to referral hospitals. J Vet Intern Med 25 (6), 1426–1430.

McAuliffe, S.B., Slovis, N.M., 2008. Colour Atlas of Diseases and Disorders of the Foal. WB Saunders, Philadelphia, PA, USA.

Ramirez, S., Williams, J., Seahorn, T.L., et al., 1998. Ultrasound-assisted diagnosis of renal dysplasia in a 3-month-old Quarter Horse colt. Vet Radiol Ultrasound 39 (2), 143–146.

Reed, S.M., Bayly, W.M., Sellon, D.C., 2009. Equine Internal Medicine, third ed. WB Saunders, St. Louis, MO, USA.

Robinson, N.E., Sprayberry, K.A. (Eds.), 2009. Current Therapy in Equine Medicine, sixth ed. WB Saunders, St. Louis, MO, USA.

Schott 2nd, H.C., 2007. Chronic renal failure in horses. Vet Clin North Am Equine Pract 23 (3), 593–612.

Schott 2nd, H.C., 2011. Water homeostasis and diabetes insipidus in horses. Vet Clin North Am Equine Pract 27 (1), 175–195.

Schumacher, J., 2007. Hematuria and pigmenturia of horses. Vet Clin North Am Equine Pract 23 (3), 655–675.

Tyner, G.A., Nolen-Walston, R.D., Hall, T., et al., 2011. A multicenter retrospective study of 151 renal biopsies in horses. J Vet Intern Med 25 (3), 532–539.

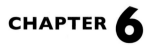

CHAPTER 6

Disorders of metabolism, nutrition and endocrine diseases

Developmental disorders

Hypocalcemia

Calcium deficiency in the horse can be acute or chronic and result from a variety of conditions (Table 6.1). Chronic deficiency presents as abnormal cartilage and bone development with or without lameness.

Acute deficiencies result in clinical signs associated with neuromuscular excitability.

The clinical consequences that are seen are varied and will be discussed individually.

Synchronous diaphragmatic flutter

SDF or 'thumps' can potentially occur in any horse with hypocalcemia but is especially common after endurance exercise where there is loss of additional electrolytes especially magnesium. Depolarization of the right atrium results in stimulation of action potentials in the phrenic nerve as it crosses over the heart. This results in diaphragmatic contractions that are rhythmic with the heart beat giving the appearance of 'hiccups'.

Hypocalcemic tetany

This again can occur in a any horse with hypocalcemia but is most commonly seen in mares as lactation tetany which can occur anywhere from 2 weeks prior to foaling to a few days after weaning. Heavy milk producers, mares on a low-calcium diet or lush pasture or those concurrently performing heavy work (draft breeds) are at increased risk.

Affected mares are depressed, sweating, ataxic or weak, and often develop marked muscle fasciculations. Pharyngeal paralysis resulting in dysphagia and/or marked inspiratory dyspnea is a frequent complication.

Hypocalcemic seizures

Decreased Ca^{2+} concentrations not only increase neuroexcitability in the peripheral nervous system but also in the central nervous sytem where it can result in seizures. This is most commonly seen in foals with hypocalcemia associated with sepsis.

Ileus

Smooth muscle cells have more voltage-gated Ca^{2+} channels than skeletal muscle, therefore any condition resulting in ionized hypocalcemia can result in ileus. This is particularly seen in horses with concurrent bowel inflammation (primary gastrointestinal disease or post colic surgery) and following transport, severe exercise or sepsis.

Retained placenta

While placental retention can occur for a number of reasons in some cases it may be confounded by hypocalcemia which results in decreased uterine tone and contractility. This has been further supported by the fact that mares treated with a combination of oxytocin and calcium borogluconate solution had a better response to therapy than mares treated with oxytocin alone.

Diagnosis and treatment of hypocalcemia

- The calculated deficit should ideally be based on the ionized calcium concentration but most laboratories measure total calcium.
- When treating hypocalcemia it is important to consider:
  - *Rate of development:* treatment is more critical in horses that have developed a rapid deficit.
  - *Ongoing losses:* lactating mares, compromised intestinal function. These horses may continue to be hypocalcemic despite aggressive replacement therapy.
- Many horses with ionized hypocalcemia may only have mild undectable signs but may progress to develop other signs such as ileus.
- Horses with functional kidneys can eliminate large amounts of calcium rapidly and it is rare to induce hypercalcemia from calcium administration but rapid administration could potentially result in cardiovascular complications. Current recommendations for speed of replacement are 1–2 mg/kg/h.

Hypercalcemic disorders

Primary hyperparathyroidism (Figs. 6.1–6.4)

An abnormality of the parathyroid gland results in excessive synthesis and secretion of PTH with no response to negative feedback from Ca^{2+}.

Table 6.1 Common clinical conditions in which hypocalcemia is reported

Acute renal failure	Colic
Post endurance	Retained placenta
Enterocolitis	Dystocia
Lactation tetany	Endotoxemia
Transportation stress	Heat stroke
Cantharidin toxicosis	Hypomagnesemia
Oxalate ingestion	Sepsis
Chronic renal failure	Pleuropneumonia

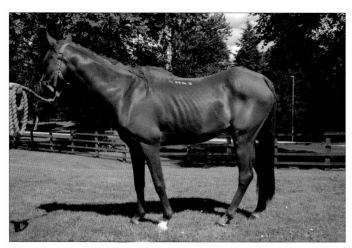

Figure 6.1 Primary hyperparathyroidism. 18-year-old Welsh pony that presented with a 6-month history of weight loss; the pony was slow to eat, had variable right forelimb lameness and exhibited weight shifting in all limbs. Blood biochemical examination revealed persistent ionized hypercalcemia, negligible concentration of PTH-related peptide and very high concentrations of PTH, consistent with primary hyperparathyroidism.

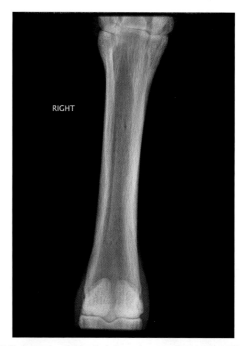

Figure 6.3 Radiographs of a forelimb (same horse as Figs. 6.1 and 6.2). Note loss of radiodensity. The mare later fractured a cannon bone and was subjected to euthanasia.

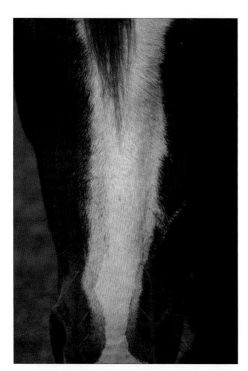

Figure 6.2 Facial asymmetry (same horse as Fig. 6.1).

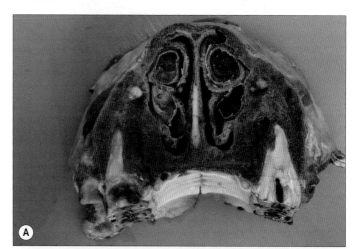

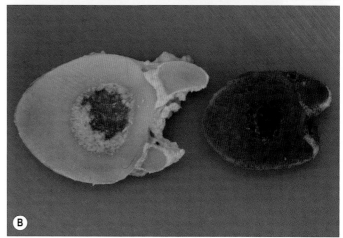

Theoretically, adenoma or hyperplasia of the parathyroid gland could result in this condition but histological examination of the gland is often complicated by the fact that it is difficult to find due to its small size and variable location.

The condition has been reported in association with osteodystrophia fibrosa. These horses have enlarged facial bones, poor body condition and lameness.

Diagnosis
- Hypercalcemia, hypophosphatemia, phosphaturia and increased intact PTH concentrations are characteristic laboratory findings.

Figure 6.4 (A, B) Necropsy (same horse as Figs. 6.1–6.3). Note changes of osteodystrophia fibrosa involving limbs and head. (B) Bone from normal pony on left and affected pony on the right.

- Additonal tests to rule out other conditions are measurement of PTHrP and vitamin D metabolite.

Secondary hyperparathyroidism (Figs. 6.5–6.7)

Excessive secretion of PTH occurs in response to hypocalcemia, hyperphosphatemia or hypovitaminosis D from renal dysfunction or nutritional imbalances. Renal secondary hyperparathyroidism does not appear to be important or common in horses, perhaps due to the fact that most horses with renal failure are actually hypercalcemic rather than hypocalemic in other species.

Nutritional secondary hyperparathyroidism (bran disease, big-head, Miller's disease)

Horses fed a diet low in calcium, high in phosphorus or both may develop this condition.

Traditionally this disorder was associated with excessive grain feeding but due to improvements in nutrition is not as frequently encountered in developed countries. However, ingestion of substances which bind out the available calcium, such as phytic acid in wheatbran or oxalate in tropical pasture grasses in Australia and North America, render the calcium less available and results in a further relative oversupply of phosphate. The most obvious manifestation of the disease is the development of a marked thickening of the flat bones of the head due to the more or less symmetrical laying down of cartilage in place of bone. Although young growing horses are most severely affected older horses are also subject to the condition. Shifting-leg lameness due to tendon and ligament avulsions, microfractures or even more serious pathological fractures are commonly the first sign of the disease. The extent of cartilage deposition and the

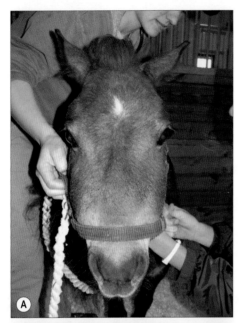

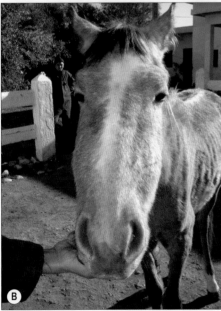

Figure 6.5 (A, B) Secondary hyperparathyroidism (osteodystrophia fibrosa, big-head, bran disease). Bilateral thickening of the flat bones of the skull.

Differential diagnosis:
- Maxillary sinusitis (usually unilateral)
- Maxillary cysts (usually unilateral)
- Edema of the head/circulation deficits. Swelling is soft issue not bone.

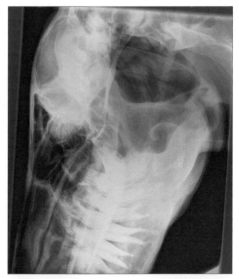

Figure 6.6 Secondary hyperparathyroidism. Radiograph of the head demonstrating generalized loss of bone density.

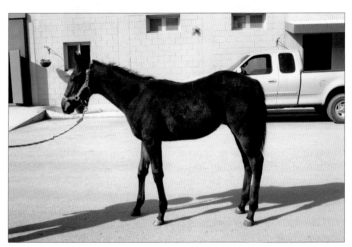

Figure 6.7 Secondary hyperparathyroidism in a 10-month-old colt. This colt had no access to pasture and was fed predominantly grain. He presented with multiple limb lameness and radiographs revealed decreased bone density and delayed closure of growth plates.

consequent weakness of the alveolar attachments of the molar teeth is a serious effect of the disease. Ultimately, cachexia develops, which is primarily a consequence of pain and physical obstructions to mastication.

Diagnosis and treatment

- History of diet and clincial signs may be suggestive. Clinical laboratory findings may include hypocalcemia and hyperphosphatemia but this is not consistent and in some cases they may be within normal ranges. Serum intact PTH concentrations are increased.
- Dietary manipulation by increasing calcium supplementation can result in rapid improvement in early cases but more advanced cases may require prolonged therapy (9–12 months). Affected animals should receive 100–300 g/day of calcium with the diet overall having a Ca:P ratio of 3:1 to 4:1.

Iron deficiency

Primary deficiency as a result of low dietary intake or poor absorption is rare but chronic blood loss, chronic infections or internal neoplasia often result in the secondary development of a dramatic, progressive and typical (microcytic, hypochromic) iron-deficiency anemia. In these horses the total body iron is invariably normal but the availability is severely impaired by the complex of inflammatory processes. Horses which suffer from a prolonged microcytic, hypochromic anemia without evidence of bone marrow activity should be investigated thoroughly for a possible underlying infectious or neoplastic disorder.

Diagnosis and treatment

- Typical cytological appearance of red blood cells. Bone marrow biopsy may be required to rule out differentials.
- Treatment is primarily aimed at identifying the cause of underlying infection or blood loss and treating it accordingly.

Thyroid disease

Thyroid gland function can be assessed by measurement of serum concentrations of thyroid hormones, either at rest or in response to thyrotropin-releasing hormone (TRH) or thyroid-stimulating hormone (TSH). Stimulation tests are regarded as more reliable but have the disadvantages of being more time-consuming and there is limited availability of TRH or TSH in an affordable form.

Bound or free forms of T_3 or T_4 can be measured in readily available assays (see Tables 6.2 and 6.3). It is best to measure levels of free hormone as changes in protein binding can alter the total level.

Certain drugs (phenylbutazone, corticosteroids), physiological events (strenuous exercise, diets high in energy, protein, zinc or copper) and pathological events (inappetance, non-thyroid disease) can alter the circulating levels of thyroid hormones without the presence of disease in the gland itself.

Hyperthyroidism

Hyperthyroidism is an extremely rare disorder in horses and the cases reported in the literature were attributed to thyroid gland neoplasias. Clinical signs in these cases included weight loss, tachycardia, hyperactive behavior, ravenous appetite and cachexia. Exposure to iodine,

such as in topical blisters, can result in a temporary increase in circulating thyroid hormones but these cases are not associated with clinical signs of disease given above.

Diagnosis and treatment

- High resting concentrations of thyroid hormones.
- Administration of exogenous T_3 failed to suppress endogenous T_4 concentrations.
- Due to the relationship with thyroid gland neoplasia further tests to rule in or out a neoplasia would include ultrasound, biopsy or nuclear scintigraphy.
- Treatment could involve removal of a portion or all of the thyroid gland followed by supplementation with thyroid hormones.

Hypothyroidism (Figs. 6.8–6.10)

Primary hypothyroidism in the horse is probably much less common than previously thought. Many of the clinical signs attributed to hypothyroidism such as obesity, abnormal fat deposits, subfertility and recurrent laminitis have now been recognized as part of the equine metabolic syndrome and many of the horses that were previously diagnosed as hypothyroid are now acknowledged to be insulin-resistant. Further supporting this is the fact that cases reported to have hypothyroidism as a result of thyroid neoplasia have predominantly presented with changes in skin/haircoat and poor exercise tolerance. Additionally, thyroidectomy in young horses results in delayed physeal closure, decreased growth rate, cold intolerance, low rectal temperature, lethargy and coarse haircoat as well as other non-specific changes in serum phosphorus, cholesterol and triglyceride concentrations.

Iodine concentrations in soil and plants in specific areas of the United States of America and in other parts of the world are known to be low. **Dietary deficiency of iodine** results in the development of goiter (chronic symmetrical bilateral enlargement of the thyroid glands which is not due to a neoplasm). Some plants, including most *Brassica* spp., are also goitrogenic through a tendency to reduce the availability of dietary iodine. The foals of iodine-deficient mares are sometimes born dead, often with an obvious goiter. Hypothyroidism has been linked to developmental abnormalities of foals including prematurity and defects of ossification of the skeleton. Hypothyroidism developing in foals early in gestation is possibly also associated with failure to establish normal respiratory function at birth, whereas if the disorder develops in later gestation, lethargy, loss of suckle, muscular weakness, long coat hair and goiter are present. Contracted tendons at birth, collapse of tarsal bones with consequent sickle-hock posture are also possibly related to the condition. In adult horses, hypothyroidism may not be accompanied by an obvious goiter.

While most cases of **goiter** in young foals are a result of iodine deficiency, some may be associated with **excessive iodine** supplementation to pregnant mares. In these, long hair, muscle weakness, flexural deformities and gross limb abnormalities may be encountered. Affected foals may be born at full term, but show characteristic

Table 6.2 Baseline concentrations of thyroid hormones in healthy adult horses

	TT$_4$ (nmol/L)	fT$_4$ (pmol/L)	TT$_3$ (nmol/L)	fT$_3$ (pmol/L)	TSH (ng/ml)
Range	6–46	6–21	0.3–2.9	0.1–5.9	0.02–0.97
Median	19	11	0.9	1.7	0.23

Table 6.3 Baseline concentrations of thyroid hormones in healthy foals

	TT$_4$ (nmol/L)	fT$_4$ (pmol/L)	TT$_3$ (nmol/L)	fT$_3$ (pmol/L)	TSH (ng/ml)
Range	238–337	46–118	3.4–10.8	2.4–20.3	0.12–0.72
Median	277	78	8.2	7.8	0.22

Adapted from Braehus BA, 2009 Thyroid disease. In: Robinson NE, Sprayberry KA (eds) *Current Therapy in Equine Medicine*, sixth ed., pp. 738–739. WB Saunders, Philadelphia, PA, USA.

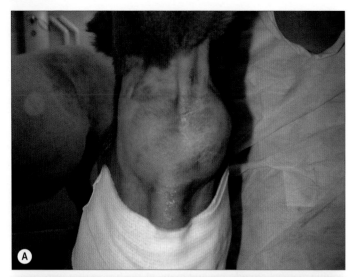

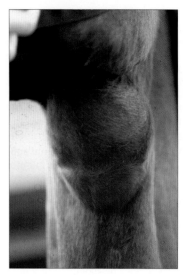

Figure 6.10 Goiter in an adult horse. Bilateral thyroid enlargement not due to neoplasia.

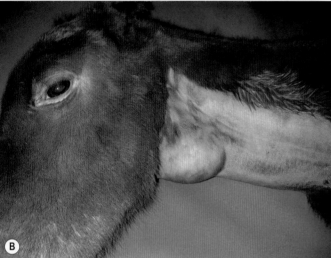

Figure 6.8 (A, B) Hypothyroidism (goiter) in a newborn foal.

Diagnosis
- Low resting concentrations of free fractions of T_3 and T_4 in a horse that is not ill, is eating normally, has not undergone recent exercise and that has not been given drugs known to lower thyroid hormone concentrations are diagnostic.
- Failure to respond to TRH stimulation provides additional support for the diagnosis.
- TSH concentration greater than 1 ng/ml is also considered diagnostic but validated TSH assays are not yet available.
- Clinical signs such as very obvious lethargy and weight gain in formerly thin (normal), energetic horses, with (or without) obvious bilateral goiter accompanied by abnormal free thyroid hormone levels, and subsequent response to the administration of thyroid hormones, is used by many clinicians to diagnose hypothyroidism.

Treatment
- Several forms of T_4 are available for administration to adult horses.
- Iodinated casein contains approximately 1% T_4 and can be given orally at 5–15 g/horse/day.
- Levothyroxine has been given at 20 mg/horse/day but this may be lower than required with some authors recommending between 50–100 mg/horse/day.
- Ideally dosages should be adjusted to normalize TSH if a reliable assay becomes readily available.
- The current dosage recommendation of levothyroxine for foals is 20–50 µg/kg/day. The suggested dose for T_3 is 1 µg/kg/day. Monitoring of serum levels is very important in foals to avoid overdosage.

Non-thyroidal illness syndrome (euthyroid sick syndrome)
Changes in thyroid function with reduction in serum concentrations of T_3 and T_4 accompany many types of illness. It is thought that these changes decrease metabolic rate and help conserve lean body mass. In humans changes in thyroid function are progressive with the severity of the disease. This is now an area of active research in horses, with recent work showing increased survival rates in post-surgical colics administered supplemental thyroid hormones.

Thyroid gland enlargement and neoplasia (Fig. 6.11)
Increased thyroid size is often encountered in older horses in particular, but these are seldom functional enlargements. Usually the enlargements are unilateral and they may reach considerable size. While

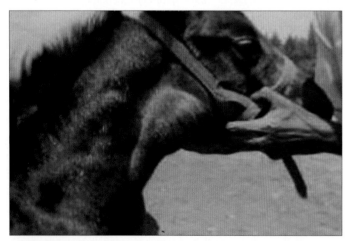

Figure 6.9 Hypothyroidism (goiter) in a young foal.

signs of prematurity, i.e. are dysmature. The similarities between foals born to iodine-deficient mares and those born to mares receiving excessive amounts are remarkable but are physiologically logical. Excessive dietary iodine depresses the stimulation of the gland and the conversion of inactive thyroid hormones to the active ones.

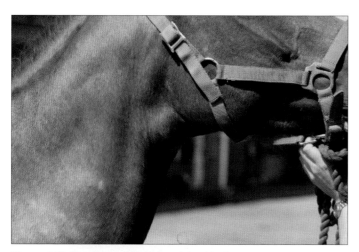

Figure 6.11 Thyroid neoplasia. Unilateral thyroid enlargement.
Differential diagnosis: Benign hyperplasia.

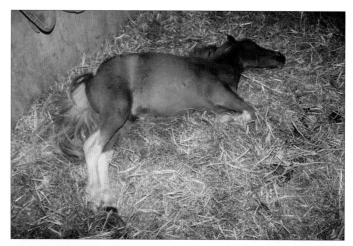

Figure 6.12 White muscle disease. Skeletal or subacute form. Affected foals frequently spend a long time in recumbency.

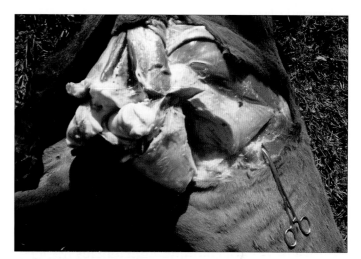

Figure 6.13 White muscle disease. (Courtesy of IEC).
Differential diagnosis:
• Polysaccharide storage myopathy (PSSM) (normally seen in older horses, but has been reported in foals as young as 1 month of age)
• Glycogen branching enzyme deficiency (signs are apparent at birth)
• Hypoxia-induced rhabdomyolysis
• Post-anesthetic myoneuropathy.

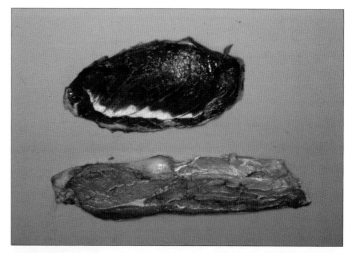

Figure 6.14 White muscle disease. Normal muscle (above) and muscle from weanling affected with WMD (below). Note the marked difference in colour, hence the name of the disorder.

most such enlargements are the result of **hyperplasia**, some are **adenomas** of the thyroid glandular tissue. Usually, very large, unilateral thyroid swellings are hyperplastic tissue and do not under most circumstances result from any goitrogenous tendency. Most adenomas are small and many are detected incidentally at post-mortem examination. Dramatic enlargements of the thyroid gland are more likely to be caused by **C-cell tumors**, which typically are small but can reach alarming size. The metabolic effect of any of the thyroid enlargements is usually minimal in spite of obvious increases in size of one of the thyroid glands. It is therefore usual to identify the changes incidentally. The cosmetic aspect of thyroid enlargements in older horses is usually of greatest concern. Functional tumors, particularly of the C-cell type, are, however, potentially of pathological and physiological significance, affecting the relevant metabolic processes, including calcium metabolism.

Diagnosis and treatment
See Hyperthyroidism above.

Nutritional and other disorders

Nutritional myodegeneration/vitamin E and selenium deficiency/white muscle disease
(Figs. 6.12–6.14)
This is an uncommon condition of young growing foals normally between 2 weeks–7 months of age. NMD is thought to result from a dietary deficiency of selenium and/or vitamin E in gestating dams with a resultant deficiency in the foal. Selenium deficiency appears to play the most important role based on prophylaxis and response to treatment. The condition has a higher than normal prevalence in Fell ponies.

Two types of the disease are seen but the classification is based on the organs affected:

1) *Skeletal or subacute form*. This form usually results in generalized muscle weakness or stiffness. It can present with asymmetric signs giving it an initial appearance of lameness and thus making diagnosis more difficult. Supporting muscle groups of the limbs (especially hindlimbs) may be swollen and painful. These foals frequently have difficulty rising and may be recumbent for prolonged periods or may become acutely recumbent following exercise. If the diaphragm and intercostal muscles are affected respiratory distress may be present. Myoglobinuria may be seen in some cases but is not consistent.

2) *Cardiac or peracute form*. In the cardiac form the predominant lesions are in the heart, diaphragm and intercostal muscles. These animals are frequently found dead or in a near-dead condition. If found alive they have a rapid, irregular heart beat and profound weakness. This form tends to occur in younger foals than the skeletal form.

Diagnosis
- Clinical signs.
- Elevated CK, AST and LDH (isoenzymes 4 and 5 are related to skeletal muscle activity and isoenzymes 1 and 2 are related to cardiac muscle activity). Elevations are usually in the thousands of IU/L. Animals which have elevations in these enzymes for other reasons rarely go past several hundred IU/L.
- Definitive diagnosis of NMD is established by determining whole blood selenium (normal range is 0.07 ppm to 0.10 ppm) and glutathione peroxidase (GSH-Px) which is selenium-dependent can also be measured (20–50 U/mg of hemoglobin/min is normal in horses).
- Response to therapy.

Treatment and prognosis
- Rest and administration of vitamin E/selenium injections. Injectable selenium should be given IM at a dose of 0.055–0.067 mg/kg (2.5–3 mg/45 kg body weight). Absorption and distribution occur rapidly and may account for the rapid improvement in clinical signs in some cases. Avoid using the neck as an injection site as pain from injection reactions may prevent nursing and injection site reactions are common. Vitamin E should also be supplemented in either injectable or oral form. The latter is easier to administer and contains 500 IU/ml; the recommended dose for NMD is 2–6 IU/kg.
- Many cases are advanced or have extensive muscle fibrosis when diagnosed and respond poorly to treatment. Those with the cardiac form that are diagnosed and treated early usually respond poorly and die within 24 hours. Full recovery of subacute cases may take a number of months.

Biotin and/or methionine deficiencies (Fig. 6.15)
Biotin and/or methionine deficiencies have become a recognized entity associated with defective horn genesis. The relationship between these two essential vitamins is unclear, but some horses having poor hoof wall quality show dramatic improvements when these substances are supplied as long-term dietary supplements.

Anhidrosis (Figs. 6.16 & 6.17)
This is the inability to sweat in response to heat or catecholamine release. It characteristically affects horses which are moved to hot climates from milder, temperate regions but it may develop spontaneously in native horses in hot humid climates such as the Gulf States of the United States of America and the coastal areas of northern Australia and the Middle and Far East. In a study in Florida 11% of

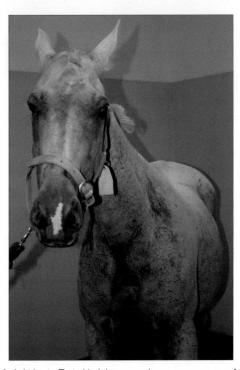

Figure 6.16 Anhidrosis. Typical lack-lustre, moth-eaten appearance of haircoat. This broodmare was imported to the Middle East and showed signs of anhidrosis following her first summer in the significantly warmer climate.

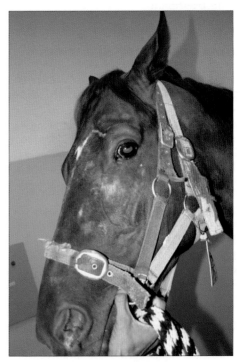

Figure 6.17 Anhidrosis. Hair loss on the face is typical in horses with anhidrosis.

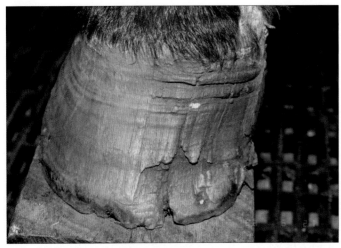

Figure 6.15 Biotin/methionine deficiency associated with hoof changes.

horses were affected, with the incidence being much greater in working/riding horses. It is caused by gradual failure of the glandular secretory cell processes, initiated by desensitization and subsequent down-regulation of the cell receptors as a result of continued adrenaline-driven hyperactivity. It progresses through secretory failure and culminates in gradual, probably irreversible, glandular dedifferentiation and ultimate degeneration.

Although there is a gradual failure of the secretory system many cases present with an 'acute' onset. These show nostril flaring, a high respiratory rate and a very high body temperature, in the absence of any sweating. In pasture-kept horses subtle changes in respiratory rate and body temperature may go unnoticed and it is the coat and skin changes that are frequently noted in these horses. The skin of chronically affected horses is dry with a 'moth-eaten' appearance, excessive scaling and some pruritus. Polydipsia, polyuria and loss of condition are sometimes found.

Diagnosis

- The condition may be suspected on the basis of suitable history and clinical signs.
- Intradermal testing with terbutaline can be used to confirm the diagnosis. Six serial ten-fold dilutions of the β2-adrenergic agonist terbutaline are prepared. One ml of each dilution is injected intra-dermally along the neck or in the pectoral region. In normal horses a localized area of sweating will be seen in association with each injection site. Some normal horses may not have response to the most dilute concentration. Sweating is seen within 5 minutes of injection in normal horses. Anhidrotic horses will not sweat at any of the concentrations. Hypohidrotic horses will only sweat at the higher concentrations or may show a delayed onset on sweating.

Treatment

- There are many anecdotal treatments for anhidrosis, ranging from electrolyte and thyroid hormone supplementation to the addition of beer to the diet!
- The role of thyroid hormone remains unclear; in one study resting concentrations of thyroid hormones and thyroid-stimulating hormone (TSH) were not different between anhidrotic and control horses. Thyroid hormone responses to TRH also were not different between the two groups of horses. However, anhidrotic horses had a significantly different TSH response to TRH compared with control horses, particularly in the winter.
- In most instances the best response to treatment is to remove the horse from the offending environment. Where it is not possible to move the horse to a cooler part of the country/different country, stabling with air conditioning during the warmer parts of the day may be beneficial but many of these horses do not return to normal.
- It is also important to remember that a history of anhidrosis is now considered in many cases sufficient reason to fail a performance horse during a pre-purchase examination.

Equine metabolic syndrome (Figs. 6.18–6.20)

The term equine metabolic syndrome (EMS) was first introduced to veterinary medicine in 2002 when it was proposed that obesity, insulin resistance (IR) and laminitis were components of a clinical syndrome recognized in horses and ponies. 'EMS' was adopted as the name for this condition because of similarities with the metabolic syndrome (MetS) in humans, which is a collection of risk factors assessed to predict the occurrence of coronary artery disease and type 2 diabetes mellitus.

The majority of affected horses have the following:

- Increased adiposity in specific locations (regional adiposity) or generally (obesity). Regional adiposity is characterized by expansion of subcutaneous adipose tissues surrounding the nuchal

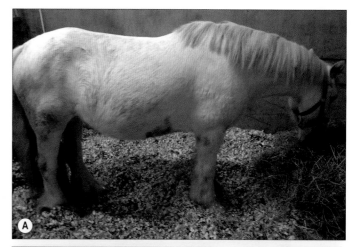
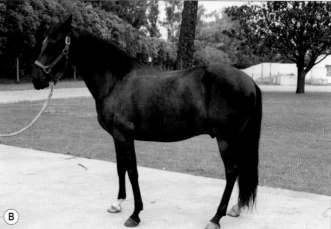

Figure 6.18 (A, B) Typical body type associated with equine metabolic syndrome.

Differential diagnosis:
- Excessive body condition associated with excessive feeding
- PPID.

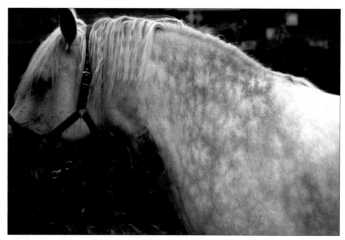

Figure 6.19 Excessive crest fat typical of regional adiposity seen with equine metabolic syndrome.

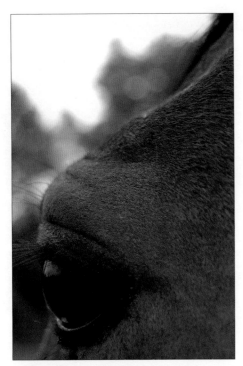

Figure 6.20 Supraorbital fat deposition which is frequently seen in horses with equine metabolic syndrome, but can also be seen in horses with PPID.

ligament in the neck (cresty neck), development of fat pads close to the tailhead, or fat accumulation behind the shoulder or in the prepuce or mammary gland region. Obesity is observed in the majority of cases, but some affected horses have a leaner overall body condition and regional adiposity, and others are normal in appearance.

- IR characterized by hyperinsulinemia or abnormal glycemic and insulinemic responses to oral or IV glucose and/or insulin challenges.
- A predisposition toward laminitis. Clinical or subclinical laminitis that has developed in the absence of recognized causes.

Additional findings in many affected horses are:

- Hypertriglyceridemia or dyslipidemia.
- Hyperleptinemia resulting from increased secretion of the hormone leptin by adipocytes in response to IR or a state of leptin resistance.
- Arterial hypertension which is recognized as a key component of MetS related to IR in humans.
- Altered reproductive cycling in mares. Loss of the seasonal anovulatory period and prolongation of the interovulatory period have been described in obese insulin-resistant mares.
- Increased systemic markers of inflammation in association with obesity.

The history often includes previous episodes of laminitis and the horse is frequently reported as being an 'easy-doer'. Anecdotally, Welsh, Dartmoor, Shetland ponies, Morgan Horses, Paso Fino, Arabian, Saddlebred, Spanish Mustang, and Warmblood breeds appear to be more susceptible to EMS. Most horses with EMS are between 5 and 15 years of age when veterinary or farrier services are first requested because of laminitis.

Diagnosis

- EMS can be diagnosed by obtaining a complete history, performing a physical examination, taking radiographs of the feet and conducting laboratory tests.

- Hyperinsulinemia in the absence of confounding factors such as stress, pain and a recent feed provides evidence of IR in horses and ponies. However, resting insulin concentrations are not found to be increased in all cases, so dynamic testing provides the most accurate diagnosis of IR. The combined glucose-insulin test (CGIT) can also be used to diagnose IR. In this test, the horse is stabled the night before and fed free choice hay only; a baseline blood sample is collected and followed by 150 mg/kg 50% dextrose solution (150 ml for a 500 kg horse); further blood samples are collected at 1, 5, 15, 25, 35, 45, 60, 75, 90, 105, 120, 135 and 150 minutes post infusion. Insulin resistance is defined as maintenance of blood glucose concentrations above baseline for 45 minutes or longer. There is a risk of hypoglycemia developing in a small number of horses and 120ml of 50% dextrose solution should be available for administration if sweating, muscle fasiculations or weakness develop.

Differentiating EMS from pituitary pars intermedia dysfunction (PPID; equine Cushing's disease)

- Regional adiposity and laminitis are clinical signs of PPID as well as EMS, so both endocrine disorders should be considered when these problems are detected.
- EMS may be differentiated from PPID by:
  - Age of onset: The EMS phenotype is generally first recognized in younger horses, whereas PPID is more common in older horses, although these disorders may coexist.
  - Further clinical signs suggestive of PPID, but not EMS, including delayed or failed shedding of the winter haircoat, hirsutism, excessive sweating, polyuria/polydipsia, and skeletal muscle atrophy.
  - Positive diagnostic test results for PPID: For example, detection of an increased plasma adrenocorticotropin hormone concentration in the absence of confounding factors such as pain and stress, and outside of the late summer/autumn period when false-positive results occur in healthy horses and ponies.

Treatment

- Most horses and ponies with EMS can be effectively managed by controlling the horse's diet, instituting an exercise program, and limiting or eliminating access to pasture. Many studies have revealed that IR in human subjects is controlled most effectively by changes in lifestyle and diet, although these strategies may fail due to lack of self-discipline. Similarly, compliance of the owner/manager is critical to the success of management changes designed to alleviate risk factors for laminitis in EMS.
- An obese horse should be placed on a diet consisting of hay fed in an amount equivalent to 1.5% of ideal body weight (1.5 lb hay per 100 lb bwt). If an obese horse or pony fails to lose weight after hay has been fed at an amount equivalent to 1.5% of ideal body weight for 30 days, this amount should be lowered to 1%. However, amounts should not fall below this minimum of 1% and it should be noted that severe calorie restriction may lead to worsening of IR, hyperlipemia and unacceptable stereotypical behaviors.

Poor body condition (Figs. 6.21–6.23)

Starvation is a common disorder of neglected horses in all parts of the world. The metabolic consequences of significant nutritional deprivation are extensive and varied. A single animal affected in a group may suffer from effective deprivation in the presence of food for social reasons, there being no physical or medical reason for the failure to ingest the food. This is relatively common in confined herds of horses which receive all their food as preserved fodder, fed particularly at irregular intervals. One animal in a group (or on its own) having access to normal quantities of food may be metabolically deprived through inability to eat, chew, swallow or make effective use of ingested food material. Horses which are in poor condition

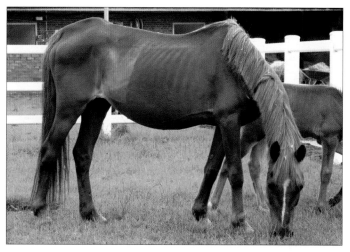

Figure 6.21 Malnutrition associated with failure to meet nutritional requirements in this nursing mare.

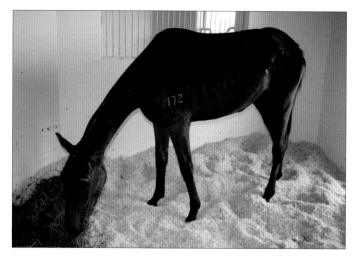

Figure 6.22 Chronic parasitism and related intestinal abscesses resulted in inability to utilize ingested food and consequent poor body condition in this horse.

may therefore not necessarily be starved. Cachexia associated with infectious or inflammatory conditions or neoplasia may also result in poor body condition in a single member of a herd. However, it is likely that where several horses in a herd are found in similarly poor bodily condition, the availability of nutritious food or any food may be limited. Individual horses in a group may, however, suffer from starvation when they are subjected to dominance behavior from more aggressive or dominant animals in the group. Horses suffering from starvation are able to tolerate considerable and prolonged deprivation without marked effects, and it is often only the extremes of nutritional deprivation which exert significant metabolic effect in terms of specific deficiencies of minerals, vitamins or other nutrients.

Neoplastic diseases

Pituitary pars intermedia dysfunction
(Figs. 6.24–6.28)
This is the most common endocrinopathy of horses and ponies with a large number of older animals affected. The clinical signs seen are a result of increased levels of ACTH, α-melanocyte stimulating hormone and β-endorphin, secreted by an adenoma or hypertrophied cells of the pars intermedia of the pituitary gland. The condition has had various names over the years including equine Cushing's disease but is now termed pituitary pars intermedia dysfunction (PPID).

It is predominantly a disease of older animals (>13 years) but there have been cases in animals as young as 7 years. It has been described in all breeds but is most common in ponies and Morgans.

Classical clinical signs associated with PPID are hirsutism, weight loss and poor muscle tone, abnormal distribution of subcutaneous fat, periorbital swelling in the absence of ocular disease, polyuria and polydipsia, laminitis and predisposition to infections. The reproductive cycles of mares are interrupted or abnormal in duration, and some affected mares even produce milk without pregnancy.

Other more rare signs associated with compression of surrounding structures in the brain include central blindness, seizures and ataxia. However, the neurological signs seen do not have a direct correlation with tumor size.

Diagnosis
- Acquired hirsutism (abnormally dense, hairy coat) is considered pathognomonic for PPID. The hair coat is abnormally long, curly, brittle and dense. Normal seasonal shedding of the coat does not occur and the horse remains hirsute in the summer months.

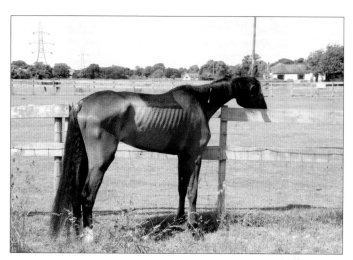

Figure 6.23 Cachexia secondary to thoracic neoplasia.

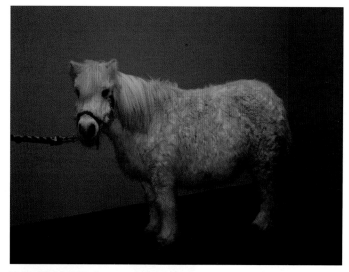

Figure 6.24 PPID. Excessive, curly coat in summer. Sweating and weight loss accompanied by polydipsia and polyuria.

Differential diagnosis:
- Metabolic syndrome (no coat-related signs)
- Diabetes mellitus (very rare)
- Acute/chronic renal failure (no coat-related signs).

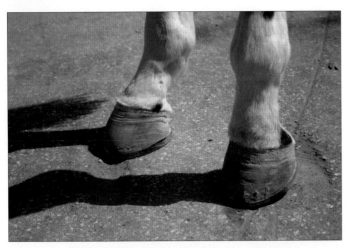

Figure 6.25 Chronic laminitis in a horse with PPID.

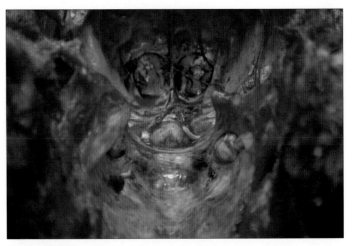

Figure 6.28 Pituitary adenoma found incidentally during post-mortem examination.

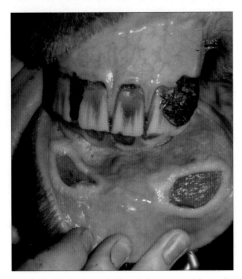

Figure 6.26 PPID (Cushing's disease). Buccal ulceration, with very limited inflammatory response.

Differential diagnosis:
- Dental abnormalities
- Neurological (sensory) disorders of cranial nerve V
- Fracture of mandible/hyoid bone
- Dysphagia (central or peripheral origin)
- Renal failure.

Table 6.4 Dexamethasone suppression test
Blood is collected for baseline cortisol levels.
40 μg/kg dexamethasone is administered IV or IM.
Blood is collected again at 12 or 15 and 24 hours post-corticosteroid administration.
In normal horses, serum cortisol levels will fall below 1 μg/dl at 12 or 15 hours and remain low at 24 hours.
In horses with PPID, cortisol remains above 1 μg/dl at 12 or 15 hours and is at least 80% of baseline at 24 hours.

Sweating and weight loss may be detectable on close examination, but may be missed under the heavy, shaggy coat. Hirsutism should not be confused with normally long winter coats in small ponies and spontaneous hirsutism seen in the Bashkir curly breed.

- Clinico-pathological findings are variable and non-diagnostic.
- The dexamethasone suppression test (Table 6.4) has long been considered the gold standard for diagnosis of PPID. The basis of the test is that normal horses are very sensitive to the administration of exogenous corticosteroid while horses with PPID are more resistant. The test is thought to be less repeatable during the autumn months and should ideally be performed at another time of the year.
- Hormone testing: MSH, ACTH and β-endorphin are generally raised in affected horses but a commercial assay is only available for ACTH. ACTH measurement is now considered the gold standard. Endogenous ACTH is increased in the fall, but many laboratories now have seasonally adjusted reference values. The laboratory should be consulted prior to testing. In general, levels >55 pg/ml are consistent with PPID. ACTH binds to glass, so samples should be taken in plastic tubes.
- Domperidone testing: when 1.5–5.0 mg/kg domperidone is administered orally, horses with PPID have a twofold increase in endogenous ACTH either 4 or 8 hours later. While potentially useful this test is not routinely performed due to the difficulties in obtaining accurate ACTH determinations.
- Resting insulin concentration, glucose and insulin tolerance testing: these tests have been popular in the past but because of abnormal responses in horses with metabolic syndrome they are no longer recommended alone.

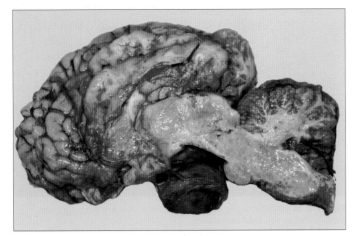

Figure 6.27 Pituitary adenoma in a 24-year-old mare. This mare was known to have Cushing's syndrome. She was euthanized during an episode of colic.

- Thyrotropin-releasing hormone: TRH administration results in increases in blood cortisol, MSH and ACTH levels. An increase in blood cortisol of 90% or greater above baseline 15–30 minutes after the administration of 1 mg of thyrotropin is considered diagnostic but TRH is expensive and difficult to obtain.

Treatment

- Therapy is aimed at increasing dopaminergic tone in the pars intermedia or decreasing circulating cortisol concentration.
- Pergolide is a dopamine agonist and is considered by many to be the treatment of choice. The initial dose is 0.002 mg/kg PO q 24 h (1 mg per 450 kg). This dose may be slowly increased if the horse becomes refractory to treatment. Adverse effects include anorexia, depression and ataxia and the dose should be decreased if any of these signs are observed.
- Bromocriptine is also a dopamine agonist but is not commonly used because of poor bioavailability.
- Cyproheptadine is a serotonin antagonist that has been widely used to treat PPID. However, reports of efficacy are lacking. Some clinicians claim a beneficial effect of using it in combination with pergolide but again there is a lack of convincing reports on this combined usage.
- Another factor in the treatment of horses with PPID is improved general husbandry including; careful feeding, early attention to infections and regular farrier care.

Tumors of the adrenal medulla (pheochromocytoma)

Tumors of the adrenal medulla (pheochromocytoma) are rare. Most cases occur in horses over 10–15 years of age. Weight loss, sweating, muscle tremors, laminitis and a high resting respiratory rate with flaring of the nostrils are encountered, as would be expected when abnormally high concentrations of endogenous catecholamines are present. One of the most significant clinical features of this condition is paroxysmal hypertension. A dramatic and unexplained increase in heart rate and force produces a hard bounding pulse and the heart beat may even be audible from a distance. Obvious mydriasis (pupillary dilatation) is usually present during these episodes and the animal may sweat profusely. The lesions responsible for this clinical syndrome are often surprisingly small, usually being well-encapsulated and nodular in appearance and located at one or other pole of one adrenal gland. Similar masses may be found incidentally at post-mortem examination apparently having no functional effect. The contralateral gland is usually normal in appearance.

Further reading

Abraham, G., Allersmeier, M., Schusser, G.F., Ungemach, F.R., 2011. Serum thyroid hormone, insulin, glucose, triglycerides and protein concentrations in normal horses: association with topical dexamethasone usage. Vet J 188 (3), 307–312.

Breuhaus, B.A., 2002. Thyroid-stimulating hormone in adult euthyroid and hypothyroid horses. J Vet Intern Med 16 (1), 109–115.

Breuhaus, B.A., 2009. Thyroid function in anhidrotic horses. J Vet Intern Med 23 (1), 168–173.

Donaldson, M.T., McDonnell, S.M., Schanbacher, B.J., et al., 2005. Variation in plasma adrenocorticotropic hormone concentration and dexamethasone suppression test results with season, age and sex in healthy ponies and horses. J Vet Intern Med 19, 217–222.

Frank, N., 2011. Equine metabolic syndrome. Vet Clin North Am Equine Pract 27 (1), 73–92.

Frank, N., Andrews, F.M., Sommardahl, C.S., et al., 2006. Evaluation of the combined dexamethasone suppression/thyrotropin-releasing hormone stimulation test for detection of pars intermedia pituitary adenomas in horses. J Vet Intern Med 20 (4), 987–993.

Graves, E.A., Schott 2nd, H.C., Marteniuk, J.V., et al., 2006. Thyroid hormone responses to endurance exercise. Equine Vet J Suppl 36, 32–36.

Jenkinson, D.M., Elder, H.Y., Bovell, D.L., 2007. Equine sweating and anhidrosis Part 2: anhidrosis. Vet Dermatol 18 (1), 2–11.

MacKay, R.J., 2008. Quantitative intradermal terbutaline sweat test in horses. Equine Vet J 40 (5), 518–520.

McEwan Jenkinson, D., Elder, H.Y., Bovell, D.L., 2006. Equine sweating and anhidrosis. Part 1, Equine sweating. Vet Dermatol 17 (6), 361–392.

Place, N.J., McGowan, C.M., Lamb, S.V., et al., 2010. Seasonal variation in serum concentrations of selected metabolic hormones in horses. J Vet Intern Med 24 (3), 650–654.

Reed, S.M., Bayly, W.M., Sellon, D.C., 2009. Equine Internal Medicine, third ed. WB Saunders, St. Louis, MI, USA.

Robinson, N.E., Sprayberry, K.A., 2009. Current Therapy in Equine Medicine, sixth ed. WB Saunders, Philadelphia, PA, USA.

Schott, H.C., 2002. Pituitary pars intermedia dysfunction: equine Cushings disease. Vet Clin North Am Equine Pract 18, 237–270.

Sevinga, M., Barkema, H.W., Hesselink, J.W., 2002. Serum calcium and magnesium concentrations and the use of calcium-magnesium borogluconate in the treatment of Friesian mares with retained placenta. Theriogenology 57, 941–947.

Skeletal disorders

Developmental disorders

Deformities of the axial skeleton (Figs. 7.1–7.4)

A wide variety of skeletal deformities occurs in horses, although individually most are rare. The importance of such abnormalities rests both in their heritability and their immediate and long-term effects upon posture and locomotion. Even if severe, the consequences of these deformities may not be life-threatening, but they may lead to significant disorders of gait as the animal grows or comes into work.

Deformities of the vertebral column

Deformities of the vertebral column are most common in the cervical (wry neck) and lumbar (kyphosis, lordosis, scoliosis) regions. **Deviations and distortions** of the skull are also encountered. While such defects are visually dramatic, there is commonly little or no material effect upon the growth or natural behavior of the horse but they will become important when ridden work is required. Severe deformities, especially of the cervical vertebrae, may result in dystocia as the fetus cannot be positioned normally for delivery. Most deviations of the axial skeleton are sporadic occurrences and there is little evidence of heritability. Such defects are thought to be the result of fetal malpositioning when, during the later rapid phases of growth, fetal

movement is naturally suppressed. However, many other factors may be involved and the more severe deviations may be the result of growth deformities, arising from a number of factors such as maternal viral or bacterial infections or toxemia during gestation.

Diagnosis and treatment

- The defects are usually obvious at birth but many may show remarkable improvement over the early weeks of life.
- Radiography can help confirm suspected lesions and further evaluate the degree and severity of the lesion.
- Treatment usually consists of conservative management with many mild cases improving. Severe cases or cases with multiple defects may require euthanasia.

Polydactyly (Fig. 7.5)

Polydactyly is a relatively common developmental abnormality with little clinical significance, although cosmetically it is generally

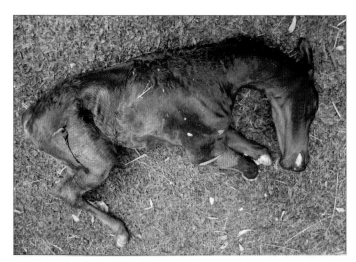

Figure 7.1 Severe torticollis in this foal resulted in dystocia.

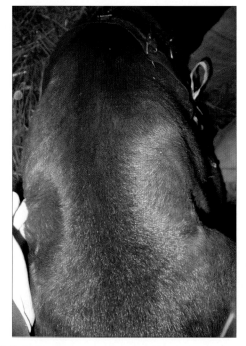

Figure 7.2 Kyphosis.

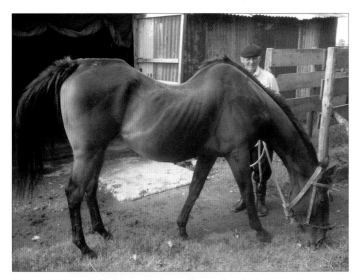

Figure 7.3 Lordosis in this mare had been present since birth.

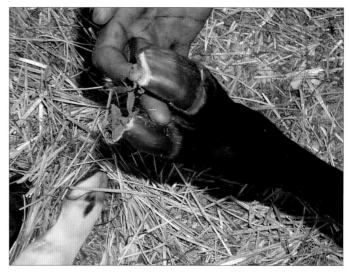

Figure 7.5 Polydactyl.

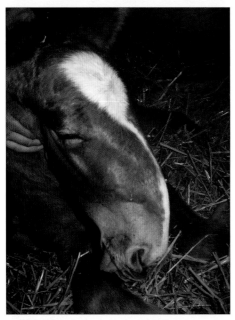

Figure 7.4 Facial deformity in this foal was accompanied by other skeletal defects.

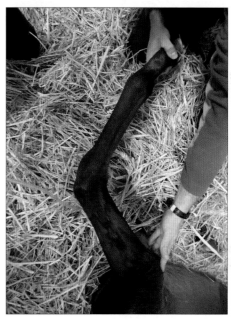

Figure 7.6 Arthrogryposis. This foal was delivered by C-section due to dystocia caused by severe contracture of three of the four limbs.

regarded as unacceptable. The extent of the defect may be variable from the presence of a small hoof-like structure on the fetlock to a full extra digit articulating with the metacarpus. It is rare for more than one extra digit to occur on one leg, but bilateral polydactyly does occur.

Diagnosis and treatment

- Visual exam but the full extent of the abnormality may need to be assessed from radiographs.
- Surgical removal for cosmetic purposes and to prevent interference injuries.

Congenital deformities of the limbs and joints (arthrogryposis) (Figs. 7.6 & 7.7)

These developmental defects are relatively common and usually obvious from birth and frequently cause significant dystocia. The extent of deformity ranges from mild deviations of limb position, resulting from relatively minor deformities in the long bones, to gross distortion of the bones, joints, ligaments and tendons of the limbs, with consequent severely restrictive, postural deformities. It is more usual for the front legs to be involved, although hind leg deviations are sometimes encountered, either on their own, or in conjunction with fore-limb distortions. It is unlikely that the disorders are the result of genetic factors, although they are more often encountered in Thoroughbred horses and in the small European draught breeds. They are generally regarded as accidents of gestation, possibly associated with developmental infections, toxins and nutritional deficiencies or excesses. In spite of their relatively high incidence, a definitive etiology and pathogenesis has not been established. In most cases no apparent cause can be identified, and fetal malpositioning is then commonly blamed for the misshapen axial or appendicular skeleton. These abnormalities are often complicated by the co-existence of

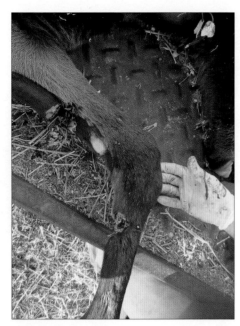

Figure 7.7 Arthrogryposis (same foal as Fig. 7.6). This is a post-mortem image demonstrating section of the tendons above and below the carpus with no change in the contracture.

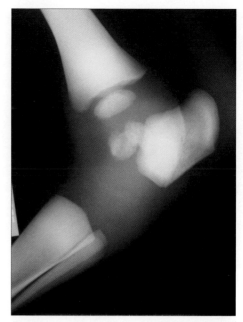

Figure 7.8 Grade 1. Incomplete ossification. Note the lack of the two distal rows of tarsal bones.

flexural and soft tissue deformities. Complex developmental deformities involving skeletal, cardiac and other defects are frequently found concurrently.

Diagnosis and treatment
- Clinical examination and radiographs.
- Radiographic changes are often marked but in some cases may appear minimal and the interpretation of the radiographic appearance may be particularly difficult as a result of both the technical difficulty of obtaining suitable projections and the immaturity of the centers of ossification.
- Cases in which joints are completely fused, having no mobility at all or those with contractions greater than 90° have a poor prognosis.

Collapse of carpal and/or tarsal bones and incomplete ossification (Figs. 7.8–7.11)

Incomplete ossification occurs commonly in premature or dysmature foals. Collapse of the tarsal or carpal bones can occur secondary to incomplete ossification and abnormal weight distribution on the developing bones. In some cases it may occur secondary to trauma or infection.

The grade of incomplete ossification may be appreciated by radiographic examination:

Grade 1. Some cuboidal bones with no ossification
Grade 2. All cuboidal bones had radiographic evidence of some ossification
Grade 3. Cuboidal bones are small and round with consequent 'wide' appearance of the joint spaces
Grade 4. Cuboidal bones are shaped like the adult counterparts.

Diagnosis and treatment
- Radiographic examination to assess degree of ossification, extent of bone compression and some cases may have concurrent infections. Assessment of white cell count and fibrinogen if there is any doubt about whether there may be a septic element.
- Foals should be restricted from excessive exercise to prevent compression of the tarsal cuboidal bones and slowly reintroduced to normal turnout even after complete ossification has occurred.

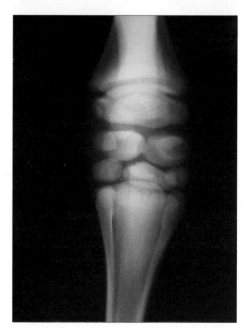

Figure 7.9 Grade 2. Incomplete ossification. All the bones are present but the small bones of this carpus have a rounded appearance.

- The tarsus should be radiographed every 10–14 days. If sepsis is suspected based on blood work and radiographic findings, foals should also be started on broad-spectrum antibiotics.
- Once collapse of the tarsal or carpal bones has occurred, the condition is easily recognized clinically by the abnormal angles adopted by the affected limb(s). Concurrent flexural deformities and other developmental defects may be found in some cases. Prognosis is usually poor for severe cases.

Congenital luxation of the patella (Fig. 7.12)

This is an uncommon condition that is most frequently identified in miniature horses and Shetland ponies. It can be unilateral or bilateral, intermittent or complete, and frequently in a lateral direction. The

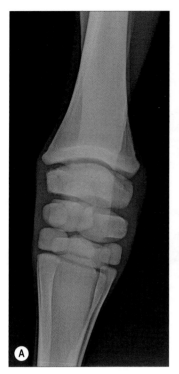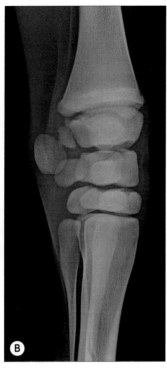

Figure 7.10 (A, B) Grade 3. Incomplete ossification. All the bones are present but there is a rounded appearance to the borders and increased joint spaces.

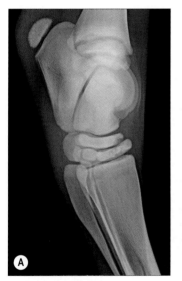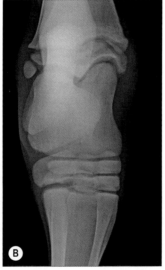

Figure 7.11 Tarsal bone collapse. (A) Lateral view: note the compression of the distal row of tarsal bones and the 'curby' appearance as a result. (B) Note that the compression in this case is more pronounced laterally (left on image), this gives the hock the appearance of bowing outwards.

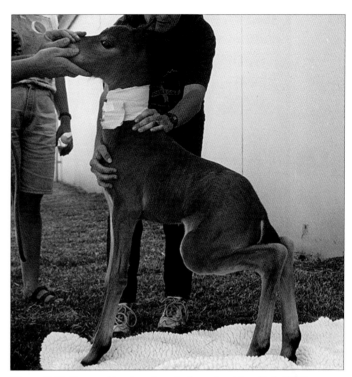

Figure 7.12 Congenital luxation of patella. Reproduced from McAuliffe SB, Slovis, NM (eds) *Color Atlas of Diseases and Disorders of the Foal* (2008), with permission from Elsevier.

- Medical management consisting of exercise restriction and manual replacement of the patella can be used as treatment in intermittent unilateral cases.
- Surgical correction is generally recommended for more persistent luxations or for foals with difficulty ambulating. A number of different surgical procedures can be used individually or combined depending on the severity of the case and surgeon preference.

Fractured ribs (Figs. 7.13–7.16)

Rib fractures are commonly found in newborn foals and minimally displaced fractures are perhaps underdiagnosed. The majority of foals with rib fractures suffer no related clinical abnormalities but moderately or severely displaced fractures can be a significant cause of death in this age group. Inappropriate or poorly timed assistance during foaling is a significant cause of rib fractures. Hospitalized patients, whether presented for rib fractures or other problems are overrepresented in numbers of mortalities. The additional manipulation of hospitalized patients may be a factor in the increased mortality rate of this group when compared with foals that have no additional abnormalities or illnesses.

Palpation of the thoracic wall should be a part of any routine neonatal examination. Signs that should direct an examiner's attention to the possibility of rib fractures include groaning or grunting in the foal, respiratory distress, plaques of subcutaneous edema overlying the ribs or along the ventrum of the thorax, especially behind the elbows, and flinching when the rib area is palpated.

Audible or palpable crepitation or a clicking sensation when the hand is gently pressed over an affected area is common with moderately to severely displaced fractures but is rarely present with minimally displaced fractures. The level of pain experienced by the foal is very variable with some showing marked pain, including grunting, while others display normal activity despite the presence of multiple fractures.

Flail chest occurs when several consecutive ribs are fractured, leading to an incompetent segment of chest wall. When a flail chest

more severely affected bilateral cases have difficulty standing or if standing carry their pelvis lower than the lumbar spine. Unilateral cases show intermittent lameness. Shetland ponies appear to be able to tolerate the condition quite well and some are even capable of mild work, although osteoarthritis usually develops over time. The etiology is not well understood but is thought to be related to a dysmaturity of the trochlear ridges and relative laxity of the femoro-patellar joint.

Diagnosis and treatment
- Clinical examination and radiographs to confirm and assess trochlear ridges.

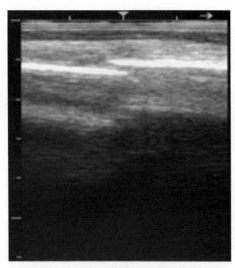

Figure 7.13 A mildly displaced rib fracture is defined as a break in the margin with displacement not more than 1 mm (corresponding to the width of the anterior echogenic line). In contrast an undisplaced fracture is defined as a break in the margin without displacement.

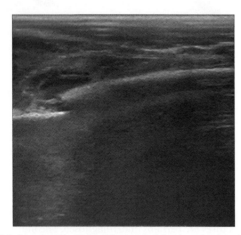

Figure 7.14 A moderately displaced fracture is defined as a break in the cortex with displacement of more than 1 mm but less than 4 mm. This moderately displaced rib fracture has an associated hematoma which is a common finding. Severely displaced fractures are defined by displacement of more than 4 mm.

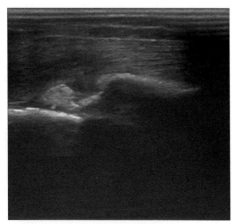

Figure 7.15 Healing rib fracture with callus formation.

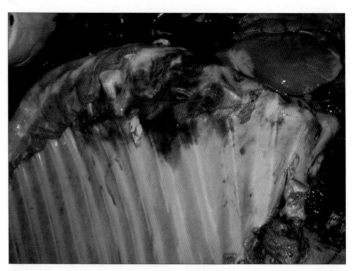

Figure 7.16 Fractured ribs. Post-mortem image of fractured ribs. Note the protruding ends of the fractured ribs and marked hemorrhage throughout the rib cage.

is present, the involved segment of chest wall will sink inwards during the inspiratory excursions of the abdomen and diaphragm.

Diagnosis

- Palpation of the costochondral junctions during physical exam can sometimes identify fractured ribs.
- The fractured ribs themselves can be well-visualized with ultrasound, even when non-displaced, and the technique requires less positioning and manipulation of the injured patient than does radiography. Ultrasound can also be used to determine the degree of fracture segment displacement and the proximity of bone ends to the heart.

Treatment

- Four to six weeks are considered to be necessary for stabilization of the thoracic wall following rib fractures. Foals are normally box rested for 2–3 weeks and then reassessed ultrasonographically before commencing paddock turnout. Administration of analgesics is generally avoided as some pain limits movement and helps avoid additional displacement of fracture segments as a result of exercise.
- The formation of a hematoma or thrombus at the broken bone ends is typical of a rib fracture injury in the acute stages. Serial examinations document the evolution of this finding to bony callus formation, and eventual smoothing and remodeling of the callus with time.
- Deformation of the lung surface and thickening of the visceral pleura may be semi-permanent to permanent findings in the long-term assessment of these foals.
- Foals that have severely displaced fractures that are adjacent to the heart or causing significant pulmonary contusions are considered surgical candidates.

Hereditary multiple exostoses (multiple osteochondroma, multiple cartilagenous exostosis, diaphyseal aclasis or endochondromatosis) (Fig. 7.17)

This is an uncommon hereditary skeletal disorder characterized by mulitple bony projections, often bilateral and symmetrical on the long bones, ribs and pelvis. A single autosomal dominant gene is thought to be responsible. Histologically the exostoses appear to be osteochondromas. They remain benign and no transformation to malignancy has been reported.

The condition may be associated with lameness if an exostosis impinges on surrounding muscle or tendon. In those cases excision of the extosis may be indicated.

Diagnosis and treatment
- The clinical appearance is highly suggestive. Radiography and ultrasonography can be used to confirm location and extent.
- No treatment is possible.

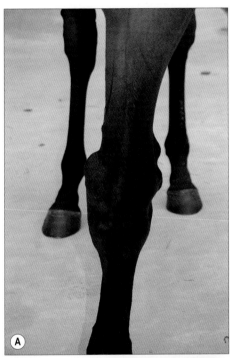

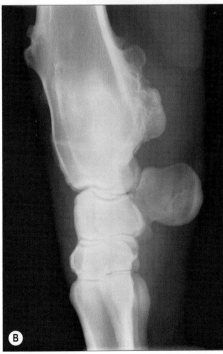

Figure 7.17 (A, B) Gross and radiographic image of multiple hereditary exostoses demonstrating multiple bony projections on the distal radius of this horse.

Developmental disorders: Acquired conditions

Osteochondrosis (Figs. 7.18–7.24)

Osteochondrosis has often been defined as failure of endochondral ossification resulting in either osteochondritis dissecans (OCD) or subchondral bone cysts. Besides defects in the process of endochondral ossification, other causes have been suggested, including loss of blood supply, genetic, gender specific, dietary, endocrine, biomechanical, traumatic and toxic. The level of exercise young horses receive has also been implicated in the development of osteochondrosis, with excessive exercise and lack of exercise in young foals both being

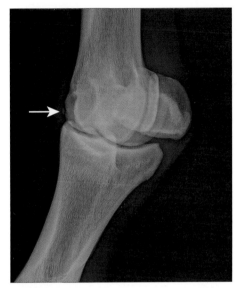

Figure 7.18 OCD lesion of the sagittal ridge of the metacarpophalangeal joint with a small chip evident (arrow).

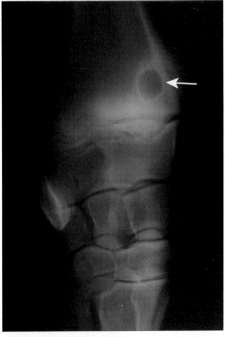

Figure 7.19 Dorso medial-palmo lateral oblique radiograph of the carpus demonstrating a large bone cyst in the distal radius (arrow).

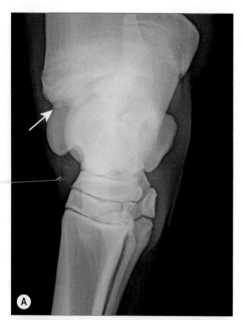

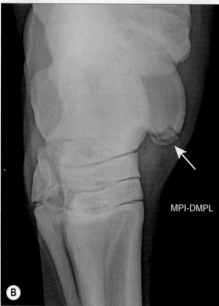

MPI-DMPL

Figure 7.20 (A) Tarsus: OCD of the distal intermediate ridge (arrow). (B) OCD of the lateral trochlear ridge (arrow).

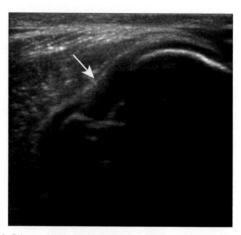

Figure 7.22 Echographic image of medial femoral condyle showing irregularity of the condylar profile consistent with a subchondral bone cyst. Notice that the overlying cartilage is intact (arrow).

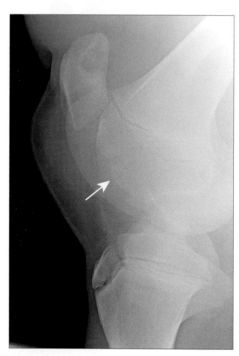

Figure 7.23 OCD lesion of the medial femoral condyle (arrow).

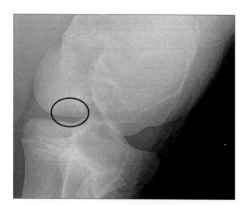

Figure 7.21 Subchondral bone cyst of the medial condyle of the femur (circle).

implicated as causing osteochondrosis. Subchondral bone cysts are now speculated to originate from possible mechanical insults when compared to osteochondritis.

Osteochondrosis commonly occurs in the tarsus, stifle and fetlock joints. Though uncommon, osteochondrosis can occur in the scapulohumeral, elbow and hip joints. Tables 7.1 and 7.2 list the most common locations of lesions within each joint. Lesions can potentially regress. In the hock, 5 months has been used as a possible cut off for lesions regressing. After 5 months, lesions will typically not regress. In the stifle, 8 months is the cut off for a lesion regression involving the lateral trochlear ridge.

Clinical signs can include joint effusion and lameness. However, in certain situations lameness and joint effusion may not be present. Joint effusion is more common with a dissecting lesion. Lameness can be present with both dissecting lesions and cysts, but cysts can often be asymptomatic until horses begin training. In some cases, joint effusion

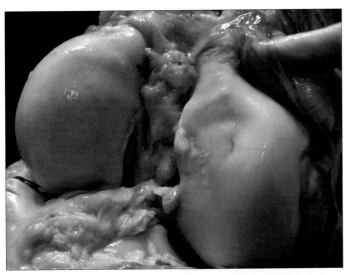

Figure 7.24 Post-mortem specimen of a subchondral bone cyst of the medial femoral condyle. Same horse as Fig. 7.21.

Table 7.1 Osteochondritis dissecans (OCD)

Joint	Location
Fetlock	Mid-sagittal ridge
	Dorsal proximal medial/lateral P1
	Palmar/plantar P1
Tarsus	Distal intermediate ridge of tibia
	Medial malleolus
	Lateral trochlear ridge
	Medial trochlear ridge
Stifle	Lateral trochlear ridge
	Medial trochlear ridge
	Distal aspect of patella
Shoulder	Glenoid cavity
	Humeral head
Elbow	Lateral/medial humeral condyle (uncommon)

Reproduced from McAuliffe SB, Slovis NM (eds) *Color Atlas of Diseases and Disorders of the Foal* (2008), with permission from Elsevier.

Table 7.2 Subchondral bone cysts

Joint	Location
Stifle	Medial femoral condyle
	Proximal tibia
Fetlock	Distal condyle of metacarpus/metatarsus
Pastern	Distal P1
Shoulder	Glenoid
	Humeral head
Elbow	Proximal radius
Coffin	Third phalanx
Carpus	Ulna, radial carpal bones (mostly commonly)

Reproduced from McAuliffe SB, Slovis NM (eds) *Color Atlas of Diseases and Disorders of the Foal* (2008), with permission from Elsevier.

is present but radiographs show no significant findings. In these cases, serial radiographs over 4–6-week intervals may be required to ensure the absence or presence of an osteochondritis lesion. It is very important to examine the contralateral joint for the presence of an osteochondral lesion as lesions are frequently bilateral.

Diagnosis and treatment

- Diagnosis of osteochondritis is often easily made based on signalment, history, clinical signs and radiographic findings. Ultrasound examination of affected joints can also help to evaluate and confirm the presence of a cartilaginous flap.
- Treatment of osteochondral lesions involves conservative or surgical management. Conservative management involves limiting exercise and chondroprotective therapy and is indicated in young foals and those which do not have any effusion or lameness associated with their OCD lesion(s).
- Surgical management of osteochondritis dissecans typically involves surgical debridement of the fragment and the fragment bed. Surgical management of subchondral bone cysts has included debridement, cartilage replacement, packing the cyst with bone marrow or injection of corticosteroids. Surgical treatment should be considered for foals with joint effusion and lameness. Prophylactic removal may also be considered in young horses intended for sale.

Prognosis

Prognosis for osteochondritis dissecans and subchondral bone cysts varies based on location, number of joints involved, size of the lesion, presence of osteoarthritis and the degree of lameness.

- ***Fetlock.*** Many fetlock lesions can improve radiographically over time with conservative management. Surgical treatment should be considered only in foals that demonstrate joint effusion and lameness. Lesions of the palmar/plantar aspect of P1 do not often require surgery.
- ***Hock (tarsus).*** The distal intermediate ridge of the tibia is the most common site of lesions and these are rarely associated with effusion and lameness. Lesions of the medial malleolus are more likely to result in joint effusion and lameness requiring surgical treatment. Lesions of the lateral trochlear ridge can be quite variable in size but if large may result in effusion and lameness. Most medial trochlear ridge lesions are incidental findings and do not require treatment.
- ***Shoulder and elbow.*** OCD lesions of the shoulder and elbow are normally only recognized when associated with lameness. The lameness in these cases may develop insidiously or acutely and identifying the site of the lesion is often difficult. Surgery should only be considered in foals less than 8–10 months of age if they are intractably lame as some cases may improve with rest. Radiography may also underestimate the size of the lesions making pre-surgical assessments of future athletic function difficult.

Angular limb deformities (Figs. 7.25–7.28)

Angular deformities of limb joints, particularly of the knee (carpus), hock (tarsus) and fetlock (metacarpophalangeal joint), are frequently encountered in all breeds. They may be congenital or acquired, and can be related to certain management and nutritional factors. Valgus deformities occur when the lower limb deviates laterally. This gives the foal a 'knock-kneed' appearance. Varus deformities occur when the lower limb deviates medially and results in a 'bowlegged' appearance. The condition may be unilateral or bilateral with single or multiple joints affected in a given limb. The forelimbs are more commonly affected but hindlimbs can also be affected. Occasionally, a foal may have a valgus deformity of one limb and varus on the other, giving a 'windswept' appearance. Although deviations occurring at the fetlock are usually less dramatic in appearance, they are regarded as being more urgent, as growth in the distal metacarpal physis ceases at an earlier age than growth in the distal radial physis. Once the growth plate has closed, the potential for therapeutic intervention involving growth acceleration/retardation is lost. Even before physeal closure, the extent of the deviation may be such that there is exceptional

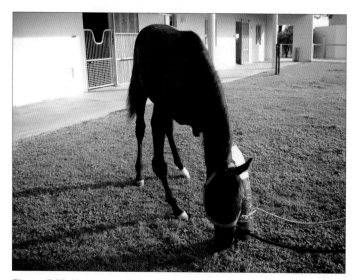

Figure 7.25 Marked carpal varus in a yearling. This horse had a mild carpal valgus initially but fractured the other limb and the excessive weight-bearing resulted in a marked carpal varus in the weight-bearing limb.

weight-bearing on the concave side and much less on the convex. This results in a slower growth rate (and often premature closure) of the physis on the 'short' side of the joint. Thus, the condition becomes progressively worse, and effective therapeutic measures are correspondingly less feasible.

Diagnosis and treatment

- Although the condition can be diagnosed visually, radiographs are used to define the extent of the deviation and physeal pathology if present.
- Conservative and surgical treatment options are available. Conservative treatment which can consist of a combination of controlled exercise, corrective trimming, application of hoof extensions and bandaging/splinting is normally attempted first, especially in newborn foals as many of these will improve considerably in the first few weeks of life.
- For severe cases or those that do not respond to conservative therapy there are a number of surgical options, all of which are based on two basic principles: growth acceleration or growth retardation. Growth acceleration (hemicircumferential periosteal transection with periosteal elevation) is aimed at speeding the growth of the physis on the concave side of the deviation and growth retardation is aimed at slowing the growth of the physis on the convex side. For growth retardation, transphyseal bridging (TPB) techniques are commonly used by many surgeons. Transphyseal bridging may be performed with staples, screws and wires, screws and a plate, or the single screw technique.

Epiphysitis and physitis (Figs. 7.29 & 7.30)

Physitis is a common problem affecting young horses. Most commonly the disease affects horses from 3–12 months of age, but horses up to 2 years of age can be affected. Typically it involves fine bone breeds on a high plain of nutrition. Most common sites of physitis include the distal radius, distal metacarpus/metatarsus and distal tibia.

Visual examination reveals swelling involving the distal radius physis, distal physis of the metacarpus/metatarsus and distal physis of the tibia.

Diagnosis, treatment and prognosis

- The diagnosis can usually be made based on history and physical examination. Digital palpation will reveal heat and pain over the affected physis. Radiographic examination reveals sclerosis of the physis and possible periosteal callus formation in severe cases.

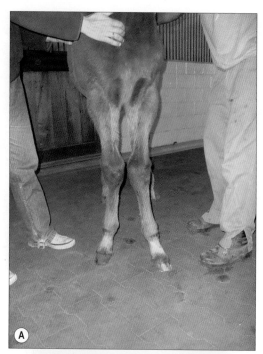

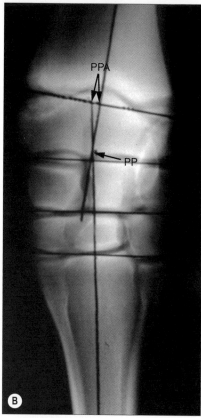

Figure 7.26 (A, B) Carpal valgus. (B) Radiograph of a carpal valgus. The origin and extent of the deviation can be defined by the location and angle of intersecting vertical lines drawn through the middle of the radius and the third metacarpal. Reproduced from McAuliffe SB, Slovis NM (eds), Color Atlas of Diseases and Disorders of the Foal (2008), with permission from Elsevier

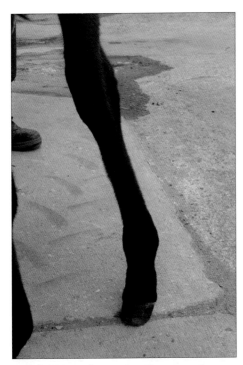

Figure 7.27 Fetlock varus in a 3 day old foal. This corrected spontaneously..

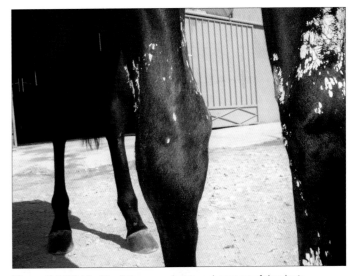

Figure 7.29 Epiphysitis of the carpus showing enlargement of the physis.

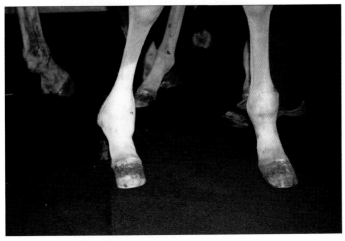

Figure 7.28 Fetlock varus secondary to Salter Harris fracture.

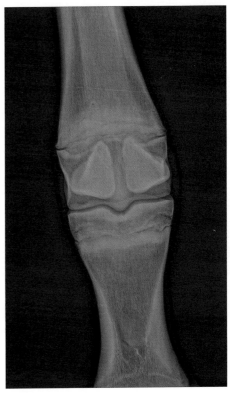

Figure 7.30 Radiograph of a fetlock with epiphysitis showing sclerosis of both physes.

- Treatment of physitis involves lowering the plane of nutrition. In foals, the mare's feed bucket should be raised, the foal could be weaned and the foal can be muzzled if the mare produces large volumes of milk.
- Anti-inflammatories and antiulcer medication should be considered in all cases. The use of topically applied poultices has anecdotal reports of benefit.
- In cases involving an angular limb deformity, the affected limb should be trimmed correctly. In severe cases, transphyseal bridging procedures may be required.
- Prognosis is good if the degree of physitis is mild and there is no evidence of an angular limb deformity.

Sesamoiditis (Figs. 7.31–7.35)

Repetitive strain, acute trauma or infection may lead to inflammation of the proximal sesamoid bones (sesamoiditis). The condition is frequently noted in Thoroughbred and Standardbred as well as in non-racing sport horses. It is also frequently noted in young Thoroughbred

not yet in race training. The clinical pathology and resultant imaging abnormalities are most often noted over the abaxial surface of the affected bone(s), or the origins of the distal sesamoidian ligaments, but axial sesamoiditis, related to sepsis or intersesamoidian ligament desmitis, has also been reported. Abnormalities noted on the abaxial surfaces have been associated with suspensory ligament desmitis and enthesopathy.

Variable degrees of lameness may be present, and in some cases it is only evident following strenuous exercise.

Diagnosis

- Mild, local swelling usually gives way to a firm, often marked, local swelling. Pain is often relatively mild, but may be more obvious with

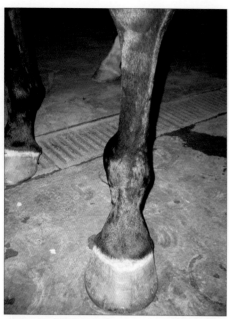

Figure 7.31 Enlargement of medial sesamoid associated with sesamoiditis in this yearling.

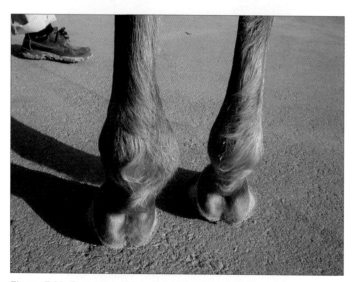

Figure 7.32 Caudal view of fetlock demonstrating enlargement of the medial sesamoid secondary to severe sesamoiditis.

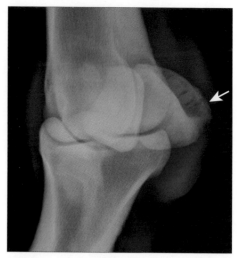

Figure 7.33 Sesamoiditis. Radiograph of the fetlock demonstrating increased vascular channels and periosteal bone reaction of the abaxial border of the sesamoid bone (arrow). Grossly this sesamoid appeared enlarged similar to Fig. 7.31.

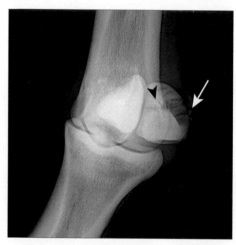

Figure 7.34 Radiograph demonstrating severe sesamoiditis with increased vascular channels, avulsion fracture of the attachment of the suspensory ligament (arrow) and a healing mid body fracture of the sesamoid (arrowhead).

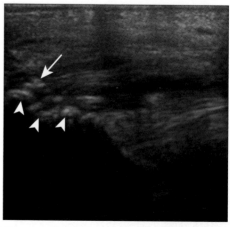

Figure 7.35 Echographic image of sesamoiditis showing irregular surface of the abaxial border of the sesamoid bone (arrowheads) with desmitis of the suspensory ligament and avulsion fracture (arrow) of the insertion of the suspensory ligament branch.

flexion, palpation and pressure, and a reduced range of motion (fetlock joint) is often encountered.

- Imaging is essential as, in addition to the proximal sesamoid bones, the fetlock joint and regional soft tissues may be involved. Radiographs may reveal the presence of fractures, or document an increase in the number or size (>2 mm) of the vascular channels, the presence of proliferative new bone (e.g. enthesopathy) or lytic bone (osteomyelitis/osteitis).
- Ultrasound is recommended to examine the associated soft tissue structures.
- MRI/CT will give a global view of both bone and soft tissue involvement and nuclear scintigraphy can be used to document inflammation.

Treatment
- Treatment is dependent on the underlying etiology but in many cases the etiology is related to the continued stress associated with

exercise. In those cases enforced rest and treatment with non steroidal anti-inflammatories (NSAIDs) for pain and inflammation are important. Many racehorses with mild sesamoiditis are helped by post-exercise icing, and altered exercise programs to include swimming or aquatread exercising.

- Other therapies include extracorporeal shock wave therapy (ECSWT) of bone and soft tissues and therapeutic ultrasound of chronic desmitis.
- If infection is associated with the etiology antibiotics are indicated.

Non-infectious/traumatic disorders

Bucked shins (Figs. 7.36 & 7.37)

Bucked shins are commonly seen in young racehorses at the start of intense training. The incidence of the condition is very high and is related to fatigue failure of bone and inadequacy of bone remodeling

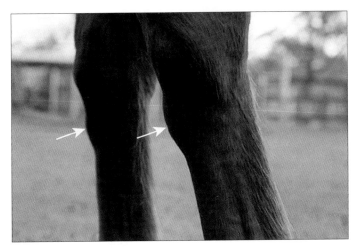

Figure 7.36 Bucked shins.

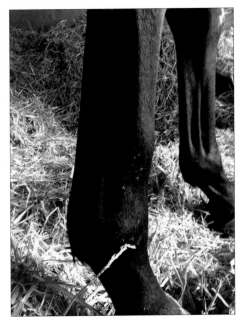

Figure 7.37 Bucked shins. All or part of the dorsal surface of the third metacarpal bone may be affected.

in skeletally immature horses. The clinical signs are very variable, varying from mild soreness or tenderness of the dorsal aspect of MCIII to extreme sensitivity and lameness and new periosteal bone formation. Much emphasis is now being placed on training programs aimed at decreasing the incidence of the condition. Bucked shins can progress to dorsal cortical (stress) fractures of MCIII if horses with periostitis are forced to continue working. Micro and saucer fractures, and subperiosteal hemorrhages are common sequels to treadmill work, particularly where the treadmill has a steel backplate on the running surface.

Diagnosis and treatment

- Heat and pain on palpation as well as appearance of a profile over the dorsal aspect of the canon bone. Radiographs may be required to determine the level of periosteal new bone formation or the presence of stress fractures if lameness is persistent or severe.
- When inflammation or tenderness is noted, NSAIDs, topical application of ice and cooling muds should be commenced in combination with modification of the exercise program.
- If the periosteum is hot, thickened and sore over a large area of dorsal MCIII then training should be stopped completely.
- Thermocautery is advocated by many as a treatment for more refractory or severe cases but is illegal in some countries.

Pedal bone fractures (Figs. 7.38 & 7.39)

Fractures involving the third phalanx are commonly observed in foals and in adults of all disciplines. They may occur as a result of trauma; kicking a fixed object, high-speed impact of hard surfaces (especially in foals), a mis-step, or following the application of acrylic hoof extensions in foals. There are eight types of fractures of the third phalanx.

In foals, the most common fracture is type VII. This type of fracture generally occurs in the front limbs and usually involves the lateral wing of the third phalanx but can also involve the medial wing and in some cases can occur bilaterally in both forelimbs.

In adults the most common is type VI. These fractures may heal, be resorbed or persist without clinical signs; therefore the identification of a fracture on an adult radiograph does not automatically indicate that it is the source of pain and a full clinical workup should be performed.

Diagnosis

- Visual examination will often reveal a non-weight-bearing and 'pointed' limb especially in foals.
- Lameness examination: lameness can be eliminated by a perineural nerve block (may not be consistent in cases involving the extensor process or articular fractures but is very useful for solar fractures in adults).
- Radiology is the diagnostic tool of choice in association with clinical signs and history, and is also useful for monitoring the healing of the fracture. In recent fractures it may be difficult to visualize the fracture line and repeat radiographs in a few days may be required.

Treatment

- Foals normally heal very well within 4–8 weeks and in many cases confinement is only required for a short period.
- Adults usually require long-term box rest, especially if there is evidence of demineralization of the solar margin. The use of a broad web shoe with a concave solar margin is often recommended.
- Lag screw fixation is recommended for articular fractures in adults greater than 3 years of age and where there is displacement of the articular margin.
- The prognosis for solar fractures in adults is good but articular fractures often have a poorer prognosis.

Fractures of the proximal sesamoids

(Figs. 7.40–7.45)

Fractures involving the proximal sesamoid bones (PSBs) are a relatively common and potentially severe injuries. The proximal sesamoid bones are a major component of the equine suspensory apparatus. Disruption of both proximal sesamoid bones could lead to a disruption in the suspensory apparatus. There are six types of proximal sesamoid bone fractures described (see Fig. 7.40).

In foals the injury can occur as a result of running after the dam and placing excessive strain on the suspensory apparatus or

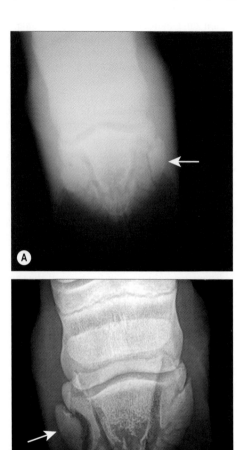

Figure 7.38 (A, B) Type VII pedal bone fractures (arrows).

Figure 7.39 Pedal bone fracture schematics.

Types of fractures:

- **Type I** is a non-articular fracture of the palmar or plantar process of the distal phalanx
- **Type II** is an oblique, articular fracture of the palmar or plantar process of the distal phalanx
- **Type III** is a midsagittal articular fracture of the distal phalanx
- **Type IV** is an articular fracture involving the extensor process of the distal phalanx
- **Type V** is a comminuted fracture of the distal phalanx
- **Type VI** is a non-articular fracture involving the solar margin of the distal phalanx
- **Type VII** is a non-articular fracture of the palmar or plantar process of the distal phalanx, but differs from type I in that the fracture line begins in and ends in the solar margin
- **Type VIII** is a non-articular fracture in the frontal of P3.

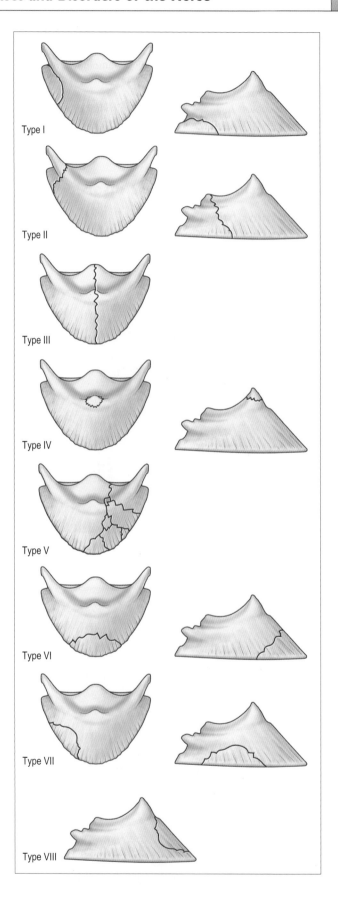

Type I

Type II

Type III

Type IV

Type V

Type VI

Type VII

Type VIII

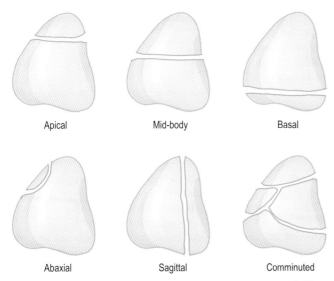

Apical   Mid-body   Basal

Abaxial   Sagittal   Comminuted

Figure 7.40 Schematic of sesamoid fractures. Reproduced from McAuliffe SB, Slovis NM (eds), *Color Atlas of Diseases and Disorders of the Foal* (2008), with permission from Elsevier.

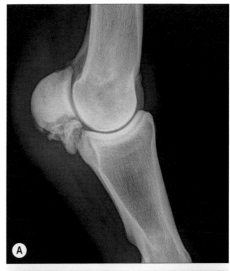

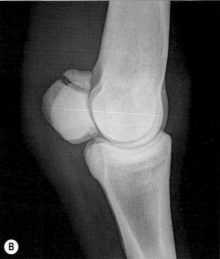

Figure 7.42 (A) Basilar fracture of sesamoid. (B) Apical fracture of sesamoid.

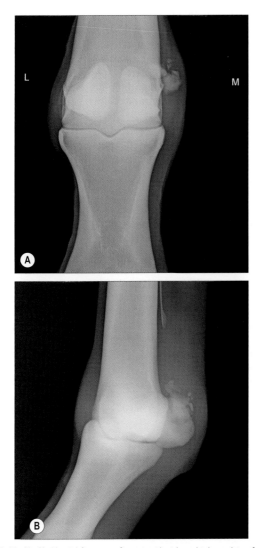

Figure 7.41 (A, B) Abaxial fracture of sesamoid with multiple avulsion fractures of the suspensory attachment to the abaxial border of the sesamoid.

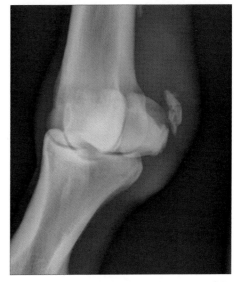

Figure 7.43 Avulsion fracture of the sesamoid at the insertion of the suspensory branch.

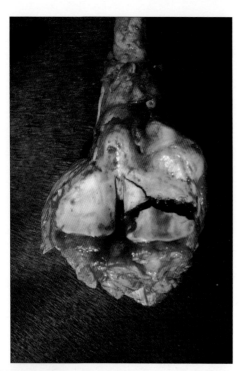

Figure 7.44 Comminuted fracture of proximal sesamoid.

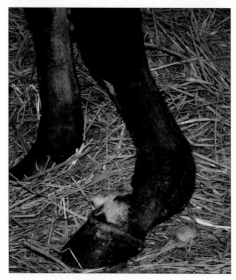

Figure 7.45 Bilateral sesamoid fractures have resulted in collapse of the suspensory apparatus.

secondary to osteomyelitis of the sesamoid bones. In adults it can occur as a traumatic event or secondary to existing pathology. Lameness depends on the site and size of the fracture. If the fracture involves both sesamoids in one limb, the degree of lameness may be more severe. There is usually obvious swelling over the affected sesamoid, although this may also be found with sesamoiditis. Joint effusion of the fetlock may also be noted due to the articulation with the proximal sesamoids. If both proximal sesamoids are affected, the fetlock may show a dropped appearance.

Diagnosis

- Visual examination: joint effusion, swelling over the affected sesamoid, dropped fetlock.

- Digital examination will often elicit pain over the affected sesamoid.
- Lameness examination.
- Radiology: this will also determine if there is underlying pathology.
- Ultrasound examination also allows concurrent assessment of the suspensory apparatus.

Treatment

Most foals with PSB fractures are treated conservatively with box rest and bandaging. Recommended treatment in adults is as follows:

- **Apical fractures**: arthroscopic removal of the fragment. If concurrent injury to the suspensory ligament (SL) is present a prolonged convalescence may be required (6–12 months). Without SL injury return to training is usually rapid (1 month).
- **Abaxial fractures**: non-displaced small fragments can be treated conservatively with box rest. Displaced fragments are generally removed arthroscopically. Very large fragments can be repaired with a screw.
- **Basilar fractures**: small fractures that do not extend more than 50–75% of the dorsopalmar width of the PSB are suitable for removal. These cases normally require prolonged rest (3–4 months) and prognosis for return to athletic function is about 50%. Horses with large basilar PSB fractures usually have a poor prognosis for return to work as there is generally considerable involvement of the distal sesamoidean ligament origin.
- **Mid body**: these fractures all require some type of therapy from casting alone to screw fixation. These are serious injuries that require prolonged rest (6 months) after surgery and although a large percentage (60%) eventually return to work, few continue to perform at their previous level.
- **Axial**: these are usually recognized in association with displaced fractures of distal MCIII or MTIII. They are usually not specifically due to inaccessibility and the likelihood that concurrent injuries will limit return to work.
- **Comminuted**: these are not usually treated as there is a very poor prognosis for a return to work.

Exostoses of the second and fourth metacarpal bones (splints) (Figs. 7.46–7.49)

The splint bones of the fore and, to a lesser extent, the hind limbs are liable to the development of exostoses in response to direct trauma, instability between MCII or MCIV and MCIII or to spontaneous inflammation arising in the periosteum and the interosseous ligaments. In most cases the result is of little clinical significance with minimal if any associated pain or lameness, but occasionally the local reaction may become sufficiently large to interfere with the tendinous and ligamentous structures of the palmar/plantar metacarpus/metatarsus resulting in pain and lameness. Such spontaneous inflammation has been related to hard training, poor conformation, malnutrition and poor hoof care. The lesions are particularly common in young, growing horses and are most common in the proximal half of the bone.

Diagnosis and treatment

- Visual examination is normally all that is required but radiographic examination may be used in cases where fractures are suspected. Diagnostic ultrasonography may be required in cases where there is suspicion of compromise of the suspensory ligament.
- Where there is no associated pain or lameness no treatment is required although some practitioners recommend rest for a clinically active exostoses as this may help to reduce the ultimate size of the splint.

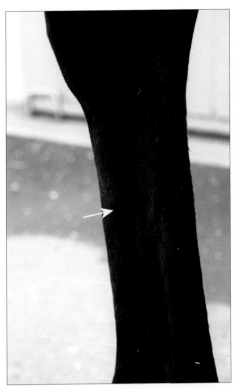

Figure 7.46 Small exostoses of splint bone in a young horse (arrow).

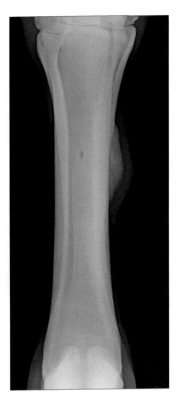

Figure 7.48 Radiograph of exostoses of splint bone.

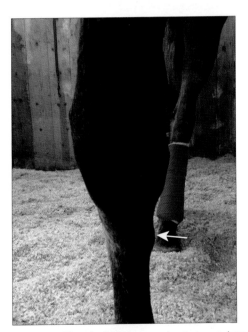

Figure 7.47 Exostoses of lateral splint bone secondary to trauma (arrow).

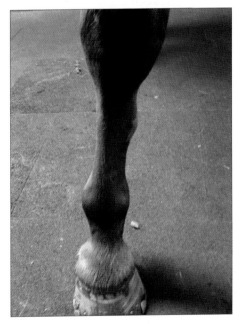

Figure 7.49 Splint bone exostoses.

- For cases with associated lameness rest is required and should be continued until firm palpation over the exostoses fails to elicit pain.
- A variety of topical and adjunct therapies are available such as local infiltration of corticosteroids, topical application of DMSO or diclofenac or shock-wave therapy.
- If impingement of the suspensory ligament occurs then surgical amputation of the bone is required.

Splint bone fractures (Fig. 7.50)

Horses may suffer from fractures of the splint bones as a result of direct external trauma or internal forces. Fractures associated with internal forces are most commonly related to concurrent suspensory desmitis which results in progressive deviation of the distal third of the bone from MCIII predisposing to fracture. Lameness associated with internal trauma is usually acute in onset and moderate. Lameness associated with external trauma is also usually acute in onset

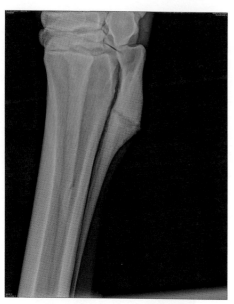

Figure 7.50 Radiographic image of splint bone fracture with large callus.

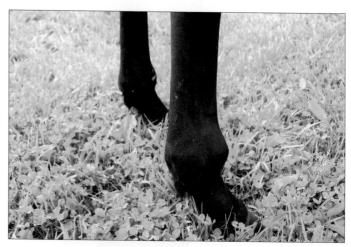

Figure 7.51 Marked enlargement of the fetlock joint as a result of villonodular synovitis. On palpation there is little effusion of the joint but palpable thickening of the joint capsule with a limited range of motion.

and can be moderate to severe. Frequently an external wound is present in such cases and the MTIV is particularly susceptible.

Diagnosis and treatment
- Clinical signs and examination may allow a presumptive diagnosis. Radiographs are required to confirm the diagnosis in addition to determining the precise location and nature of the fracture.
- Fractures of the distal third usually heal satisfactorily in 4–6 weeks with conservative management but in some cases or depending on surgeon's preference removal of the distal fracture fragment may be recommended.
- Fractures of the proximal third (especially MCII) may require surgical stabilization to prevent carpal instability.
- It is important to remember that fractures associated with external trauma are particularly prone to infection and early efforts to control and eliminate infection are important.

Chronic proliferative synovitis (villonodular synovitis) (Figs. 7.51 & 7.52)
Chronic repetitive trauma to the dorsal aspect of the fetlock joint from hyperextension leads to hyperplasia of the synovial pad over the sagittal ridge, which results in the development of a soft-tissue mass within the dorsocranial aspect of the joint. It is most commonly seen in racehorses and predisposing conditions are the presence of dorsopalmar P1 fragments and long pasterns.

Diagnosis
- There is a palpable thickening over the dorsal aspect of the affected joint with or without joint effusion.
- Lameness commonly worsens following exercise and joint flexion.
- Radiography may show a crescent-shaped radiolucency on the dorsal aspect of the distal third metacarpus due to cortical lysis. It can also reveal other evidence of osteoarthrosis and dystrophic mineralization.
- Ultrasound demonstrates thickening of the synovial pad (>10 mm) and may reveal other changes of the dorsal aspect of the joint.

Treatment and prognosis
- Intra-articular medication with hyaluron and corticosteroids combined with rest is the initial treatment and in most cases is all that is required.

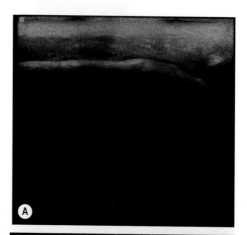

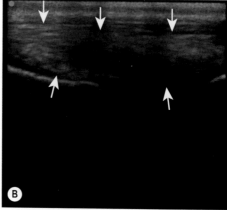

Figure 7.52 (A) Echographic image of a normal fetlock joint. (B) Echographic image of a fetlock joint with villonodular synovitis demonstrating marked thickening of the joint capsule (arrows).

- Changes in training may be required in the management of individual cases. Arthroscopic surgical excision has been performed in some cases.
- The prognosis is variable but generally is regarded as guarded to poor.

Pelvic fractures (Figs. 7.53–7.59)

Pelvic fractures are being increasingly recognized as a cause of lameness with young horses (<4 years) being predisposed. Stress fractures associated with repetitive bone fatigue and complete fractures are seen. Complete fractures can occur as a result of trauma or develop from untreated stress fractures.

The clinical signs seen depend on the location and extent of the fracture. The most common signs are unilateral hindlimb lameness and asymmetry of the pelvis. Initially asymmetry may not be obvious due to soft tissue swelling and with time may become more apparent due to additional muscle atrophy.

- **Tuber coxae fractures.** Moderate to severe lameness that decreases to mild lameness within 48 hours, with a 'knocked-down' hip appearance. External wounds, hematomas or draining tracts associated with sequestra may all be evident depending on the time of examination and extent of the injury.

- **Ilial wing fractures.** Stress fractures of the wing of the ilium are most commonly found in Thoroughbred racehorses. There may be a mild to moderate lameness that resolves in 24–48 hours. Complete fractures may result in ventral displacement of the ipsilateral tuber sacrale and there may be resentment to palpation of the displaced tuber sacrale.

- **Ilial shaft fractures.** Ilial shaft fractures produce the most marked clinical signs with a non-weight-bearing lameness and intense muscle spasms. The fracture ends can result in laceration of the internal iliac artery with consequent exsanguination. Hematoma or crepitus may be evident on rectal examination. The affected limb may appear shorter.

- **Acetabular fractures.** Acetabular fractures are also extremely painful. Crepitus may be palpated externally or during rectal or vaginal examination in addition to soft tissue swelling.

- **Pubic and ischial fractures.** These are the least common forms of pelvic fractures. Pubic fractures result in bilateral hindlimb

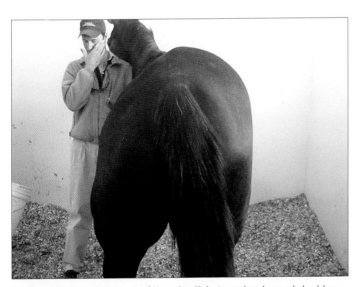

Figure 7.53 Multiple fractures of the pelvis (ilial wing and neck, acetabulum) have resulted in marked pelvic disparity. Note also the tail deviation which is frequently found in association with pelvic fractures.

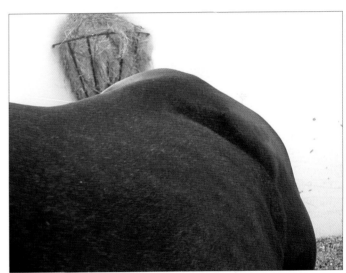

Figure 7.55 Multiple displaced fractures of the ilial wing have resulted in marked pelvic disparity in this mare. Such changes can be anticipated to be likely causes of dystocia in pregnant mares.

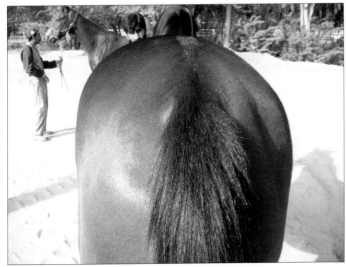

Figure 7.54 Pelvic disparity as a result of a fractured ilium.

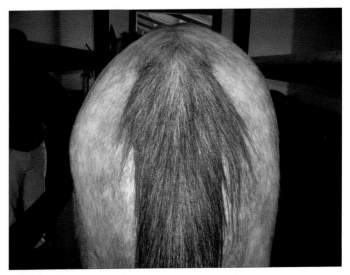

Figure 7.56 Pelvic disparity as a result of a fractured ischium.

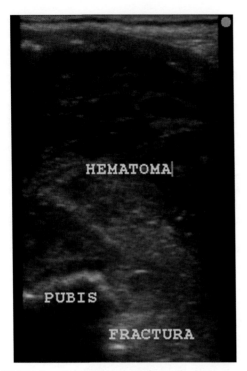

Figure 7.57 Pelvic hematoma associated with fractured pubis.

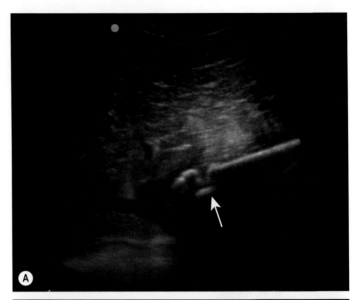

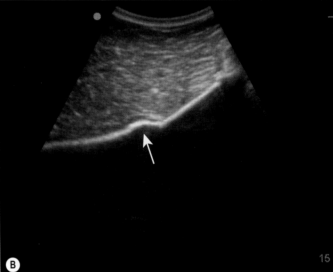

Figure 7.58 Ultrasonographic image of the ilial wing. (A) Recent fracture showing bony irregularity with fragmentation (arrow). (B) Bony irregularity associated with a healed fracture (arrow).

lameness while ischial fractures result in unilateral lameness and swelling over the tuber ischi.

Diagnosis
- Clinical examination is the mainstay of initial diagnosis with localization and assessment of the extent of the fracture generally requiring further diagnostics.
- Ultrasonography is useful for diagnosis of ilial wing and shaft fractures with the advantage that it is easily performed with a little practice and it can be performed in situ.
- Radiography is generally limited to ventrodorsal projections and has the disadvantage of requiring general anesthesia with associated complications of recovery in an already injured horse.
- Scintigraphy is currently the most sensitive means of assessing pelvic fractures but requires experienced staff and special techniques.
- In many instances the goal is salvage of the horse and thus exact determination of the location of the fracture is unnecessary.

Treatment and prognosis
- The majority of cases are treated conservatively with restriction of movement, pain management and contralateral limb support.
- Surgical debridement and removal of sequestra may be required in some cases of tuber coxae fractures.
- The prognosis largely depends on the location and extent of the fracture. Overall survival rates vary from 50–77%. A good prognosis is associated with tuber coxae and ilial stress fractures. Fractures of the ilial wing and acetabulum have the poorest prognosis and are also most likely to compromise future reproductive function in mares.

Sacroiliac disease (Figs. 7.60–7.63)
Sacroiliac disease can result from injury or inflammation to any of the following structures: pelvic bones, vertebral column, sacroiliac joints, ventral sacral ligaments, dorsal sacroiliac ligaments (long or short), muscles of the caudal portion of the vertebral column and pelvis

(semimembranosus, semitendinosus and psoas muscles). It is important to remember that even though the range of motion of the sacroiliac joint is small, any pain that results from alterations in this motion is magnified by the lever distance between the point of rotation (the sacroiliac joints) and the distal portion of the limb, which can consequently result in marked changes in gait and lameness when lesions are present.

Horses with sacroiliac disease can present with a wide range of complaints. Signs of lameness may be subtle or there can be severe lameness (associated with rupture of the sacral ligaments or acute dislocation of one of the sacroiliac joints). Lameness or altered gait may in some cases only be detectable when the horse is ridden. Frequently noted complaints are:

- Changes in the rhythm or quality of the walk
- Reduced stride length of the affected side
- There may be no clear signs at the trot but signs are often most marked at a canter with a classical 'bunny-hop' gait and frequent changes of leads or cross cantering

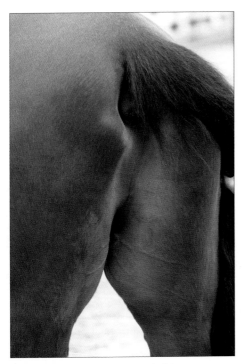

Figure 7.59 Muscle wastage secondary to an ischial fracture.

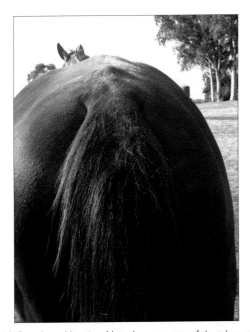

Figure 7.60 Sacroiliac subluxation. Note the asymmetry of the tuber sacrale.

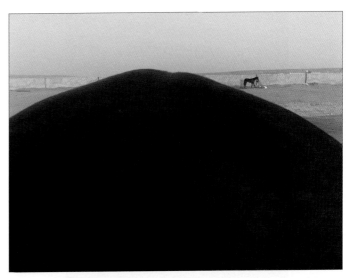

Figure 7.61 Craniocaudal view of sacroiliac subluxation, again demonstrating asymmetry of the tuber sacrale.

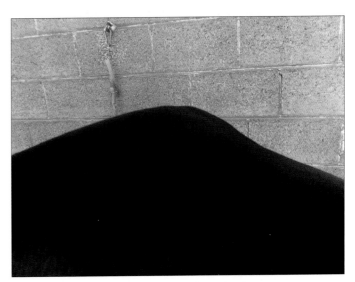

Figure 7.62 'Hunter's bump', chronic bilateral sacroiliac disease.

- Downward transitions can be of lower quality than normal and any type of downhill movement may be difficult
- There may be a refusal to jump in jumping or eventing horses
- Pain may be more notable when one hind leg is raised for farrier work
- Exercise riders of Thoroughbreds frequently note an unwillingness to go forward when asked for acceleration
- There may be a notable change in the position of tail carriage with the tail held 'straighter' than normal and with reduced mobility

- Behavioral changes such as kicking, bucking or striking may also be noted.

Diagnosis and treatment
- The basis of diagnosis is a good lameness examination with emphasis placed on observation of the gait at the walk and canter, work in serpentines and where appropriate work under saddle. There may be reduced dorsal and ventral flexion as well as reduced lateral flexion on the affected side.
- Manipulation of the tuber ischium can be used to identify pain originating from the sacroiliac joints and application of pressure to the tuber sacrale elicits signs of pain at the site of insertion of the dorsal sacral ligaments.
- Ultrasound examination can be used to assess the dorsal sacral ligaments and their attachment to the tuber sacrale. Scintigraphy allows evaluation of the sacroiliac joints as well as identification of enthesopathy of the tubera sacrales.
- The treatment given depends on the location and degree of injury present. There is much author difference with regard to treatment

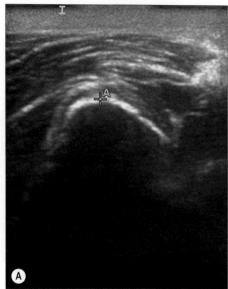

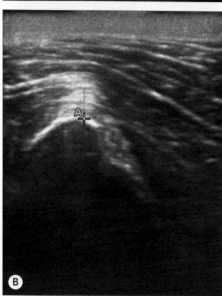

Figure 7.63 Echographic image of the sacroiliac ligament. (A) Normal dorsal sacroiliac ligament. (B) Thickening of the dorsal sacroiliac ligament and the thoracolumbar fascia above the ligament.

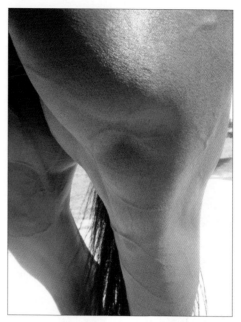

Figure 7.64 Effusion of medial femorotibial joint secondary to traumatic injury in this case.

Diagnosis
- Careful clinical and lameness examination.
- Analgesia of the joint is usually required to confirm the origin of the pain but may not completely alleviate the lameness.
- Crepitus may be present with severe cruciate injuries.
- New bone formation on the medial intercondylar eminence is associated with meniscal and cruciate injury but is only present in about one-third of cases. Other changes found on radiography are dystrophic mineralization and osteoarthritic changes.
- Radiographic changes of cruciate injury are variable with no changes found in 50% of cases. Cranial displacement of the tibia may be seen radiographically with cranial cruciate ligament injury.
- A definitive diagnosis of meniscal injury requires arthroscopy. Arthroscopic diagnosis is limited by the fact that only the cranial and caudal poles of the menisci can be seen.

Treatment
- Horses with acute stifle lameness that are either diagnosed as having meniscal or cruciate injuries or have an undiagnosed cause of lameness should be rested and treated with anti-inflammatories.
- Arthroscopy is indicated in horses that have a poor response to conservative therapy or for horses in which severe lameness fails to improve with rest.
- Fifty to sixty percent of horses will regain full function.

recommendations with some advocating initial rest of up to 2 months followed by controlled rehabilitation programs and others claiming that there should be no rest given and treatment should focus on exercise programs to strengthen the supporting muscles.

Stifle joint (Figs. 7.64–7.66)

Meniscal, cruciate and collateral ligament injuries of the stifle are common. A combination of crushing forces with rotation of the tibia combined with flexion or extension of the stifle may result in meniscal injuries. Cruciate injuries can result from direct trauma to the joint, degenerative changes in the ligament or twisting of the stifle while the joint is flexed.

Lameness is often acute and severe in onset but frequently becomes low grade after a short period of time. Distension of the femoropatellar or medial femorotibial joints will be present in two-thirds of the cases. Lameness will be exacerbated by joint flexion in 90% of cases.

Tibial stress fractures (Fig. 7.67)

This is the most common cause of crus-related lameness and is seen most frequently in 2–3-year-old Thoroughbred racehorses. The caudal tibial cortex appears prone to stress-related bone injury due to compressive forces when loaded.

The lameness seen is usually unilateral and the horse typically presents acutely lame following a period of work or post-racing. This is followed by the lameness improving over the next 3–5 days with the result that the horse becomes reasonably sound only to become lame again after further work. Other overt clinical signs such as swelling are normally lacking. In rare cases severe non-weight-bearing lameness may be present which is frequently indicative of spiral fractures.

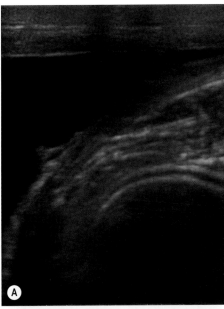

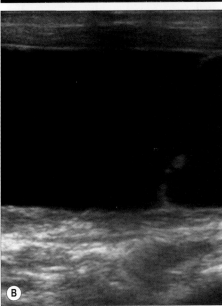

Figure 7.65 (A, B) Echographic images of the stifle joint showing marked effusion (anechoic fluid) of the femoropatellar joint. This horse had a traumatic injury to the joint when he became hung up at the stifles while jumping a paddock fence.

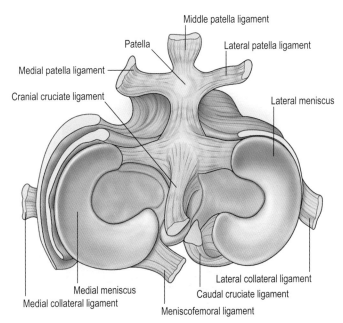

Figure 7.66 Schematic representation of the stifle cruciate ligaments.

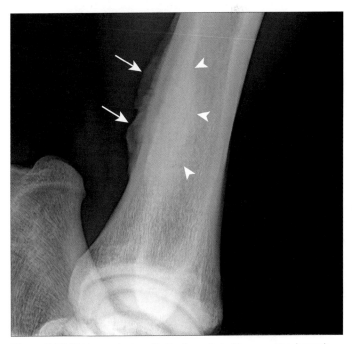

Figure 7.67 Tibial stress fracture. Notice the periosteal bone reaction (arrows) and endosteal sclerosis of the cortex (arrowheads) of the tibia associated with this chronic healed stress fracture.

Diagnosis and treatment

- Clinical examination and history may be suggestive but further diagnostics are usually required to confirm the diagnosis.
- Radiography and ultrasonography can be used.
- Scintigraphy is the most sensitive means of diagnosis with the intensity of increased radiopharmaceutical uptake (IRU) being inversely proportional to the amount of radiographic change.
- An initial period of 4 weeks box rest is given followed by a further 4 weeks of box rest with hand walking and then a 2-month period of turnout in a small paddock before a gradual return to training.

Condylar fractures of the third metacarpal bone (Fig. 7.68)

These fractures occur almost exclusively in racehorses at racing speed. There is marked lameness but the degree of lameness is not correlated with the degree of fracture displacement. Some horses may have pre-existing subchondral bone damage but many have no previous history of lameness. Medial condylar fractures are more significant due to their tendency to extend further along the length of MCIII with frequent subsequent failure of the mid-diaphysis.

Diagnosis, treatment and prognosis

- Good-quality radiographs are essential. Dorsopalmar views with the beam directed 15–200 degrees downward allow best visualization of the distal articular surface.

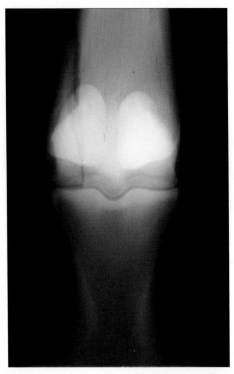

Figure 7.68 Fracture of lateral condyle of the cannon bone (MCIII).

- In some non-displaced fractures it may be difficult to identify the fracture in the acute stages and repeat radiographs in 2–3 days following demineralization along the fracture line make diagnosis easier.
- Most cases are best treated with lag screws but medial fractures may require a bone plate in addition to lag screws. The prognosis is better for non-displaced lateral fractures but is guarded to poor for a return to previous athletic performance.

Salter Harris fractures (Figs. 7.69–7.73)

Salter Harris fractures are fractures that involve the physis. There are six types with type 1 and type 2 being most common. Foals present markedly lame and there is frequently a previous history of osteoarthritis.

Diagnosis and treatment

- Radiographs are required for a definitive diagnosis and also to determine what type of fracture is present which dictates the surgical correction required.
- Surgical correction by internal fixation is required in most cases but type 1 fractures can in some cases be treated with external coaptation alone.
- The prognosis is much poorer for cases that occur secondary to infection as failure of surgical implants is common in this group. Extensive articular involvement can also result in early degenerative joint disease.

Osteoarthritis (Figs 7.74–7.80)

Osteoarthritis (OA) is a common disorder that in advanced cases can mean the end of an athletic career. Early recognition and treatment can significantly improve outcomes but early identification is not always straightforward. Osteoarthritis can occur as a result of numerous factors, continual 'trauma' associated with training and competition, injuries, sepsis and other traumatic injuries can all be involved.

All joints can be affected but the hock and fetlock are the most commonly affected.

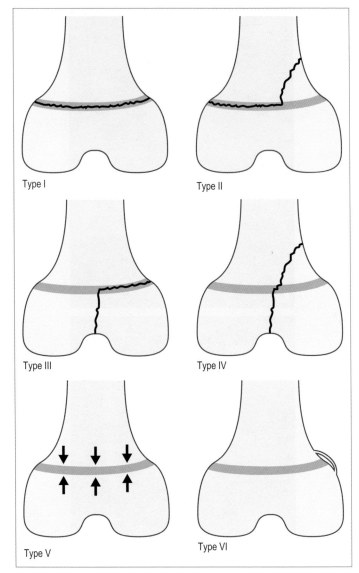

Figure 7.69 Salter Harris fractures (schematic).

- **Type I**. The fracture is through the physis with no involvement of the epiphysis or metaphysis. The germinal cells remain on the epiphyseal side.
- **Type II**. The fracture is through one side of the physis and also breaks through the metaphysis. This is a common fracture observed in foals. This fracture is seen in the proximal tibia, distal femur and distal metacarpus/metatarsus.
- **Type III**. The fracture courses through one side of the physis and then breaks through the epiphysis into the joint. This fracture is articular, and is not very common in foals.
- **Type IV**. The fracture extends from the joint surface through the epiphysis and physis and then breaks through the same side in the metaphysis. The fracture is articular, and is also rare in the foal.
- **Type V**. This injury is due to a crushing or collapsing of the growth plate involving either the medial or lateral side of the growth plate. This is possibly observed in foals involving the medial aspect of the distal metacarpus in foals. Collapse of the medial side of the distal metacarpus growth plate is possibly the reason for the fetlock varus deformities noted in foals at 3–4 months of age.
- **Type VI**. This type of injury is a result of the development of a periosteal bridge between the metaphysis and epiphysis. This results in growth retardation on the side with the periosteal bridge. This type of injury has been noted following removal of transphyseal bridge implants such as staples and screw and wires. Placement of a transphyseal bridge on the opposite side can help correct growth discrepancies associated with this type of injury. Surgical removal of the periosteal bridge could also be performed, but there is the potential for the bridge to reform.

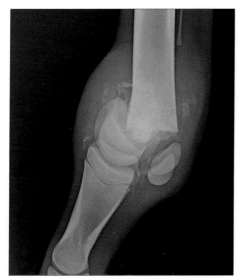

Figure 7.70 Salter Harris type I fracture.

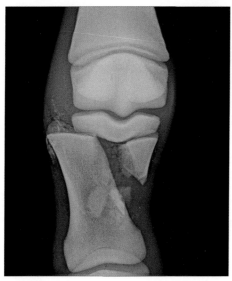

Figure 7.71 Salter Harris type II fracture.

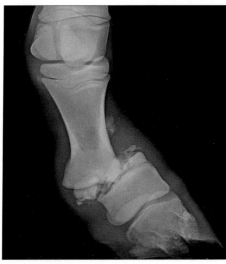

Figure 7.72 Salter Harris type IV fracture.

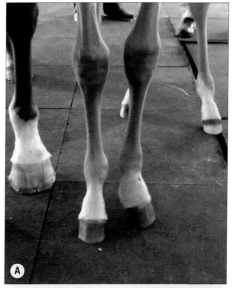

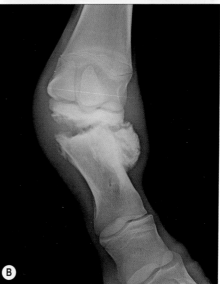

Figure 7.73 (A, B) Salter Harris type I fracture that was left untreated for 4 weeks. Note the large callus development; this resulted in a marked angular limb deformity.

The earliest signs of OA are evident in the synovial fluid with joint effusion being the first notable sign. This may be noted as a mild palpable increase in effusion in early stages. Acute inflammatory effusions result in marked joint distension, pain and lameness. The severity of lameness seen is dependent on the inciting cause and the time of examination. OA associated with infection or severe trauma would as expected result in severe lameness while OA associated with progressive low-grade trauma may present as a mild lameness or reduction in performance.

Diagnosis

- Thorough lameness examination which may include intra-articular blocks.
- Analysis of synovial fluid. As joint inflammation occurs the protein content and neutrophil count of synovial fluid can be expected to increase (for normal values see Table 7.5 p. 270).
- Radiographic signs of osteoarthritis can include changes in soft and bony tissue.

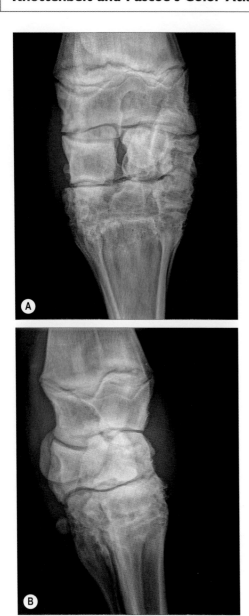

Figure 7.74 (A, B) Severe osteoarthritis of the carpal joint resulting in fusion of the carpal-metacarpal joint (same foals as Fig. 9.28). This occurred secondary to a snake bite.

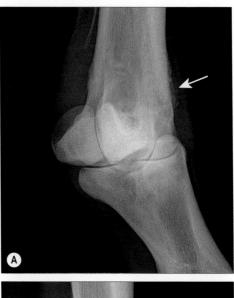

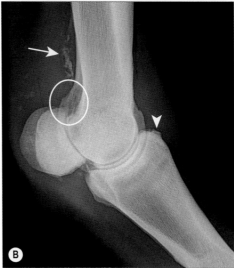

Figure 7.75 Osteoarthritis of the fetlock joint.(A) Periosteal bone reaction of the dorsomedial attachment of the joint capsule (arrow). (B) Calcification of the suspensory branch (arrow). Subchondral lysis of the caudal aspect of the cannon bone (circle). Bony reaction of craniodorsal P1 (arrowhead) and multiple bone fragments visible caudoventrally (*).

Treatment

- If there is an acute injury the horse should be rested, cold-therapy applied and anti-inflammatories administered. Horses with low-grade disease may respond to as-needed administration of anti-inflammatories. Administration of hyaluronan can be achieved by systemic administration of sodium hyaluronate.
- Other treatments include polysulphated glycoaminoglycans (PSGAG), oral supplements and feed additives, topical NSAIDs and intra-articular therapy, including stem cell therapy, platelet rich plasma (PRP) and interleukin.

Tarsus

The hock is particularly sensitive to pain, and even minor injury to bones or synovial structures results in gross joint distension and marked pain. The pain may be sufficiently severe, even as a result of relatively minor intra-articular inflammation, to lead to severe lameness.

Tarsocrural synovitis (bog spavin)

Effusion of the tibiotarsal (hock) joint (commonly referred to as bog spavin) is a response to a wide range of intra-articular lesions. These include fractures, bone cysts, osteochondrosis, inflammatory arthritides or degenerative joint disease. Other causes include recurrent cartilage microtrauma predisposed by poor hock conformation, joint capsule sprain and box rest, especially in older competition horses (this should disappear on the return of exercise). The level of lameness seen depends on the underlying cause. Distensions can be severe with only mild if any lameness in early OCD lesions; traumatic injuries may have severe lameness. Horses with osteoarthritis or synovitis may be progressively more lame over time.

Diagnosis

- Horses that are lame require careful examination.
- Arthrocentesis in chronic cases or horses that are sound is often unremarkable. In acute cases a wide range of changes are possible

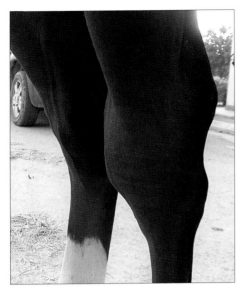

Figure 7.76 Hock bog spavin. Reproduced from McAuliffe SB, Slovis NM (eds), *Color Atlas of Diseases and Disorders of the Foal* (2008), with permission from Elsevier.

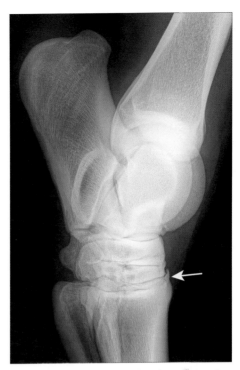

Figure 7.78 Osteoarthritis of the hock with large bone spur on the proximal MTIII (arrow).

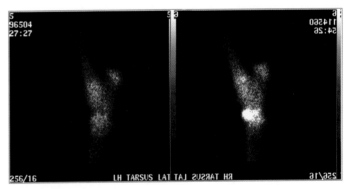

Figure 7.79 Scintigraphy image of normal and abnormal hock joints demonstrating increased uptake evident on the area of the tarso-metatarsal joint consistent with osteoarthritis of the hock.

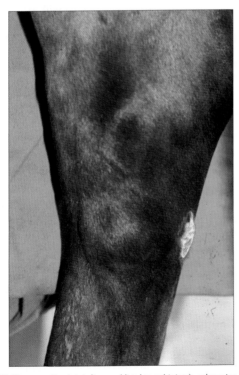

Figure 7.77 Degenerative joint disease (distal tarsal joints), otherwise known as hock bone spavin. Note the distinctive bony enlargement over the distal intertarsal and tarso-metatarsal joints. On the medial aspect of the hock.

depending on the cause, including hemarthrosis and increase in WBCs and proteins.

- Standard radiographic views frequently reveal an underlying cause such as OCD. If no changes are found additional radiographic views or other imaging techniques should be employed.

Intertarsal synovitis/osteoarthritis (bone spavin)

The distal intertarsal and tarso-metatarsal joints are classified as low-motion joints, and these bear the brunt of the concussive forces transmitted up the limb. They are subjected to compression, torsional and tensile forces during normal movement. This not only makes them more liable to fracture, but also to osteoarthritic degeneration. Osteoarthritis and periostitis of the low-motion, distal intertarsal and tarso-metatarsal joints of the hock is referred to commonly as 'spavin'. Initially, the lameness is mild. The affected horse has a tendency to drag the foot, producing prominent wear at the toe. Concurrent strain of the superficial digital flexor tendon (SDFT) and deep digital flexor tendon (DDFT) may be present as well as sacroiliac or lumbar muscle pain and in some cases proximal muscular atrophy is seen. Progressive joint deterioration results in radiographically apparent narrowing of the joint spaces and periarticular new-bone production. Ultimately this may lead to an obvious bony swelling known as **bone spavin** on the medial aspect of the hock, which is readily identified radiographically by use of appropriate (dorso lateral-planteromedial oblique 45°) projections. While most cases of tarsal osteoarthritis result in this characteristic bony change, some show little or no overt

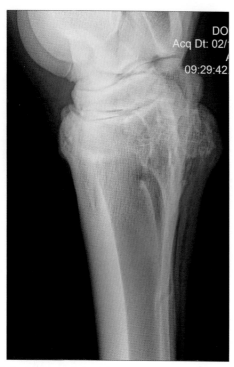

Figure 7.80 Severe osteoarthritis of the hock has resulted in fusion between the distal row of tarsal bones and the metatarsus.

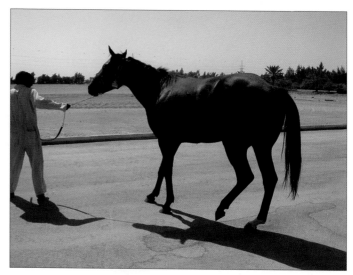

Figure 7.81 Laminitis. Two-year-old filly with acute laminitis; note the typical reluctance to walk.

evidence of any physical abnormality in spite of moderate or severe lameness. The latter condition is commonly referred to as **occult spavin**. Such cases show irrefutable clinical evidence of hock lameness following the use of intra-articular analgesia, and the cause of the problem may (or may not) be identifiable radiographically. Radiographically some lesions are found to be of a predominately lytic character, in which the joint space is wide and irregular and there is an irregular loss of radiodensity in the subchondral bone of the affected tarsal bones. Uncommonly, the talocalcaneal joint may be affected with radiographic evidence of sclerosis, lysis and joint margin irregularity. Once osteoarthritic changes have resulted in ankylosis of the affected joints, lameness is usually no longer detectable. The presence of a large bony swelling on the medial aspect of the distal tarsal region is usually indicative of spontaneous ankylosis, and, while it may appear unsightly and somewhat alarming, paradoxically the prognosis for such animals is good.

Diagnosis

- Lameness examination including a positive response to the 'Churchill' (medial splint bone pressure) and/or 'spavin' tests, although not specific to the tarsus, gives additional subjective support to the differential diagnosis. The increased (convex) silhouette of the distal medial tarsus can be pathognomonic for new bone formation and joint remodeling.
- Intra-articular blocks are also of use but one must be aware of the effects on plantar soft tissues (e.g. origin of the suspensory ligament) as well as the rare communication to the tarsocrural joint. All radiographic views should be assessed and occasionally the flexed lateral and skyline views (tuber calcaneous) are indicated. Caution must be used in over-interpreting radiographic abnormalities such as central or third tarsal bone sclerosis or proximodorsal MTIII 'spurs' (osteophyte).
- Other imaging techniques (ultrasound, computed tomography [CT] and nuclear scintigraphy) may be required in individual cases to determine the extent of the disease process.

Treatment and prognosis

- Treatment for osteoarthritis whether resulting in bog spavin or bone spavin is described below.
- Newer approaches to medicating the synovitis/arthritis include intra-articular interleukin receptor antagonist protein (IRAP) or platelet rich plasma (PRP), and (in cases of bone lysis) bisphosphonates (e.g. tiludronate).
- Surgical and chemical (e.g. ethyl-alcohol) athrodesis of the distal joints is necessary in chronic cases that have not responded to medical therapies.
- Physical therapy (e.g. ECSWT, icing, etc.) may be of benefit.
- Prognosis depends on the severity of the process and the adjunct tissues involved (e.g. concurrent collateral ligament desmitis).

Non-infectious disorders

Laminitis (Figs. 7.81–7.88)

One of the most serious and most frequently encountered conditions affecting the equine foot is laminitis. Inflammation, laminar destruction or pressure from either third phalanx displacement onto the sole or laminar pressure as a consequence of edema result in the characteristic clinical syndrome. Laminitis can be classified broadly into three forms.

1) **Acute laminitis related to systemic septic diseases.** This is commonly seen as a consequence of a septic disease process such as gastroenteritis, enterocolitis, pleuropneumonia, endometritis and grain overload. These horses typically have clinical signs indicative of a systemic inflammatory response including tachycardia, fever and leukocytosis. The exact pathophysiology has been clarified but is likely to be multifactorial, including such factors as: systemic activation of leukocytes, increase in concentration or activation of matrix metalloproteinases, inflammatory injury of basal laminar epithelial cells and disruption of laminar blood flow, in addition to oxidative injury to cells resulting in inability of cells to use oxygen ('cellular dysoxia').

2) **Acute laminitis caused by excessive forces placed on the digit.** This can be seen as a bilateral condition in horses that have been exercised on a hard surface: 'road founder'. However, it is more commonly seen in a supporting limb when there is severe lameness or disease resulting in non-weight-bearing in the contralateral

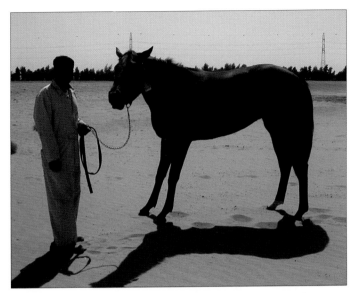

Figure 7.82 Laminitis. Same filly as Fig. 7.81. Note the typical stance with every effort being made to remove weight from the front feet.

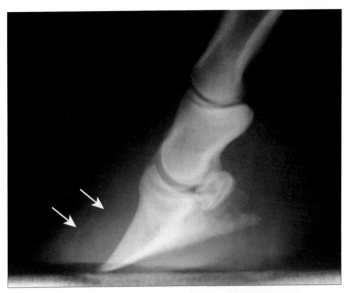

Figure 7.84 Laminitis. Radiograph of acute laminitis demonstrating rotation of the pedal bone and edema of the laminae (arrows).

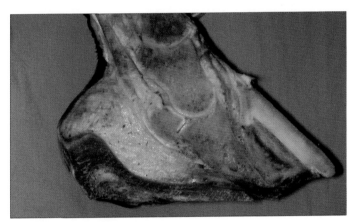

Figure 7.83 Laminitis. Post-mortem image of cut section of front hoof from filly in Fig. 7.81, note the marked rotation of the pedal bone.

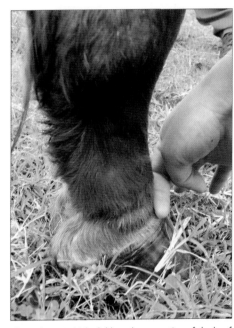

Figure 7.85 Acute laminitis 'sinker'. Note the separation of the hoof at the coronary band.

limb. The pathophysiology in these cases is thought to result from excessive shear forces and strain being placed on the dermal–epidermal interface. Additionally there may be decreased laminar blood flow due to compression of solar vessels.

3) **Laminitis associated with metabolic or endocrine diseases.** This most commonly presents as a chronic form but can be seen acutely. The pathophysiology of this type of laminitis has not been well elucidated but may involve systemic and local cellular glucose dysregulation in addition to increased levels of inflammatory cytokines found in many horses with metabolic syndrome.

In addition to the acute forms noted above chronic forms are also encountered; the chronic form may develop insidiously although most chronic cases are recovering or recovered acute cases.

Regardless of the different etiological or pathophysiologic possibilities, the clinical signs are very similar and are easily recognized. In its acute phases severe pain is usually present. Usually both front feet, or all four feet, are affected with equal severity, although the extra weight carried by the forelimbs makes the disease more obvious in these. Where the fore feet are more severely affected the horse will usually

lean back onto its hindlegs with its forelegs stretched out in front. Where all the feet are severely/equally affected the horse may adopt a 'rocking-horse' stance with all four feet brought together under the abdomen. In severe cases, the horse may lie down for long periods and show a marked reluctance to rise. All cases are extremely reluctant to move. Shifting weight from one foot to the other and resting the feet in turn are commonly seen. Mild cases may be made to walk with relative ease, but their action has a characteristic heel–toe movement where the heel is placed down first and the foot is lifted quickly, giving a shuffling, stilted gait. Mild cases will often walk without much encouragement, but are very reluctant to trot.

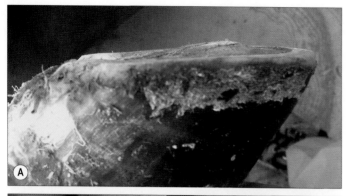

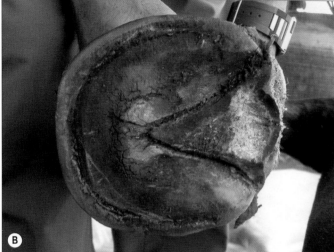

Figure 7.86 Acute laminitis. Note bulging of the sole of hoof consistent with rotation of the pedal bone and impending sole penetration.

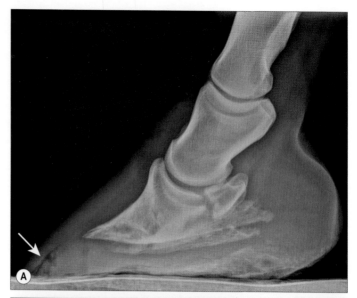

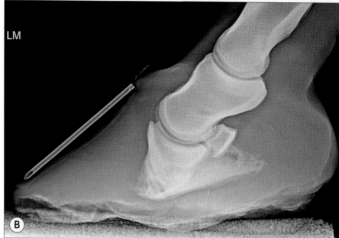

Figure 7.87 Radiographs of chronic laminitis. (A) Note the change in shape of the pedal bone and white line disease evidenced by the presence of air (arrow), which is common in chronic cases of laminitis. (B) Note the rotation of the pedal bone, resorption of the tip of the pedal bone, concavity of dorsal hoof wall, bulging of the sole and excessive toe length.

Clinical examination in the acute stage reveals the affected feet to be hot and painful, and a characteristic bounding pulse can usually be palpated in the palmar digital arteries. Progressive necrosis and disruption of the laminae result in separation of the hoof from the underlying pedal bone. Downward rotation of the pedal bone within the hoof results from a combination of dorsal laminar separation and continued tension on the deep flexor tendon. The action of the horse while moving exerts even greater tension on the flexor tendon as the animal attempts to take more and more weight on the heels. Once the pedal bone starts to rotate the process is continued by the persistent flexor tension and the force of weight applied to the dorsal aspect of the distal interphalangeal joint. Continued pressure applied to the foot may drive the dorsal, solar margin of the pedal bone through the sole of the foot but, even without this, some distortion of the sole, showing either a focal bulging of the sole dorsal to the point of the frog, or a general solar convexity, is apparent. Paring of the sole will invariably reveal extensive subsolar bruising and hemorrhage.

Gross disruption of the laminar attachments in the most acute cases (usually those suffering from severe toxemia) allows the pedal bone to sink without much rotation, within the hoof. Cases in which this occurs have a distinctive depression at the coronary band. In severe cases the hoof may separate completely, or there may be separation of the coronet over limited areas.

The chronic form is characterized by pedal bone rotation, a compensatory thickening of the dorsal hoof wall caused by excessive growth of laminae to form a laminar wedge, a convex sole and dramatic widening of the white line at the toe. Diverging rings on the hoof wall, in which the spaces between the rings at the heel are wider

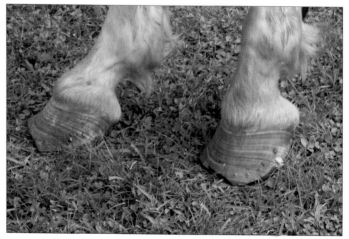

Figure 7.88 Chronic laminitis. Note the marked 'growth rings', the 'slipper' appearance to the hooves and in this case very poor compensatory farrier work.

than those at the toe, will often be found. A typical heel–toe gait is present, although the extent of this depends largely upon the severity of the disease at the time of examination. Persistent heel walking, together with a faster hoof growth at the heels than at the toes, often results in the development of long overgrown 'Turkish-slippers', in which the walls of the hoof adopt a tubular form. There may be preferential hoof placement laterally or medially, indicating more severe injury on the side from which the horse tries to relieve weight.

Diagnosis

- In most instances of laminitis the diagnosis is obvious although in acute cases there may be little radiographic changes or subtle changes in the early stages despite marked pain.
- The radiographic features of acute and chronic laminitis have been well described elsewhere. It is important that good-quality lateral, dorso-palmar and dorso-palmar oblique projections are obtained. Radio-opaque markers are important to evaluate the position of the third phalanx within the hoof.

Treatment and prognosis

- Treatment of laminitis can be frustrating for the veterinarian and owner as many of the available treatments are poorly effective in controlling the processes that cause edema, ischemia and consequent separation of the dermal and epidermal laminae. In many cases the pathological processes are well established by the time clinical signs are noted.
- Pharmacological agents used in the treatment and control of laminitis are largely justified on the basis of the proposed pathological mechanisms involved (inflammatory, vasoactive, thrombotic, ischemic and reperfusion injury).
- There are few studies that illustrate demonstrable and repeatable benefits of many of the agents used and there is large variation in anecdotal reports of their benefit also. Thus the treatment in many cases is largely dependent on clinican preference and available resources. The following are some of the agents commonly used:
  - *Anti-inflammatory medications.* NSAIDs are widely used due to their anti-inflammatory and analgesic properties in addition to the anti-endotoxic properties of flunixin meglumine. Non-selective Cox inhibitors are generally used preferentially due to the concern that specific Cox 2 inhibitors may result in some vascular compromise. Other anti-inflammatories include dimethylsulfoxide (DMSO).
  - *Systemic and local analgesia.* In addition to the above, many clinicians now use constant-rate infusion and epidural administration of a variety of drugs to assist in pain management. Commonly used drugs for continuous rate infusion (CRI) are outlined in Table 7.3. These may be used alone or in combination with a sedative such as detomidine (0.02 mg/kg) or acepromazine (0.2 mg/kg). The addition of a sedative counteracts some of the potentially excitatory effects of opioids and the analgesic benefits are increased by combination therapy. Epidural administration of morphine is reported by many to be beneficial. Perineural opioid administration is also being used by some clinicians.
  - *Vasoactive drugs.* Acepromazine (0.02 mg/kg IM q 6 h) remains a widely used treatment to enhance laminar blood flow despite a lack of studies that clearly demonstrate benefit. Isoxuprine and nitroglycerin have also been used but are currently less popular due to failure to demonstrate effectiveness in clinical studies.
  - *Alteration of blood viscosity.* Aspirin, heparin and pentoxifylline have all been used for this purpose. The benefits of these drugs may not only be related to their effects on microthrombi (which have not been consistently demonstrated in cases of laminitis), but to other broad-ranging effects such as the inhibition of pro-inflammatory cytokine production by pentoxifylline.
  - *Osmotherapy.* This is a relatively new area of treatment based on the aim of reducing digital edema and the improvement seen in some horses following the administration of contrast media locally for radiographic studies. Local or systemic administration of hypertonic saline is a possible therapy to achieve these effects.
- An important consideration of therapy is supportive farrier/foot care with raising the heels in the acute stages being an important consideration. This is frequently achieved by the use of pads or special boots with incorporated frog support.
- The severity of clinical signs and response to therapy in addition to the ability to control the underlying disease process is often the best indicator of prognosis in acute cases.

Navicular (Figs. 7.89 & 7.90)

Navicular disease is one of the commonest causes of lameness in adult horses, and while Thoroughbreds, Dutch Warmbloods and Quarterhorses are most often affected, the disease may affect all types and ages of horse, including ponies. It is however particularly rare in heavy horses. Although the hind legs may be affected, the disease principally is a condition of the fore feet.

The condition is associated with pain arising from the navicular bone, distal sesamoid or related structures such as the collateral ligaments of the navicular bone, the distal sesamoidean impar ligament,

Table 7.3 Commonly used drugs for CRI

Drug (IV)	Dose	Approximate rates of administration in a 500-kg horse
Lidocaine	1.3 mg/kg over 15 min (loading dose) 0.05 mg/kg/min (maintenance)	650 mg over 15 min 9 g in 1 L balanced electrolyte solution over 6 h
Butorphanol	0.02 mg/kg (loading dose) 0.013 mg/kg/h (maintenance)	10 mg loading dose 39 mg in 1 L balanced electrolyte solution over 6 h
Ketamine	0.4–1.2 mg/kg/h (maintenance)	1.2–3.6 g in 1 L balanced electrolyte solution over 6 h

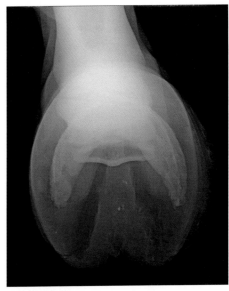

Figure 7.89 Radiographically normal navicular bone.

the navicular bursa and the deep digital flexor tendon (DDFT). The etiopathology is not well understood and the disease has not been reproduced experimentally. It is thought that Dutch Warmbloods may have a genetic predisposition.

Affected horses often have a history of an insidious onset of progressive bilateral lameness, which is characteristically intermittent in the early stages. Rarer cases may present with an acute unilateral forelimb lameness. Lame horses which are rested after exercise display an increased lameness on further exercise, but, at least in the early cases, lameness will often be noted to work-off with exercise. There is a tendency to rest the affected foot in a slightly flexed position with the toe pointed. Pressure applied to the heel region is resented. During movement, the toe tends to land first and the anterior phase of the stride is reduced, possibly in an attempt to avoid heel pressure. Bruising of the sole at the toe and increased vascularity of the sole are common findings, resulting from the abnormal foot placement. Heel contraction, as a result of reduced heel pressure, is a common sign, and longstanding cases may show marked foot contraction with increased concavity of the sole in both dorsopalmar and lateromedial planes.

Diagnosis

- While the condition can be suspected on the basis of history and clinical signs it can in some instances be more difficult to confirm definitively through diagnostic techniques:

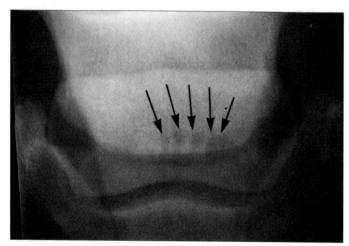

Figure 7.90 Navicular disease (podotrochleosis) (60 degrees dorsoproximal projection radiograph). Enlarged lollipop and flask-like vascular channels (arrows).

- **Local analgesia.** Perineural analgesia of the palmar digital nerves performed axial to the cartilages of the foot may result in improvement in the lameness but rarely leads to complete alleviation. Palmar digital analgesia performed at the base of the proximal sesamoids frequently results in complete alleviation of pain. Intra-articular analgesia of the distal interphalangeal joint will result in improvement in horses with pain associated with the navicular bone but false-negatives can occur. False positives can also occur in horses with solar pain, disease of the joint itself or conditions of the DDFT not associated with navicular syndrome. A positive response to analgesia of the navicular bursa is sensitive for disease associated with the navicular bursae but correct positioning of the needle is imperative to avoid blocking other sites and is best performed under radiographic or ultrasound guidance.
- **Radiographic examination.** A grading system (see Table 7.4) has been applied to the radiographic changes that can be seen. In general the greater the number of radiographic changes seen in all radiographic projections, the greater the likelihood that the horse has clinical navicular disease. The most significant changes likely to reflect disease are cyst-like lesions within the medulla, medullary sclerosis, reduced corticomedullary demarcation, new bone on the flexor surface and erosions of the flexor cortex of the bone. However, in some horses the development of significant radiological features precedes the development of clinical disease. Conversely, the absence of radiographic findings does not definitely rule out navicular syndrome.
- **Nuclear scintigraphy.** There is a significant number of horses with clinical signs and local analgesia findings compatible with navicular pain that have no radiographic abnormalities but do have increased uptake of radiopharmaceutical associated with the navicular bone. Therefore nuclear scintigraphy is a sensitive method of diagnosis but the specificity of the technique is probably not as good.

Impingement of dorsal spinous processes (kissing spines/overriding dorsal spinous processes) (Figs. 7.91–7.93)

This is a common cause of thoracolumbar pain in the horse. The spaces between the dorsal spinal processes (DSPs) in the mid-thoracic or lumbar vertebral column narrow dorsally and the opposing bone surfaces remodel. The incidence is highest in the saddle region (T12–T18). The exact pathophysiology is unclear and there appears to be a large number of subclinical cases according to survey studies.

Table 7.4 Radiographic findings of the navicular bone

Grade	Condition	Radiographic findings
0	Excellent	Good corticomedullary demarcation. Fine trabecular pattern. Flexor cortex of uniform thickness and opacity. No lucent zones along the distal border of the bone, or several (fewer than six) narrow conical lucent zones along the horizontal distal border. Right and left navicular bones symmetrical in shape
1	Good	As above but lucent zones on the distal border of the navicular bone are more variable in shape
2	Fair	Slightly poor definition between the palmar cortex and the medulla as a result of subcortical sclerosis. Crescent-shaped lucent zone in the central eminence of the flexor cortex of the bone. Several (fewer than eight) lucent zones of variable shape along the horizontal border of the navicular bone. Mild enthesiophyte formation on the proximal border of the navicular bone. Navicular bones are asymmetrical in shape
3	Poor	Poor corticomedullary definition as a result of medullary sclerosis. Thickening of the dorsal and flexor cortices. Irregular opacity of the flexor cortex of the bone. Many (more than seven) radiolucent zones along the distal horizontal or sloping borders of the navicular bone. Lucent zones along the proximal border of the bone. Discrete mineralization within a collateral ligament of the navicular bone. Radiopaque fragment on the distal border of the navicular bone
4	Bad	Large cyst-like lesion within the medulla of the navicular bone. Lucent region in the flexor cortex of the navicular bone. New bone on the flexor cortex of the navicular bone

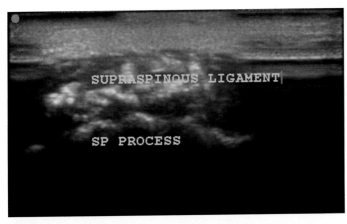

Figure 7.91 Echographic image of the supraspinous ligament and dorsal spinous process of T6 in a horse with a history of pain on saddling and palpation of the area. Note thickening and irregular mixed echogenicity of the supraspinous ligament and concurrent irregularity of the dorsal spinous process.

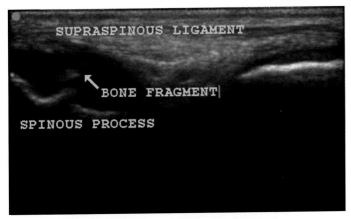

Figure 7.92 Echographic image of lumbar vertebrae showing bone reaction of the spinous processes and the presence of a bone fragment.

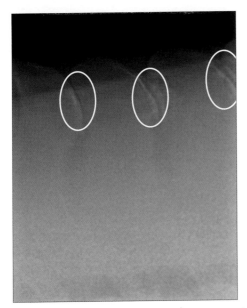

Figure 7.93 Radiographic image of 'kissing spines'. demonstrating impingement of spinous process with loss of intrerspinous space and sclerosis of the involved processes (circles)

Thoroughbred, Thoroughbred crosses and horses used for jumping seem to be predisposed. It is reasonable to assume that certain back conformations (lordosis) may predispose to the condition and in some cases there is known history of trauma such as a fall.

Clinical signs are variable perhaps in part due to the fact that many horses may have had the condition for a considerable period of time before being presented for examination. Reports of decreased or poor performance are most common. Signs are most pronounced when more than two spinous processes are affected.

Diagnosis

- Clinical examination including palpation may detect narrowing of the interspinous spaces.
- Ultrasonography may also demonstrate narrowing of spaces.
- Radiography is used to determine the extent of lesions and secondary changes but the presence of changes does not necessarily confirm the diagnosis as these changes may be present in normal horses.
- Local analgesia is then used on the affected spaces to determine if they are in fact a source of pain. If the pain is normally only demonstrated under saddle it is important to include this as part of the examination.
- Scintigraphy is also a useful diagnostic tool with increased uptake being more indicative of problem areas.

Treatment

- A percentage of these horses will recover spontaneously over a period of months or following rest. Other conservative therapies such as local anti-inflammatories or counter inflammatories may provide relief in individual cases.
- For more severe cases or cases that fail to respond to conservative therapy surgical removal of the involved DSP tips can be performed with success rates for a return to work reported to be as high as 70%.

Ringbone (Figs. 7.94 & 7.95)

Periarticular bone formation associated with the pastern joint (P1–P2) is called 'high ringbone' and that which occurs at the coffin joint (P2–P3) interface is defined as 'low ringbone' or 'pyramidal disease'. The latter is encountered with extensor process fractures of the coffin bone and in extensive degenerative joint disease (DJD). In high ringbone, the etiology is thought to be initially periarticular soft tissue strain followed by joint region fibrosis and asymmetrical and increased loading of the articular cartilage and subchondral bone leading to DJD. Horses with high heels and short toes, and particularly where these are present with a stilted or 'choppy' stride, are at increased risk. Draft horses that are used for pulling heavy loads are particularly susceptible to the condition in the hindlimbs. Both forms are painful osteoarthritic conditions generally leading to overt lameness. Low ringbone presents as new bone formation in and around the extensor process and this often extends onto the dorsal aspect of the second phalanx creating the so-called '**buttress foot**'.

Diagnosis, treatment and prognosis

- Clinical examination and radiography are usually sufficient for a diagnosis. Intra-articular or regional anesthesia can be used if the diagnosis is unclear after radiography as may occur in some early cases.
- Treatment depends on when the diagnosis is made. If early, rest, systemic PSGAG and intra-articular injections of corticosteroids with hyaluron combined with shoeing may yield good results.
- Spontaneous fusion of the proximal interphalangeal joint may occur but rarely occurs with the distal interphalangeal joint. Surgical arthrodesis of the proximal joint may be selected in some cases

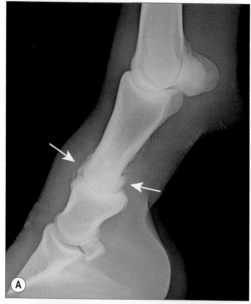

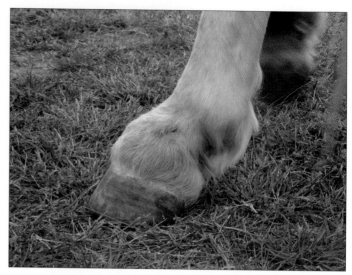

Figure 7.95 Ringbone. Typical 'buttress foot' appearance.

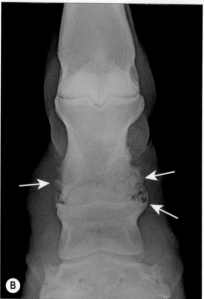

Figure 7.94 (A, B) Ringbone. Periarticular bone formation (arrows).

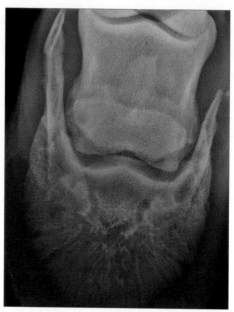

Figure 7.96 Dorsoproximal palmarodistal 60° oblique of the pedal bone demonstrating ossification of the lateral cartilages.

but is generally not recommended in draft horses due to the prolonged surgery time required and difficulty with anesthesia recovery in large horses. Contralateral laminitis is a possible complication in all cases but especially in the post-surgical period.

- The prognosis is poor for a return to the previous level of athletic function with progressive degeneration in the face of medical intervention. Horses which respond well to initial medical therapy may continue to perform without lameness.

Sidebone (Figs. 7.96–7.98)

The cartilages of the foot, also referred to as collateral cartilages, ungular cartilages and lateral cartilages, may undergo extensive ossification which is described as 'sidebone'. It is most often encountered in horses with poor digit conformation, but is a common finding in apparently normal, heavy-draught horses. Direct damage to the cartilages by wire cuts or over-reaching injuries may also result, ultimately, in the development of sidebone. Sidebones are rarely

encountered in the hind feet except following traumatic injuries. Ossification of the cartilages itself is unlikely to be a primary cause of lameness, but the changes may arise as a consequence of underlying pathology of which lameness is an integral feature. Occasionally a fracture of the ossified cartilage may be associated with lameness.

Diagnosis

- Clinically, affected horses have prominent collateral cartilage(s) on the affected side(s) of the foot. Ossification extending as far dorsally as the proximal interphalangeal joint is more likely to be associated with lameness or alterations in stride length.
- Radiography can be used to establish the degree of ossification. Lateromedial and weight-bearing dorso-palmar views should be obtained. Radiography can also be used to detect fractures but care should be taken in interpretation as some horses may have a radiolucence present due to separate centers of ossification.

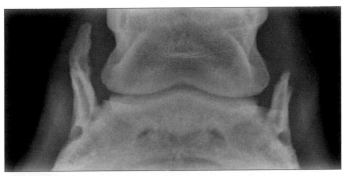

Figure 7.97 Dorsopalmar radiograph of the pedal bone demonstrating ossification of the lateral cartilages, 'sidebone'.

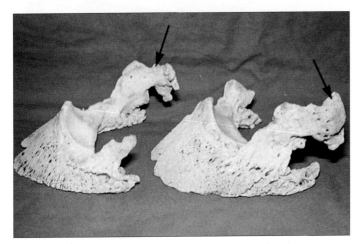

Figure 7.98 Sidebone (bilateral). Lateral cartilages (arrows) affected worse in a heavy draught horse with a base narrow posture. Condition very easily palpated and obvious radiographically.

Ischemic necrosis of the medial femoral condyle (Figs. 7.99 & 7.100)

This is an infrequently seen condition. It is thought to result from an ischemic process secondary to septicemia but the exact etiology is not understood. Affected foals present with moderate to severe lameness and marked effusion of femorotibial and femoropatellar joints, normally between 3–4 weeks of age.

Diagnosis, treatment and prognosis

- Analysis of the synovial fluid generally fails to indicate osteoarthritis.
- Plantar-dorsal radiographs may reveal thin fragments of bone displaced from the medial condyle into the femorotibial pouch with minimal subchondral bone changes. Repeat radiographic examinations may be required in some cases. Ultrasonography can also be useful in foals that have separation of the cartilage without accompanying bone fragments.
- Post-mortem examination of these foals reveals a large area of exposed subchondral bone with separation of osteochondral fragments over 60–70% of the medial condyle.
- There is no specific treatment available. The author has treated a number of affected foals with systemic and intra-articular hyalurone. These foals however have remained lame but were useful for breeding purposes.
- Prognosis is hopeless for athletic performance.

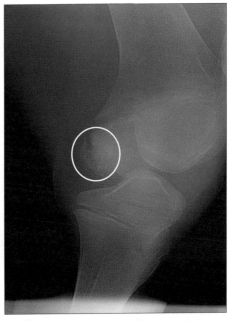

Figure 7.99 Ischemic necrosis of medial femoral condyle. Radiograph demonstrating irregularity of medial femoral condyle and thin bone fragment which has detached with the cartilage (circle).

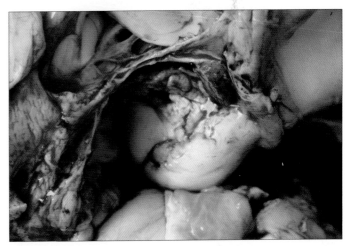

Figure 7.100 Necropsy of foal with medial femoral necrosis. Note a distinct cleft between the affected and non-affected areas. The cartilage of the medial condyle could be peeled away from the bone.

White line disease and seedy toe
(Figs. 7.101 & 7.102)

White line disease (WLD) and 'seedy toe' are common terms for a powdery disintegration of the hoof wall, external to the white line, at the toe and quarter regions. The condition is readily recognized during routine farrier care or podiatry/soundness/purchase examinations. WLD occurs secondary to mechanical damage to the hoof wall, acquired or conformational hoof imbalances, laminits, hoof cracks, i.e. any disease or defect that allows microbes and organic matter to invade the junction between statum medium and statum lamellatum. 'Seedy toe' is a circumscribed, focal area of WLD located on the solar surface mid-toe. Numerous species of bacteria, yeast and fungi (generally considered opportunistic or secondary pathogens) have been cultured from WLD-affected hooves. Environmental conditions (e.g. excessive moisture) and nutritional deficiencies of copper, zinc,

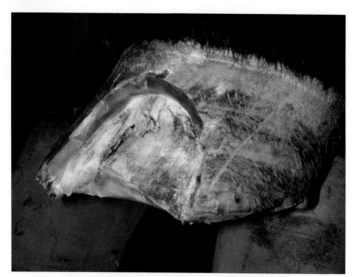

Figure 7.101 White line disease as a result of a fungal infection. The affected part of the hoof has been resected.

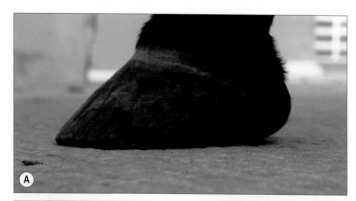

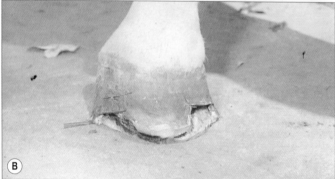

Figure 7.102 (A) Seedy toe, early case, note breaking away of dorsal hoof wall. This is followed by introduction and impaction of foreign material between the sensitive and horny laminae as in (B). (B) More advanced case of seedy toe with extensive breakage of the dorsal hoof wall and impaction of foreign material.

selenium, methionine, lyseine and/or biotin have also been implicated as causal factors, but a definitive single or set of etiologies has not been determined. Lameness is generally not evident, or is mild (III/X), but may be severe (VII/X) when laminitis is present. With extensive hoof involvement, shoes may be difficult to nail on or are easily lost.

Diagnosis
- The external appearance is distinct and diagnostic, but may underestimate the disease process. Underlying hoof imbalances or defects should be documented.

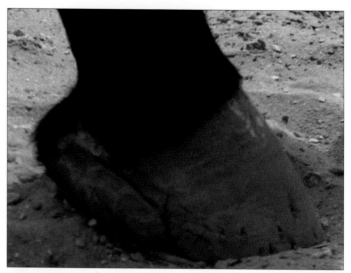

Figure 7.103 Full-length quarter crack.

- Radiographs are essential to determine the extent of hoof involvement, to define the region of debridement and to document the presence of laminitis.
- Cultures are generally non-specific.

Treatment and prognosis
- The hoof imbalance or hoof wall defects should be corrected, and the entire region affected should be debrided (to 'normal' hoof wall). Failure to completely remove the necrotic debris frequently leads to treatment failure.
- Topical medications (e.g. betadyne or nolvasan soln; sodium oxychlorosene) may be beneficial, but systemic medications are generally not indicated.
- Environmental modifications (i.e. a dry area) should be instituted. Acrylic compounds (with or without antimicrobial powders) covering the region of debrided hoof and shoes may be applied when the condition appears under control, but the patient must be monitored for recurrence.

Hoof wall cracks (Figs. 7.103–7.106)
Hoof wall cracks occur from improper hoof balance, coronary band defects, excessive hoof growth, excessively wet or dry environmental conditions, nutritional deficiencies and there is also a suspected genetic predisposition.

Hoof cracks are described on the basis of location (toe, quarter, heel or bar), length (complete or incomplete), depth (superficial or deep), site of origin (ground surface or coronary band) and whether there is infection or hemorrhage present. Lameness is variable and depends largely on the depth of the crack with involvement of deeper structures and whether or not infection is present.

Damage to the germinative tissue at the coronet is a common consequence of trauma at this site. Although the coronary band injury may seem relatively innocuous the resultant hoof defect ('**sand crack**') may extend from the coronet to the solar margin and persist for life.

Quarter and heel cracks are often incomplete and low-heel, long-toe conformation with underslung heels predisposes to their development.

Diagnosis, treatment and prognosis
- Visual and clinical examination. The depth of the crack and associated instability of the regional hoof wall is determined by careful palpation and hoof tester examination.

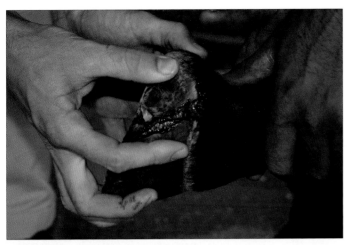

Figure 7.104 Full-length infected quarter crack with purulent material exuding from the site. It is obvious that there is marked instability of the hoof wall upon manipulation.

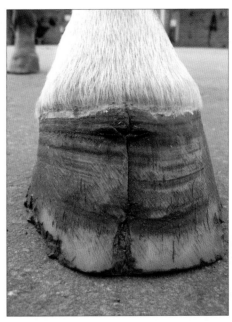

Figure 7.106 Full-length toe crack. Note the rasping of the hoof wall that has been performed in an attempt to prevent the crack extending dorsally to the coronary band. In this case it has not worked as the rasping was likely performed too late.

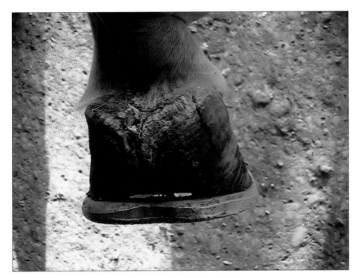

Figure 7.105 Quarter crack. Notice the marked mediolateral imbalance of the heel bulbs and high heels which are contributing factors in the development of such cracks.

- Radiography may be useful to determine involvement of deeper structures.
- Treatment varies with the type of hoof crack present and the involvement of deeper structures in addition to the use of the horse. Treatment involves a combination of veterinary and farrier care and consultation with an experienced farrier is in many cases advisable, especially where a rapid return to use is the goal in athletic horses.
- The goals of therapy are treating any infection present, providing good hoof balance and appropriate shoeing (in most cases a full bar shoe).
- Quarter and heel cracks are frequently treated by the placement of sutures in the hoof wall to stabilize the crack.
- The prognosis for horses with hoof cracks is good with appropriate treatment, but in many cases the cracks recur and recurrent lameness and infections are common.

Coronary band and hoof wall avulsions
(Figs. 7.107 & 7.108)

The foot of the horse is subject to a wide range of traumatic disorders. The horn of the hoof is frequently **avulsed**, as a result of **wire injuries** in particular, and while the appearance of such an injury is often alarming, provided that the coronary band and underlying structures of the foot are unaffected, the outlook is generally fair. Over-reach injuries in the region of the bulb of the heel may tear the heel away from the underlying tissue, but in many cases the area is only bruised. Repeated damage of this type results in marked thickening of the skin, and often some degree of ossification of the underlying collateral cartilages. Damage to the horn and skin over the heels often results in separation and the ingress of infection.

Diagnosis, treatment and prognosis

- The diagnosis is usually obvious but the extent of involvement of deeper structures usually requires radiographic examination. Contrast radiography may be required to identify involvement of synovial structures and ultrasonography can be used to assess damage to the soft tissues.
- Treatment varies with duration, severity and type of injury. Incomplete hoof wall lacerations without coronary band involvement are treated with excision of the separated hoof and bar shoe placement.
- Incomplete, clean hoof avulsions can be treated by cleaning the affected area and suturing the avulsed segment in place. Immobilization is also required and this is achieved by placement of a foot cast.
- Horses with complete avulsions can be treated with daily cleaning and bandaging until healing occurs.
- Treatment in many cases is prolonged (6 months or longer).
- Incomplete avulsions that heal by first intention carry a good prognosis but complete avulsions or those involving deeper or synovial structures carry a guarded prognosis.

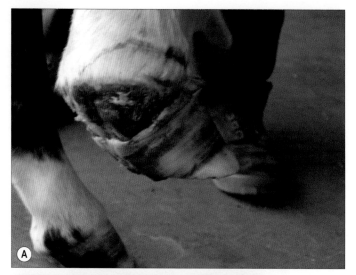

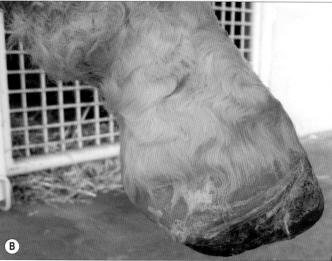

Figure 7.107 (A, B) Coronary band avulsion. This foal had suffered a severe wire laceration of the limb which resulted in compromise of the digital vessels. In this case the hoof regrew over a period of 5 months. In these cases of complete avulsions, the abnormal weight bearing during the recovery phase results in abnormal hoof growth with a smaller contracted hoof (B).

Hypertrophic osteopathy (Marie's disease, pulmonary osteopathy) (Figs. 7.109–7.111)

This is an unusual disorder of the horse characterized by proliferative, periosteal new bone formation. The long bones of the limbs are most often and most obviously affected, but the axial skeleton and skull may also show similar changes, although these are often more difficult to demonstrate. While the disease is well recognized in other domestic animals, as a result of pulmonary or other intrathoracic pathology, often the condition in the horse is not accompanied by any detectable underlying disease. However, some cases are found to have longstanding abdominal or thoracic, neoplastic or inflammatory foci; pulmonary tuberculosis or other intrathoracic infections, such as pleuritis, and abdominal or thoracic neoplasia, such as lymphosarcoma, are the most common instigating factors. The clinical signs are related to the underlying cause (if this can be established) and to the periosteal hyperostoses. The condition is often painful, and particularly so to palpation of the bones. Local edema of soft tissues is commonly present.

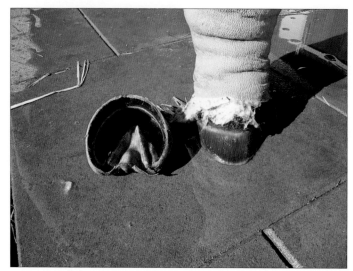

Figure 7.108 This filly suffered a severe wire injury of the caudal aspect of the pastern which lacerated the digital arteries resulting in an ischemic necrosis and hoof slough.

Diagnosis, treatment and prognosis

- The radiographic appearance is characteristic with palisading new bone formation perpendicular to the cortices, although the extent of the changes is not always marked and some areas may be more affected than others.
- Every effort should be made to identify an underlying cause and the diagnostics involved may be extensive.
- Some cases apparently resolve spontaneously, while others resolve following satisfactory treatment of any underlying disease processes. However, as many cases have no detectable concurrent disorder which might be responsible, or have serious, untreatable underlying disease, many affected horses gradually, or sometimes rapidly, deteriorate and are then euthanized.

Nail blind

A close nail is defined as a horseshoe nail that has been placed close enough to the sensitive structures of the hoof as to exert pressure on the sensitive tissues. This may result in immediate or delayed pain.

A pricked or quickened nail is when the nail has actually been placed through the sensitive structures and usually results in immediate pain but in some cases the onset of pain may be delayed until infection is present.

Diagnosis and treatment

- Depending on the position of the nail, lameness may be mild or severe and diagnosis often relies upon eliminating other causes of hoof pain in combination with a history of recent shoeing (usually within 1 week).
- Treatment for a close nail involves removal of the offending nail. Frequently no other treatment is required but in some cases poulticing of the affected hoof may be recommended.
- If a quickened nail is recognized at the time of shoeing the offending nail should be removed and the nail hole irrigated with povidone-iodine solution or hydrogen peroxide.
- If infection is present the shoe should be removed and the foot soaked in Epsom salts or povidone-iodine solution for 20–30 minutes twice daily. Between soaking the foot should be bandaged

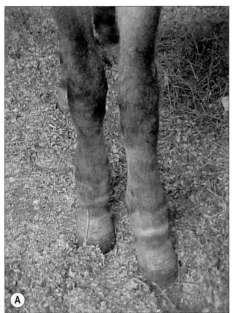

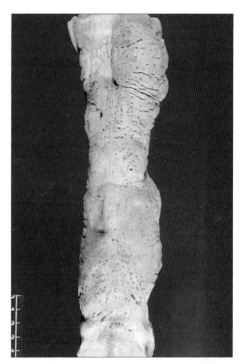

Figure 7.110 Hypertrophic osteopathy (Marie's disease). Irregular new bone growth particularly at the distal and proximal ends of the cannon bone. No joint involvement.

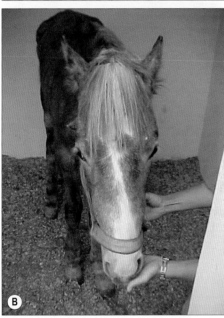

Figure 7.109 (A, B) Hypertrophic osteopathy (Marie's disease). (A) Marked thickening of the cannon bones. (B) Thickening of maxillary bones (same horse as (A)).

or poulticed. Improving drainage by enlargement of the nail hole is usually required.

• Systemic antibiotics may be required in cases with widespread infection.

Solar bruising

A bruise is an impact injury that causes focal (or generalized) damage with subsequent hemorrhage of the solar corium. It occurs commonly in all types of horses. The basic cause is abnormal focal weight-bearing. This may be due to improper shoeing or trimming. Horses with long toes and low heels are particularly susceptible to bruising, as are horses with flat feet. Flat feet may be congenital or the result of

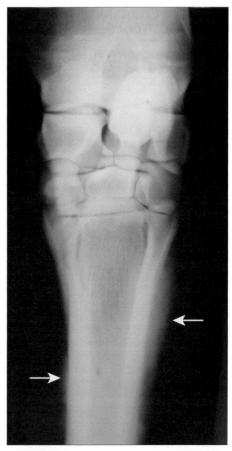

Figure 7.111 Radiograph of metacarpal III (cannon bone) demonstrating new bone formation (arrows) typical of hypertrophic osteopathy.

overtrimming. Additionally, exercise or turnout on hard or rocky surfaces can result in bruising.

Ill-fitting shoes, or an over-long interval between shoeing, may result in excessive pressure being applied over the 'seat-of-corn' (that portion of the sole between the bars and the wall of the hoof) and the development of a foot 'corn'. As the hoof grows, the heel of the shoe is drawn forward and medially, to lie directly over the sensitive tissue rather than over the wall of the hoof. Pressure at this site frequently causes bruising (bruised heel/corn), which may be obvious when the foot is cleaned and prepared. Sustained damage, associated with the accumulation of foreign matter such as sand particles and bedding between the sole and the shoe, may allow the site to become infected (infected/septic corn). Typically, these 'corns' are very painful. If they are neglected, infection may result in extensive tracking into the soft tissues of the foot and ultimately present with a discharging sinus at the coronet or, as is more often the case with 'corns', over the bulb of the heel.

The degree of pain present is variable from intermittent and mild to severe. Solar bruises frequently become infected and result in abscesses or can in rare chronic cases result in osteolytic lesions or solar margins of the distal phalanx.

Diagnosis and treatment

- Examination with a hoof tester usually elicits a focal response. Discoloration of the solar surface may be evident but where bruising is chronic, deep or there is heavy hoof pigmentation, it may be difficult to identify.
- Initial treatment with NSAIDs and hoof soaking is sufficient for most bruises. Hoof balance problems, trimming or shoeing issues should be addressed.

Infectious disorders

Septic arthritis/osteomyelitis/osteitis
(Figs. 7.112–7.120)

Bacterial infections of the bones, as a result of hematogenous spread or direct introduction of bacteria, result in osteomyelitis when the infection involves the cortex and the medullary cavity or infective osteitis when it arises from the outer surface of the bone.

Infection of joints and other synovial structures, such as tendon sheaths and bursae, represents a very serious and common clinical problem. Gross, open articular wounds are an obvious site for entry of bacteria as a result of damage to joint capsule pouches and tendon sheaths. However, relatively small innocuous-looking wounds at sites which might not, ordinarily, suggest involvement of the joint or tendon sheath, may result in an extremely serious synovial infection. Egress of synovial fluid, even in very small amounts, indicates that a synovial structure is open, and is therefore almost certainly infected.

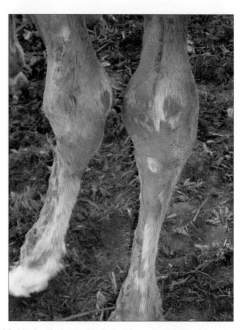

Figure 7.113 Hock effusion in this foal with septic arthritis. Note the extensive hair loss associated with recent diarrhea.

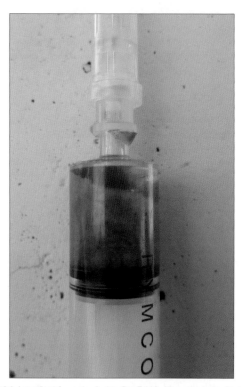

Figure 7.114 Joint fluid from the foal in Fig. 7.113. Note the large fibrino-purulent clots within the fluid.

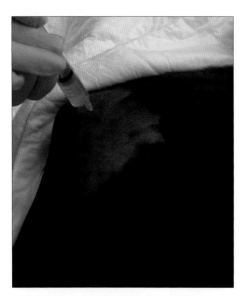

Figure 7.112 Marked effusion of the right hock in a foal with septic arthritis. Note the difference with the contralateral hock

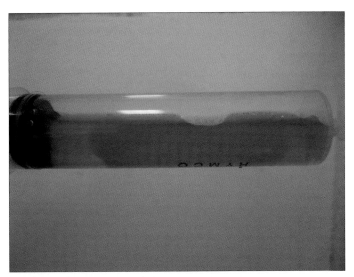

Figure 7.115 Joint fluid from a foal with type S septic arthritis. Note the intense straw color which is normally indicative of a high white cell count and the high fibrin content as indicated by the rapid development of a large clot. Type S septic arthritis is defined as infection arising from inoculation of the synovial membrane and there is no evidence of bony involvement.

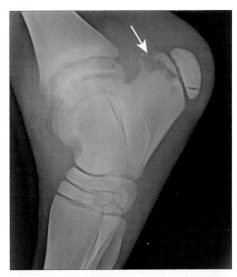

Figure 7.117 Type T (tarsal/cuboidal) septic osteoarthritis is defined as infection involving the tarsal or cuboidal bones. Note the lytic and reactive lesion of the calcaneus in this foal (arrow).

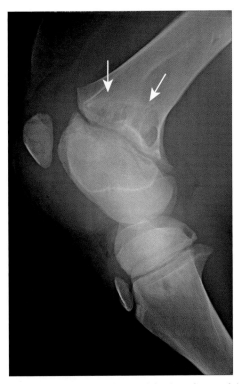

Figure 7.116 Type P (physis) osteoarthritis is defined as infection of the physis on the metaphyseal side of the growth plate. Note the osteolytic lesions along the physis of the distal femur in this foal (arrow).

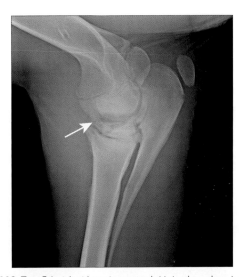

Figure 7.118 Type E (epiphysis) septic osteoarthritis is where there is subchondral bone infection present. In this case there is infection of the scapulohumeral joint with extensive destruction of subchondral bone (arrow).

Sequestration of blood-borne bacteria into the synovial structures is relatively common, particularly in the foal. Iatrogenic septic arthritis or tenosynovitis are common sequels to contaminated intrasynovial injections (particularly when these include corticosteroids or local anesthetic drugs) and/or aspiration of synovial fluid. Infection of synovial structures is always extremely serious, and without prompt, aggressive treatment the prognosis for return to normal function is,

at best, poor. The identification of synovial fluid in the discharge from a wound is not always easy and it may be confused with partially clotted plasma and serum.

Heat, pain and swelling are the cardinal signs of joint infection. These signs may not be quite so obvious in cases of bone infection alone. Initially, lameness associated with joint infection may be mild, but it rapidly progresses to a total, non-weight-bearing lameness. Infected joints become grossly swollen by synovial effusion, hot and painful, and, in foals, systemic illness with fever, inappetence and depression are common.

Swelling of the periarticular soft tissues is frequently present, which may be somewhat misleading unless the underlying synovial structure can be assessed accurately.

Diagnosis

- History and clinical signs. Complete blood count and fibrinogen assessment in addition to synovial fluid assessment (see Table 7.5).

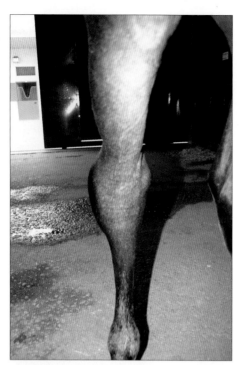

Figure 7.119 Hematoma on lateral aspect of the hock as a result of direct trauma. This is not to be confused with joint effusion associated with septic arthritis.

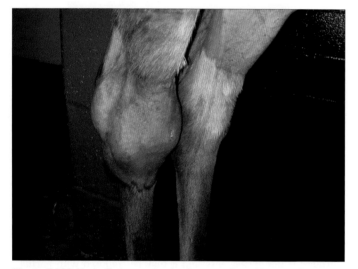

Figure 7.120 Hock effusion associated with septic arthritis. Note the effusion of medial and lateral aspects of the joint as compared with Fig 1.119 in which only the lateral aspect of the joint demonstrates swelling.

Radiographs to assess the level of bony involvement. Ultrasound is particularly useful in characterizing the quantity and cellularity of the fluid within the affected structure. It allows the visualization of fibrin within the structure.

- Longstanding cases show extensive periarticular fibrosis and new bone formation with destruction of articular surfaces and underlying bone which is obvious radiographically.

Treatment

- Treatment is aimed at controlling and eliminating infection. Antibiotics and anti-inflammatories are used in all cases. Anti-ulcer medication may be required concurrently in most cases. Ideally antibiotic selection is based on culture and sensitivity testing but while awaiting culture results or if the culture is negative but an infective process is believed to be present on the basis of clinical signs and synovial fluid cytology, broad-spectrum antibiotics should be used. Many infections are Gram-negative but mixed infections are common.
- Where synovial structures are involved through-and-through lavage of the structure is recommended. This is normally combined with intra-articular infusion of antibiotics.
- Regional limb perfusion is now frequently performed, especially in cases of bone infections. It can be used alone or combined with hyperbaric oxygen therapy.
- Intraosseus injection of antibiotics can also be used for bone infections if the site can be easily accessed.
- In more severe cases of osteomyelitis, removel of necrotic bone or bone sequestrums may be required.
- In cases of joint infections which are unresponsive to lavages and other therapies an arthroscopy or arthrotomy may be required to remove fibrin from the joint.

Sequestrum (Figs. 7.121–7.123)

Disruption of the periosteal blood supply to an area of bone, through direct trauma or local infection, may result in the development of a **sequestrum** or a piece of dead bone. Initially the extent of bony damage may appear to be minimal, with apparently insignificant damage to the periosteum, but the consequent sequestrum is often surprisingly large. The separation of the piece of necrotic bone may be slow and this is a common possible explanation for failure of apparently minor wounds to heal satisfactorily. Wounds complicated by the presence of necrotic pieces of bone fail to heal, leaving a chronic discharging sinus and/or extensive overlying exuberant granulation tissue in which deep clefts can often be seen.

Diagnosis and treatment

- The history of trauma or infection combined with clinical appearance may be suggestive that radiography is required to determine location and extent of the sequestrum.
- The characteristic radiographic findings consist of a radiopaque dead bone surrounded by an area of lucent granulation tissue (involucrum). This may be surrounded by an area of more

Table 7.5 Synovial fluid cytology for various clinical conditions

Parameter	Normal	Mild synovitis (e.g. OCD)	Osteoarthritis	Infectious arthritis
Total leukocytes (per μl)	50–500	20–250	$\leq 1 \times 10^3$	$20–200 \times 10^3$
Neutrophils (%)	<10	<10	<15	>90 (variable toxic changes)
Mononuclear cells (%)	>90	>90	>85	<10
Total protein (g/dl)	0.8–2.5	0.8–3.0	0.8–3.5	4.0–8.0 +

Reproduced from McAuliffe SB, Slovis NM (eds) *Color Atlas of Diseases and Disorders of the Foal* (2008), with permission from Elsevier.

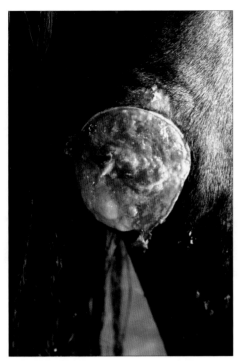

Figure 7.121 Sequestrum following fracture of the calcanus in this mare resulted in a chronic discharging wound on the lateral aspect of the hock.

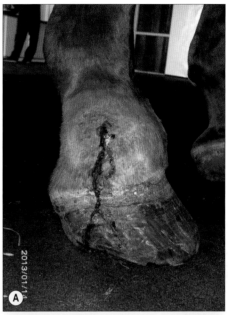

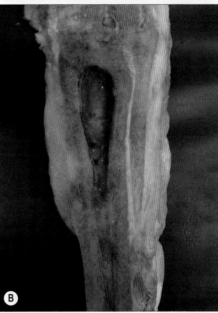

Figure 7.122 (A) Sequestrum/ intramedullary abscess. Note the marked swelling of pastern area and an associated discharging sinus tract; such chronic discharging tracts are typically encountered with sequestrums. (B) Intramedullary abscess post-mortem specimen demonstrating a large cavitary lesion within the medulla containing purulent material.

radiopaque bone which is laid down in an attempt to wall-off infection. If a sinus is present it is visualized as a radiolucent tract.

- Unless the offending sequestrum is sloughed out naturally or removed, the wound will continue to discharge. Therefore in most cases the treatment of choice is surgical debridement. However, if the area of bone involved is large this may be technically difficult. Frequently long-term antibiotic therapy is required in addition to surgery.

Foreign body penetration of the sole

(Figs. 7.124 & 1.125)

This is a very common problem in the horse. The consequences range from insignificant to life-threatening and such penetrations are almost always infected. The specific location of the foreign body, its length and its nature have an important bearing upon the prognosis and subsequent treatment. Puncture wounds of the sole may cause osteitis, fracture or necrosis of the digital cushion or third phalanx (with possible sequestration). Penetrations at the white line are frequently associated with infections which track up the wall and produce a discharging sinus at the coronet. The middle third of the sole and particularly the area around the frog at this site is perhaps the most dangerous area for penetrations by sharp foreign bodies such as nails, thorns and glass shards. The underlying deep digital flexor tendon and its sheath and the navicular bone and its bursa are most liable to infection as a result. Deeper penetration results in infective contamination of the distal interphalangeal (fetlock) joint. The only protective mechanism for these structures is the dense fibroelastic digital cushion and the frog itself. Penetrations may appear to be innocuous initially but the consequences are possibly extremely serious. These include infectious tenosynovitis of the digital sheath and infection of the navicular bursa and/or the coffin joint. Infection within any of these synovial structures carries a poor or very poor prognosis. This is often associated with infective osteitis of the navicular bone or fractures of the navicular bone. Horses with serious penetrating wounds of the sole usually show immediate lameness but, particularly where the

foreign body is no longer present, this may be slight or even inapparent until infection is well established and is by then, commonly life-threatening. Severe lameness with or without draining sinuses at the coronet following sole penetration(s) should be regarded extremely seriously and every effort should be made immediately to explore the full extent of the problem.

Diagnosis and treatment

- In cases where the foreign body is still present or there is a clear history, the diagnosis is obvious, but this is rarely the case.
- Diagnosis often relies on trying to identify a foreign body tract and elimination of other causes of pain. Radiography, and in cases of

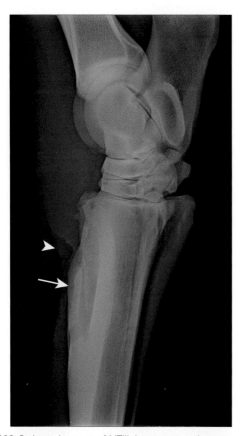

Figure 7.123 Radiographic image of MTIII demonstrating a large sequestrum on the proximo-cranial aspect of the third metatarsal bone (arrow) associated with a large soft tissue injury as shown by the disruption of the soft tissue (arrowhead) evident on the radiograph.

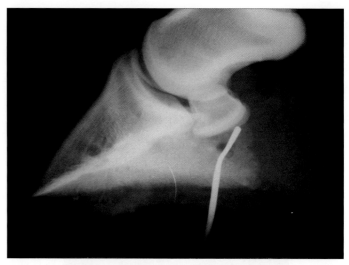

Figure 7.125 Radiographic image of wire foreign body that has the solar surface of the hoof through the frog and terminates adjacent to the navicular body. This image demonstrates the importance of taking radiographs in these cases as the trajectory of the foreign body is not always predictable and treatment may vary depending on the structures involved.

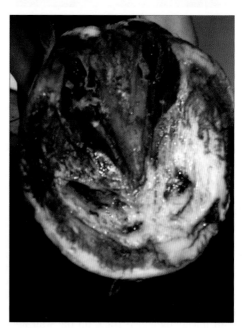

Figure 7.126 Subsolar abscess. Note the under-run sole has been removed to reveal purulent material.

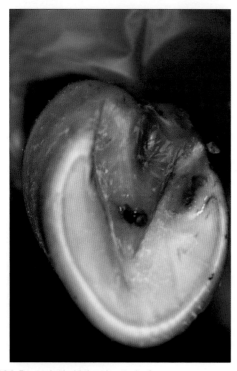

Figure 7.124 Foreign body. Nail evident in the frog.

frog penetration, ultrasonography may be useful to delineate the extent of the tract and associated structures.

- Basic therapy consists of NSAIDs, antibiotics and hoof soaking/ poulticing. Depending on the site and level of infection it may be necessary to improve drainage by enlarging the tract. Tetanus prophylaxis is also required.

Subsolar abscess (Fig. 7.126)

Subsolar abscesses (gravel) are perhaps the commonest cause of acute lameness in horses. They result from penetrating wounds, white line infections or subsolar bruising. Affected horses are frequently

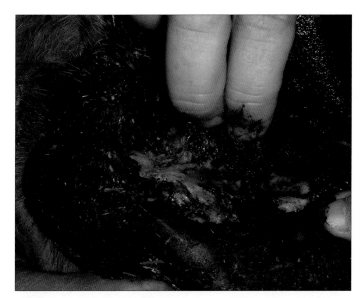

Figure 7.127 'Thrush', bacterial infection of the clefts of the frog.

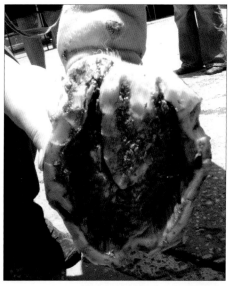

Figure 7.128 Canker. Note the marked undermining of the sole in this case that has been trimmed back revealing a granulation-like tissue that bleeds easily.

non-weight-bearing and may point the affected limb. Distal limb swelling occurs frequently with severe abscessation or abscesses that have not drained. Systemic signs of infection such as fever may be apparent in more severe cases.

Thrush (Fig. 7.127)

Poor hoof care and persistently wet conditions underfoot, particularly associated with wet, deep-litter bedding systems, often permit the development of a necrotic, foul-smelling bacterial infection of the clefts and central sulcus of the frog known as '**thrush**'. The region is poorly ventilated and bacteria, such as *Fusobacterium necrophorum*, multiply readily in the deepest crevices of the clefts of the frog. The infection may ultimately penetrate into the soft tissues of the foot, and result in a dramatic lameness and extensive under-running and separation of the sole. More serious deep infection, involving the deep structures of the foot, may also develop, resulting in severe foot sepsis. Infection of the deeper structures of the foot, such as the distal interphalangeal (coffin) joint, and extensive bone degeneration, may develop as a result of extension of the infection leading to even more serious consequences.

Diagnosis and treatment

• Characteristically, affected horses are not lame in the early stages, but foul-smelling black or gray necrotic hoof material can be found deep in the clefts. If there is underlying structural damage, severe pain may be present.
• Identification and removal of the inciting cause is imperative. The horse should be moved to a clean, dry environment and the feet cleaned daily. Any necrotic debris and undermined tissue should be removed.
• Subsequent bandaging may be required if debridement is extensive. Antibiotics may be required in cases with infection of deeper structures.

Canker (Fig. 7.128)

Canker is an infrequent proliferative pododermatitis of the frog that may extend to undermine the sole and heel bulbs. The condition can occur in one or more feet and there is no predilection for fore or hind feet. Lameness is variable depending on the number of feet involved

and severity of the condition. The condition is frequently misdiagnosed as thrush but differentiating features are a foul odor and the presence of granulation-like tissue that bleeds easily when manipulated. Thrush and canker can occur simultaneously.

Diagnosis, treatment and prognosis

• Diagnosis is done through visual and clinical examination.
• Treatment is normally quite involved and prolonged and requires commitment on the part of the owner. Initial debridement is followed by topical antibiotic application (metronidazole, tetracycline or sulfapyridine), gauze packing and application of a hospital plate shoe. The bandaging is changed daily for the first 10–14 days.
• It may be necessary to place a tourniquet at the fetlock when debriding is performed as bleeding can be extensive. Complete debridement may require several different sessions to avoid exposing uninvolved deeper structures. Systemic antibiotics are concurrently administered with a treatment course of at least 3 weeks normally being required. Healing may take several months.
• The prognosis with aggressive therapy is good but in many cases the occurrence of the condition is related to management and environmental factors and unless these can be changed the condition may recur.

Quittor (Fig. 7.129)

Bacterial infection and/or necrosis of the lateral cartilages ('quittor') results in a chronic discharging sinus above the coronet on the affected side. Draft breed horses are most frequently affected. Gross foot deformities with coronary band defects result from a very longstanding, non-healing damage to the cartilages, with severe consequences upon the other structures of the foot. In spite of a relatively small drainage sinus, the extent of damage to the cartilage may be considerable and in some cases the entire cartilage is affected. Palpation of the affected area is usually painful, but in longstanding cases this may not be so. Likewise lameness may be mild or marked, and some cases may show little or no evidence of the condition for months or even years. The prognosis for horses affected by necrotic infected lateral cartilages depends largely upon the extent of the infection. They seldom resolve without aggressive surgical treatment and indeed may extend quickly into the underlying distal interphalangeal (coffin) joint and/or digital sheath.

Diagnosis and treatment

- Clinical examination is sufficient for initial diagnosis but radiographic examination of the area with a metal probe inserted into the draining tract and by sampling fluid from the adjacent synovial structures may determine the extent of damage.
- Aggressive surgical debridement is required. Post-surgical care will depend on the other structures involved.

Neoplastic disorders (Figs. 7.130–7.132)

Neoplastic conditions of bones and joints in horses are rare and there are few descriptions of treatment available, possibly because of the advanced nature of the neoplasm at the time of diagnosis in some cases, or surgical inaccessibility in others.

Chondrosarcoma and undifferentiated sarcoma have been seen in the distal radius and associated with carpal lameness. Neoplasia of other tissues that can extend to involve joint structures include fibromas, hemangiosarcomas, synovial cell sarcomas and melanosarcomas. Neoplastic diseases of the hoof of the horse are particularly rare. Keratomas are most frequently encountered but malignant melanomas, squamous cell carcinomas and hemangiomas have been reported.

Keratoma

These are defined as benign neoplasms originating from the coronary dermis. The growth may vary in diameter from a few millimeters up to 2–3 centimeters. While some are regular and cylindrical in shape, others are triangular, and still others are irregular. They may be the result of chronic irritation at the coronary band or within the laminae, but some develop without any apparent reason. As the mass grows distally hoof wall deformation normally occurs which may result in

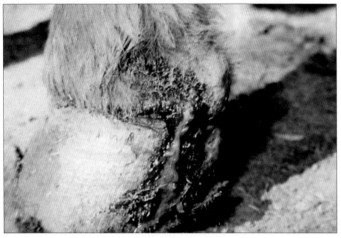

Figure 7.129 Quittor (infection/necrosis of larteral cartilage). Lesion was present without alteration after 12 months. No apparent lameness.

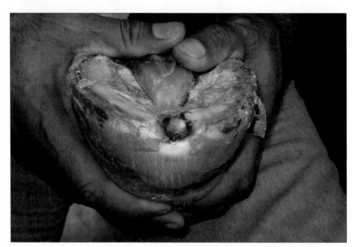

Figure 7.130 Keratoma. Note the well-defined keratoma that had resulted in bulging and deformity of the dorsal hoof wall.

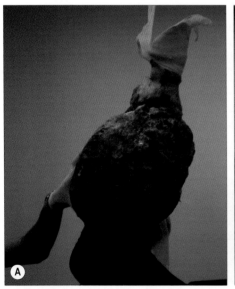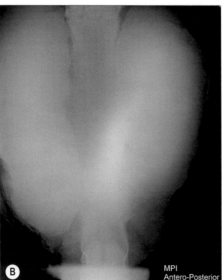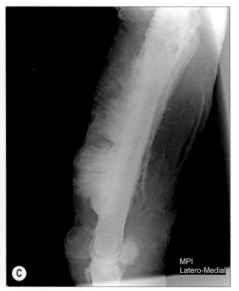

Figure 7.131 (A–C) This mare was presented with a history of rapidly developing granulation tissue. The extent of bony involvement was difficult to determine from initial radiographs due to the large amount and density of soft tissue present. Following removal of a large amount of the soft tissue, radiographs revealed the presence of new bony formation consistent with neoplasia. Post-mortem examination confirmed the presence of an osteoma.

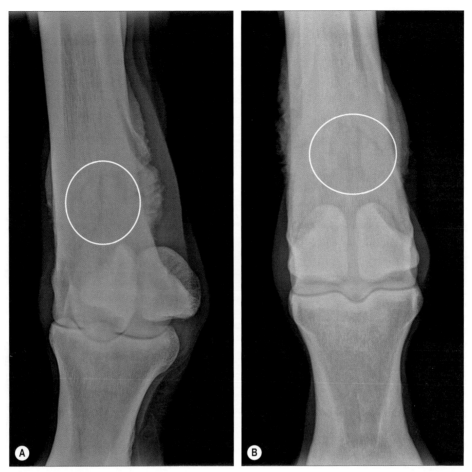

Figure 7.132 (A, B) This 5-year-old racehorse was presented with lameness and swelling of the distal aspect of MCIII. He was treated initially with anti-inflammatories in addition to rest. Note on the radiographs that not only is there irregular new bone formation but areas of patchy sclerosis within the medulla and cortex (circles). The lesion progressed rapidly and was confirmed to be a neoplastic change at necropsy.

separation of the white line and entry of infection. Expansion of the mass also results in pressure on the underlying sensitive laminae and ultimately pressure necrosis of the distal phalanx.

Diagnosis and treatment
- They are frequently difficult to identify clinically, and relatively innocuous distortions of the white line at the site may be the only indication of a problem. In some cases fistulous tracts extend between the coronet and the toe along the lesion and these are the animals which show the most dramatic consequent lameness.
- Radiographically, a characteristic appearance is seen, with a well-defined, smoothly demarcated radiolucent defect in the margin of the pedal bone. However, a keratoma may be present without evident radiographic changes with only distortion of the hoof capsule or disruption of the white line evident. Nuclear scintigraphy can be used to help differentiate keratomas from other space-occupying lesions as keratomas are usually associated with increased focal uptake of the radiopharmaceutical. Ultrasonography can also be used by experienced operators to identify keratomas at the coronary band.
- Treatment for keratomas and other benign space-occupying lesions is excision. Such lesions usually have a good prognosis following excision. A hoof wall rather than solar approach is generally preferred. Neoplastic lesions of the hoof usually have a guarded prognosis.

Tendons, ligaments and bursae: Developmental disorders

The tendons, ligaments and bursae of the horses are subjected to considerable forces in the course of natural movement, and the uses to which the horse is put and its management make diseases and disorders of these structures relatively common. Many of the conditions relate directly to trauma or to excessive tension, and there is, therefore, an almost infinite variety of injury possibilities. The clinical consequences of the traumatic rupture or straining of a tendon or ligament are directly dependent upon the function of that structure and the extent of the damage.

Flexural laxity (Fig. 7.133)
Newborn foals of all breeds are frequently born with laxity of one or more of the major limb tendons. **Flexor laxity** is particularly common in heavy breeds such as the Shire, Percheron, Suffolk Punch and Clydesdale, but is by no means restricted to this class of horse The hindlimbs are usually more severely affected than the forelimbs. The extent to which individual foals are affected varies markedly, but it is usual for both left and right limbs to be affected more or less equally. Some show only a very slight dropping of the fetlock while others may walk on the palmar aspect of the pastern with the palmar fetlock on the ground. Flexor laxity is particularly common in premature foals (gestational age of less than 320 days), or dysmature foals.

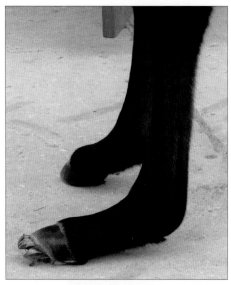

Figure 7.133 Flexor laxity. This newborn full-term foal has severe laxity of the flexor tendons. Heel extensions were applied and the foal progressed well.

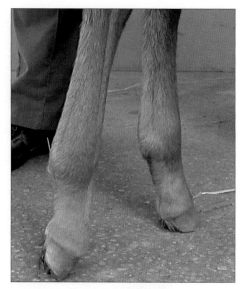

Figure 7.135 Congenital contracted tendons. Contracture can occur in one or more limbs. In this case only the left limb is affected.

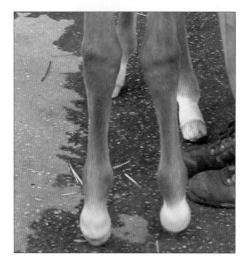

Figure 7.134 Congenital contracted tendons. This newborn foal has contracture of the tendons of both forelimbs. The right foot is pivoting on the toe whereas the left is knuckling forward onto the dorsal hoof wall.

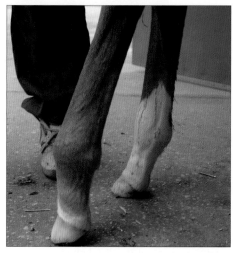

Figure 7.136 Congenital contracted tendons. In some instances the hoof can be placed in full contact with the ground and the contracture appears to affect the proximal joints more severely.

Diagnosis and treatment

- Visual examination. Radiographs are useful in many cases as skeletal ossification is often found to be poor.
- Most cases improve rapidly, resolving spontaneously within days of birth, although controlled exercise is usually recommended to avoid secondary injuries. Foals with concurrent systemic disease or prematurity may take longer to resolve (up to a few weeks).
- Severe cases benefit from the application of heel extensions. Bandaging is generally contraindicated as it results in further relaxation and laxity of the soft tissues.

Congenital contracted tendons (Figs. 7.134–7.136)

This occurs, not uncommonly, where there is a discrepancy between the relative lengths of bone and soft tissue. The pathogenesis is not entirely understood and a number of factors are thought or proven to be involved including: uterine malpositioning, genetic defects, toxic or infectious insults during gestation and hypothyroidism. Forelimbs are

more commonly affected and one or more limbs can be affected. The clinical signs seen depend on the structure(s) affected and degree of deformity.

Diagnosis and treatment

- These deformities are grossly evident but further examination is usually required, especially in more severely affected cases or cases with multiple limbs affected to differentiate between joint and tendon contracture.
- This includes careful examination and, in some cases, radiographs, although it is important to note that even with well-taken radiographs and careful clinical examination it is not always possible to differentiate between joint and tendon contracture.
- The treatment given depends on the severity of the deformity and number of limbs affected but normally includes a combination of splints/casts/bandages, physiotherapy (generally in the form of controlled exercise) and intravenous oxytetracycline.

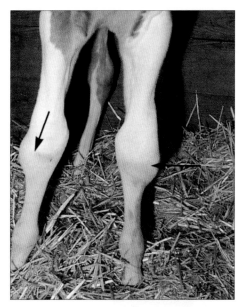

Figure 7.137 Common extensor tendon rupture (bilateral). Characteristic swelling on dorso-lateral aspect of carpus (arrows).

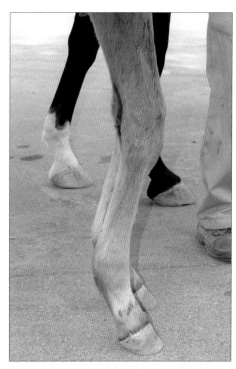

Figure 7.138 Acquired contracted tendons. Note the forward bowing of the knee which is typical of acquired tendon contracture. At this point these animals need box rest and dietary restriction.

Rupture of the extensor tendons (Fig. 7.137)

This can occur as a primary condition or secondary to other flexural deformities of the carpus. Many of these foals will have a normal stance with an over-at-the-knee appearance and characteristic swelling over the dorsolateral aspect of the carpus at the level of the distal carpal joint. Some foals will have a dramatic over-flexion of the fetlock, especially those that are affected bilaterally.

Diagnosis and treatment

- Careful examination should permit identification of the disrupted and distracted ends of the extensor tendon in the sheath. Ultrasonographic examination may be particularly useful in identifying the site of the disruption.
- Foals with primary rupture (no associated flexural deformities) should be box rested and may need bandages to avoid abrasion injuries.
- Foals with secondary rupture may require the placing of splints on the palmar aspect of the limb (from elbow to fetlock).

Acquired contracted tendons (Figs. 7.138–7.140)

Acquired flexural deformities can also occur due to growth discrepancies between the normal longitudinal bone growth and the flexor tendon elongation. Foals which are developing rapidly or being fed excessively can develop both fetlock and carpal contracture. Foals growing rapidly will often show evidence of very mild carpal contracture (over at the knees) multiple times during the first 6–12 months of age. These cases respond well to managing the foal's energy and protein intake.

Acquired flexural deformities are sometimes found in association with other developmental and growth disorders such as osteochondrosis and physitis or occur **secondary to a traumatic insult**. It is believed that pain causes reduced weight-bearing and a reduction in the stretching of soft tissues which culminates in tendon contractures on the painful limb and over-stretching on the normal limb from excessive weight-bearing. Foals showing any form of flexural deformity should be carefully examined to establish whether there are any underlying reasons for the condition.

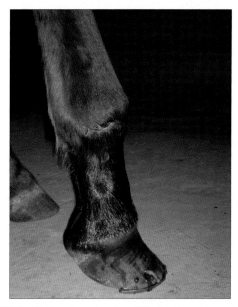

Figure 7.139 Acquired contracted tendons. This chronic case has a change in the fetlock angle and abnormal hoof growth. At this point any treatment given (including surgery) is unlikely to result in a competitive career for this animal.

The clinical signs seen depend on the structure(s) affected:

- **Superficial flexor contracture** results in an upright distal limb but a normal hoof ground contact.
- **Deep flexor contracture** results in an upright 'ballet dancer' posture. It can be further subdivided into two types: type I is when the dorsal surface of the hoof wall is less than 90 degrees; type II is when the dorsal surface is greater than 90 degrees.

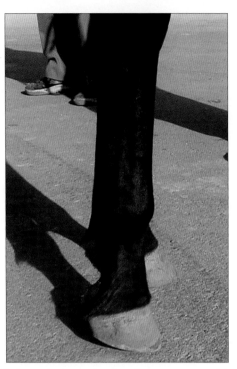

Figure 7.140 Acquired contracted tendons. Severe contracture of the flexor tendons has resulted in a 'ballet-dancer' pose in this yearling.

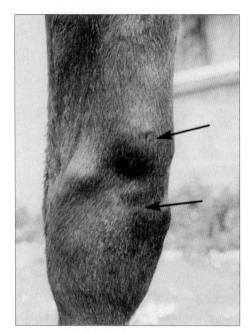

Figure 7.141 Extensor carpi radialis tendon rupture (old). Disrupted ends of tendon visible (arrows) (and palpable) and atrophy of the extensor carpi radialis muscle giving a hollow appearance to the forearm.

- *Combined contracture* results in an upright pastern and upright hoof.

Diagnosis, treatment and prognosis
- Diagnosis is done mainly through visual examination. Digital examination may help distinguish tendon contracture from joint contracture.
- Radiology is useful in making an initial diagnosis and serial radiographs are helpful in monitoring the progress of the condition.
- The condition can be managed medically or surgically:
  - *Medical management*. Growth discrepancies due to excessive nutrition potentially respond to decreasing and monitoring the nutrition in the affected foal. Controlled exercise programs and potentially exercise restriction is required in some cases. Low-dose non-steroidal anti-inflammatory agents can be used to help control mild levels of pain. Regular trimming to gradually lower the heel and shoeing or application of toe extensions in some cases. Bandaging/splinting/casting can be utilized to help provide soft tissue laxity.
  - *Surgical management*:
    - *Distal interphalangeal joint contracture.* Inferior check ligament desmotomy; deep digital flexor tenotomy.
    - *Fetlock contracture.* Superior check ligament desmotomy.
    - *Carpal contracture.* Ulnaris lateralis tenotomy.
- Prognosis in mild cases is fair to good, but poor in severe cases.

Tendons, ligaments and bursae: Non-infectious disorders

Rupture of the extensor carpi radialis tendon (Fig. 7.141)
Rupture of the extensor carpi radialis tendon in adult horses also occurs. Rupture may be partial or complete and is most commonly seen in jumping horses. Many cases are the direct consequence

of trauma, with repeated over-flexion of the carpus being the most likely factor. Partial rupture has been reported to be a consequence of tendon damage caused by exostoses on the distal radius. Others may be a residual effect of rupture at a younger age but often no etiology can be established.

Acute rupture is characterized by pain and fluid distension of the tendon sheath. In chronic cases the distension of the tendon sheath persists but there is less or no pain present. Complete rupture is characterized by excessive flexion of the carpus during limb protraction and a double movement of the carpus during limb extensions as the carpus suddenly snaps into extension. Longstanding cases show a marked and distinctive atrophy of the *extensor carpi radialis* muscle on the dorsum of the forearm.

Diagnosis, treatment and prognosis
- Diagnosis is by careful palpation, ultrasonography and contrast radiography. Plain radiographs should also be obtained to evaluate for associated osseous lesions.
- There are different opinions as to what is the best treatment. Some advocate surgical intervention in acute complete ruptures with suturing of the tendon ends. Tendon anastomosis with the carpi obliquus tendon has also been reported.
- Others advocate tenoscopy for identification of the damaged ends of the tendon with debridement, tenolysis and lavage of the sheath. Casting of the limb for 2–4 weeks post-surgery is recommended with rehabilitation exercises introduced thereafter to minimize adhesion formation and fibrosis of the carpal joint capsule.
- The prognosis for return to athletic performance in horses with complete ruptures is unfavorable. Those with partial ruptures have a better prognosis for return to function.

Rupture of the peronius tertius tendon (Fig. 7.142)
The rupture of the peroneus tertius tendon produces a classical clinical syndrome in which the integrity of the reciprocal apparatus, which ensures the normal coordinated flexion of the hock and stifle, is lost. The hock may be extended while the stifle is flexed. Whilst this

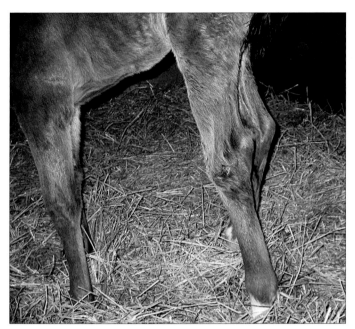

Figure 7.142 Rupture of the peroneus tertius. Note the classical extension of the hock. Reproduced from McAuliffe SB, Slovis NM (eds), *Color Atlas of Diseases and Disorders of the Foal* (2008), with permission from Elsevier.

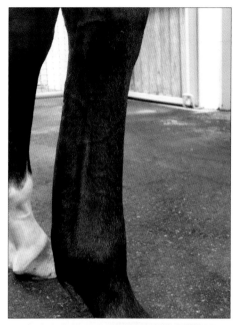

Figure 7.143 Typical 'banana bow' of the superficial digital flexor tendon (SDFT).

manipulation is performed, a characteristic dimpling of the common calcanean tendon is visible. The condition is encountered after falls at speed, following violent struggles to free a trapped leg or following traumatic injuries to the cranial region of the limb below the stifle. It also occurs relatively frequently following the use of casts extending up to the mid tibia. Horses with a ruptured peroneus tertius tendon have a characteristic shuffling gait, in which the foot consistently fails to clear the ground as a result of reduced hock flexion. There is often marked wearing of the toe of the affected leg. In chronic cases little or no pain is usually encountered.

Superficial digital flexor tendon injury
(Figs. 7.143–7.149)
The superficial digital flexor tendon (SDFT) is the most frequently injured soft tissue structure in (flat) racehorses (7–43%), national hunt horses, and event horses, but it is less likely to be injured in other disciplines. Repetitive speed cycles over distance and possible genetic predisposition in Thoroughbreds are thought to be important factors in injury. Other important factors that may predispose to injury are conformation, working surface, shoeing training and readiness for the level of exercise being performed. Most injuries caused by athletic use are in the mid-metacarpal region (zones 2B–3B) but injuries are also frequently seen at the musculotendinous junction of the antebrachium, in the carpal canal, subcarpal region and in the pastern. The plantar hock region is the most common site of injury in the hindlimb, especially in Standardbred racehorses.

Clinical signs
These vary considerably depending on the location, severity and duration of the injury:

- *Lameness.* Lameness is very variable and usually not correlated with the severity of the tear. Some horses will have extensive core lesions with no lameness and other small lesions will cause the horse to be lame.
- *Swelling.* The typical swelling associated with SDFT injury is in a bowed appearance. Swelling can also be associated with subcutaneous or peritendinous accumulation of fluid. Subcutaneous

accumulation is found in acute injuries and can also be seen in 'bandage-bows' related to malpositioned or too-tight bandages or exercise boots.
- *Thickening.* Thickening or enlargement detected by palpation or visually may be related to an acute injury or can represent end-stage repair from a previous injury. In cases of mild or diffuse injuries, thickening may be difficult to appreciate on palpation. Injuries in the subcarpal region where the tendon is enveloped by retinaculum or injuries associated with significant tenosynovitis result in difficulty detecting thickening by palpation. Assessing the flexibility of the DSFT is also useful as stiffness may be a reflection of previous injury.
- *Heat.* The presence of heat in the region may be the earliest detectable sign of injury.
- *Sensitivity to palpation.* A painful response to direct digital palpation is frequently used clinically to detect tendon injury and is usually quite specific to a tendon problem.
- *Tendon profile.* Evaluation of the profile of the tendon with the limb in a full weight-bearing position can also provide valuable information. The profile should be examined from all angles. With slight injuries the tendon may have a normal profile when viewed from one angle but abnormal when viewed from another. Acute total ruptures may, in the initial few hours after injury, have little changes in profile but a hyperextension of the metacarpophalangeal joint may be noted when compared to the contralateral limb.

Diagnosis and treatment
- Clinical examination and palpation as outlined above are important aspects of initial diagnosis and in many cases it is the initial clinical examination that is used to select horses for further diagnostic tests such as ultrasonography.
- Initial management of acute-phase injuries includes administration of anti-inflammatories and physical therapy including icing and application of poultices or support bandages. Other therapies such as systemic or perilesional corticosteroids or administration of polysulfated glycosaminoglycans is largely dependent on clinician preference.

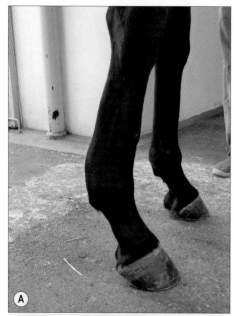

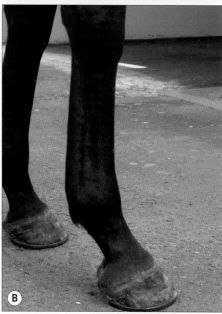

Figure 7.144 (A, B) Tendonitis 'bow' of both the upper and lower sections of the SDFT. (B) Acute tendonitis 'bow' of the SDFT. The development of the 'banana' profile of a bowed tendon is due to the hemorrhage/edema and inflammation. This may take a number of days to reach its maximum and in the acute stages there may be minimal changes to be observed grossly.

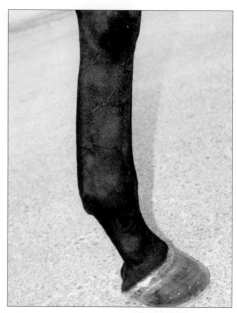

Figure 7.145 Bandage bow. Notice that the swelling is less defined than what is normally seen with a typical tendonitis of the superficial digital flexor tendon and is quite prominent below the knee. This occurred after the horse was shipped with tight bandages.

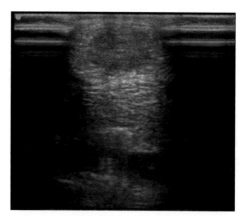

Figure 7.146 Echographic image of a large core lesion of the SDFT. This lesion involves more than 80% of the total tendon area. This 2-year-old was noted with acute swelling the morning after a fast work. Due to the severity of the lesion and the poor prognosis the horse was retired from racing.

- Therapy thereafter may be medical or surgical. Medical therapies include controlled exercise and time out of training, hyaluron, PSGAG, stem cells and plasma rich platelets. External Blister is still used despite lack of scientific data that proves its benefits.
- Surgical therapies include tendon splitting, transection of the accessory ligament of the SDFT and annular desmotomy.
- It must be said that the way the horse is rehabilitated and managed once it gets back to training is possibly the most important aspect in the success rate of a horse with this type of injury despite the treatment.
- Also the success largely depends on the use and discipline of the horse. Horses that perform at lower-level or slow-speed sports (i.e.

dressage, show jumping) have a much higher chance of recovery than the sports where speed is predominant (i.e. racing).

Suspensory desmitis (Figs. 7.150–7.158)

Suspensory ligament desmitis is a frequently encountered condition in all breeds. It is a common cause of forelimb lameness in Thorough-bred racehorses, fore- and hindlimb lameness in Standardbreds and hindlimb lameness in sport horses. Clinical presentation differs depending on the location of the injury and therefore each condition is discussed separately.

The pathophysiology of the suspensory desmitis is similar to that of SDFT tendonitis. Branch injuries may be associated with a single asymmetrical or excessive weight-bearing event. Branch injuries can also be related to sesamoid injuries or sesamoiditis. Poor conformation may predispose to the condition.

In the hindlimb, proximal desmitis is suggested to be associated with a compartment syndrome.

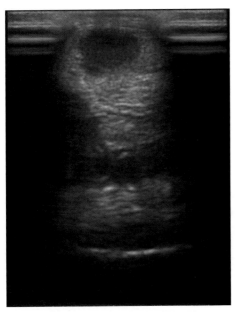

Figure 7.147 Echographic image of a severe acute SDFT bow. The lesion started at zone 1A and extended distally to zone 3A. It is important to notice the completely anechoic pattern of the lesion indicating a very severe tear with complete fiber disruption.

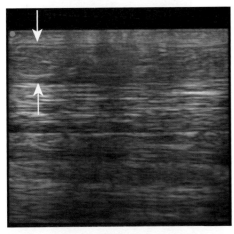

Figure 7.148 Longitudinal image of a severe bowed SDFT. Note the demarcation of the lesion (arrows) and the lack of normal fiber (compared with deep digital flexor tendon below).

Proximal suspensory desmitis

Lameness can be mild to severe and frequently worsens with exercise. Lameness is frequently acute in onset in the forelimb but may be more chronic or insidious in onset in the hindlimb. Mild lameness may be accentuated on a circle or when the horse is ridden. Occasionally there is a non-specific swelling of the palmar/plantar cannon region and digital pressure applied to the proximal suspensory ligament may elicit a painful response.

Diagnosis

- The diagnosis can be challenging, especially in cases where there is only mild lameness present. A thorough systematic lameness examination including diagnostic analgesia is essential. The lameness is usually not altered by distal metacarpal/metatarsal analgesia (lower six-point block). The lameness may or may not improve to proximal analgesia (high six-point block).

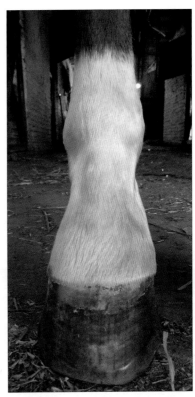

Figure 7.149 Tear of medial branch of the SDFT. Notice the change in profile on the right side of the leg (medial).

- Lameness should be abolished by application of local anesthetic around the origin of the ligament or by antebrachial or crural regional analgesia. A deep lateral plantar nerve regional block can be diagnostic in the hindlimb. It is important to remember however that false-negatives and false-positives can both occur. Some cases may only respond to analgesia of the carpometacarpal or tarso-metatarsal joints.
- Radiography may show sclerosis with loss of trabecular pattern and thickening of the cortex of the palmaro- or plantaro-proximal third of the metacarpal or metatarsal bone. Cortical fissures or avulsed fragments may be visible near the origin of the ligament.
- Ultrasonographic lesions can be subtle and may include enlargement of the ligament, poor definition of ligament margins, hypoechogenic or hyperechogenic (in chronic cases) areas within the ligament, and irregularity of the palmar or plantar surface of the bone. Scintigraphy shows increased uptake over the origin of the ligament and can be useful to rule out joint disease.

Treatment and prognosis

- **Forelimb.** Conservative management with initial rest/hand-walking only for 5–10 minutes, 2–4 times daily for 4 weeks. Then 20 minutes walking for the next 4 weeks. Follow-up ultrasonography is performed at 8 weeks. Acute injuries may require 3–6 months of management before a full return to work. Chronic cases may be more difficult, and absence of evolution of the lesion over a 3-month period is required before a return to work. Intraligamentous medication does not appear to improve the outcome.
- **Hindlimb.** The same conservative treatment is applied but generally a longer management period is required as frequently lesions are more chronic when recognized. Surgical fasciotomy combined with neurectomy of the lateral plantar metatarsal nerve may help in some chronic cases. It should however be combined with a

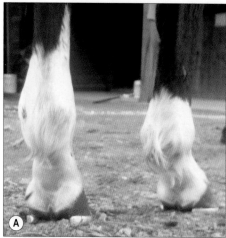

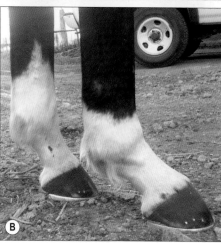

Figure 7.150 (A, B) Suspensory desmitis in the right hind leg. The tear was severe and involved the proximal area of the ligament, resulting in the dropping of the hind fetlock.

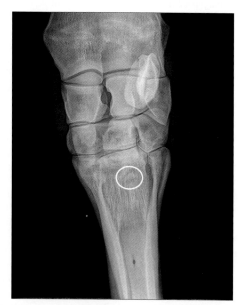

Figure 7.151 Radiograph demonstrating an avulsion fracture (circle) of the insertion of the proximal suspensory ligament 'high suspensory'.

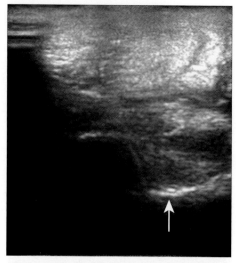

Figure 7.152 High suspensory desmitis echographic image. Notice the heterogeneous echogenicity and the small avulsion fragment of the plantar aspect of the metatarsal bone (arrow).

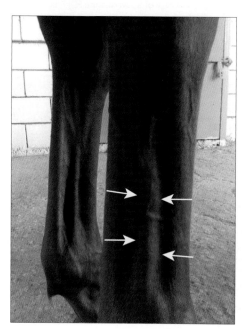

Figure 7.153 Mid suspensory desmitis. Markedly enlarged suspensory ligament (arrows).

period of rest and in many cases corrective foot trimming and shoeing.

- Shock-wave therapy improves clinical signs in up to 50% of cases without improving the ultrasonographic findings. It is thought to work by providing analgesia through destruction of nerve endings.
- The prognosis for return to the same level of performance is good in the forelimbs (90%) but poorer in the hindlimbs (22%). Chronic injuries do not respond as well to treatment and recurrence is common.

Desmitis of the suspensory ligament body

Lameness is very variable; it can be severe at the outset but tends to decrease over the next 3–6 weeks. The condition is normally unilateral in the forelimbs. There is obvious swelling and edema in the area. As the edema recedes, thickening of the suspensory body becomes obvious. Pain may be elicited on digital palpation.

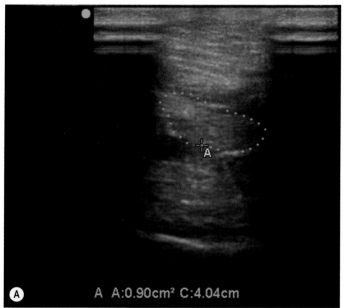

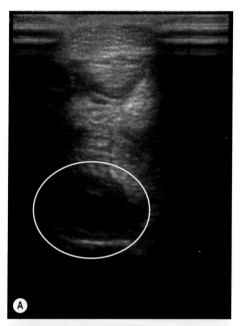

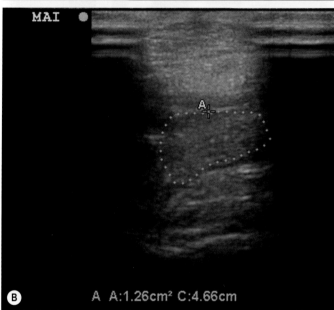

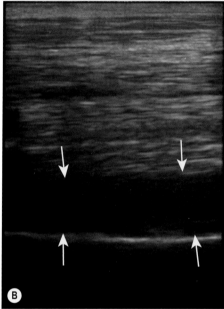

Figure 7.154 (A, B) Echographic image of a desmitis of an inferior check ligament. Notice the thickening of the ligament when compared with the normal leg (A).

Figure 7.155 (A, B) Severe core lesion of the high portion of the suspensory ligament (circle). (B) Notice the absence of normal tissue on the longitudinal image (arrows).

Diagnosis, treatment and prognosis

- Clinical examination with palpation is highly suggestive and regional anesthesia is rarely required. Ultrasonography is useful to characterize the lesion and determine if there is interference from the splint bones.
- Lesions are variable from an increased cross-sectional surface to discrete anechoic or hypoechoic lesions. Diffuse lesions are more common and hyperechoic areas can be seen in chronic cases.
- Treatment is often conservative and follows the same medical management as for SDFT tendonitis.
- The lesions frequently persist despite clinical improvement and recurrence is common.

Suspensory branch desmitis

This is the most common injury of the suspensory ligament. The condition can be unilateral or bilateral with bilateral lesions more common in the forelimbs. Lameness is variable but is generally more severe in acute and bilateral cases.

Diagnosis, treatment and prognosis

- There is marked thickening and pain on palpation of the affected branches. There can be concurrent injuries of the sesamoids, fetlock joint or digital sheath. Severe bilateral cases can result in a marked fetlock drop.
- Ultrasonography can reveal lesions similar to those found in body injuries. Chronic cases may have ectopic mineralization within the ligament and irregularity at the distal insertion of the sesamoid bone may be present.
- Conservative and medical management are conducted as for SDFT lesions. Lesions can be difficult to treat. Shock-wave therapy can be used and is reported to improve clinical signs.

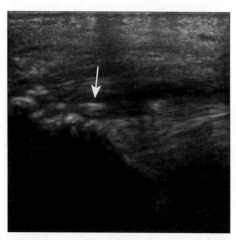

Figure 7.156 Echographic image of the branch of the suspensory ligament showing tearing of the fibers and avulsion at the attachment of the sesamoid bone (arrow). This filly was a 2-year-old when the problem was diagnosed. Rest and controlled exercise were recommended and she made a full recovery.

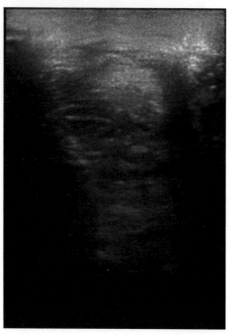

Figure 7.157 Chronic suspensory branch desmitis with heterogeneous appearance of the fibers. Notice the thickening of the ligament and the periligamentous tissue.

- The prognosis is related to the severity of the lesion, being worsen with more severe or bilateral lesions. Interligamentous mineralization is related to a poorer prognosis. Re-injury is common and leads to a poorer prognosis.

Deep digital flexor tendonitis

(Figs. 7.159 & 7.160)

Injury to the deep digital flexor tendon (DDFT) occurs most frequently within the foot or within the digital sheath. It has also been associated with carpal canal syndrome, thoroughpin and desmitis of the accessory ligament of the DDFT.

Injuries within the tendon sheath are usually a spontaneous sprain injury or as a result of overextension. Direct trauma and puncture wounds can also occur and can result in severe lesions despite minimal outward signs.

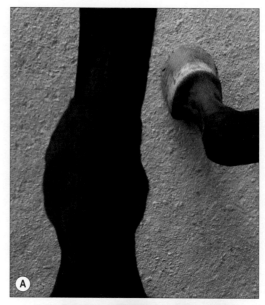

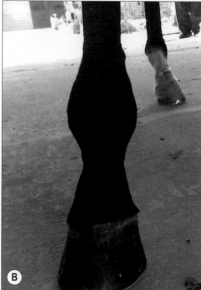

Figure 7.158 (A, B) Lateral suspensory branch chronic desmitis. Notice the thick aspect of the branch when leg is flexed and tension is relieved.

DDFT tendonitis within the digital sheath (Fig. 7.160)

Lesions within the tendon sheath are always associated with distension and inflammation of the sheath, and are most commonly seen in the hindlimb. Sheath distension may precede lameness or lameness may be acute in onset concurrent with sheath distension. Pain may be elicited by applying pressure to the tendon but this may be difficult in cases of extreme distension.

Diagnosis and treatment

- Clinical signs are suggestive. Ultrasonography of the digital sheath region normally reveals one of four typical lesions: enlargement and change in shape of the tendon; focal hypoechoic lesions; mineralization within the DDFT; marginal tears. More chronic cases may also have adhesion formation and synovitis changes.

Medical and surgical treatments are both options. Conservative treatment as for SDFT tendonitis. Surgical treatment with tenoscopy has been used to debride tears and adhesions but healing is typically slow and success rates are low.

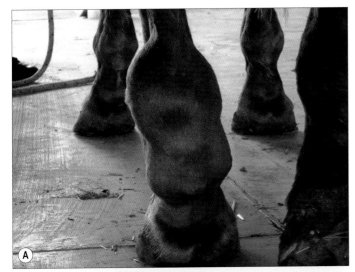

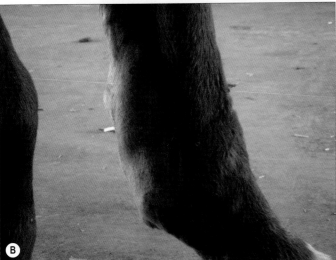

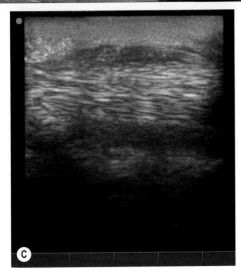

Figure 7.159 (A–C) This polo mare had severe tenosinovitis of the digital tendon sheath of the right hind. The mare was lame and an echographic study showed a tear of the DDFT.

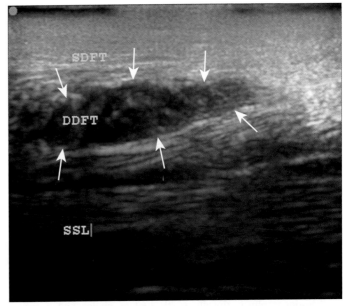

Figure 7.160 Echographic image of a severe tear of the DDFT (arrows). This yearling was found lame in the paddock and had swelling around the pastern area.

DDFT injuries within the foot

Since the advent of more advanced forms of diagnostic imaging it has become clear that injuries to the DDFT within the foot are a greater cause of lameness than previously thought. Tendonitis of the distal portion of the DDFT can occur alone or can occur in conjunction with navicular bone pathology, or with multiple soft tissue injuries.

The pathophysiology is not clearly understood and is likely to be multifactorial. Possible causes and predisposing factors are repetitive overload stress, acute traumatic tearing, poor conformation, use of the horse (jumping horses have a higher incidence) and previous palmar digital neurectomy.

The lameness seen is variable even within an individual horse. There is a tendency, however, to disimprove with hard work and improve with rest. Some cases will be sound when trotted in a straight line but all are lame when trotted in a circle with the affected leg on the inside on hard ground. Rarer individual cases may be lame on soft ground or when the affected limb is on the outside.

Sixty percent of horses are affected unilaterally. Of those that are affected bilaterally the lameness in the second limb may only become obvious following analgesia of the other limb.

Diagnosis

- Clinically there are no visual or palpable abnormalities of injuries of the distal portion of the DDFT. If the lesion extends proximally to the level of the digital sheath, distension may be obvious. Flexion and extension tests yield variable results and are not specific for DDFT injury.
- Regional anesthesia with palmar digital nerve blocks, coffin joint blocks or intrabursal blocks only results in complete ablation of lameness in about 10–30% of cases. An abaxial sesamoid block is usually required to abolish lameness.
- Radiography is generally normal but changes that can be found include focal osteolysis of the distal phalanx in chronic severe cases and dystrophic calcification of the digital portion of the DDFT.
- Ultrasonography can be used to visualize the distal part of the DDFT to the level of the proximal border of the navicular bone. Transcuneal echography can also be used to visualize the distal

portion of the DDFT but can be limited by the shape and hardness of the frog. False-negative results are common.

- Scintigraphy may demonstrate focal increased radiopharmaceutical uptake in bone-phase images of the region of the DDFTs insertion on the distal phalanx.

Inferior check ligament desmitis (accessory ligament of the deep digital flexor tendon)

Partial or complete tears of the inferior check ligament are common causes of lameness in sport and pleasure horses and incidence increases with age. It is more common in the forelimb but can also be seen in the hindlimb.

It is most likely related to age-related degeneration although overextension of the distal interphalangeal joint may result in acute injuries. It results in acute lameness with diffuse swelling in the proximal and middle metacarpal (metatarsal) region. Chronic cases show thickening of the tendon area with some horses developing persistent lameness and/or postural deformities resembling acquired contracted tendons.

Diagnosis, treatment and prognosis

- The condition can be suspected on the basis of clinical appearance. Ultrasonography is the diagnostic tool of choice and common changes are decreases in echogenicity and increases in the crosssectional area of the ligament. Adhesions between the ligament and DDFT/SDFT are commonly found, especially in chronic cases.
- Conservative therapy as for SDFT injuries is employed in acute cases with lesions healing more rapidly than SDFT lesions.
- Physiotherapy consisting of controlled exercise and passive manipulation can be useful in reducing adhesion formation.

Sesamoidean ligament desmopathy

Deep distal sesamoidean ligament (DDSL) injuries may be a component of fracture of the base of the sesamoids. Oblique distal sesamoidean ligament (ODSL) and straight distal sesamoidean ligament (SDSL) injuries may be seen as a result of overreach injuries or as a component of suspensory apparatus breakdown. It is thought that most injuries occur as a result of a single traumatic event. The clinical signs are variable but there is usually marked lameness. There may be distension of the digital sheath. Injuries to the ODSL can result in pain on digital flexion and hyperextension. Thickening may be palpated over the distal abaxial aspect of the affected sesamoid bone.

Diagnosis

- Lameness examination will localize lameness to the pastern area but is not specific for sesamoidean ligament injury.
- Ultrasonography of this area is difficult and requires some experience. Lesions that can be recognized are as follows:
  - **DDSL.** The ligaments may appear hypoechogenic and there may be bone remodeling at the sesamoidean and phalangeal insertions.
  - **ODSL.** Thickening and decreased echogenicity most commonly near the sesamoidean origin.
  - **SDSL.** Core lesions in the mid ligament are most common and are seen as discrete hypoechoic to anechoic areas.
- Radiography should be performed in all cases to determine if there is associated sesamoid bone pathology.
- Advanced imaging terchniques (CT and MRI) may be especially useful for not only diagnosing such lesions but determining the extent of the lesion.

Treatment and prognosis

- Conservative management as for suspensory ligament desmitis.
- The prognosis is variable and there may be persistent or recurrent lameness. The increased availability of advanced imaging is likely to provide more information on true incidence and prognosis.

- Chronic cases can be more difficult to treat and may require resection (desmotomy) of the check ligament.
- Corrective farrier work is an important part of therapy, especially in chronic cases.
- The prognosis is fair to good in acute mild cases but recurrence is common and chronic cases have a poorer prognosis.

Tenosynovitis of the tarsal sheath (thoroughpin)

The tarsal sheath is the synovial sheath of the lateral digital flexor tendon (LDF). This tendon runs over the medial aspect of the hock and sustentaculum tali of the calcaneus to join the medial flexor tendon in the proximal metatarsus to form the DDFT. Distension from whatever cause is known as thoroughpin and is visible as swelling of the proximal pouch in the distal crus, laterally and medially between the tibia and common calcaneal tendon. Idiopathic distension is the most common cause but other possible causes are direct trauma or spontaneous injury to the tendon. Injuries to the medial aspect of the hock frequently result in concurrent injury to the sustentaculum tali. Open injuries may result in septic tenosynovitis. Chronic cases frequently have adhesions within the sheath which may undergo tearing due to the large range of motion of the tendon over the sustentaculum tali. Tearing of the adhesions results in repeated hemorrhage and inflammation.

Lameness may be variable depending on the cause. Idiopathic cases are not associated with lameness. Tenosynovitis causes a moderate to severe lameness, with restricted hock flexion and decreased foot flight arc.

Diagnosis

- The swelling should be differentiated from joint or bursal swelling but clinically this is normally apparent. Pressure applied to the swelling on one side will result in corresponding enlargement of the other, confirming that the two are interconnected. 'Thoroughpin' is significantly different from the swelling found in chronic distension of the tibio-tarsal joint (bog spavin), in which the swelling is lower and pouches anteromedially. Intrathecal anesthesia of the sheath is useful to confirm pain originating from the sheath.
- Radiography including four standard views and a skyline view of the calcaneus should be obtained to assess sustentaculum tali fragmentation or erosion. It can also be used to detect the presence of lytic lesions associated with osteitis.
- A range of lesions can be found on ultrasonographic examination similar to lesions of the digital sheath.
- Adhesions when present can be large and fibrous.
- Large synovial masses may be present in chronic cases of tenosynovitis.
- LDF tendon lesions are variable and are often diffuse and longitudinal.
- Erosion of the fibrocartilage and fragmentation of the sustentaculum tali may be apparent.

Treatment and prognosis

- Conservative management is tried initially and is similar to treatment for digital tenosynovitis.
- Chronic cases are frequently unresponsive to treatment and surgical treatment may be required in these cases.
- Surgical therapy including debridement of erosive lesions and partial synovectomy can be successful in many cases.
- Horses that do not respond to this surgical therapy have a guarded prognosis.

Curb (Fig. 7.161)

The term 'curb' is used to describe any swelling of the distal, plantar aspect of the tarsus, i.e. the area affected excludes the calcaneal bursa

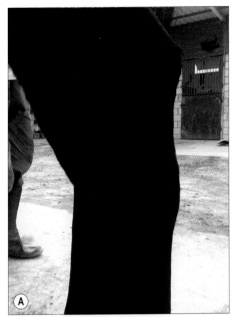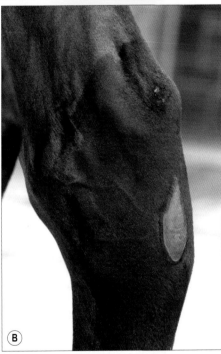

such as the SDFT, DDFT, as well as peritentinous and periligamentous structures can be involved.

Considerable variation in clinical signs can be seen depending on the structures involved and the extent of the injury. Lameness can range from none to severe. Some affected horses will show no pain on palpation or when trotted in hand but show lameness at speed. Frequently horses with curb have concurrent osteoarthritis of the hock and differentiation of the source of pain is important.

Diagnosis, treatment and prognosis

- History, clinical appearance and lameness examination are all useful but ultrasonographic examination is generally required to identify the structures involved and the extent of injuries. Radiography and scintigraphy may be useful to help differentiate other sources of pain.
- The treatment chosen depends largely on the structure involved but for clinical lesions typically involves a period of rest that may be as long as 6 months in cases of DDFT injury. Peritendon and periligamentous injury may require minimal rest and respond to local injection of corticosteroids. Due to frequent difficulty in convincing trainers that a curb that is palpably painful is the cause of their horse's lameness, some practitioners advocate the use of blisters or pin-firing as a means of enforcing rest.
- The prognosis for horses with injuries to the SDFT or DDFT is guarded for a return to previous athletic performance.

Traumatic injuries to flexor tendons and suspensory apparatus (Fig. 7.162)

Traumatic severance of both deep and superficial flexor tendons occurs quite frequently in both fore- and hindlimbs, and is usually the result of lacerations in the mid-cannon region. In the hindlimb, severance above the point of the hock has the same result, and additionally it will result in a loss of hock extension ability. Injuries below the carpus or hock result in a combination of the expected signs, with dropping of the fetlock (which in the absence of simultaneous division of the suspensory ligament does not fall to the ground under load) and lifting of the toe under weight-bearing conditions.

Complete severance or disruption of all the supporting structures of the palmar/plantar cannon results in complete collapse of the distal limb. The fetlock falls to the ground when the animal takes weight on the limb and the toe is lifted.

Spontaneous disruption/collapse of the suspensory apparatus alone in the absence of concurrent flexor tendon rupture, with or without concurrent proximal sesamoid fractures, is a common cause of acute breakdown in racing Thoroughbreds and in foals, particularly of heavy breeds. It is usually the result of extreme over-extension of the fetlock, especially where this occurs in conjunction with weakness or disease of the proximal sesamoids or their ligaments. Clinically, the fetlock is grossly swollen, and the horse is severely lame. Weight-bearing results in immediate sinking of the fetlock to the ground with obvious over-extension but the foot remains in its natural position. In some cases, the breakdown can result from rupture of the distal sesamoidean ligaments. The loss of the supporting ligaments may result in concurrent subluxation of the pastern joint. Radiographically the condition has a distinctive appearance and is often associated with (bilateral) abaxial fractures of the sesamoid bones. Concurrent rupture of the digital arteries carries a poor or hopeless prognosis.

Extensor tendon injury (Fig. 7.163)

The extensor tendons of both fore- and hindlimbs are liable to **traumatic division**, often due to wire-laceration injuries, which occur most often on the dorsal aspect of the cannon. While the clinical appearance may be dramatic, the injury has less long-term effect on the gait of the horse than flexor tendon injuries. The inability of the horse to extend the digit may result in stumbling and toe-dragging

Figure 7.161 (A, B) Image of a curb. Notice the distinct profile of the plantar aspect of the hock.

and proximal aspect of the calcaneus. There is a characteristic convex profile to the distal plantar hock that is best appreciated from the side.

Much confusion can arise due to the common use of the term 'curby hocks' which refers to a convex appearance to the distal plantar aspect of the hock associated with conformational changes. Horses with 'sickle-hock' conformation will frequently have 'curby' appearance, as will foals that have experienced crushing of the distal tarsal bones or foals with incomplete ossification of the tarsal bones. These animals may have a curby appearance without actually having a curb or they may have both concurrently. In clinical terms curb is restricted to lesions involving the soft tissues of the area. Traditionally this was thought to only involve the long plantar ligament but the increased use of ultrasonography has shown that other soft tissue structures

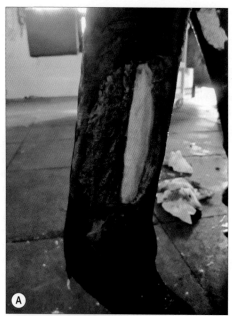

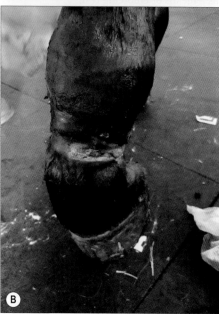

Figure 7.162 (A, B) Traumatic injury. This filly was caught in a wire fence. She sustained degloving injuries to both hindlimbs in the region of MTIII, resulting in exposure of the bone and soft tissues. However, in this case the most serious injury was sustained at the level of the pastern with complete transaction of the digital arteries. The resultant ischemic necrosis resulted in sloughing of the hoof.

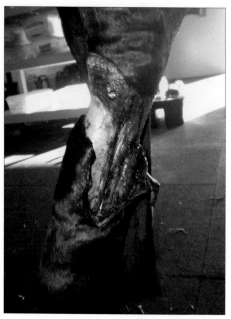

Figure 7.163 Traumatic transection of the extension tendons as a result of a wire laceration.

and the animal may even 'knuckle-over' at the fetlock. Weight-bearing is normal once the foot is placed in its natural position, and animals soon learn to compensate for the loss of extensor function by developing a 'flicking' action of the foot during motion.

Diagnosis and treatment

- The diagnosis is normally obvious and commonly associated with severe injury to other structures such as skin, subcutaneous tissues and even bone.
- Treatment is primarily aimed at control of infection by careful cleaning and debridement of the injury followed by administration of antibiotics and anti-inflammatories in addition to bandaging.

- The type of bandage used will depend on the injury present and extent of tissue contamination. It may be necessary in the early stages to have frequent bandage changes.
- Limitation of exercise will speed healing and limit the formation of granulation tissue at the site.

Dislocation of the superficial flexor tendon
(Fig. 7.164)

Dislocation of the superficial flexor tendon from the summit of the tuber calcis (luxation of the superficial flexor tendon) is a common injury, particularly of jumping horses. The dislocation occurs when the medial attachments of the tendon over the point of the hock (which appear to be weaker than the lateral attachments) rupture and allow the tendon to move laterally. Severe swelling, particularly over the point of the hock, occurs immediately, and it may be difficult to establish the diagnosis in the early stages without recourse to ultrasonography. The condition may be confused with a severe 'capped hock' but, when the swelling subsides, the tendon can always be identified visually or by palpation, lying over the lateral aspect of the calcaneus. The tendon can usually be restored to its normal position with the hock in extension, but it immediately displaces again on flexion. Initially, affected horses may be severely lame, but with prolonged rest they may regain some semblance of normality. The condition is sometimes accompanied by fractures of the calcaneus (fibular tarsal bone), and both radiographic and ultrasonographic examination should be employed to establish the extent of the damage in acute cases. Occasionally the lateral supporting band is affected, and the displacement is medial and these cases have a markedly worse prognosis.

Annular ligament syndrome (annular ligament constriction, stenosis of the fetlock canal, stenosing palmar ligament desmitis)
(Fig. 7.165)

The palmar (plantar) annular ligament of the fetlock (PAL) is a tough, fibrous and thickened portion of the fascial sheath and forms a tight retaining structure around the palmar (plantar) aspect of the fetlock.

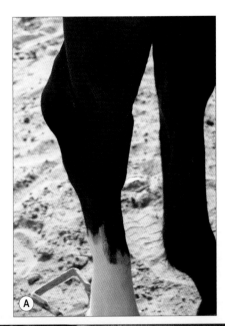

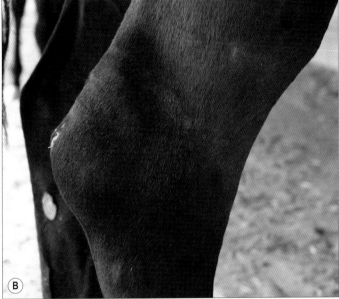

Figure 7.164 (A, B) Slipped SDFT. This occurs when the SDFT slides to the lateral aspect of the calcaneous.

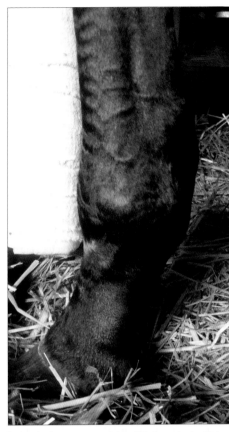

Figure 7.165 Annular ligament constriction. This horse had a thickened annular ligament that caused lameness. The horse was rested and the condition did not recur.

of the fetlock is considered pathognomonic for the disorder. This notch is due to the inability of the DFTS to distend at the site of intimate attachment between the SDFT and the dorsal surface of the thickened inelastic PAL.

Diagnosis
- Although clinical signs and lameness examination can lead to a diagnosis of the syndrome, further diagnostics are required to determine the extent of thickening of the annular ligament and determine the presence or absence of other lesions.
- Local anesthetic agents injected aseptically into the digital sheath often result in a temporary abolition of most of the lameness.
- Adhesions between the tendons, the digital sheath and the annular ligament are commonly found. In nearly all cases there will be an obvious distension of the digital sheath proximal to the annular ligament, and in some cases the superficial flexor tendon will be thickened (either as a result of the condition or as part of its etiology). These changes can often be identified by ultrasonographic examination.
- Entheseous new bone may be present at the insertions of the PAL on the palmar border of the PSBs and can be identified radiographically.

Treatment
- Acute cases can be treated with rest and topical and systemic anti-inflammatories.
- Many chronic cases require desmotomy of the PAL but the selection of cases depends somewhat on what other lesions are present as determined by ultrasonographic findings and the intended use of the horse.

The PAL functions to counteract the tendency of the PSBs to move dorsally and abaxially during weight-bearing.

Thickening and desmitis of the PAL have been associated with a number of different etiologies. Direct impact, laceration, overextension of the fetlock, excessive swelling of the DFTS and chronic inflammation of the DFTS have all been implicated as causes. Thickening of the PAL is the response to inflammation; this results in a relative stenosis within the fetlock canal leading to increased pressure from the tendons and leading to further inflammation, fibrosis and thickening. There is an increased incidence in association with age, certain breeds (Peruvian Pasofino) and location (hindlimbs).

The condition can present as an acute lameness with localized heat, pain and swelling. The chronic condition is more common with a mild to moderate lameness that fails to improve with rest and worsens with exercise. A fetlock flexion test exacerbates lameness and distension of the DFTS with a notch in the palmar (plantar) outline

- The prognosis after desmotomy for soundness is good in horses with desmitis alone but less favorable in cases with concurrent tenosynovitis.
- **Swelling of the flexor tendons in the carpal sheath or contraction of the carpal retinaculum** (often secondary to an accessory carpal bone fracture) may result in a similar problem on the palmar aspect of the carpus. This is frequently referred to as the **carpal tunnel syndrome**.

Upward fixation of the patella (Fig. 7.166)

Upward fixation of the patella occurs when the stifle joint is fully extended and the medial patellar ligament hooks over the medial trochlea of the femur, thus locking the reciprocal apparatus with the limb in extension. The condition is frequently seen in horses having a 'straight' hindleg conformation and in stabled horses which on rising, extend one or other leg backward in a stretching effort. However, in some cases, trauma, lack of muscular fitness and poor body condition may also be significant. The disorder is characterized by an abrupt, momentary or complete, recurrent locking of the limb in an extended position. The stifle and hock cannot flex but the fetlock is normal, although usually the fetlock is flexed with the toe resting on the ground. Momentary, milder forms of the condition are manifest by an apparent 'catching' or clicking of the stifle during movement without the limb becoming fixed in extension. These cases will often be noted to drag the toe and will invariably be reluctant to walk up and down slopes. At the trot, the foot may be seen to hesitate momentarily, as it leaves the ground. In some cases the signs are very intermittent and/or subtle. The 'locking' may only be shown for limited numbers of strides, the gait then becoming quite normal. In cases of complete fixation release of the entrapped medial patella ligament from the medial trochlear groove is often accompanied by an audible snapping sound. The condition is commonly bilateral, although one side may be more severely affected than the other.

Diagnosis

- The clinical features of the disorder are almost pathognomonic but careful clinical and lameness examination should be performed in order to determine if there is an accompanying stifle disease such as osteochondrosis.
- Radiographic examination of the stifles is generally recommended to determine the existence of any predisposing factors or secondary conditions such as fragmentation of the patella.

Treatment and prognosis

- In those young horses in which the condition develops as a result of loss of muscular condition a conservative approach involving muscle toning and fitness, is sometimes effective. These programs generally involve limiting box rest combined with increasing exercise such as lunging. A large number of horses respond to conditioning programs.
- Surgical sectioning of the medial patellar is indicated in young horses or poorly conditioned horses which have not improved following conservative therapy, and in horses in which lameness has developed as a result of the condition.

Synovial bursae (Figs. 7.167 & 7.168)

Synovial bursae occurring naturally or those acquired in response to persistent insult act as cushions between two moving parts, or at points of unusual pressure, such as between bony prominences and tendons. Naturally formed bursae are present in constant positions and are present before birth, while the acquired bursae are usually formed subcutaneously over bony prominences such as the olecranon and the calcaneus (tuber calcis). The formation of an **acquired bursa** is usually in response to persistent pressure over bony prominences and, although they may be large, they are seldom inflamed under normal circumstances.

Occasionally they arise without any obvious predisposing cause at sites in which traumatic injuries are not common and no surface evidence for trauma can be found. These may be a result of leakage of synovial fluid from adjacent joints or tendon sheaths, and may reach considerable size. Acquired superficial bursae are seldom painful and, unless they attain great size, or become infected, they remain cold and painless.

Acquired subcutaneous bursae commonly develop over the olecranon of draught breeds in particular, a condition known as 'capped elbow'. In some cases, the skin over the area is traumatized and the acquired bursa may become infected ('shoe boil'). In most cases these are formed in response to direct trauma, often from the shoe or hoof when the animal is lying down. Horses which remain recumbent for any reason are also liable to the development of this

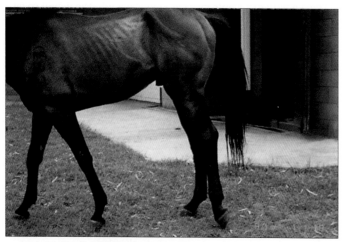

Figure 7.166 Upward fixation of the patella. The limb is locked in extension as the horse attempts to draw the limb forward. Note the flexed fetlock and pastern while stifle and hock joints are fixed in extension.

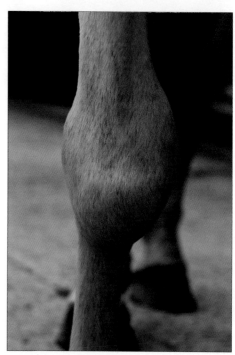

Figure 7.167 Carpal bursitis 'hygroma'.

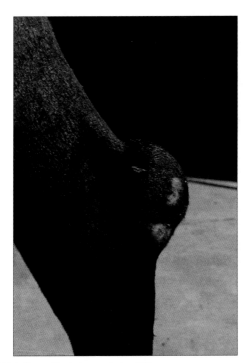

Figure 7.168 Capped hock (traumatic bursitis).

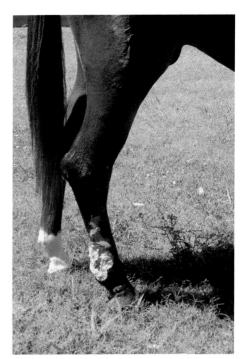

Figure 7.169 Severe cellulitis in this horse occurred following an intralesional injection of the SDFT. The cellulitis which was untreated for a number of weeks resulted in sloughing of large areas of the soft tissue.

bursa. Gaited or Standardbred horses may cause damage to this area during exercise.

A large acquired **carpal bursa** often develops as a result of direct and repeated trauma, associated with lying down on hard surfaces such as concrete or from habitual banging of the knee on stable doors. At this site the skin overlying the bursal swelling is usually thickened, and the lining of the bursa may become thickened giving a firm, rather than a fluid-filled, texture.

Another common site for acquired bursa formation is over the point of the hock ('**capped hock**'). Again, this is usually the result of trauma from kicking out against a wall or trailer tailgate, and may develop very rapidly. Although in some cases there is a transient mild lameness, most are not lame.

Diagnosis and treatment
- Diagnosis is usually obvious visually but occasionally additional diagnostic techniques such as radiography may be required to eliminate differentials, especially in cases in which there is infection present.
- Uncomplicated cases are frequently treated with topical applications of anti-inflammatories in addition to improving management such as deeper bedding, padding on doors and walls, etc.
- In the event that they become infected and/or burst, they often fail to heal, discharging copious amounts of infected fluid and may then become significant causes of lameness. Exuberant granulation tissue is a common sequel.

Non-infectious bursitis
Non-infectious bursitis can occur with tendonitis of the biceps brachii or osteitis of the humeral tubercles. Bicipital bursitis is most often encountered in draught horses with ill-fitting collars, and is probably the result of direct trauma and persistent pressure. The lameness seen is variable and generally improves with local analgesia.

Diagnosis and treatment
- The diagnosis is confirmed by ultrasonography that demonstrates an increased amount of fluid within the bursa.

- Intrathecal administration of hyalurone and triamcinalone combined with controlled exercise and elimination of predisposing factors normally yields good results.

Tendons, ligaments and bursae: Infectious disorders

Infectious bursitis (Fig. 7.169)
Inflammation of bursae, in response to infection or trauma, results in bursitis. Infection of natural bursae is more unusual because they usually have deeper locations. However the **atlantal bursa**, which lies between the ligamentum nuchae and the rectus capitis dorsalis major muscle, is liable to both aseptic inflammation and to infection, either spontaneously or more commonly from wounds in the poll area, a condition known as '**poll evil**'. Initially the bursa is swollen, the head is held extended, and movement of the head and neck is strongly resisted. Persistent inflammation of the bursa results in progressive thickening of the bursal membrane. Ultimately this extends to the funicular portion of the ligamentum nuchae, and the bursa ruptures onto the surface. Necrosis and infection of the ligament and the bursa result in a non-healing, chronic, discharging, fistulous condition. This has a characteristic appearance, and discharges a clear serosanguineous exudate or (in older lesions) a creamy, yellow purulent material. Historically, this condition (and fistulous withers) was often associated with primary systemic infection with *Brucella* spp. or *Actinobacillus* spp. bacteria, but once the affected bursa ruptures, secondary, complicating bacteria are often involved.

The **supraspinous bursa**, which lies between the dorsal spines of the third and fourth thoracic vertebrae and the *ligamentum nuchae*, in the withers, may, similarly, become infected by hematogenous spread or by direct inoculation via a wound in the area. *Brucella abortus* has been identified as being the major cause for this infection, but this is probably less significant nowadays and a wide variety of bacterial species may be involved. The inflamed bursa increases in size and, with the considerable forces applied to the surface by the ligamentum nuchae, enlarges into the tissues of the withers. The horse is usually reluctant to move, and marked pain and swelling are evident on palpation of the withers. Eventually the bursa bursts onto the skin. **Fistulous withers** is characterized by the presence of chronic discharging sinus tracts between the bursa and the skin, most often producing profuse quantities of cloudy, serosanguineous and purulent exudate.

Diagnosis and treatment
- Diagnosis is generally made on clinical appearance but radiographic studies (+/– contrast) may be used to identify the full extent of the problem and the possibility of concurrent osteomyelitis or sequestra arising from traumatic damage to the spines of the thoracic vertebrae.
- Care must be taken in interpretation, as separate centers of ossification of the dorsal spinous processes of the cranial thoracic vertebrae are usually irregular in appearance, and this should not be misinterpreted as a sign of bone infection.
- In the treatment of these conditions meticulous surgical debridement and drainage are paramount.

Tendons, ligaments and bursae: Neoplastic disorders

There are no significant neoplastic disorders of the tendons and ligaments of the horse and secondary tumors within these are also not reported.

References and further reading

Ball, M.A., 2000. White line disease. J Equine Vet Sci 20 (2), 114.

O'Grady, S.E., 2002. White line disease. An update. Equine Vet Educ 14 (1),51–55.

Robinson, N.E. (ed.), 1992. Current Therapy in Equine Medicine, third ed. WB Saunders, Philadelphia, PA, USA.

Ross, M.W., Dyson, S.J. (eds.), 2010. Diagnosis and Management of Lameness in the Horse, second ed. WB Saunders, St Louis, MO, USA.

Stashak, T.S., 1985. Adams Lameness in Horses, fourth ed. Lea & Fabiger, Philadelphia, PA, USA.

Turner, T.A., 2000. White line disease. Equine Vet Educ 2, 73–76.

CHAPTER 8

Muscle

CHAPTER CONTENTS

Congenital/developmental disorders

Hyperkalemic periodic paralysis (HYPP) (Fig. 8.1)

This is a disease of Quarterhorses and their crosses. To date it has only been traced to descendants of the stallion 'Impressive'. It is transmitted as an autosomal dominant trait. Most cases are seen in 2–3-year-old well-muscled males but cases have been seen in foals as young as 4 months.

Heterozygotes and homozygotes show clinical signs, with signs often being more severe and detected earlier in the latter. The most common sign is muscle fasciculations. This can be followed by muscle spasms, weakness and recumbency. Death can occur due to cardiac or respiratory failure. Increased respiratory rates are common during attacks. The pharyngeal and laryngeal muscles can also be affected resulting in stridor or dyspnea.

Attacks may be precipitated by stressors such as transport, showing, change in weather and general anesthesia. Hyperkalemia is common during an attack although episodes without hyperkalemia have been reported.

Diagnosis and treatment

- Definitive diagnosis is by genetic testing. This can be performed on whole blood or hair root. The American Quarter Horse Association (AQHA) will accept HYPP test results only if performed through a licensed laboratory. Testing kits for non-registration purposes are available from the AQHA.
- Diagnosed subjectively by clinical signs and signalment.
- Post-mortem samples that can be collected if a horse has died during a suspected attack are: hair samples for DNA testing and aqueous humor for potassium concentration.
- Mild cases can be treated with light exercise, by feeding a readily absorbable source of carbohydrate (oats), and/or with acetazolamide (3 mg/kg orally).
- For severe cases, the following treatment is recommended: intravenous administration of 5% dextrose with sodium bicarbonate (1–2 mEq/kg) and intravenous administration of 23% calcium gluconate (0.2–0.4 ml/kg) diluted in 5% dextrose (4.4–6.6 ml/kg).

Control

- Management is an important feature of control and should include regular exercise and ideally frequent paddock turnout. Wholegrain feeds should be fed instead of sweet feed. Avoid feeds with high potassium content such as alfalfa and replace with timothy or Bermuda grass hay. Give several small feeds daily at regular intervals.
- Avoid stressors such as rapid changes in diet, exposure to cold or overexertion.

- Acetazolamide (2–4 mg/kg q 8–12 h) has been recommended to decrease the frequency and severity of episodes. The daily dose can be decreased over time until the lowest effective dose is reached.

Prognosis

The prognosis for normal activity is considered good. Counseling about breeding such horses should be offered.

Myotonia congenita (Fig. 8.2)

Myotonia congenita is a rare condition of Quarterhorse (QH) and QH cross foals that results in periods of involuntary muscle contractions following stimulation or start of exercise. Affected animals usually show clinical signs within the first year and often have well-developed musculature and a pelvic limb stiffness/lameness. The well-muscled appearance is similar to that seen in HYPP-affected animals.

Only the skeletal muscle is involved in myontonia congenita which means that progression of clinical signs is not seen beyond 12 months of age. A separate condition known as myotonic dystrophy has also been reported in a QH foal. This condition progresses to severe muscle atrophy and involvement of other organs.

Diagnosis

- Frequently a tentative diagnosis can be made on the basis of breed, age and clinical signs.
- Definitive diagnosis requires EMG examination. The pathognomonic finding is described as crescendo-decresendo, high-frequency repetitive bursts with a characteristic 'dive-bomber' sound.
- Muscle biopsies are not useful for diagnosis as they may be normal.

Treatment

- Most treatment modalities have poor efficacy. Phenytoin has been used in a number of affected horses with reported success.
- Other drugs that may be beneficial are quinine and procainamide. These are used to treat a similar condition in man and dogs.

Prognosis

- Depends on the severity of signs but is considered poor in most cases.
- Some cases are mild and show a decrease in signs with age. Other more severely affected animals may develop extensive fibrosis with resultant restriction of movement.
- Some cases have also had concurrent HYPP.

Glycogen branching enzyme deficiency

This is an autosomal-recessive glycogen storage disorder that affects neonatal Quarterhorses or Paint horses and has been identified in

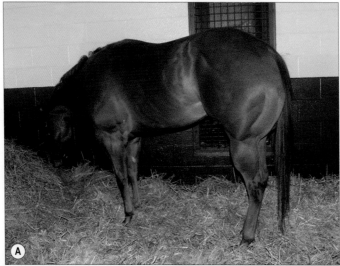

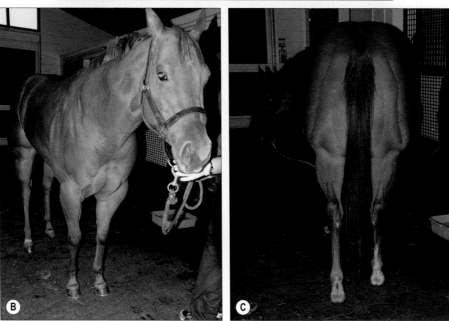

Figure 8.1 (A–C) Typical heavily muscled body type associated with hyperkalemic periodic paralysis.

Differential diagnosis:
- Weakness, muscle fasciculations and collapse
- Generalized muscle weakness of neurological origin (e.g. equine degenerative myeloencephalopathy) or neuromuscular origin (e.g. botulism)
- Encephalitis (e.g. West Nile virus infection) (can cause muscle fasiculations)
- Electrolyte disorders (e.g. hypocalcemia)
- Exertional rhabdomyolysis
- Narcolepsy/cataplexy
- Syncope
- Seizures
- Nutritional myopathy
- Dyspnea
- Obstruction of the respiratory tract (e.g. foreign body)
- Pharyngeal/laryngeal paralysis (e.g. secondary to nerve damage in strangles cases).

aborted fetuses. As a result of the specific mutation certain tissues such as the brain, liver, cardiac and skeletal muscle cannot store and mobilize glycogen to maintain normal glucose hemostasis. Approximately 8% of both Quarterhorses and Paint horses are carriers of GBED. In one study 2–4% of aborted fetuses were homozygous for GBED. The condition is likely underdiagnosed due to the lack of readily available testing and the similarity in clinical signs between this and many other neonatal conditions.

The most frequently encountered clinical signs are weakness, hypothermia, hypoglycemia, flexural limb deformities and ventilatory failure. None of these signs is pathognomonic and all are easily confused with other conditions.

Diagnosis and treatment
- The most accurate form of diagnosis is through genetic testing but there is currently limited availability.

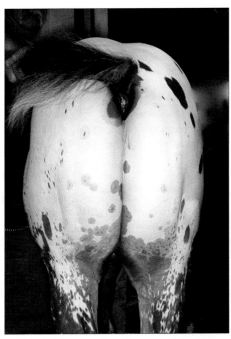

Figure 8.2 Myotonia congenita. Typical double muscled appearance. Many of the affected horses are quarter horses which may also be affected with HYPP. Reproduced from McAuliffe SB, Slovis, NM (eds). *Color Atlas of Diseases and Disorders of the Foal* (2008), with permission from Elsevier.

Differential diagnosis:
• HYPP
• Myotonic dystrophy
• PSSM type 1.

• Other findings are not consistent but include:
  • Basophilic globules and eosinophilic crystalline material in hematoxylin and eosin stains
  • Periodic acid-Schiff (PAS) staining of cardiac and muscle sections may contain PAS-positive globular inclusions.
• There is no effective treatment and therefore early identification and euthanasia are is essential to avoid unnecessary costs in neonatal care untis.

Polysaccharide storage myopathy (PSSM)

(Figs. 8.3 & 8.4)
This disorder is characterized by higher glycogen concentrations and abnormal granular amylase-resistant inclusions in skeletal muscle. There are two types of PSSM: type 1 PSSM refers to horses with a specific glycogen synthase 1 gene (GYS1) mutation. This is commonly found in Quarterhorses, draft horse breeds and their crosses; type 2 PSSM is not related to a mutation in GYS1 and occurs in Quarter-horses and a large number of Warmblood breeds.

The clinical signs seen are somewhat breed-dependent:

• ***Quarterhorses.*** The most common signs are firm, painful muscles, stiffness, fasciculations, weakness, sweating and reluctance to move. The hindquarters are most commonly affected but other muscles can also be involved. Signs of pain can be severe and long-lasting. Signs can be seen with minimal work especially in horses that have been rested for several days or are on a high-grain diet. There is no specific association to gender, body type or temperament. Average age of onset of clinical signs is 5 years but signs have been seen in horses as young as 1 year of age. Serum CK and AST activities are often persistently high in affected horses with median values reported at 2 809 and 1 792 U/L, respectively.

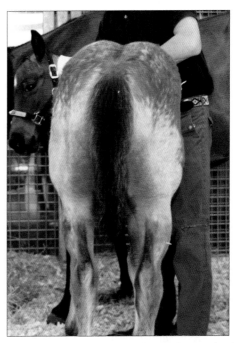

Figure 8.3 Polysaccharide storage myopathy. Note the firm muscles of the hindquarters in this young Quarterhorse with type 1 PSSM.

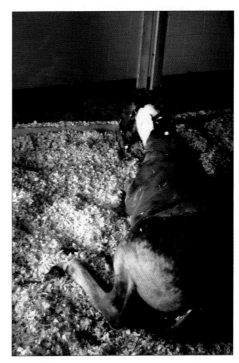

Figure 8.4 Polysaccharide storage myopathy. Generalized weakness and inability to stand.

• ***Draft horses.*** Many affected horses do not have clinical signs. Rhabdomyolysis and myoglobinuria can be seen in horses that are fed high-grain diets, exercised irregularly or have little turnout. Signs can also be seen with general anesthesia. Again there is no gender predilection and the mean age of onset of clinical signs is 8 years. The median CK and AST levels in affected horses are reported to be 459 and 537 U/L, respectively.

- *Warmbloods.* Warmbloods may have either type 1 or type 2 PSSM depending on the crosses from which they are derived. The most common clinical signs noted are painful, firm back and hindquarter muscles. Overt rhabdomyolysis is not that commonly seen. The mean age of onset is 8–11 years of age and the median CK and AST activities are 323 and 331 U/L, respectively.

Diagnosis and treatment

- Type 1 PSSM can be diagnosed through genetic testing which is available through the University of Minnesota. Muscle biopsies can also be used with the characteristic findings of amylase-resistant granular polysaccharide in amylase periodic acid-Schiff (PAS) stains.
- There is no genetic test available for type 2 and muscle biopsies demonstrate increased or abnormal PAS-positive material that is usually amylase-sensitive.
- However, because the diagnosis of PSSM based on muscle biopsies alone is quite subjective it is important that the horse is thoroughly evaluated to rule out other conditions.
- Episodes of rhabdomyolysis need specific treatment.

Management

- Horses with PSSM should ideally have some form of turnout available.
- Exercise regimens should only be implemented after there has been adequate time allowed for dietary changes (2 weeks). The duration and not just the intensity of exercise is important and exercise should be gradually introduced and consistently performed. It is also important to minimize the number of days without some form of exercise.
- Dietary management is very important in affected horses and should first consist of reaching the ideal body weight for the horse. Once this has been done the dietary modifications should combine reducing glucose load and providing fat as an alternative energy source. There are now a wide variety of commercially produced diets available for horses with PSSM. The basic dietary principle is that less than 10% of digestible energy (DE) be provided in the form of starch and at least 13% in the form of fat.

Recurrent exertional rhabdomyolysis (RER)

There are many causes of exertional rhabdomyolysis in horses. The term recurrent exertional rhabdomyolysis is used to describe one form that appears to have a heritable basis in Thoroughbred horses. The specific cause has not however been identified although it is believed that there is abnormal regulation of intracellular calcium in skeletal muscle. Clinical signs are more common in fillies especially those with a nervous temperament. These signs include hindlimb pain and lameness, high respiratory rate, sweating, a reluctance to move and colic signs such as repeated pawing. These signs may last several hours without treatment. Clinical signs are more frequently seen in horses fed high-grain diets and concurrent lameness. The type of exercise is also important with episodes being more common in racehorses restrained to a slow canter, while post-race episodes are infrequent. In some cases episodes can be seen without any exercise or after transportation and in these cases may be more related to temperament and nervousness associated with anticipated work or racing.

Diagnosis

- Evaluation of serum CK and AST levels is used by many to identify poor performance in association with subclinical episodes of RER. In doing such tests it is important to be consistent with regard to sampling times. The ideal is 4–6 hours after exercise but in many cases due to yard management this is not possible and then samples should be routinely collected at a standardized time in relation to the previous day's work.
- If serum muscle enzymes are normal but RER is still believed to be a cause of poor performance an exercise test can be performed with samples taken before and 4–6 hours after exercise. Exercise for such tests should consist of 15 minutes of collected trotting. A 3–4-fold rise in serum ck activity is indicative of subclinical muscle damage.
- While there is currently no genetic testing available for RER horses it is an area of active research and such a test may be available in the near future.

Treatment

- The goals of therapy for specific episodes of exertional rhabdomyolysis are relieving pain and anxiety, replacing fluid and electrolyte losses and maintaining renal function.
- Non-steroidal anti-inflammatories are frequently used to relieve pain and in mild cases may be the only treatment necessary. However, they should be cautious or combined with intravenous fluid therapy in dehydrated horses.
- Severely affected horses, dehydrated horses or horses with myoglobinuria should receive intravenous fluids. Hyperkalemia can occur in some horses and can be treated by the administration of isotonic sodium chloride. Some horses will be hypocalcemic and will require supplementation with calcium.
- Other drug therapies include dantrium sodium (4 mg/kg PO q 4–6 h) which decreases muscle contracture and may help prevent further muscle necrosis. Methocarbamol (a muscle relaxant) (5–22 mg/kg IV slowly) produces variable results perhaps as a reflection of the dose used. Corticosteroids are advocated by some especially if the horse is recumbent. DMSO has been used as an anti-oxidant, anti-inflammatory and osmotic diuretic. Tranquilizers may help relieve anxiety and the perpetuation of an episode.

Management

- Efforts to minimize stress for individual horses should be made; this may include regular turnout perhaps with a companion, a regular routine with regard to feeding and exercise and tailoring other management factors for specific needs, e.g. some horses find the use of mechanical walkers stressful while others may get overexcited if handwalked.
- Exercise should be consistent and daily, avoiding trigger factors such as fighting to maintain a certain speed.
- Feed programs should also be individually tailored with the recommendation that less than 20% of DE be supplied by starch and at least 15% be supplied by fat. Increasing the frequency of feeding may help reduce anxiety associated with feeding and may also encourage increased caloric intake in fussy feeders.
- Exercising horses require daily dietary supplementation with sodium and chloride. This is provided in most cases by commercial feeds but can also be provided by loose salt. Other electrolytes may also be required, especially if horses are exercising in hot, humid climates. Historically there have been supplements given with a sodium bicarbonate base based on the former belief that lactic acidosis contributed to exertional rhabdomyolysis. Given current knowledge that this is not actually the case there is no basis for the administration of such supplements.
- Various other medications such as tranquilizers, dantrium sodium, phenytoin, hormones and thyroid supplements have been given to horses with RER. The need for such medications should be evaluated on an individual basis but it is important to remember that many of these may result in positives in post-competition doping tests.

Malignant hyperthermia

This is a rare autosomal-dominant mutation of the skeletal muscle ryanodine receptor gene (RYR1) that results in marked hyperthermia and metabolic acidosis during inhalational anesthesia.

Diagnosis and treatment

- To date the condition has only been reported in Quarterhorses and could be suspected in any horse of that breed showing classical signs of lactic acidosis and hyperthermia (rectal temp >40°C).
- There is a genetic test available from the University of Minnesota.
- Pre-treatment with oral dantrolene sodium (4 mg/kg) 30–60 minutes prior to anesthesia is ideal but requires recognizing at-risk horses.
- Once an episode is underway there is little effective therapy; despite efforts to cool horses and treat acidosis with intravenous sodium bicarbonate the two reported cases both died of cardiac arrest.

Non-infectious/traumatic disorders

Gastrocnemius muscle rupture (Fig. 8.5)

Rupture of the gastrocnemius muscle can occur in young foals as a result of overextension while chasing the dam or as a foaling injury. It can also occur secondary to severe flexor tendon laxity or tarsal contracture.

Rupture of this muscle results in a typical crouched stance and inability to bear weight on the affected limb. The gastrocnemius may be markedly swollen secondary to hemorrhage. It is not uncommon to see anemia secondary to blood loss. Foals have died acutely secondary to a severe gastrocnemius rupture and hemorrhage.

Treatment and prognosis

- Treatment most commonly involves placing a Thomas-Schroeder splint for 1 month while confining the foal to stall rest. Following removal of the splint box rest is required for a further month.
- Care should be taken in constructing the splint to ensure it is a correct fit for the foal in question.
- Careful padding and regular reassessments are required to ensure that pressure sores do not develop.
- Tube casts can also be used but must be changed frequently and cast sores are inevitable.

- The prognosis for athletic function is guarded, but is reported to be better in foals which respond well to initial therapy.

Exertional rhabdomyolysis (Figs. 8.6 & 8.7)

Although most horses that will experience episodes of exertional rhabdomyolysis have an underlying myopathy overexertion can lead to rhabdomyolysis in any horse. It is particularly seen as part of the exhausted horse syndrome in 3-day event and endurance horses. Many of these horses will have multiple organ failure in addition to rhabdomyolysis as a result of a combination of factors including exertion past their fitness level, fluid and electrolyte losses, depletion of energy stores and extremes of environmental conditions.

Diagnosis and treatment

- The signs of rhabdomyolysis may be overshadowed by other signs in exhausted horses where there is frequently a marked tachycardia and tachypnea. Synchronous diaphragmatic flutter may be seen in some cases as well as marked depression, dehydration, anorexia, elevated body temperature, poor sweating response, ileus and muscle cramps.

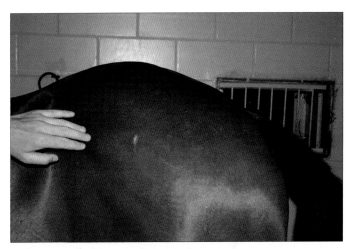

Figure 8.6 Exertional rhabdomyolysis. This is the sporadic form where this mare was temporarily separated from her foal and ran her paddock for 20 minutes before they could be reunited. Soon afterwards the mare showed stiffness, myoglobinuria and extreme hardening of the gluteal muscles.

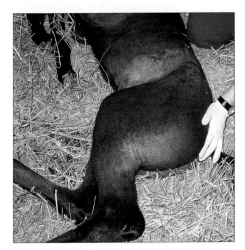

Figure 8.5 Gastrocnemius muscle rupture. Reproduced from McAuliffe SB, Slovis, NM (eds). *Color Atlas of Diseases and Disorders of the Foal* (2008), with permission from Elsevier.

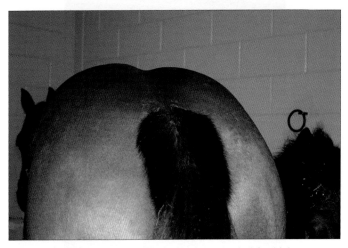

Figure 8.7 Hardening of the muscles (more obvious on the left side) (same horse as Fig. 8.6).

- Non-exhausted horses that have experienced exercise beyond their fitness level will show pain and firmness of the back and hind leg muscles in particular. There can be marked sweating and signs of anxiety or colic.
- Laboratory findings in the exhausted horse can include metabolic alkalosis, paradoxical aciduria, hypokalemia, hyponatremia, hypochloremia, increases in CK, AST, LDH, proteinuria, azotemia, lipidosis and elevations of serum creatinine and hepatic enzymes.
- In non-exhausted horses treatment is the same as other cases of rhabdomyolysis (see p. 298).
- In exhausted horses early and aggressive fluid therapy is required. Careful attention should be paid to electrolyte imbalances and their correction and it is important to offer feed. Cooling of hyperthermic horses is also important and is often best achieved by the use of cold water body spray fans.

Post-anesthetic myelopathy (Fig. 8.8)

Post-anesthetic myelopathy has been reported in several young, heavy horses. Halothane anesthesia was used in all cases. Signs ranged from difficulty standing, to tetraplegia with flaccid paralysis and anesthesia of the pelvic limbs. Affected horses became recumbent or remained in lateral recumbency until euthanasia 1–8 days later. The syndrome is thought to involve a number of factors including systemic arterial hypotension, local venous congestion caused by halothane anesthesia and compression of the caudal vena cava by abdominal viscera.

Diagnosis is based on history and clinical signs. The prognosis is hopeless in the cases that have been described but milder cases may not be recognized.

Post-anesthetic myopathy

Myopathy due to prolonged recumbency is relatively common, and represents a complication of general anesthesia, in heavy horses in particular. Characteristically the condition affects the dependent muscles. Thus, heavy animals maintained in dorsal recumbency develop an ischemic myopathy in the lumbar muscles, while the muscles of one fore- or hindlimb (or both) may be affected in those held in lateral recumbency for extended periods. The clinical features of such a myopathy are obviously related to the specific muscles affected and the extent of the damage. Affected muscle masses may be hard, hot and grossly swollen but may, equally, be normal in

appearance while being extremely painful and non-functional. In the forelimb, the triceps mass is the most commonly affected and although it is seldom grossly swollen as a result, muscle function is severely compromised. Affected horses present with a lameness and weakness which is very similar in appearance to radial paralysis. In some cases there may also be components of neurological dysfunction at the same time due to local nerve compression.

Diagnosis and treatment

- Typically, the onset of the clinical effects of these myopathies is immediately or shortly after recovery from anesthesia and this aids diagnosis.
- Muscle enzyme levels are almost always very elevated.
- Supportive care results in most horses responding well to therapy and making a full recovery within 1–2 days.
- In rarer cases, especially where there has been local nerve damage, some muscle atrophy may develop.

Traumatic injuries to the muscles (Figs. 8.9–8.15)

These are many and varied. Disruption of muscle masses without concurrent breaks in the skin presents two major clinical syndromes.

Where the muscles of the abdominal wall are ruptured, an **acquired hernia (rupture)** may develop. While in many cases these appear to cause little difficulty, complications may arise when abdominal viscera become entrapped within the hernia and more particularly when these become incarcerated therein.

Rupture of muscles, occurring as a result of excessive or violent contraction, may cause obvious distortion of the muscle belly itself when there is simultaneous rupture of the muscle sheath (epimysium). More often such disruption causes little overt swelling, with the hemorrhage and disruption remaining within the sheath. Under these circumstances, healing is accompanied by scarring, fibrosis and possibly by calcification. Individual muscles undergoing fibrous metaplasia following this type of injury may ultimately become severely wasted.

Diagnosis

- Clinical signs are sufficient for a diagnosis in cases of hernias but ultrasonographic examination of the hernia contents may be

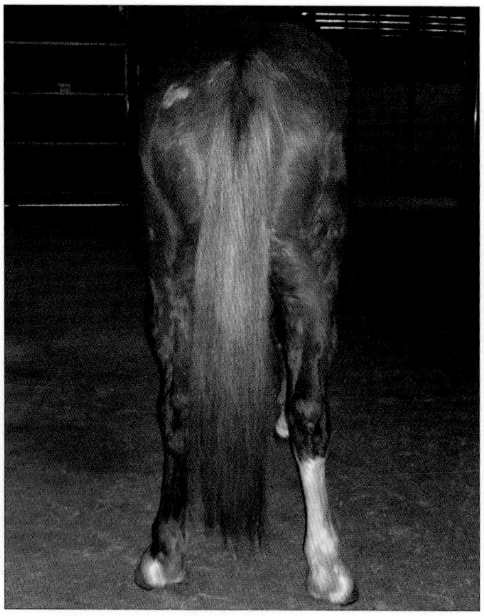

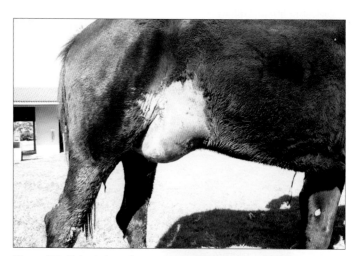

Figure 8.9 Abdominal muscle tears are most commonly traumatic in origin or can be related to increased abdominal weight associated with late pregnancy or hydrops of the fetal fluids. This mare had unsuccessfully tried to jump a gate, on which she became hung from the backlegs with a resultant extensive tear of the abdominal musculature and related hernia of abdominal contents. This photo was taken 3 weeks after the initial injury.

Figure 8.8 Post-anesthetic myopathy. Note the swelling of the gluteal muscles on the right side.

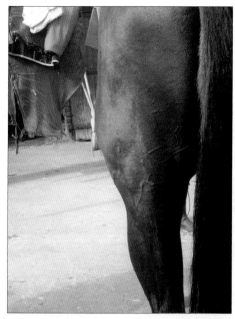

Figure 8.10 This horse presented with swelling over the lateral aspect of the stifle. Ultrasound revealed a tear and hematoma of the quadriceps. The horse was not lame. He was limited to hand walking for 2 weeks and made an uneventful recovery.

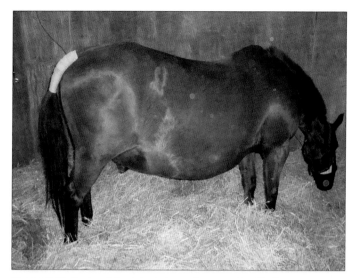

Figure 8.12 Tearing of the abdominal musculature may be difficult to differentiate from tears of the prepubic tendon in mares in advanced pregnancy; also, in many cases, both may co-exist. Cranial movement of the mammary gland (as seen in this image) may help with differentiation, but ultrasonography should be performed to determine the extent of involvement of the musculature.

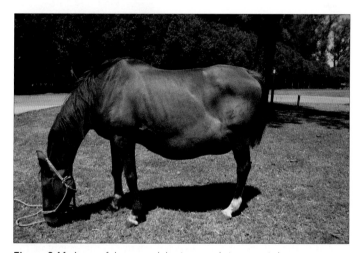

Figure 8.11 A tear of the rectus abdominus muscle in a mare in late pregnancy. There is a large amount of associated edema that makes the affected area appear much larger than it actually is. Ultrasonographic imaging localized the tear to an area of 20 cm in diameter. This mare was treated with placement of a belly band, exercise restriction and anti-inflammatories. She later foaled with minimal assistance.

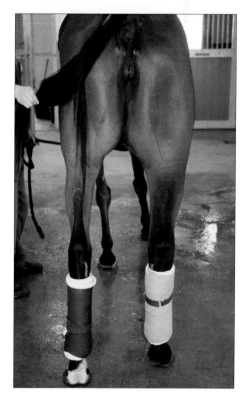

Figure 8.13 Muscle tear with large intramuscular hematoma formation.

required, especially if the horse suddenly becomes painful or the hernia dramatically increases in size or there is associated edema.

- Muscle rupture without herniation or swelling can be diagnosed ultrasonographically. Depending on the stage at which the horse is examined there may be obvious hemorrhage within the muscle body or there may be evidence of fibrosis.

Treatment

- Treatment for individual cases varies. Hernias may be closed surgically either with sutures or with a mesh, depending on the size and location of the hernia.

- Muscle tears or ruptures of other muscle masses may require specific physical therapy to avoid excess restriction associated with fibrosis especially in competitive horses.

- More dramatic wounds, involving the laceration of skin and underlying muscles, are common in the horse. While the damage may look dramatic, the consequences are often surprisingly limited, with healing and wound contracture occurring rapidly in the absence of complicating factors such as sequestration of bone or foreign

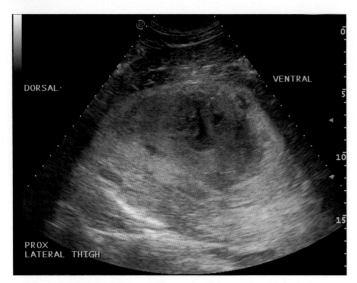

Figure 8.14 Ultrasound image of the horse in Fig. 8.13 demonstrating a large intramuscular hematoma.

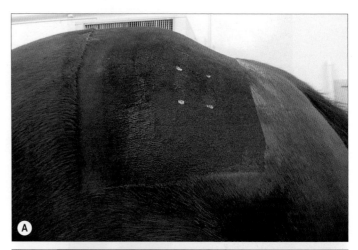

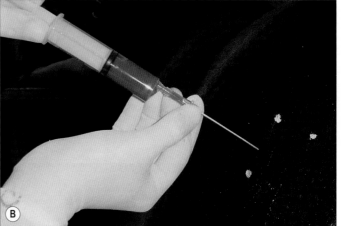

Figure 8.16 (A, B) Injection site abscess. (A) Swelling over the affected area. (B) Aspiration of abscess contents.

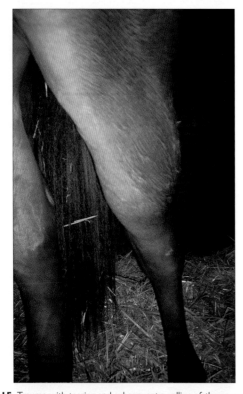

Figure 8.15 Trauma with tearing and subsequent swelling of the common digital extensor muscle.

matter, infection and/or excessive movement. Generally, wounds involving large amounts of muscle are better prospects for spontaneous healing than those occurring in areas where no, or limited, underlying muscle is present, such as the distal limb and those wounds complicated by other damage such as to tendons and joints.

Muscle necrosis (Figs. 8.16–8.19)

There are many possible causes of muscle necrosis. These include: infectious, toxic, nutritional, ischemic or in a large number of cases idiopathic. The necrosis itself may be focal or generalized. Focal

necrosis is commonly seen in foals after intramuscular administration of drugs or following snake or spider bites.

Venomous snakes and spiders occur world-wide and the effects of their toxins are varied. Many have profound neurological and/or circulatory effects but many also have strong cytotoxic properties. Most such bites are also infected by pathogenic bacteria and lead to localized myonecrosis. As the effects of envenomation are closely related to the volume of toxin injected relative to the weight of the animal, few snake bites are capable of killing a horse directly but the secondary effects of clostridial myonecrosis and swelling may have a fatal result.

Necrosis and bacterial infection of muscle masses usually occur as a result of infected wounds, or from iatrogenic damage following the injection of irritant or caustic drugs. The injection of antibiotics seldom results in local infection, but quite frequently intramuscular injections result in local myonecrosis and infection subsequently develops. The injection of other drugs more commonly results in infected sites, and the most serious of these infections are those due to *Clostridium* spp. bacteria, in which gas production and extensive myonecrosis produce a life-threatening situation. Local damage of this type within a muscle may have very serious immediate toxic consequences, and affect the function of the specific mass of muscle, adjacent nerves and blood vessels and other structures.

Muscle has a great capacity to regenerate, especially in young animals and frequently a complete recovery is made. Extensive or severe lesions may result in fibrosis of the muscle and permanent

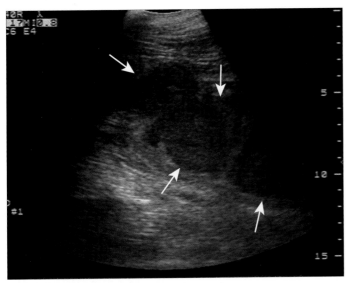

Figure 8.17 Ultrasound image of the horse in Fig. 8.16 showing a large intramuscular abscess (arrows).

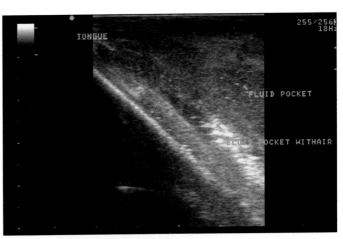

Figure 8.19 Ultrasound image of clostridial infection of the tongue secondary to a wire foreign body. Note the hyperechoic gas echoes scattered through a pocket of fluid which was consistent with a local anaerobic abscess.

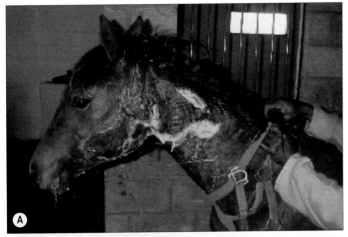

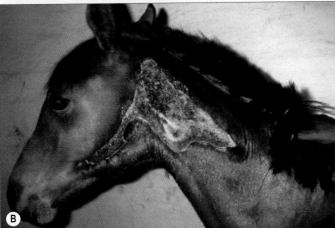

Figure 8.18 (A) Clostridial myonecrosis of the neck and head of a foal following a poorly administered intramuscular injection. (B) The same foal imaged a number of weeks later showing good healing but extensive scarring of the area.

deformity. Localized swelling and pain will be evident. If associated with a limb there may be profound lameness.

Diagnosis and treatment

- A diagnosis can often be reached on the basis of history and clinical signs. Imaging of the area affected, radiography or ultrasonography depending on the site, reveals soft tissue swelling and may demonstrate the presence of gas/air within the soft tissue. Culture any discharge from draining tracts.
- Treatment involves supportive care, anti-inflammatories and antimicrobials. In cases where anaerobic infections are thought to be involved such as clostridial myonecrosis, fenestration of the area is recommended.

Fibrotic myopathy

Traumatic damage to the semitendinosus, abscesses or local inflammation of the semitendinosus or tearing of the insertion of the semitendinosus which may occur for example during sliding stops in reining horses can result in fibrotic myopathy. Damage to the semimembranosus or gracilis can also result in the condition but these are less common. Another cited cause is degenerative neuropathy causing denervation of the distal semitendinosus. This is regarded as the most likely cause in horses which have fibrotic myopathy in one hindlimb with a progression to involve the other limb.

It is most often a unilateral condition and is not associated with any pain or stress for the horse. The abnormal gait that accompanies the condition is characteristic and diagnostic. There is a shortened cranial phase of the stride with an abrupt 'catching' of the forward swing, a slight caudal swing and a marked 'slapping' of the hoof to the ground. This gait abnormality may be much less apparent at the trot and canter. Affected horses may have a palpable thickening of the semimembranosus or semitendinosus muscles or an obvious dimpling or depression of the affected area. Some horses will have an area of osseous metaplasia that will be readily palpable.

The condition has also be seen in young foals and the etiology in this group is unknown, although theories include traumatic insult before, during or soon after delivery. Cases in foals are less likely to be associated with palpable fibrosis.

Treatment

- There is no effective medical therapy.
- Surgical treatments include semitendinosus myotomy (resection of the affected semitendinosus muscle), semitendinosus myotenectomy (resection of affected muscle and tendon of insertion), or

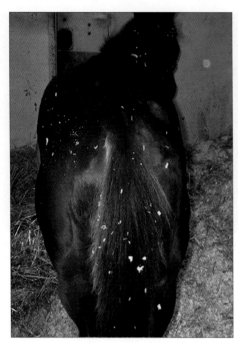

Figure 8.20 Immune-mediated polymyositis. Note the extensive muscle wastage over the gluteal area.

Differential diagnosis:
• Other myopathies
• Neurogenic wastage from local nerve trauma
• Cachexia
• Poor nutrition.

semitendinosusectomy at the tibial insertion. All will result in immediate gait improvement although myotomy and myotenectomy are associated with a higher percentage of complications. At least partial recurrence of the condition occurs in 30% of horses. If a progressive neuropathy is involved in the pathogenesis then a recurrence of signs is likely.

Immune-mediated myopathies (Fig. 8.20)

Three distinct myopathies with an apparent immune-mediated etiology are recognized in horses:

• Acute rhabdomyolysis caused by *S. equi*
• Infarctive purpura hemorrhagica
• Immune-mediated polymyositis.

Acute rhabdomyolysis caused by S. equi

The majority of reported cases have been in Quarterhorses <7 years of age. Affected horses usually have other concurrent evidence of *S. equi* infection such as lymphadenopathy or guttural pouch empyema. Initial clinical signs include a stiff gait that rapidly progresses to firm swollen and painful gluteal and epaxial muscles. Recumbency follows quickly and most horses are euthanized within 48 h of presentation.

The exact pathogenesis is not known but may be related to a toxic-shock-like syndrome caused by *S. equi* superantigens or local bacteremia with production of exotoxins or proteases.

Diagnosis

• The condition should be suspected based on clinical signs alone and treatment instituted early.
• There are marked elevations of CK and AST. Titers to the M protein of *S. equi* are low in affected horses unless there has been recent

vaccination for strangles. Titers to myosin-binding protein are typically high. Post-mortem examination reveals large areas of pale necrotic lumbar and hindlimb muscles.

Treatment and prognosis

• There has been a high mortality rate in cases to date despite antibiotic therapy. A combination of rifampicin (which inhibits protein synthesis) and penicillin is thought to be the best treatment although reports are lacking.
• Additional treatments include non-steroidal anti-inflammatories and high doses of short-acting corticosteroids, both of which may help to control the inflammatory response.
• Because of the severe pain noted in affected horses constant rate infusion of lidocaine, detomidine or ketamine may help reduce anxiety and provide additional pain relief.

Infarctive purpura hemorrhagica

Affected horses present with painful lameness, muscle stiffness and/or colic signs. There is normally a history of known exposure to *S. equi* within the previous 3 weeks or elevated serum M-protein titers. Classic signs of purpura hemorrhagica (PH) are present such as limb edema and petechiation. Laboratory changes include marked elevations in CK and AST. Gastrointestinal infarction may result in elevation of WCC, RBC and total protein in peritoneal fluid. Biopsies of abnormal muscle reveal diffuse acute coagulative necrosis. Post-mortem examination shows extensive infarction and leukocytic vasculitis of skeletal musculature, skin, gastrointestinal tract and lungs. The pathogenesis is thought to involve the deposition of immune complexes in vessel walls. These complexes are primarily composed of IgM, IgA and streptococcal M protein.

Diagnosis, treatment and prognosis

• Clinical signs combined with laboratory findings are used for diagnosis initially while awaiting biopsy results. Early recognition and aggressive therapy may lead to a better outcome.
• High-dose methylprednisolone is used to treat a similar condition in humans and could be combined with immunosuppressive agents such as cyclophosphamide or azathioprine.
• While the prognosis with classic PH is normally good, cases of infarctive PH have a poor prognosis. There is a report of successful treatment of a horse with penicillin, non-steroidal anti-inflammatories and corticosteroids.

Immune-mediated polymyositis

This condition is being increasingly reported in horses. Most affected horses to date have been Quarterhorses with horses <8 years of age or >16 years of age over-represented. Approximately one-third of cases have had a history of previous exposure to *S. equi*. Clinical signs include rapid-onset muscle atrophy of the back and croup muscles. This atrophy may involve up to 50% of the affected muscle mass within 1 week. Stiffness, malaise and weakness are also common non-specific findings. In contrast to other immune-mediated myopathies there are only mild to moderate elevations in muscle enzymes. The pathogenesis of the condition remains unclear.

Diagnosis, treatment and prognosis

• Clinical signs and biopsy specimens of affected muscles which reveal lymphocytic vasculitis, lymphocytic myofiber infiltration, fiber necrosis with macrophage infiltration and regeneration.
• Horses with concurrent streptococcal infection should be treated with antibiotics.
• Administration of corticosteroids normally results in rapid improvement of clinical signs and prevents further muscle atrophy. Treatment is required for at least 10 days and recurrence of muscle

atrophy requiring reintroduction of corticosteroids may be necessary in some cases.

• The prognosis with treatment is good.

Atypical myopathy/pasture-associated myopathy

This has been most frequently reported from the UK but has been seen in other European countries and is also present in the US. The etiology is an area of active investigation that is currently thought to be related to a toxin produced by Box elder and *Acer* species of trees. There is usually a history of recent (within the previous 4 days) grazing for at least 6 hours a day. Several co-grazers may be affected simultaneously. Clinical signs are acute in onset and include depression, weakness, stiffness, recumbency, trembling, sweating and myoglobinuria.

Diagnosis and treatment

• The condition should be expected in any horse with suitable clinical signs, history and geographical location. There are marked increases in CK activity along with hypocalcemia, hyperglycemia and hyperlipemia. Histology reveals multifocal Zenkers necrosis. Urine of affected horses has increased levels of acylcarnitines.

• Treatment is largely supportive in affected horses with mortality rates of up to 85%. Unaffected grazing companions should be removed for the pasture and fed concentrates/hay.

• Horses that have recovered have either made rapid full recoveries or have had prolonged recoveries with marked muscle wastage.

Masseter myopathy (Fig. 8.21)

Masseter myopathy in which the masseter muscles become grossly swollen and intensely painful is a rare disorder, affecting adult horses kept under poor management and nutritional conditions. Affected horses have an abrupt onset of anorexia; the masseter muscles are obviously swollen and are intensely painful. Manipulation of the mandible is resented strongly, and the lower jaw may be held slightly open or firmly closed. Simultaneous cardiac and diaphragmatic dysfunction (including synchronous diaphragmatic flutter) are frequently seen.

Diagnosis and treatment

• Diagnosis is usually obvious clinically.

• Treatment involves improving the plane of nutrition and client counseling in addition to anti-inflammatories and supportive care if there is difficulty eating. Recovered horses may seem relatively normal for a limited time, but profound masseter atrophy is a common sequel.

Muscle atrophy (Fig. 8.22)

Loss of muscle mass in the horse may be a consequence of starvation when the loss is general, but specific groups of muscles may undergo atrophy in response to trauma, myopathy, denervation and chronic disuse. **Disuse atrophy** is generally slow to develop whereas **neurogenic atrophy**, following total neurectomy, is much more rapid and would be expected to affect all the muscles supplied by a particular nerve. Disuse atrophy of muscles usually relates to underlying pain or disability syndromes, often associated with a musculo-skeletal disorder. The identification of the cause of obvious and severe, longstanding muscle atrophy may be particularly difficult.

Neoplastic disorders (Fig. 8.23)

Neoplastic conditions involving the muscles of the horse are rare, but possible conditions include spindle cell tumors and primary sarcoma. Occasionally individual muscles become affected by slow-growing defects of structure which may resemble neoplastic changes. The gross proliferation of a normal tissue type in an abnormal site such as this is called a hamartoma. Their significance is usually related to space-occupying compression of adjacent structures. A relatively common site for muscle hamartoma formation is the semimembranosus and semitendinosus muscles, and massive enlargement of these may have secondary effects on bowel and urogenital function.

Diagnosis and treatment

• May be suspected on the basis of clinical appearance but biopsies are generally required for a definitive diagnosis.

• Depending on the site and size, removal can be considered but normally their location and proximity to local vital structures preclude removal.

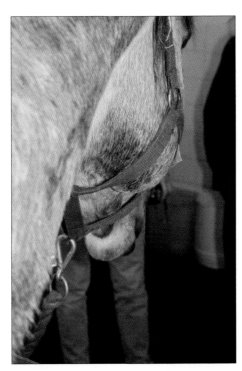

Figure 8.21 Masseter myopathy.

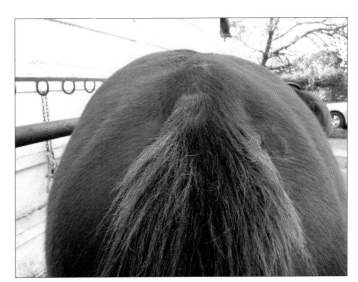

Figure 8.22 Disuse atrophy of muscle associated with a pelvic fracture.

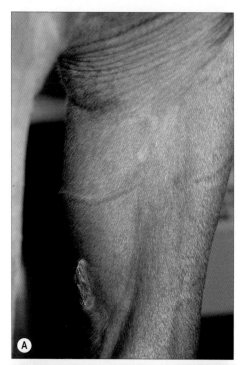

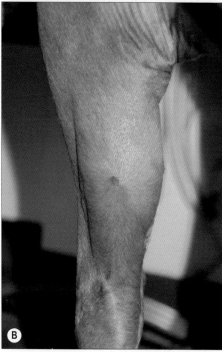

Figure 8.23 (A, B) Neoplasia. Muscular hamartoma.

References and further reading

Aleman, M., Brosnan, R.J., Williams, D.C., et al., 2005. Malignant Hyperthermia in horses anesthesized with halothane. J Vet Intern Med 19, 363–366.

McAuliffe, S.B., Slovis, N.M., 2008. Colour Atlas of Diseases and Disorders of the Foal. WB Saunders, Philadelphia, PA, USA.

Reed, S.M., Bayly, W.M., Sellon, D.C., 2009. Equine Internal Medicine, third ed. WB Saunders, St. Louis, MO, USA.

Robinson, N.E., Sprayberry, K.A. (eds.), 2009. Current Therapy in Equine Medicine, sixth ed. WB Saunders, St. Louis, MO, USA.

Valberg, S.J., 2006. Polysaccharide storage myopathy: indepthmuscle disorders. In: Proceedings. 52nd American association of Equine Practitioners, pp. 365–372.

CHAPTER 9

The integumentary system

CHAPTER CONTENTS

The skin is a large, diverse organ, and diseases and conditions may be primarily of dermatological origin or may be secondary manifestations of disease in other organs. Whilst the clinical signs may be obvious on the surface of the skin some are the result of underlying disorders of metabolism and organ dysfunction. Of all equine diseases, those of the skin are amongst the most difficult to diagnose and treat.

Congenital/developmental disorders

Epitheliogenesis imperfecta (Figs. 9.1 & 9.2)

In this condition there is complete or partial absence of one or more dermal components. Defects on the limbs are the most common and the condition is frequently confused with epidermolysis bullosa. Many severely affected foals are aborted or stillborn.

Diagnosis and treatment

- Clinical signs are diagnostic (there are no other disorders with these signs evident at birth).

- If the affected area is small treatment with repeated surgery may have a satisfactory result. However, most cases involve extensive lesions with resulting secondary infections and septicemia a common problem.
- Euthanasia is frequently recommended if the condition involves large areas.

Epidermolysis bullosa (Fig. 9.3)

This is a rare junctional mechanobullous disease which is found principally in Belgians and Saddlebreds of both sexes. It is characterized by severe blister formation of the skin of newborn foals. Lesions at mucocutaneous junctions are usually visible at birth and lesions at other sites shortly thereafter. Secondary infections are common.

Diagnosis and treatment

- History and clinical signs.
- Histopathology shows cleavage and bulla formation at the epidermal–dermal junction.
- Positive Nikolskys sign; finger pressure causes the epidermis to 'slip' off the dermis.
- There is no treatment available.

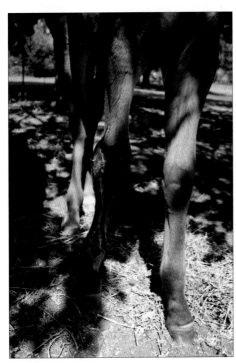

Figure 9.1 Epitheliogenesis imperfecta affecting the right front limb of this foal.

Differential diagnosis:
- Epidermolysis bullosa
- HERDA. Largely restricted to Quarterhorses and usually delayed until skin is subject to trauma with lesions most commonly seen over the trunk
- Obstetric trauma/savaging or predation.

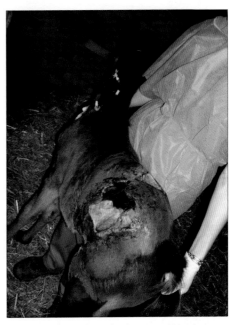

Figure 9.2 Large areas of wounds on the dorsum and lateral aspect of pelvis on this foal that was attacked by a stallion. Traumatic injuries occuring soon after birth should not be confused with epitheliogenesis imperfecta.

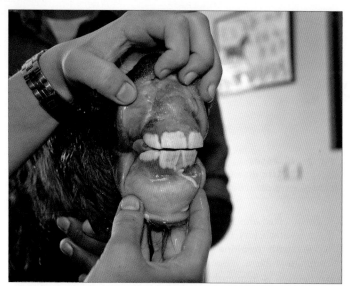

Figure 9.3 Epidermolysis bullosa with collapsed bullae in the mouth. This condition is largely restricted to Belgians but rare cases have been seen in other breeds and donkeys.

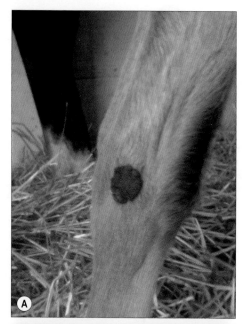

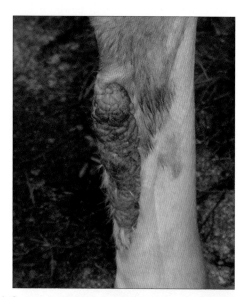

Figure 9.4 Congenital vascular hamartoma/cavernous hemangioma. This was a localized lesion on the caudal aspect of the cannon of this young foal.

Differential diagnosis:
- Viral papilloma
- Equine congenital cutaneous mastocytosis. Rare condition with lesions found mainly on the trunk
- Epidermal nevus: benign, usually flat hyperkeratotic popular lesions.

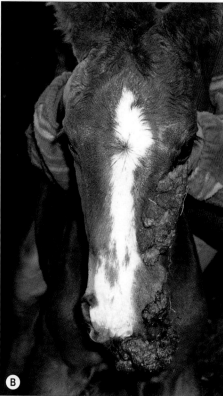

Figure 9.5 (A, B) Congenital papillomas are normally found as single discrete small masses with the characteristic papilloma appearance. (B) Occasionally more severe cases are encountered with multiple papillomas covering a large area.

Congenital equine cutaneous mastocytosis

This is a rare form of mast cell tumor that is present at or shortly after birth. It presents as multiple small, focal nodules along the trunk and lateral aspect of the hindlimbs. Larger nodules may have a soft fluctuant center and skin ulceration.

Diagnosis and treatment
- Biopsy and histopathology.
- Many of these lesions regress spontaneously with time; those that do not can be treated with surgical removal or radiation therapy, but some are difficult to remove due to location.

Congenital vascular hamartoma/cavernous hemangioma (Fig. 9.4)

Rare, spontaneous (usually singular) tumor of vascular endothelial cells that is most frequently seen on the distal limbs and abdomen. It is most commonly reported in Arabians and Thoroughbreds. They appear as fleshy, papilloma-like lesions. More aggressive forms may expand to involve underlying structures.

Diagnosis and treatment

- Histopathology of biopsy specimens.
- Surgical removal which may need to be followed by skin grafting.
- Radiation teletherapy and brachytherapy have been useful in some cases.

Congenital papillomatosis (neonatal wart/epidermal nevus) (Fig. 9.5)

Papovavirus has been associated with the development of papillomatous skin lesions on newborn foals and these show as warty growths on any body location. Lesions are usually singular but multiple lesions can occur.

Diagnosis and treatment

- Clinical signs.
- Spontaneous resolution does not occur but surgical excision is curative and recurrence does not occur.

Linear keratosis/alopecia (Figs. 9.6 & 9.7)

This is a relatively common but poorly recognized disorder in which a focal keratinization defect manifests as one or more linear, usually vertical, bands of crusting and alopecia. Normally only a few linear bands of alopecia and/or hyperakeratinization are seen. The condition is not associated with pain or pruritis. Lesions may remain static over long periods of time or may progress slowly.

Lesions are most often located on the sides of the neck or over the buttock, but may be found elsewhere. Most cases are seen in Quarterhorses but other breeds can be affected and a heritable form has been demonstrated in Belgians and Quarterhorses.

Diagnosis and treatment

- Histopatholgy can be used but generally the diagnosis is based on clinical signs with clipping of the area making lesions more obvious.
- There is no treatment available and usually none is necessary.

Hereditary equine regional dermal asthenia (HERDA; hypoelastosis cutis; cutaneous asthenia/Ehlers-Danlos syndrome) (Figs. 9.8 & 9.9)

This is an inherited defect of connective tissue which results in abnormal folding of the skin, particularly of the shoulders, body and upper limbs. This usually causes considerable, abnormal local folding of the skin which is noticeably thin on palpation. The skin is excessively fragile and is liable to trauma. Healed lesions involving this skin show abnormally prominent scarring. The condition is most frequently seen in Quarterhorses (especially descendants of Poco Bueno) but has been seen in other breeds.

Diagnosis and treatment

- DNA testing is available and will also differentiate carriers.
- Affected horses have an elevation of their urine deoxypyridinoline (DPD):pyridinoline (PYD) ratios which is diagnostic of the disease, from birth, but this testing may not be readily available.
- Currently, there is no effective therapy for HERDA. Affected horses are often euthanized due to the severity of lesions and associated discomfort.

Dermoid cysts (Fig. 9.10)

Single or multiple dermoid cysts are found on the skin of the dorsal midline, particularly in Thoroughbred horses between 6 months and 3–4 years of age. These contain coiled hair and a cheesy, caseous, sterile material. They are seldom painful unless they burst and become infected.

Diagnosis and treatment

- Close examination is usually sufficient for diagnosis and differentiation from inflammatory, neoplastic and parasitic lesions which sometimes occur in the same vicinity.

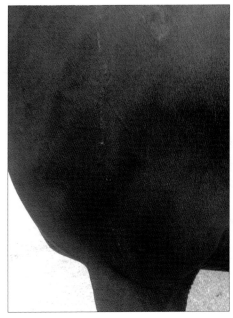

Figure 9.6 Linear keratosis/alopecia in a single well-defined line.

Differential diagnosis:
- Chronic hyperkeratosis from irritant chemicals
- Dermatophilosis (usually more extensive and found on the dorsum of horses maintained in wet conditions; it resolves with treatment whereas linear keratosis does not)
- Clipper rash, recent trauma or scarring from previous injury
- Verrucose sarcoid (these are rarely linear).

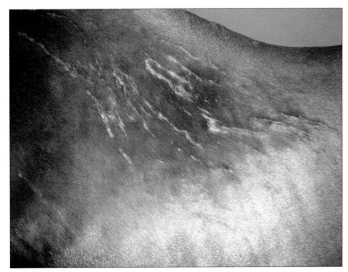

Figure 9.7 Linear keratosis/alopecia in numerous lines across the side of the withers and lateral trunk.

- Incision and removal of the contents is normally all that is required to treat this condition with minimal aftercare.

Hypotrichosis/mane and tail dystrophy (follicular dysplasia) (Fig. 9.11)

This is a rare condition in which there is less than normal density of hair. It is most commonly seen affecting mane and tail hair but can affect other areas of the body. It is frequently seen in Arabians and Appaloosas.

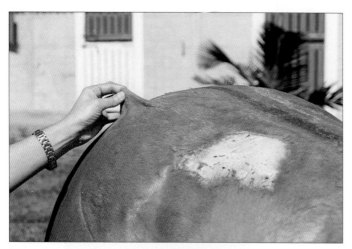

Figure 9.8 Hereditary equine regional dermal asthenia (HERDA), showing residual skin scarring after trauma and typical 'loose' skin.

Differential diagnosis:
- Epitheliogenesis imperfect/cutaneous agenesis
- Persistent irritation/self trauma
- Rapid weight loss/dehydration resulting in loss of skin elasticity.

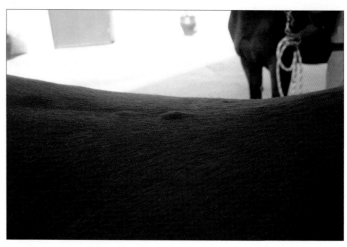

Figure 9.10 Two dermoid cysts on the dorsal midline of this Thoroughbred yearling.

Differential diagnosis:
- Epidermoid cysts (confined to the nasal region)
- Dentigerous cysts (confined to ear and lateral calvarium)
- Hypodermiasis (usually isolated, seasonal and painful)
- Eosinophilic granuloma (commonly found in adult horses)
- Insect bite (localized hypersensitivity)
- Nodular sarcoid fibroma.

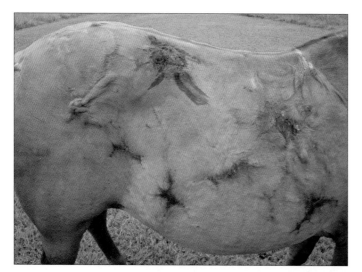

Figure 9.9 Hereditary equine regional dermal asthenia (HERDA), showing extensive areas of skin scarring following minor trauma.

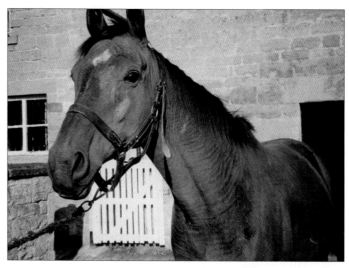

Figure 9.11 Hypotrichosis showing poor hair density and quality, especially over the face and neck. This had been present since birth but became increasingly evident with age. The mane and tail are more frequently affected.

Differential diagnosis:
- Selenium poisoning (affects mane and tail initially and is frequently accompanied by sloughing of hooves)
- Chronic anhidrosis (history of lack/reduced sweating)
- Ectoparasites (pruritis results in damage and loss of hair especially of mane and tail)
- Zinc, copper and iodine deficiencies (rare causes of hair loss; body hair is affected before the mane or tail)
- Alopecia areata (mostly affects the skin of the body and head)
- Mimosa poisoning (rare condition and history of access).

Diagnosis and treatment
- Diagnosis is usually made based on clinical signs and breed, but histopathology of biopsy samples may help to demonstrate the lack of functional hair follicles.
- It is important to differentiate from selenium poisoning.
- No treatment is possible and it does not affect the horse clinically, being more of a cosmetic defect.

Arabian fading syndrome (pinky Arab syndrome) (Fig. 9.12)
This is a common condition that primarily affects gray Arabian horses but has also been seen in Welsh Mountain ponies and Clydesdales. The skin in affected areas loses its pigmentation and may also lose the hair. It is found most frequently on the face and in the perineal region.

Diagnosis and treatment
- Diagnosis is normally based on clinical signs, but biopsy will confirm the loss of melanocytes.
- There is no effective treatment.
- Tattooing has been used in some Arabian show horses in which the loss of pigmentation is regarded as undesirable cosmetically.

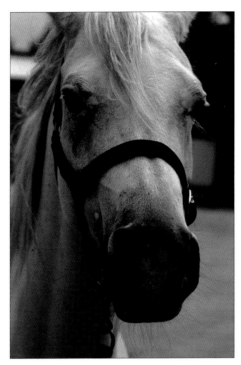

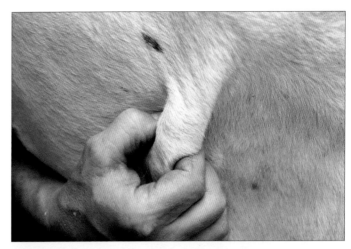

Figure 9.13 Calcinosis circumscripta. Typical firm, non-painful, non-pruritic subcutaneous nodule.

Differential diagnosis:
- Calcification following trauma
- Foreign body (calcification of the area can make differentiation difficult)
- Acquired bursa (fluid-filled and ultrasonographically distinctive).

Figure 9.12 Arabian fading syndrome. Other than the pigment changes the skin is normal in appearance.

Differential diagnosis:
- Systemic lupus erythematous-like syndrome (pigmentary incontinence and multisystemic involvement)
- Vitiligo (loss of pigmentation on the face and perineum)
- Appaloosa parentage syndrome (appaloosa cross-bred foals frequently do not have color change until 3–4 years of age, at which time a fading in coat color and development of white spots can be seen)
- Leukoderma/leukotrichia following trauma or radiation therapy
- Discoid lupus (photo-exacerbated condition with discoid epidermal lesions on the face and limbs).

Non-infectious disorders

Calcinosis circumscripta (Figs. 9.13 & 9.14)

This is a rare condition of young horses (1–4 years) of unknown etiology although it is thought that in many cases there may be a relation to previous trauma. It presents as a firm swelling which is sometimes mobile over the underlying tissue and is most frequently seen over the lateral aspect of the stifle.

Diagnosis and treatment
- Clinical signs are usually diagnostic, but radiography or ultrasonography can be used to confirm.
- Biopsy shows multinodular deposits of minerals within fibrous and granulomatous tissue.
- Complete surgical removal is the treatment of choice, but depending on the area affected and the size of the lesion may be difficult to achieve.

Equine axillary nodular necrosis (Fig. 9.15)

This is a rare disorder that is characterized by the development of an irregular number of firm, well-defined skin nodules of varying size which are particularly distributed in the girth and axillary regions. The lesions do not at first involve the loss of overlying hair but latterly they may become larger and usually show a focal area of alopecia. The lesions are painless and are not associated with local inflammatory responses.

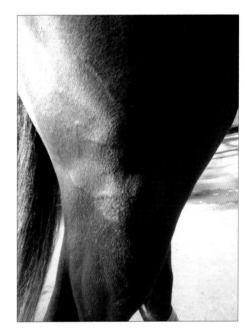

Figure 9.14 Calcinosis circumscripta.

Diagnosis and treatment
- Clinical signs are suggestive but definitive diagnosis requires biopsy (excisional biopsy is required).
- Eosinophilic granulomatous inflammation is detected histologically.
- Surgical excision is curative but diagnosis should be definitive prior to excision. In many cases no treatment is pursued due to the benign nature of the condition.

Wounds

The scope for damage to the skin of horses is extensive. An almost infinite variety of injuries may occur. Trauma to the skin of horses is frequently directly attributable to their lifestyle or to their excitable

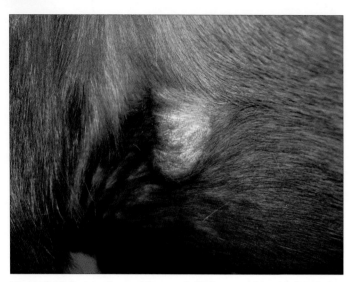

Figure 9.15 Equine axillary nodular necrosis. Single non-painful nodule in typical position.

Differential diagnosis:
• Traumatic damage/scarring
• Nodular sarcoid
• Lymphosarcoma/lymphoma
• Nodular panniculitis/steatitis (painful inflammatory changes in the panniculus or subcutaneous fat; commonly affects the girth and lower chest walls)
Other differentials which rarely affect the girth area include: mastocytoma, amyloidosis, hypodermiasis, epidermoid and dermoid cysts.

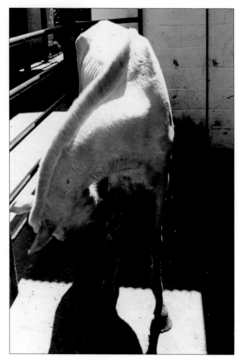

Figure 9.16 Severe self-inflicted wound on the forearm.

Differential diagnosis:
• Neurological self-mutilation (viral neurological pruritis, rabies and other encephalitides, neuritis, peripheral neuropathy)
• Pruritis due to ectoparasites, atopy, dermatophytosis.

nature when confronted by unusual events such as storms, transport, strange horses, new paddocks, etc. In many cases the more serious consequences of the injury involve underlying structures such as tendons, ligaments, nerves or blood vessels.

Healing of limb wounds is often slow, particularly if the injury, such as deep wire cuts, involves deeper tissues. Where the periosteal blood supply is disrupted sequestration of the underlying bone frequently occurs (see Fig. 7.121). Failure of even relatively minor wounds to heal at sites subjected to trauma involving (even minor) periosteal damage should be investigated carefully in case such sequestration has occurred. These wounds invariably completely fail to heal until either the sequestrum has been spontaneously reabsorbed or surgically removed. Other reasons for the failure of wounds to heal include excessive movement at the site, inadequate wound contraction, infection (bacterial and parasitic), poor or interrupted blood supply, foreign bodies, excessive blood loss and underlying systemic disease.

Wounds in some areas such as the thorax and neck often heal rapidly, relying on a combination of wound contracture and effective spontaneous drainage of exudates and inflammatory debris. Wounds involving the eyelids (see p. 358) or the margins of the mouth, nose and vulva, may heal effectively by second intention healing but may result in a possibly more serious secondary effect after cicatrization (scarring) has taken place.

Non-healing wounds of the lower limb (or elsewhere) which produce large accumulations of exuberant granulation tissue (proud flesh) create a considerable problem for the clinician. Repeated debridement of the granulation tissue and subsequent skin grafting (usually pinch grafting) is required, but such wounds should first be explored by all possible means (including radiography and ultrasonography) to ensure that there is no obvious reason for the failure to heal. Careful handling of wounds in these areas will ensure that healing when it finally occurs will contain the minimum amount of

unsightly fibrous and/or osseous tissue. Wounds which fail to heal should also be examined carefully for the possibility that the apparent granulation tissue is not in fact sarcoid.

Foreign body wounds

Foreign bodies which are introduced through skin wounds may lead either to a persistently discharging non-healing wound or to discharging sinuses in the skin. The latter may discharge a considerable distance from the original site and this may be misleading when such wounds and sinuses are examined. Radiography (using probes and/or contrast media if necessary), ultrasonography and careful exploratory surgery under general anesthetic may be required in order to locate and remove such foreign bodies.

Self-inflicted trauma (Fig. 9.16)

Self-inflicted injury also occurs as a result of irritation from biting insects such as *Stomoxys* spp. Skin mutilation can also occur as a result of the self-mutilation syndrome in stallions; horses bite severely at flanks, ribs and pectoral areas, causing patchy alopecia, leukotrichia and scarring. The use of aluminum muzzles or neck cradles, which allow the horse to eat and drink normally but prevent self-molestation, may be necessary in this and in other skin conditions accompanied by self-mutilation. It is unusual for horses to chew or lick at open wounds unless they are associated with nerve damage or foreign bodies, but they do occasionally chew dressings and bandages where these are poorly applied or where there is an excessive exudation.

Pressure sores (Fig. 9.17)

A more chronic type of skin trauma occurs from poorly applied plaster casts or from localized pressure over bony prominences during prolonged recumbency. These wounds and decubital (pressure) sores are notoriously slow to heal. Residual slow healing occurs only if the pressure is relieved and appropriate treatment applied.

Where skin trauma is prolonged but intermittent, and/or is not severe enough to cause circulation problems, the skin reacts to form a callus. These are common over joints and bony protuberances, especially at the knee, fetlock, elbow, hock and tuber ischia. False or acquired bursae are often encountered where the pressure is applied, such as over the carpus in horses which habitually kneel. Skin thickening and lichenification are common sequels to such injuries. Embedded foreign bodies are also a possible cause of such thickened skin but the history of the lesion is notably different. In all these conditions the lesions are usually cold and non-painful. Prevention of pressure and local irritation may improve the condition but, again, the total resolution is often disappointing.

Thermal injury (Fig. 9.18)

Thermal injury may occur as a result of either heat loss as in frost bite, cryotherapy or heat excess such as sunburn, photosensitization, thermocautery or accidental fire burns. Skin injury caused by

exposure to extremely cold environmental conditions appears to be particularly unusual in horses and where it does occur it primarily affects the tail and ears. Even very low environmental temperatures appear to have little effect upon the limbs. Application of severe heat, such as used in the firing of horses' legs, causes swelling, exudation and residual scarring in much the same fashion as freezing injuries.

Horses trapped in fires may sustain very severe skin damage. The most common sites for severe burns are around the head and dorsum. Horses with burns which cover more than 50% of the body surface almost invariably die from the secondary circulatory, renal and cardiovascular effects. The extent of involvement of the layers of the skin is used to classify burns into four degrees with the most severe, fourth-degree burns involving the entire depth of the skin and underlying tissues. The deeper the skin involvement the more plasma protein is lost in the acute stage and the more severe the consequent scarring. The typical thick, coagulated crusts which develop following thermal (or chemical or physical) cauterization of the skin are called eschars. Severe exudation, loss of body fluids and extremely slow healing of up to 12 months or more, with extensive hairless scarring commonly follows burns of third or fourth degree. The treatment of extensive or localized burns of any degree should be oriented toward controlling the loss of plasma as well as toward pain relief and the limitation of subsequent sloughing. Skin grafting may be an effective method of speeding the naturally slow healing process. Secondary complications, including severe pneumonia due to inhalation of smoke and/or noxious chemicals released from fires (such as burnt plastic), may result in death during the 24–48 hours after the incident.

Endocrine diseases with cutaneous manifestations

Horses with **equine Cushing's disease** (see Chapter 6, p. 227) have a wide range of endocrine abnormalities but frequently the first signs to be noted by owners are the changes in coat (hirsutism), excessive sweating and abnormal fat deposits.

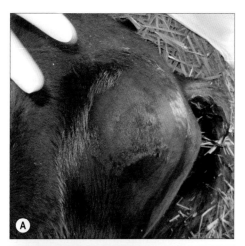
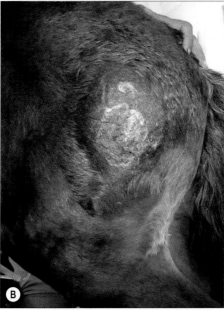

Figure 9.17 (A) Early pressure sore showing swelling and change in texture of the skin over the affected area. (B) Same foal a number of weeks later. The affected area of skin sloughed and the remaining wound healed with time.

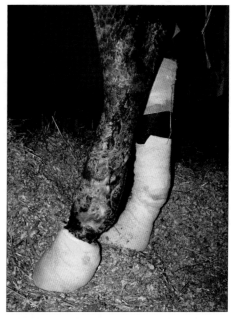

Figure 9.18 Thermal injury sustained during a barn fire. Second- and third-degree burns showing edema, serum exudation and sloughing of superficial layers of skin.

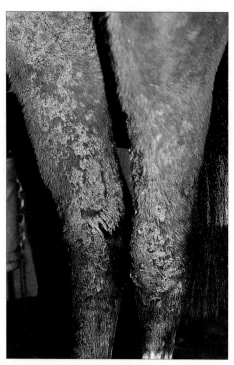

Figure 9.19 Zinc deficiency with severe exfoliative non-inflammatory shedding of the hair and hyperkeratosis. Reproduced from Knottenbelt D, *Pascoe's Principles & Practice of Equine Dermatology*, second ed. (2009), with permission from Elsevier.

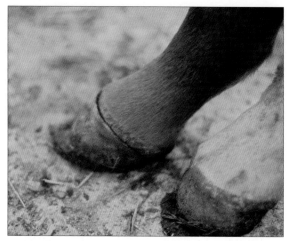

Figure 9.20 Selenium. Separation of coronary band with slippering of hoof.
Differential diagnosis:
- Laminitis (idiopathic and other)
- Arterial occlusion (neuroma)
- Infection within hoof.

Nutritional diseases with cutaneous manifestations

These are infrequent conditions in horses. Nutritional diseases are poorly differentiated and have non-specific skin changes more related to general health than specific deficiency. However, specific mineral deficiencies including zinc, iodine and copper may be associated with skin disorders.

- **Zinc** (Fig. 9.19). Zinc has a major influence on skin health and adult daily requirements are 500 mg. Deficiency causes a generalized alopecia and flaking of the superficial skin layers giving a dandruff-like appearance. Dietary supplementation with zinc methionine or other zinc salts is curative over a number of weeks.
- **Iodine**. Young foals born to mares with sub-optimal iodine diets during pregnancy may be born with an obvious **goiter** (see p. 221) and such foals are often weak and have a very poor coat quality. On occasion they may be almost hairless. Iodine poisoning (iodism) results from ingestion of abnormal amounts of iodine (usually from supplements). Cutaneous findings are heavy surf/seborrhea mostly on the mane and tail base but it can also be seen on the body. Diagnosis is normally based on a history of iodine supplementation and treatment involves removal of the supplement.
- **Copper**. Copper deficiency is particularly unusual in horses, even in areas with a primary copper-deficient soil or in areas with high soil molybdenum concentrations, but in the event that the animal is unable to maintain its copper status, alteration in the color of the hair (hypochromotrichia) is usually all that is seen. Dark-pigmented hair may become obviously russet in color. Other more serious consequences of copper deficiency are a tendency to arterial rupture and chronic anemia. Diagnosis can be made by blood and liver analysis of copper levels but frequently response to supplementation is used. It is important to remember that not all

forms of copper are bioavailable and if deficiency is suspected consultation with an equine nutritionist is valuable in selecting or developing supplementation.

- **Selenium poisoning** (Fig. 9.20). Selenium causes toxicity either in metallic base form (usually following over-enthusiastic feed supplementation) or from plants which either concentrate selenium or have increased selenium levels as a result of seleniferous soils. Loss of mane and tail hair occurs, as well as the prominent signs of laminitis. In some cases the laminitis may be severe enough to result in separation of the coronary band and sloughing of the hoof. Long-term toxicity or repeated episodes may result in obvious laminitic deformities of the hoof walls with converging growth lines.

Diagnosis, treatment and prognosis of selenium poisoning

- Diagnosis is usually based on history. Skin biopsy changes and changes in the hoof wall are non-specific.
- This condition is treated by removing the source of selenium combined with a dietary adjustment to include high-protein supplement.
- The overall prognosis is guarded with full recoveries difficult to achieve.

Chemicals, toxic plants and heavy metals
Chemical trauma (Fig. 9.21)

Inappropriate application of topical medications, blisters or counterirritants is a common cause of exudative or necrotizing dermatitis. Where irritation is mild, there may be only wrinkling of the skin. With more severe irritation, such as occurs with irritants like phenols and wood preservatives, there may be obvious destruction of the skin. 'Therapeutic' blistering (counter-irritation) of the skin using mercurial compounds or extracts of cantharides is commonly practiced and results in moderate or severe caustic burns to the skin. Particularly severe reactions may arise if these chemicals are accidentally transferred to the lips and mouth, or eyes. The skin lesions heal particularly slowly at these sites and may even lead to permanent scarring. Milder forms of blister treatment, such as mustard, applied to the skin of horses usually induces swelling and scale formation, without any significant permanent effects.

Skin lesions are usually confined to the area of application but systemic effects may also be induced depending on the chemical used.

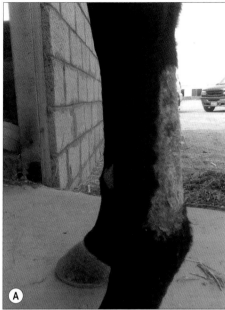

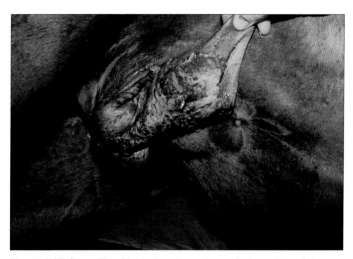

Figure 9.22 Skin scalding. Urinary incontinence has resulted in scalding of the perineum of this horse.

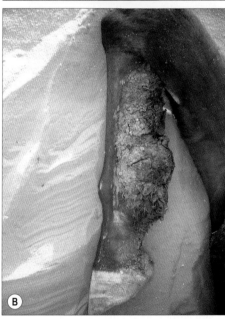

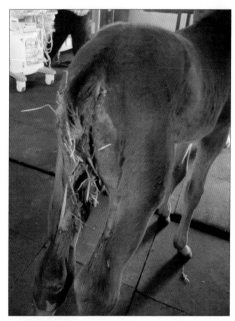

Figure 9.21 (A, B) Chemical trauma from overzealous application of a blister product.

Figure 9.23 Skin scalding. Alopecia and excoriation as a result of diarrhea.

Diagnosis, treatment and prognosis

- Diagnosis is usually made based on history, but may be difficult in some cases if the owner or caretaker does not admit the application of the chemical.
- Treatment should start by removing the irritant if application was recent, followed by appropriate wound management. Systemic effects may require specific therapy and supportive care depending on the chemical applied.
- Prognosis depends on the extent of the injury, the chemical applied and the degree of systemic effects, but consequences can be severe in many cases.

Skin scalding (Figs. 9.22 & 9.23)

Skin scalding from persistent bathing in body fluids is a common occurrence. Diarrhea, urine, serum/plasma, milk or lacrimal secretions can result in marked alopecia and dermatitis if they remain in contact with the skin for prolonged periods. Matting of the hair is often seen initially and secondary infections are common.

Diagnosis, treatment and prognosis

- Diagnosis is usually based on the history and clinical signs.
- The most important factor in therapy is cessation of the contact between the fluid and skin. The affected area should be cleaned thoroughly but gently and then emollients applied with fluid-repellent creams.
- Prognosis is generally good though longstanding cases may have persistent changes in skin thickness and flexibility. Healing may be prolonged if the area affected is extensive.

Table 9.1 Actinic dermatitis

Sunburn Excessive exposure to UV light with an expected response	Severity of damage is related to degree of exposure and sensitivity of the skin with pale-skinned horses being more liable to damage
Photosensitization Normal exposure to UV light with an unexpected or exaggerated response	Even mild exposure may generate a severe response. Requires: • Presence of a photodynamic agent in the skin • Exposure to sunlight (or other UV light) • Cutaneous absorption of the UV light

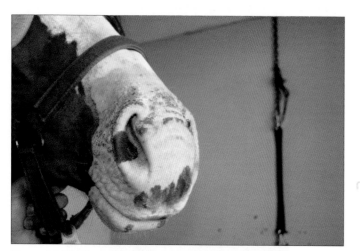

Figure 9.24 Sunburn. This is a typical pattern affecting only unpigmented areas and the animal was otherwise healthy.

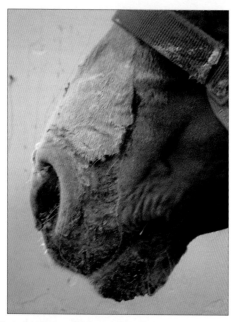

Figure 9.25 Actinic dermatitis (photosensitization) affecting the non-pigmented areas of the face in a horse with liver failure.

Actinic dermatitis (Figs. 9.24 & 9.25)

Actinic dermatitis can be divided into two categories (Table 9.1).

There are three types of photosensitization; type 1 (primary) and type 3 (secondary) occur in horses.

Type 1: This occurs as a result of ingestion of preformed photodynamic substances such as those found in certain plants (*Polygonum fagopyrum, Thamnosma texans, Hypericum perforatum, Loliumperenne, Sphenociadium capitellatum, Heracleum mantegazzianum, Trifolium hybridum/pretense*).

Type 3: This type is more common than type 1 and is related to hepatic failure. The photodynamic substance phylloerythrin (a derivative of plant chlorophyll), which is normally removed by the liver, is allowed into the circulation and is then deposited in the skin.

Diagnosis

- All horses showing evidence of photosensitive dermatitis should, even when they are known to have ingested a photodynamic plant or chemical, be carefully investigated for hepatic failure, whether or not there are other supportive signs.
- History is critical as it may indicate other signs of hepatic failure or grazing patterns associated with ingestion of toxic plants.
- Physical examination with localization of lesions to pale-skinned areas. In photosensitization all white areas of the body will be affected. In sunburn cases it is common that only the face (especially muzzle) is affected.
- Lithium heparin blood samples for detection of alkaloid on red cells. However, this will only be positive if ingestion is current or ongoing.

Treatment and prognosis

- Removal of all sources of UV light; stabling bandaging, rugs, etc.
- Glucocorticoids and/or non-steroidal anti-inflammatories to reduce inflammation but in cases of liver failure may exacerbate hepatoencephalopathy.
- Symptomatic treatment of liver failure (if present).
- Prognosis is poor in cases of type 3. Type 1 respond well to therapy but there may be residual scarring.

Arsenic poisoning (chronic)

Arsenic compounds in small quantities are still used in some parts of the world to improve coat quality and most chronic intoxications are due to prolonged use of these supplements or inadvertent dosing. Rarely arsenical dips can be responsible but these are now rarely used.

It is important to remember that acute poisoning has no dermatological effects and chronic poisoning results in generalized hair thinning and seborrhea in addition to poor body condition.

Diagnosis and treatment

- Diagnosis is through history of feeding arsenic-containing compounds or contact with arsenic-containing compounds.
- Arsenic assay of hair. Most laboratories provide a heavy metal panel and will test for mercury at the same time.
- Removal of the causative supplement should be enough, but recovery may be prolonged.

Mercury poisoning

Historically this was caused by ingestion of seed corn treated with organic, mercurial fungicides. These are rarely used now and as such this condition has largely disappeared but may occasionally be seen associated with topical application of mercurial-containing compounds such as mercury blisters. Similar to arsenic, acute poisoning has no dermatological consequences. Chronic poisoning results in progressive loss of body hair followed by loss of mane and tail hair. Oral ulceration can also be seen resulting from direct contact.

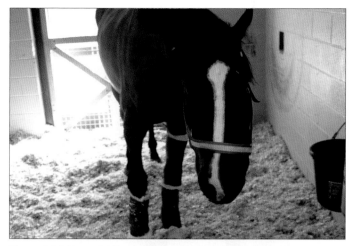

Figure 9.26 Severe facial swelling as a result of a snake bite. Site of bite is not always obvious but its character may help to identify the type of snake involved. Secondary effects of myonecrosis, coagulation defects and neurological signs may develop.

Differential diagnosis:
• Spider/scorpion bites, bee stings (these can all appear very similar and be near impossible to differentiate without visual observation of the bite or sting)
• Vasculitis (usually more generalized or affecting multiple areas).

Diagnosis and treatment
• Diagnosis is through history of exposure/ingestion and/or hair analysis.
• Treatment starts by removing the source of mercury. Many cases also have organ failure due to mercury accumulation, e.g. liver and/or kidney.

Plant poisoning (leucaenosis/mimosine toxicity)
Leucena spp. trees including *Leucena leucocephala* and mimosa (*Mimosa pudica*), which are found in Australasia, New Guinea, the Philippines and the West Indies, contain a potent depilatory alkaloid and are readily ingested by horses. The toxicity is characterized by patchy alopecia, which particularly affects the mane and tail hair, and laminitis. Both the hair and hoof disorders may develop within 7–10 days following ingestion.

Diagnosis and treatment
Diagnosis is made looking at the location (access to the plants) and the elimination of other differentials.

Treatment starts by removing the horse from the source.

Zootoxicosis (Figs. 9.26–9.29)
Zootoxicosis is caused by the bite or sting of venomous snakes, arachnids and insects. While in most cases the effects of envenomation remain localized, some toxins are potentially lethal and have significant effects upon the nervous system or upon blood coagulation, or both. Venoms are also usually highly allergenic and previously sensitized animals may show severe anaphylactic reactions. In the horse the ratio of body weight to the volume of toxin introduced makes systemic effects unusual. In most cases the bites induce localized erythema, edema, exudation and necrosis of skin and underlying muscle and sloughing of the skin. The biting parts of many noxious animals such as snakes are often heavily contaminated with bacteria and localized infections frequently follow such bites. Permanent damage to the blood vessels, veins and lymphatics can also occur, particularly from spider bites. Usually the prevalent dangerous snakes, spiders and scorpions, etc. are well known in their respective regions of the world.

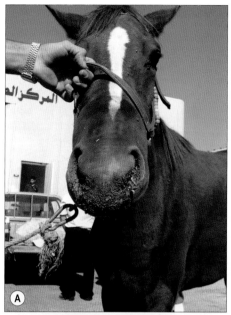
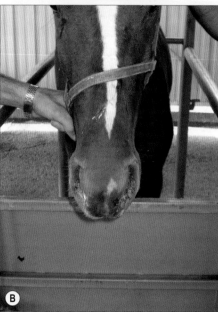

Figure 9.27 (A) Snake bite: edema of the muzzle in this young horse as a result of a snake bite. Horses frequently are bitten on or near the muzzle; this type of severe edema can threaten breathing and may require an emergency tracheostomy. (B) Same horse following treatment with steroids.

Disorders of pigmentation and hair density
Acquired persistent leukoderma/leukotrichia (Fig. 9.30)
This is an acquired depigmentation of hair **(leukotrichia)** or skin **(leukoderma)** that occurs following traumatic insult or injury to the skin. Common causes included freeze branding, thermal injuries, trauma, surgery or radiation. The insult does not necessarily have to be severe to result in leukotrichia but leukoderma is generally associated with more severe injuries.

Diagnosis and treatment
• Clinically obvious.
• No treatment is available and the condition in most cases is cosmetic, unless the original injury also resulted in severe scarring.

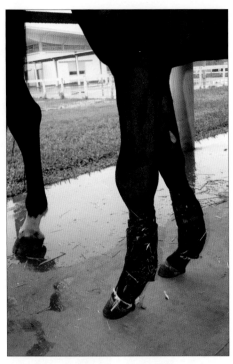

Figure 9.28 (A, B) Snake bite to the foreleg of this young foal resulted in local necrosis and severe arteritis.

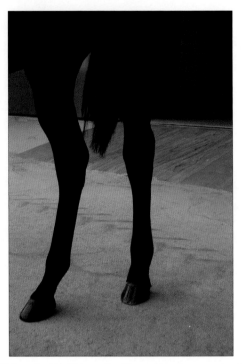

Figure 9.29 Scorpion bite. This yearling filly was bitten by a scorpion. These bites typically result in severe local effects with slow healing and in many cases a persistent lymphangitis.

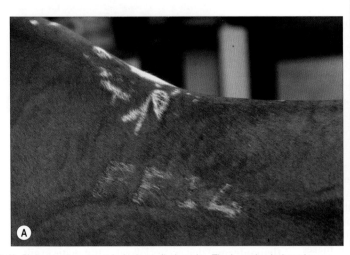

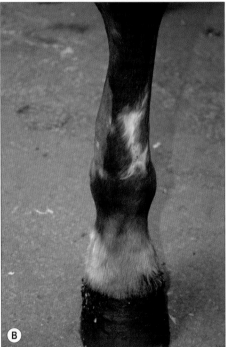

Figure 9.30 (A, B) Acquired persistent leukoderma/leukotrichia. This horse has leukotrichia as a result of a freeze brand and also as a result of tack placement (A). The horse in (B) has leukoderma and leukotrichia following inappropriate (too tight) bandage placement.

Differential diagnosis:
- Vitiligo (usually around eyes, face and perineum)
- Spotted leukotrichia/leukoderma (isolated white spots that may come and go)
- Coital exanthema (perineum only)
- Arabian fading syndrome
- Reticulated leukotrichia (linear pattern, characteristically along the back)
- Systemic lupus erythematous-like syndrome (multisystemic disorder)
- Discoid lupus
- Transient trauma-related depigmentation.

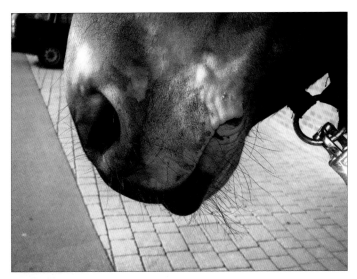

Figure 9.31 Vitiligo (idiopathic depigmentation) of the muzzle.

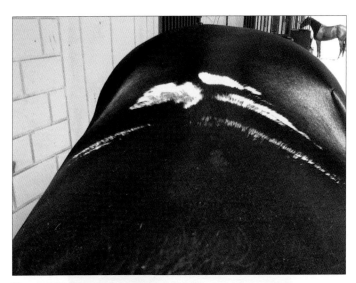

Figure 9.33 Variegated leukotrichia.

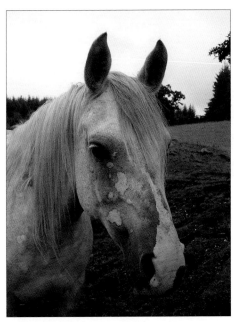

Figure 9.32 Leukoderma. Idiopathic depigmentation of the face.

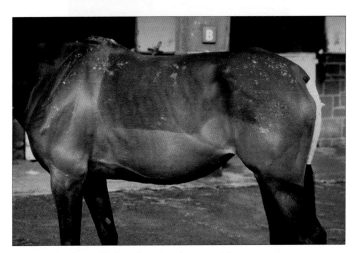

Figure 9.34 Spotted leukotrichia. Idiopathic spotted form.

Idiopathic depigmentation or vitiligo (Figs. 9.31 & 9.32)

This is an acquired depigmentation disorder of limited areas (most commonly around the eyes and face) and may be related to an autoimmune condition involving anti-melanocyte antibodies. Usually there are no other signs and the condition is most frequently seen in Arabians, Thoroughbreds and Shire horses, and horses of all ages can be affected.

Diagnosis

Clinical signs are usually sufficient for a diagnosis but biopsy can confirm the sparcity of melanocytes.

Treatment

None is available and as the condition is largely aesthetic none is usually warranted.

Variegated or reticulated leukotrichia (Figs. 9.33 & 9.34)

This is a rare condition that affects the dorsum of mainly young (1–3 years) Standardbreds and Quarterhorses more commonly than other

breeds. The initial linear crusting, which develops in a characteristic lace-like fashion over the back between the withers and tail, and over the sides of the neck, sheds leaving a transient alopecia which is followed by the permanent growth of white hair in the same pattern. Leukoderma is not usually present. There may be some discomfort or pain initially but long-term discomfort is rare.

There is a suggested heritable cause but this has not been clearly established and the condition is usually sufficiently mild as to not preclude breeding from affected individuals.

Diagnosis and treatment

Clinical signs are used for diagnosis as histology of biopsy specimens is normal.

There is no treatment for this condition.

Hyperaesthetic leuko(melano)trichia

This is a rare disorder of unknown etiology. It may have an immunological basis or may represent a more severe form of reticulated leukotrichia. The distribution of lesions is similar to the reticulated version but early lesions are associated with more pain and obvious inflammation. The initial crusting lesions can be present for up to 3 months and the areas then develop white hair growth.

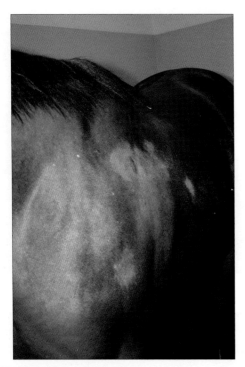

Figure 9.35 Anhidrosis. Typical patchy alopecia.

Diagnosis, treatment and prognosis
- History and clinical signs are diagnostic. Biopsy findings are generally non-specific with evidence of inflammatory responses.
- Treatment is largely symptomatic with non-steroidals administered during the inflammatory phase.
- Some cases may recur.

Anhidrosis (Fig. 9.35)
Anhidrosis (see Chapter 6, p. 224) has skin manifestations with patchy loss of hair and thinning of the hair coat. Longstanding cases show more prominent hair coat abnormalities with a harsh, staring, dry and thin coat quality.

Immune-mediated skin diseases

Urticaria and angioedema (Figs. 9.36–9.39)
These may have both immunologic and non-immunologic etiologies and cause pruritus and edema. It may be transient, prolonged or chronically recurring, and may arise from several possible stimuli. These include stimulation of immune processes, typically involving type I (immediate/anaphylactic) and type III (immune complex) hypersensitivities. Non-immunological causes include physical factors such as heat, exercise, sunlight or even rug pressure, as well as various drugs and chemicals either applied locally or ingested.

Urticaria has also been associated with a wide range of other disorders including viral, bacterial, fungal and protozoal infections. Insect bites, contact with noxious chemicals such as phenol-based wood preservatives and pour-on insecticides may also induce an urticarial rash. A wide variety of systemic medications including penicillin and/or streptomycin, oxytetracycline, phenothiazine, potentiated sulfonamides, iron dextrans, various vaccines and sera have also been blamed for its development.

Changes in dietary components including sudden access to fresh hay, green grass or 'new' grain and other noxious animal bites (snakes, spiders, bees), toxic plants such as nettles and inhaled pollens, stable dust and chemicals from fires and sprays may also produce urticaria. The wide variety of possible factors makes the

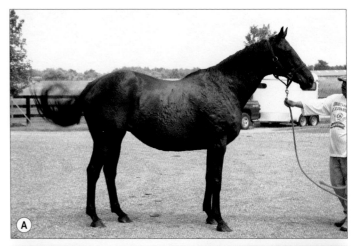

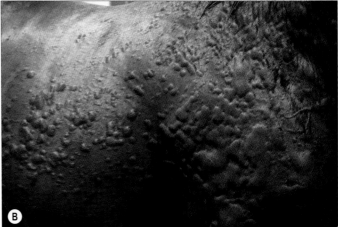

Figure 9.36 (A, B) Urticaria with a mixture of annular and papular wheals.

Differential diagnosis:
- Insect bites or stings
- Nettle rash
- Dermatophytosis (especially early lesions)
- Folliculitis (usually painful and exudative)
- Vasculitis
- Purpura haemorrhagica (usually has a specific history of respiratory disease, presence of petechiae and variable fever)
- Erythema multiforme.

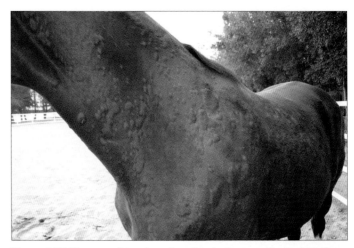

Figure 9.37 Urticaria with annular and papular wheals as a result of multiple fly bites.

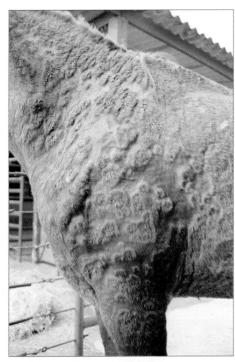

Figure 9.38 Focal but extensive lesions of angioedema with serum exudation.

Differential diagnosis:
• Urticaria
• Amyloidosis
• Mastocytoma
• Cutaneous histiocytic lymphosarcoma
• Vesicular dermatoses.

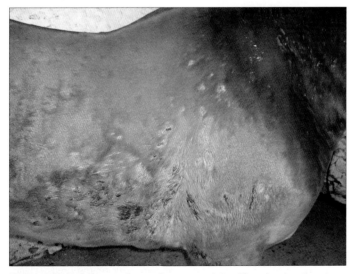

Figure 9.39 Diffuse angioedema with serum exudation. Note that the edema is diffuse and ill-defined but it will still pit on pressure. Reproduced from Knottenbelt D, *Pascoe's Principles & Practice of Equine Dermatology*, second ed. (2009), with permission from Elsevier.

interpretation of the disorder very difficult and an accurate and complete history is vital to the investigation of the condition which appears in all cases, regardless of the specific etiological factor, to be clinically the same. A thorough clinical examination will also help to eliminate some of the possible causes.

Urticaria is variously described as 'heat rash', 'hives', 'feed-lumps' and no-doubt many other colloquial names. The clinical signs may be

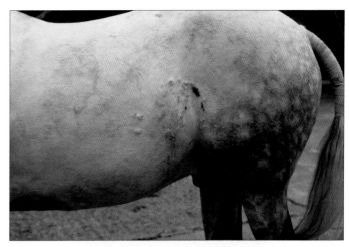

Figure 9.40 Atopy. Generalized variable pruritis was present in this pony for which no cause could be established. Hyperpigmentation and lichenification were present in the skin of the flank areas in particular as a result of self-inflicted damage.

acute or, more rarely, chronic and in either case recurrent episodes are relatively common. Urticarial reactions are characterized by localized or more generalized raised skin wheals. There may be multiple small wheals or more extensive plaques which may occur on the neck, trunk or legs. A less well-defined edema and swelling of the face, eyelids and nose may be present. The lesions themselves pit on pressure and, usually, individual lesions are not longlasting. In some cases the extent of the local edema is such that serum or even blood exudes through the skin at the site.

Angioedema is a subcutaneous form of urticaria in which there is massive intracellular protein loss and plasma exudation. It tends to be more diffuse than urticaria due to the spread of fluid through the subcutis. It most commonly affects the head and extremities and is frequently a reflection of more severe disease than urticaria alone. Pruritis is usally not present and in many cases may be difficult or impossible to distinguish from vasculitis.

Conditions in which vasculitis is a presenting feature, such as **immune-mediated vasculitis, systemic lupus erythematosus, equine viral arteritis and photoactivated vasculitis,** may produce lesions which are almost identical in clinical appearance but generally have other significant clinical signs.

Diagnosis and treatment

• Diagnosis of the condition is generally easily made based on clinical signs but identification of the causative agent(s) may be somewhat more difficult.
• Corticosteroids (dexamethasone) are rapidly curative in most cases. Horses which have recurring episodes may become somewhat more refractory to treatment.
• Removal of the causative agent prevents recurrence.

Atopy (Fig. 9.40)

Atopy is a rare, multifactorial, genetically programmed pruritic disease probably associated with sensitization to environmental antigens. There is little known in horses about the heritability of the condition but Arabian and Thoroughbred breeds are most often affected with signs commonly seen in early adulthood. Specific antigens presumably trigger the release of IgE, possibly IgG, and reaginic antibodies in the production of a type I (anaphylactic) hypersensitivity.

Clinical signs are those of intense pruritus, usually with self-mutilation to the face, limbs and body. This can be so intense as to cause actual skin tearing and bleeding. During repeated attacks the horse usually mutilates a different area of the body and therefore

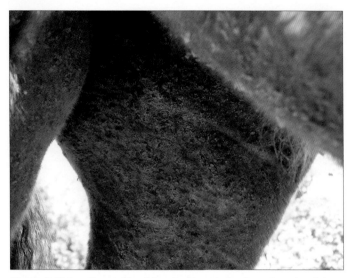

Figure 9.41 Juvenile pemphigus foliaceus with marked scaling and crusting of the inner thigh region.

Differential diagnosis:
- Dermatophilosis
- Dermatophytosis
- Folliculitis
- Bullous pemphigoid
- Exfoliative eosinophilic dermatitis
- Epitheliogenesis imperfecta/epidermolysis bullosa (usually seen in newborns whereas pemphigus foliaceus is seen in older foals)
- Seborrhea (rare).

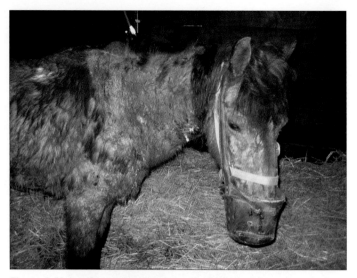

Figure 9.42 Juvenile pemphigus foliaceus with a marked exfoliative dermatitis has resulted in extensive areas of alopecia.

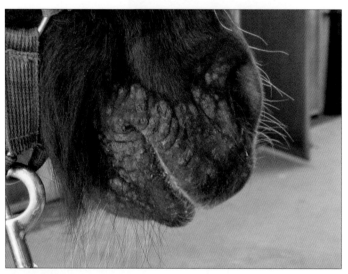

Figure 9.43 Pemphigus foliaceus. Early lesions confined to the muzzle area.

Differential diagnosis: (see Fig. 9.41)
- Chemical dermatoses; history of application of chemicals
- Drug eruptions; history of drug administration
- Coronary band dystrophy
- Papular dermatitis
- *Culicoides* spp. dermatitis
- Onchocerciasis.

scarring or evidence of previous attacks are usually not obvious. Typically the horses do not seem able to stop the frenzied biting and rubbing once an attack begins.

Predisposing causes include changes in environmental temperature such as extra rugs or in other instances, increased cold rather than heat.

Diagnosis
- Elimination of all other possible causes of pruritis
- Elimination of insect and food hypersensitivities
- Intradermal testing in many cases is of limited use due to the lack of availability of local antigens
- Skin biopsies are not useful as they indicate non-specific changes
- Serum testing is not recommended as it has poor sensitivity and specificity.

Treatment
- If the allergen can be identified it should be removed from the horse's environment.
- Systemic glucocorticoids generally form the basis of treatment, but treatment may need to be maintained at high levels for prolonged periods.
- Hyposensitization may be possible in some cases, but requires commitment from the owner to prolonged dosing regimens. Complete resolution is rare but in many cases a partial resolution with resultant reduction in drug use to control the condition is often acceptable.
- Other novel therapies such as cyclosporin A have been tried in some cases.

Autoimmune skin conditions

Pemphigus foliaceus (Figs. 9.41–9.46)

This is an autoimmune skin disease characterized by an exfoliative dermatitis due to a type II hypersensitivity, with autoantiboides directed against the cell membrane of epithelial cells.

It can be seen in horses of all ages, although juvenile onset (<6 months) is often related to a better prognosis. It has been identified in many breeds although Appaloosas are over-represented. Trigger factors such as drug administration, neoplasia, allergens and ill-defined stressors have been proposed as initiating factors but none have been specifically identified.

- *Advanced/chronic lesions.* Diffuse, severe crusting and scaling with extensive alopecia, which is often present over large areas of the body. The exfoliating dermatitis may result in the epidermis peeling off in sheets.
- *Paraneoplastic pemphigus.* This is an aggressive rapidly progressive form that has been seen in horses with solid neoplastic disorders. Systemic signs such as lethargy, anorexia, edema, fever and weight loss which can be seen in all forms of the disease are often more marked in this form.

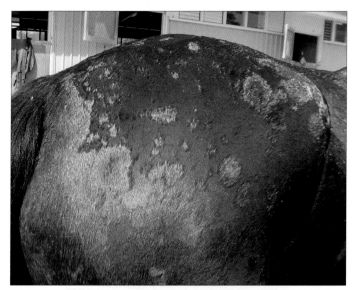

Figure 9.44 Pemphigus foliaceus. Lesions of an extensive exfoliative dermatitis, with no perceptible blistering, had been present for 6 months. Similar lesions were present over the neck and inside the ear.

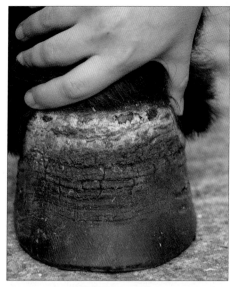

Figure 9.46 Pemphigus foliaceus. Severe lesions around the coronary band. This is frequently the first site at which lesions are noted.

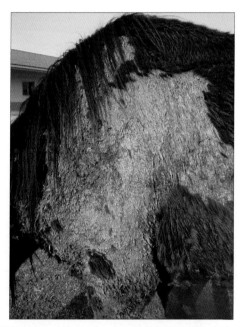

Figure 9.45 Pemphigus foliaceus can occur as a paraneoplastic syndrome. Severe peracute pemphigus foliaceus in a mare with a hepatic neoplasm.

Clinical signs

- Early/mild: A persistent urticaria-like eruption commonly over the head or limbs is usually the first sign noted. Scaling and crusting then becomes evident with variable alopecia. Inflammation of the coronary band is particularly common and the limbs may feel hot to touch.
- Pruritis is not commonly present in early cases but it is variable.
- Lesions spread over the entire body over a course of days/weeks.

Diagnosis

- History and clinical appearance are usually suggestive.
- Biopsy is characteristic with acanthocytes in the superficial crusts and scale.

- Note: biopsy sites should not be clipped or scrubbed prior to biopsy. Multiple biopsies are often required (6–8) and surface scabs should be included as far as possible.
- Direct immunofluorescence is also diagnostic but requires samples with intact vesicle or pustules. Additionally the test may not be routinely available in many laboratories.

Treatment

- The first line of treatment in most cases is prednisolone.
- Dexamethasone can also be used but is less preferred due to greater effects on the pituitary–adrenal axis.
- There are many different treatment protocols described for both of these drugs but all involve high initial doses followed by a decreasing dose regimen until a control dose can be achieved.
- Cases that fail to respond to corticosteroids can be treated with gold salts such as sodium aurothiomyolate.

Bullous pemphigoid (Figs. 9.47 & 9.48)

This is a rare vesiculo-bullous, ulcerative disease of the mucocutaneous junctions and the skin. Autoantibodies are directed against the basement membrane resulting in deeper lesions than those seen with pemphigus foliaceus. Although the disease has an autoimmune basis, it is thought that trigger factors such as stress, other infections or neoplastic disease may play an important role.

Clinically, sub-epidermal vesicles and erosions occur around the mouth, eyes, nose, tongue and vulva. Chronic lesions in advanced cases show crusting and ulceration with epidermal collarettes. Severely affected horses lose condition, become depressed and may be febrile. Systemic signs which are non-specific include pyrexia, anorexia and weight loss.

Diagnosis and treatment

- Diagnosis is made from carefully collected biopsies and similar to diagnosis of pemphigus foliaceus it is important not to clip or prep the biopsy site.
- The condition is characterized histologically by dermoepidermal vesicle formation and immunologically by auto-antibody at the basement membrane of the skin and mucosa.
- Treatment is unrewarding, requiring high doses of corticosteroids and/or other immunosuppressive drugs.
- Euthanasia is invariably indicated.

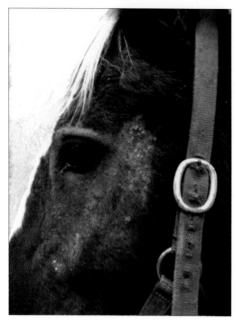

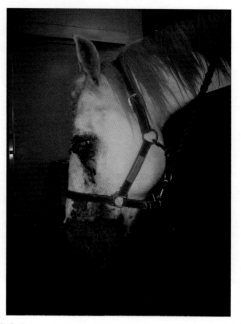

Figure 9.47 Bullous pemphigoid with early crusting lesions evident around the eyes.

Figure 9.48 Bullous pemphigoid with typical lesion distribution around the muzzle and eyes.

Differential diagnosis:
- Viral skin diseases (such as poxvirus and coital exanthema)
- Systemic lupus erythematous-like syndrome
- Drug eruptions
- Granulomatous enteritis syndrome
- Pemphigus foliaceus
- Vesicular stomatitis
- Chronic dermatophilosis
- Chronic chorioptic mange
- Oral irritation and toxic burns
- Renal failure.

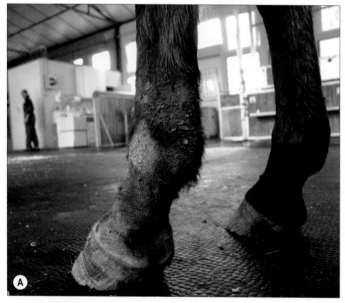

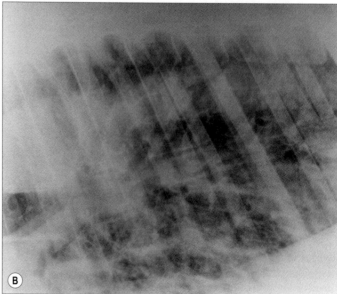

Figure 9.49 Equine sarcoidosis. Heavy scurf, crust and exfoliative dermatitis with areas of alopecia. Weight loss and epidermal folding were evident. Similarly to the human form of the disease, pulmonary lesions are common (B); this horse also had diffuse infiltration of both lungs giving a marked interstitial pattern on radiographic examination.

Differential diagnosis:
- Dermatophilosis
- Dermatophytosis
- Pemphigus foliaceus
- Seborrhea
- Systemic lupus erythematosus-like syndrome
- Exfoliative eosinophilic dermatitis
- Arsenic and mercury poisoning.

Equine sarcoidosis (Fig. 9.49)

This is a rare systemic idiopathic granulomatous disease with no age, breed or sex predilection. The cause and pathogenesis are unknown although a multifactorial etiology is suspected. It is thought to be similar to the human condition of the same name with an abnormal immunological response to an undefined antigen(s). Most cases present initially for skin disease although commonly multiple internal organ involvement is present and clinically horses show loss of appetite, persistent low-grade fever and severe loss of body condition. Cutaneous signs include generalized scaling and crusting with variable alopecia of the head and limbs. Some horses may have nodules or tumor-like masses and in some cases both skin forms may be present simultaneously.

Diagnosis

• History and clinical signs may be suggestive but as the condition is rare it may be overlooked as a differential for skin disease.

• Hematology and serum biochemistry findings show non-specific changes such as leukocytosis, hyperfibronogenemia, hypergamma-globulinemia and increased renal and hepatic enzymes. Although non-specific these indicators of a more extensive systemic involvement combined with cutaneous lesions may also be suggestive of the disease.

• Skin biopsy shows the presence of sarcoidal granulomatous perifollicular and mid-dermal dermatitis.

• Organ biopsies may reveal sarcoidal granulomas.

Treatment

• Dietary changes can be helpful for identification and removal of other possible antigens.

• Systemic corticosteroids are usually prescribed (prednisolone) but may be required for prolonged periods.

• Similar to the the human condition some cases resolve spontaneously over a period of months or years while others are progressive.

Multisystemic eosinophilic epitheliotropic disease/generalized eosinophilic disorder (Figs. 9.50 & 9.51)

This is a rare but significant disorder that primarily affects young horses (3–6 years) but can also be seen in older horses. The etiopathogenesis is poorly understood but is thought to be related to a hypersensitivity reaction to a variety of possible antigens including toxins, concurrent disease or neoplasia, viruses or parasites.

The principal cutaneous sign seen is an exfoliative dermatitis with intracutaneous nodules or linear cutaneous thickenings. Ulceration of the cutaneous nodules may occur. Secondary bacterial infections are common. Ulceration of oral mucosa especially along gingival margins is also commonly encountered. Diarrhea, weight loss and mutli-organ failure usually occur.

Diagnosis

• Clinical signs are highly suggestive.

• Lymph node, skin or rectal biopsy may be supportive but specific stains may be required so the pathologist should be informed if the condition is suspected.

• It is important to bear in mind that concurrent infectious or neoplastic conditions may be present.

Treatment

• High-dose corticosteroid therapy is required and may lead to useful remission although continuation of corticosteroid therapy at a reduced dose is required.

• Relapses are common when steroids are withdrawn or the dose is reduced below an effective level, and deterioration can be rapid.

• Overall the prognosis for affected horses is poor.

Systemic lupus erythematosus-like syndrome (SLE) (Fig. 9.52)

This is a rare, multisystemic autoimmune disorder with ill-defined etiopathogenesis. The syndrome has features of both discoid lupus erythematosus (DLE) and systemic lupus erythematosus (SLE). Trigger factors are usually reported and may include viral infections, changes in environment, extremes of temperature, drugs or stressful events such as pregnancy or heavy work. Multiple organs are usually involved although cutaneous signs are the most obvious. However, these are non-specific and include symmetrical alopecia, seborrhea, edema of extremities and pigmentation loss. Signs associated with involvement of other organs are lameness (polyarthritis), uveitis, pyrexia, weight loss, petechiation of mucous membranes, hypopyon and hyphaema.

Diagnosis

• Diagnosis is difficult and usually requires the interpretation of a number of tests together.

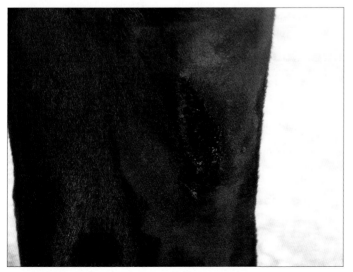

Figure 9.50 Multisystemic eosinophilic epitheliotropic disease/generalized eosinophilic disorder.

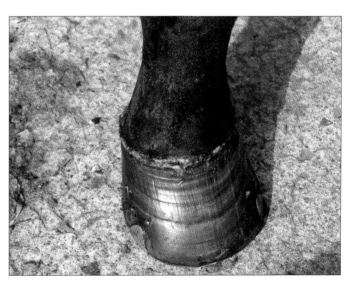

Figure 9.51 Coronitis is a frequent finding of multisystemic eosinophilic epitheliotropic disease.

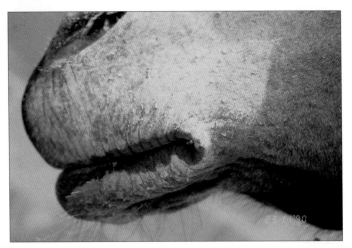

Figure 9.52 Systemic lupus erythematosus-like syndrome. Skin scaling is common and depigmentation of the muzzle is common. In many cases it may be difficult to differentiate from sunburn when depigmented areas are affected.

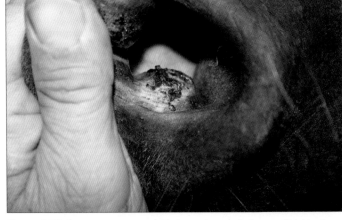

Figure 9.53 Equine cutaneous amyloidosis; nasal mucosal plaques which bleed easily were present.

- The combination of systemic and cutaneous signs may be suggestive but each sign is not consistently present and none is pathognomonic.
- Skin biopsy for immunofluorescent studies which show a characteristic hydropic interface dermatitis.
- Serum can be tested for antinuclear antibody (ANA) but may not be positive in all cases. The Coombs test may be positive in some cases.
- Serum hematology and biochemistry may reveal hyperfibrinogenemia, hypergammaglobulinemia and elevated white cell counts, but none of these are specific for SLE.

Treatment
- Where possible trigger factors should be identified and treated. Antibiotic therapy should run concurrently with corticosteroid therapy and prolonged treatment times may be required.
- The course of the disease is notoriously unpredictable; remissions have been reported, but where general wasting and other systemic abnormalities such as thrombocytopenia, polyarthritis, monoclonal gammopathies and recurrent fever have occurred, the prognosis is unfavorable.

Immune vasculitis
This is a not uncommon small-vessel immune-mediated vasculitis that is most frequently associated with drug reactions (penicillin) and streptococcal bacterial proteins. Petechial hemorrhages and necrotizing cutaneous vasculitis are the main signs. Marked limb edema may be the first sign noted by the owner. Concurrent hematuria, protein loss and anemia may reflect non-cutaneous involvement. High fevers are frequently seen.

Diagnosis
- Clinical signs while characteristic in the later stages may be non-specific initially.
- Historical exposure to a causative antigen is suggestive but it is important to remember that a previous streptococcal infection may have gone unnoticed.
- Biopsy of the early lesions shows neutrophilic (leukocytoclastic), eosinophilic, lymphocytic or mixed vasculitis. Immunohistochemistry and fluorescent antibody confirmation is definitive but only available at a limited number of laboratories.

Treatment
- Initial treatment involves immunosuppressive doses of corticosteroids.

- It is generally advised to remove all other drugs in case they are the causative antigen. However, if no drugs were being concurrently administered and there is a concurrent infection that is suspected of being the cause antimicrobial treatment may be warranted.
- Many cases experience full remission, others may relapse and some have a rapid deterioration.

Equine cutaneous amyloidosis (Fig. 9.53)
This is a rare papulonodular disorder of skin and nasal mucosa, which presents clinically as nodules and plaques in the skin and the mucosa of nasal passages. The lesions often appear suddenly and are slowly progressive. Epistaxis may be the earliest sign of the condition. Systemic forms of amyloidosis rarely have cutaneous involvement.

Diagnosis, treatment and prognosis
- Diagnosis is frequently based on clinical signs and history, which often reveal repeated immune stimulation, underlying neoplasia or a chronic organic infectious process.
- Histopathology of lesions shows the presence of amyloid.
- This condition is treated through surgical excision, but depending on location this may be difficult.
- Spontaneous remissions and improvement following corticosteroid administration are usually temporary.

Infectious diseases

Important infectious skin disease may be caused by viral, bacterial or fungal agents. Commonly they all cause hair loss and variable epidermal exfoliation and exudation. In the case of deeper tissue diseases such as pythiosis and other systemic mycoses, excessive fibrous tissue formation and more copious exudation are typically present. Pruritus may be intense or may be absent. Secondary physical damage can occur from self-inflicted trauma, which in turn encourages continued self-mutilation.

Virus diseases
Equine genital herpes virus (coital exanthema) (Fig. 9.54)
This is a viral venereal disease which is caused by equine herpes virus-3. It occurs throughout the world and while transmission is, in most cases venereal, it can also be transmitted iatrogenically by contaminated veterinary equipment. Following an incubation period of between 7 and 10 days, papules and vesicles develop on the affected skin of the penis and prepuce or vulva. These rapidly develop into

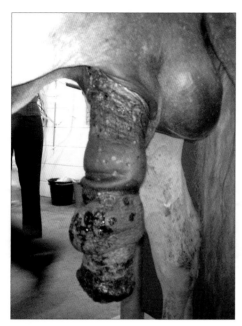

Figure 9.54 Equine coital exanthema (EHV 3). Typical circular lesions found in the early stages of the disease. Initially vesicles are present which rupture to leave small crater-like lesions (seen here) many of which will have a pustular center.

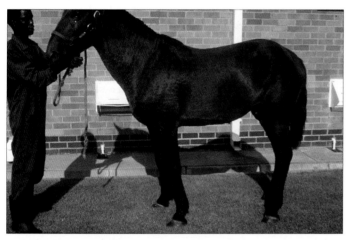

Figure 9.55 Equine molluscum contagiosum. Typical waxy raised papules.

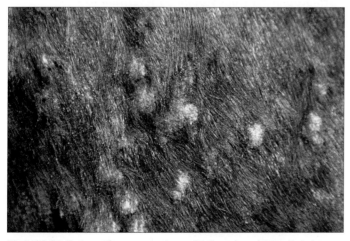

Figure 9.56 Equine molluscum contagiosum. Small pearly, umbilicated papular epithelial lesions.

pustules in the penile skin and vulva. There may be localized pain and fever. Infection may extend to the anus and skin of the tail. Spontaneous regression occurs with developing immunity over 3 weeks and during this time the affected horse is potentially infective. Healed lesions are depigmented.

Diagnosis, treatment and prognosis

- History and clinical signs are usually diagnostic.
- No treatment is generally required but soothing antibiotic creams may heal recovery and local anesthetic creams may ease discomfort. Breeding horses should be rested until lesions are completely healed.
- While immunity in most cases is permanent following recovery, recurrence of lesions can occur in both stallions and mares due to lowered resistance such as might be caused by other generalized disease, over work and parturition.

Horsepox virus

This is a rare condition that is likely caused by an unidentified equine pox virus or vaccinia (cowpox-derived attenuated virus used for human smallpox vaccination). Infection occurs directly through the skin or the respiratory tract although localized forms are the commonest with the muzzle/mouth affected most commonly. Pox lesions have a typical clinical appearance of macules, papules and vesicles which then develop into pustules with a depressed center. Lesions can be painful but are usually transient.

Diagnosis and treatment

- Diagnosis is rarely required as most cases may not even be presented to a vet.
- There is no treatment available and usually none is required but there is a potential zoonosis.

Equine molluscum contagiosum (Figs. 9.55 & 9.56)

This is caused by another unclassified pox virus, with a clinical appearance of circumscribed, raised, smooth, often umbilicated, papules with a waxy surface. A caseous plug may be found in the center of the oldest lesions. The lesions most frequently occur around the genital organs of mares and stallions, and the axilla and muzzle.

Diagnosis and treatment

- Diagnosis may be confirmed by biopsy.
- There is no treatment available or usually necessary. Resolution may be slow in some cases and rare cases may have persistent lesions.

Viral papular dermatitis

This is due to another unclassified pox virus, and initially shows papules which develop crusts and after some 10 days the lesions develop an annular alopecia with scaling. Spontaneous resolution occurs over 2–4 weeks.

Diagnosis and treatment

- Diagnosis is frequently presumptive based on clinical appearance of lesions but viral isolation from papular lesions is possible.
- No treatment is usually required.

Viral papillomatosis (Figs. 9.57 & 9.58)

This is a common skin disease of young (1–4 years), grazing horses caused by papovavirus infection. The condition can occur in older horses which are immunologically naive to the virus. The characteristic lesions show as single or multiple small verrucose warts, principally around the nose, lips and eyes. They may occur singly or form tight groups and may extend over a wide area of the face at an alarming rate. Lesions almost invariably regress spontaneously after 3–4 months. The virus appears capable of survival from season to season with each succeeding crop of weanling foals developing the condition at approximately 10–12 months of age each year on affected farms.

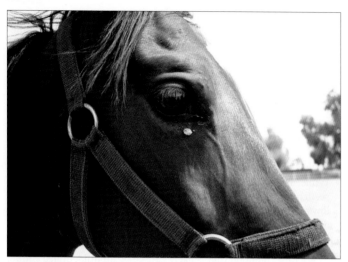

Figure 9.57 Viral papillomatosis. These lesions are commonly seen around the eyes and muzzle in young horses.

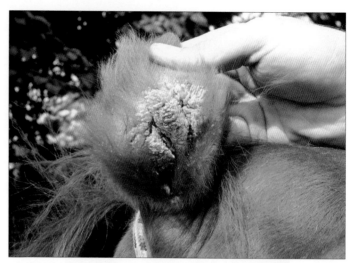

Figure 9.59 Pinnal acanthosis. In this advanced case there are multiple coalescing lesions of thickened hyperkeratotic skin.

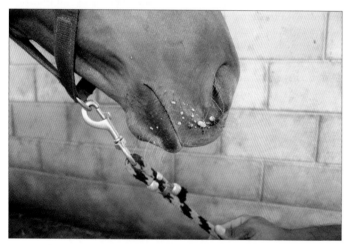

Figure 9.58 Viral papillomatosis.

The adult-onset form may not regress but likewise has no clinical significance but should be differentiated from the verrucose forms of sarcoid which are clinically much more significant.

Diagnosis and treatment
- Clinical signs are usually all that is required although biopsy may be required for differentiation in adult-onset cases.
- Treatment is not generally required due to spontaneous regression. However in cases where a more rapid recovery is required due to upcoming sales/shows, surgical excision with topical anti-wart applications can be helpful.
- Autogenous vaccines can also be helpful but should not be used on other horses even though they may appear to be similarly affected.

Pinnal acanthosis (hyperplastic aural dermatitis/aural plaques/fungal plaques) (Fig. 9.59)
This is a common condition in horses over 2 years of age. It is probably a clinically distinct form of papillomatosis caused by an unidentified papilloma virus. These commence as small, smooth depigmented papillae and progress to large, often extensive hyperkeratotic plaques on the inner surface of the pinna. Lesions may also be found on the groin and inner thighs. Most cases have a summer onset leading to the suspicion of an insect vector.

Diagnosis and treatment
- Clinical signs will help diagnosis, but biopsy and electron microscopy can be needed in some cases
- These lesions seldom regress spontaneously and although they have little or no harmful effect they may become unsightly.
- Treatment options are limited as topical applications rarely result in a cure and frequently lead to ear resentment.

Bacterial diseases
Normally, horse skin is highly resistant to bacterial infection unless constantly exposed to factors which cause lowering of the natural skin defense mechanisms. This will occur with excessive wetting, friction, physical trauma, biting insects and arthropods, injurious topical treatments and self-mutilation. Bacterial skin disease may be primary or secondary to infection elsewhere in the body.

Diagnosis of (primary) bacterial dermatitis is confirmed by the identification of bacteria obtained by skin scrapings or smears, but must be interpreted in conjunction with the clinical signs, due to the wide variety of organisms present as commensals on normal skin and the rapid secondary infection of wounds. In order to establish the true significance of a bacterial species with respect to its role in skin disease, such smears or samples should be taken from intact pustules, nodules or deep swabs from abscesses, preferably by needle aspiration or by direct culture from biopsy samples.

Dermatophilosis (rain scald/mud fever/rain rot)
(Figs. 9.60–9.62)
This is a common infectious and contagious bacterial dermatitis that occurs worldwide due to the Gram-positive actinomycete *Dermatophilus congolensis*. It is characterized by a moist exudative dermatitis and pustular crusting of the hair. Repeated soaking of the skin results in breaks in the physical integrity of the skin allowing for the entry of infection. As a result affected areas are those that are continually soaked such as the dorsum and lower legs. Extensive crusting and exudation with hair loss, or hair matted with exudate and bare skin areas showing patchy hypopigmentation are common developments. Early cases of the disease in horses with long winter coats often show a matted, tessellated coat over the affected areas, which, on being plucked, reveals a purulent undersurface. The lesions may be painful but are rarely, if ever, pruritic. As the matted hair is shed, it may leave long, linear, hyperkeratotic scabs. In short-haired horses (including summer-coated animals), lesions are smaller and occur as multifocal skin 'bumps' covered

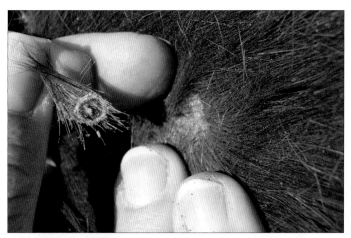

Figure 9.60 Dermatophilosis. Typical paint brush appearance of freshly removed scab.

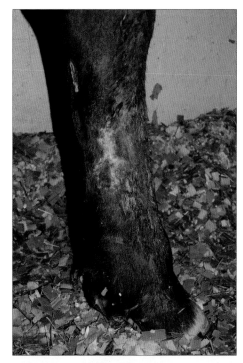

Figure 9.61 Dermatophilosis confined to the legs.

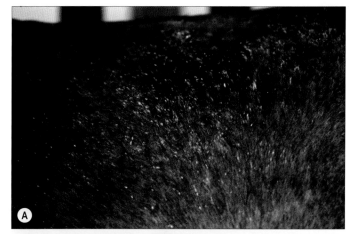

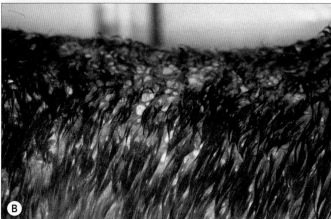

Figure 9.62 Dermatophilosis. (A) Hair matted in a tessellated pattern. (B) Extensive hair loss leaving hyperkeratotic linear scabs and skin denuded of hair.

Diagnosis
- Clinical signs are diagnostic.
- A diagnosis of dermatophilosis is sometimes difficult as a result of prolonged, heavy, secondary bacterial contamination, but Giemsa, methylene blue or Gram-stained smears of the exudate from fresh lesions show typical branching filaments or rows of coccoid bodies having a 'railway-line-like' appearance.

Treatment
- In most cases dermatophilosis is a self-limiting condition, provided that all inciting factors such as wetness, skin trauma, sweating and ectoparasites are eliminated and the micro-environment for the organism is thereby altered to preclude its multiplication.
- Severe cases may require antibiotics.
- It is important to remember that the condition is contagious and affected horses should be isolated.

Bacterial folliculitis and furunculosis (Fig. 9.63)

Folliculitis is inflammation of the hair follicle with accumulation of inflammatory cells within the follicle lumen. It is most frequently caused by coagulase-positive **Staphylococcus spp.** and less commonly by **Streptococcus spp.** Most cases are related to poor hygiene or cutaneous immunity problems. Infection is most frequently seen in the groin and saddle area but can also affect the sides of the face. A painful localized papule can be felt in the skin. This progresses to an exudative and edematous lesion. Most then form individual pustules while others may coalesce to form abscesses or furunculosis. Lesions occurring in the saddle area, girth and the withers often induce

with crusts or scale. Although the lesions are obvious in severely affected horses they are often more apparent by palpation than by visual inspection in mildly affected horses. Examination of tufts of hair plucked from these lesions reveals typical dermatophilosis scabbing at the roots of the hair giving a paint-brush effect. Denudation of hair is common in this 'summer/short-coat' form. Interestingly, white-skinned areas appear to be particularly sensitive/susceptible to the condition and it is therefore commonly encountered on white areas of the distal limbs, particularly if the horse is maintained in long wet grass. Continued serum exudation provides ideal conditions for replication of the bacterium and other secondary pathogens such as *Staphylococcus* spp. Lesions of dermatophilosis may also occur on the head and again, at this site, white-skinned areas are more susceptible.

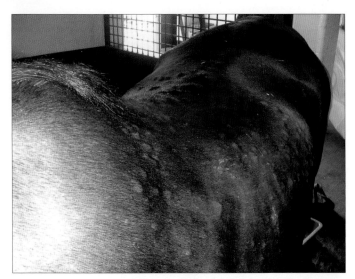

Figure 9.63 Extensive raised lesions of bacterial folliculitis on this yearling.

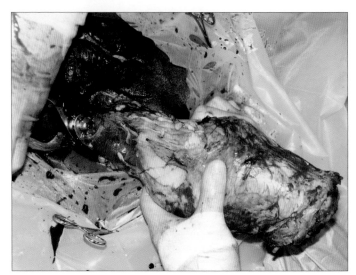

Figure 9.64 Marked thickening and pyogranulomatous areas of this spermatic cord following infection of the cord after castration. This is known as botryomycosis.

Differential diagnosis:
- Exuberant granulation tissue
- Cutaneous habronemiasis
- Fungal granuloma/mycetoma
- Sarcoid
- Neoplasia.

marked and permanent leukotrichia, producing the so-called 'saddle marks'.

Diagnosis, treatment and prognosis
- While clinical examination will usually lead to a diagnosis of folliculitis/furunculosis the changes seen are not pathognomonic for a particular bacteria and early lesions can be confused with various forms of dermatophytosis.
- Treatment can be difficult, especially in severely affected cases. Antiseptic washes, systemic antibiotics, anti-inflammatories are all frequently required.
- Stable hygiene is of the utmost importance.
- The prognosis is fair to good but lesions may take a long time to resolve with prolonged therapy. Healed lesions may have permanent alterations to hair color and quality.

Botryomycosis (Fig. 9.64)
This is a chronic bacterial (*Staphylococcus* spp.), pyogranulomatous disease of the skin most often associated with skin trauma such as laceration, puncture or surgery. A more severe form involving spread to regional lymph nodes can occur in immunocompromised horses. The most common clinical entity is that which follows contamination of limb or scrotal wounds. The lesions are non-pruritic, non-healing, granulomatous nodules which sometimes develop into larger tumor-like growths. Botryomycosis occurring at the site of contaminated castration wounds results in a non-healing, discharging mass of fibrous tissue at the end of the spermatic cord, containing myriads of small septic foci. These wounds seldom, if ever, heal spontaneously and a chronic discharging sinus is usually present at the scrotal incision which is known as a scirrhous cord.

Diagnosis, treatment and prognosis
- Although history and clinical signs may be suggestive, a diagnosis is only confirmed histologically from surgical sections or biopsy which show a nodular to diffuse dermatitis with tissue granules.
- The goal of therapy is to remove all infected tissue. Thereafter control of further infection is important and may involve administration of antibiotics and dressings.
- Prognosis depends on the feasibility of removal of all infected tissue.

Streptococcal dermatitis/folliculitis (Figs. 9.65 & 9.66)
Streptococcal skin infections occur widely amongst the horse population and are probably the commonest secondary bacterial invaders of skin wounds in horses. The clinical syndromes seen are widely

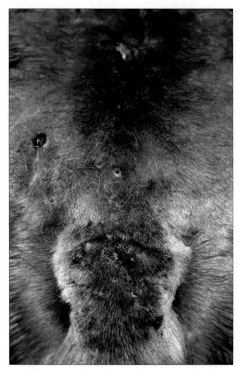

Figure 9.65 Folliculitis of the tailhead and rump.

variable from folliculitis (*S. equisimilis, S. equi* var. *zooepidemicus*), to disseminated abscessation (*S. equi* var. *equi*). Ulcerative lymphangitis and focal abscesses are other common presentations.

Diagnosis, treatment and prognosis
- Definitive diagnosis requires culture ideally from fine-needle aspirates as *Strep.* spp are common contaminants.

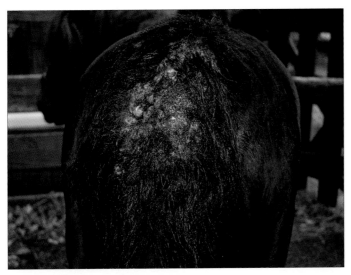

Figure 9.66 Streptococcal dermatitis.

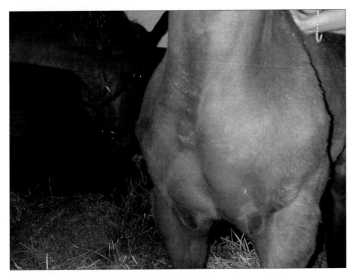

Figure 9.67 Pigeon fever. Pectoral swelling associated with *Corynebacterium pseudotuberculosis* abscess.

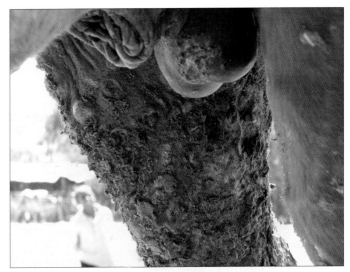

Figure 9.68 Glanders. Extensive ulcerating cutaneous nodules are frequently found, especially on the inner thigh. Reproduced from Knottenbelt D, *Pascoe's Principles & Practice of Equine Dermatology*, second ed. (2009), with permission from Elsevier.

- The affected area should be cleaned and clipped if required. Localized mild folliculitis can be treated with topical antibiotic creams.
- Immature abscesses may benefit from hot packing to speed maturation. When mature abscesses can be drained it is important to always dispose carefully of abscess material and keep affected horses isolated until a definitve diagnosis can be reached.
- Antibiotics may be required (see section on Strangles p. 137).

Pigeon fever (pigeon chest, Wyoming strangles or false strangles) (Fig. 9.67)

Large pectoral or ventral abdominal abscesses can develop as a result of infection with *Corynebacterium pseudotuberculosis*. Transmission is thought to be by biting flies and the condition is limited to areas of the United States of America and in Brazil. The abscesses characteristically contain (and discharge) a creamy or caseous white to greenish pus.

Clostridium *species infection* (see Chapter 8, p. 300)

Localized infections with *Clostridium* spp. are capable of acute and dangerous wound infection at sites of injections, trauma and/or surgery. Abscesses may develop over a period of days and result eventually in a hot painful swelling and severe lameness (depending on the site of injection). Many require surgical drainage to release their purulent to serosanguineous gassy contents; necrosis of overlying skin and adjacent muscle is not uncommon.

Glanders (farcy) (Fig. 9.68)

This is a highly contagious zoonotic disease that occurs in Eastern Europe, Asia and North Africa, caused by *Burkholderia mallei* (*Pseudomonas/Malleomyces mallei*). Both acute and chronic forms of the infection are encountered and there are occasional subclinical carriers.

- *Acute.* This form is rare in horses but more common in donkeys and mules. There is an acute respiratory tract infection with rapid death as a result of septicemia.
- *Chronic.* This form is characterized by skin disease as well as a more protracted respiratory disease. Horses are often debilitated with ulcerative cutaneous nodules that occur most commonly on the medial aspect of the thigh, face and neck. The lesions begin as subcutaneous nodules which rapidly ulcerate and discharge a honey-like exudate. Corded lymphatics and swollen lymph nodes are common.

Diagnosis

- History including geographical location and clinical signs
- The 'mallein' (intradermo-palpebral) test is definitive in most horses, but rare cases may not show a clearly positive result
- Bacterial culture or polymerase chain reaction (PCR)
- Complement fixation.

Treatment

- No treatment is available and the disease is reportable in most countries with a slaughter policy.
- Note: The disease can be fatal to humans and is highly contagious. Extreme care must be taken in handling samples and the laboratory advised of the potential agent involved.

Fungal diseases

Fungal dermatoses in horses range from common superficial disorders such as dermatophytosis (ringworm) to more exotic disorders such as pythiosis (Florida leeches). Classification is based on location of the infection. These include superficial (cutaneous), subcutaneous and systemic mycoses.

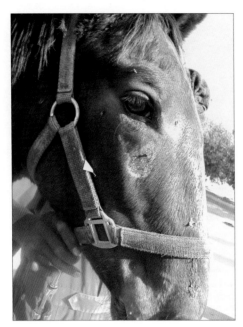

Figure 9.69 Dermatophytosis. Typical roughly circular appearance of dermatophyte lesion.

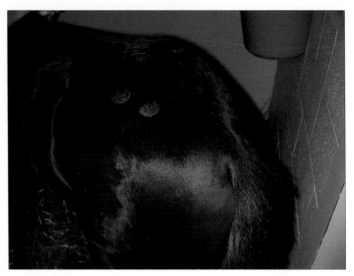

Figure 9.70 Dermatophytosis.

- **Superficial mycoses** are the most common and include the diseases known as ringworm (dermatophytosis, dermatomycosis) which is a fungal infection of the superficial keratinized layers of the epidermis. Tissue penetration is limited only to actively growing hair follicles. Broadly, only two fungal species affect the skin of horses in this way. These are *Trichophyton* spp. and *Microsporum* spp., but other fungi such as *Candida* spp. and *Malassezia* spp. may occasionally induce skin disease.
- **Cutaneous mycoses** affect all keratinized tissue including hair, horn and skin.
- **Subcutaneous/deep mycoses** involve subcutaneous tissues in addition to dermis and epidermis. Some remain localized while others spread to contiguous tissue or spread along lymphatics. Seroconversion occurs but is rarely protective.

Dermatophytosis (Figs. 9.69 & 9.70)

The most common organisms are *Trichophyton equinum* var. *autotrophicum* (TE-vA) and *Trichophyton equinum* var. *equinum* (TE-vE). *Trichophyton verrucosum* may occur in horses with direct contact with infected cattle. Transmission of the pathogen is usually through indirect contact (grooming brushes, rugs, saddles, girths, etc.), with only occasional cases being acquired through direct contact with other affected horses. A much higher incidence of the disease is encountered in hot humid climates but sunshine appears to have a strong inhibitory effect on most of the species concerned. The spores are notoriously long-lived and may survive for several years in the environment in a viable form. Furthermore, they are highly resistant to many disinfectants and antiseptics. The spores must have access to skin abrasions for the clinical condition to develop and this is the reason for its development in sites where skin friction occurs, such as the girth, saddle and face.

Young horses under the age of 4 years are particularly susceptible and show a more prolonged course than older horses. The incubation period varies between 1 and 4 weeks, depending upon the immune status of the host and the ambient temperature and humidity. *T. equinum* lesions are typically ringworm-like in appearance, initially being well-defined, circular areas of erect, raised or short hair. The hair is then lost and the lesions enlarge centrifugally, developing crusts and scabs; new hair growth resumes between 35 and 55 days following infection and characteristically starts in the center of the lesions. Alopecia and scaling are usually associated with limited inflammation. *Trichophyton equinum* var. *autotrophicum* (TEvA), which is the more common pathogen in the southern hemisphere, produces a more diffuse and scaly appearance. Plucked hair from areas affected with TEvA reveals underlying gray, glistening skin, which scales over within 1 or 2 days. In both forms the larger, less well-defined areas represent the more protracted lesions. Pruritus is usually only present in the earliest stages. As each fresh batch of yearlings enters the contaminated environment, they are soon exposed to rapid and predictable infection. This may take the form of face infection from contact with contaminated feeders, or body infection, usually from contaminated grooming equipment or tack.

Should infection not occur during the initial handling period, horses usually become infected during breaking-in or training, usually from contaminated girths, jockey's boots or from the use of contaminated tack such as rugs. The location of the primary lesions is entirely predictable in areas of physical damage and indirect contact with infective material. Further rapid spread may occur from the initial lesions by the use of contaminated grooming brushes, to the extent that generalized infection is relatively common. Horses can become accidentally infected with **Trichophyton verrucosum** through contact with infected cattle or a contaminated environment where cattle have been stabled. In these cases lesions are more commonly found on the lower limbs, appearing initially as raised hair with a thick, closely adherent crust. The hair is gradually shed, usually leaving a large alopecic area with dense hyperkeratotic scaling.

Horses affected with **Microsporum gypseum** generally have smaller well-defined lesions, usually over the buttocks and neck. The hair, in these lesions, plucks noticeably less-readily than that in *Trichophyton* spp. lesions. *Microsporum gypseum* is a soil saprophyte gaining entry to the horse's skin by abrasion and contact, or by biting insects such as *Stomoxys* spp. and mosquitoes, and the siting of the lesions reflects this mode of transmission. Contact with contaminated soil or bedding or horse transporters also spreads the disease; soils from yards containing infected horses yield *Microsporum gypseum* on culture. Other less common organisms which have been isolated include *Microsporum equinum* which produces small annular lesions with light scurf; lesions are usually found on harness pressure areas, and the organism is only weakly infective.

Subcutaneous mycoses occur in horses relatively commonly, particularly in tropical environments. They are usually characterized by localized swellings, draining tracts, and the presence of visible granules in the exudate. Clinically, most present as a chronic abscess which is refractory to normal medical treatment. Most of these fungal diseases need to be diagnosed accurately by means of fungal culture and biopsy. The causative agents may occasionally be identified with the help of specific fungal stains on direct microscopic examination of smears from exudates. In the case of sporotrichosis immunological tests can be used.

Diagnosis
- History and characteristic clinical signs are all that is usually required.
- Hairs plucked from the margins of fresh lesions can be examined microscopically for the presence of hyphae or cultured on Sabourauds fungal medium. Cultures provide the only practical means of identifying the species concerned but they usually take a long time to grow in culture.

Treatment and prognosis
- The majority of ringworm infections in horses will ultimately resolve spontaneously if left without treatment, but the epidemiological factors involved with such a highly contagious disease make its early recognition and treatment important.
- Topical washes with fungicidal compounds (natamycin, enilconazole, miconazole) are the best form of treatment. The whole horse should be washed then the defined lesions washed again. These treatments are normally applied twice weekly until healing is evident.
- Other treatments include daily scrubbing (1–2 min) for 7–10 days with any of the following:
  - 10% povidone-iodine solution
  - 2.5% lime sulfur in water
  - 10% thiabendazole in water
  - 2.5–10% tincture of iodine (not scrubbed, painted on)
  - 0.3% Halamid
  - Tertiary amine disinfectant scrub solution.
- Griseofulvin is not an effective treatment.
- Additionally, all the species responsible for disease in horses have the potential to infect humans.

Eumycetic mycetoma
Eumycetic mycetoma is caused by several different fungi (*Curvularia geniculata*, *Helminthosporium spiciferum*, *Pseudoallescharia boydii* and *Madurella* spp.), which invade body tissues following skin injury. The disease may occur at any site where the organism is introduced into traumatized skin. Clinically, the lesions which are usually on the body trunk, external nares or the legs resemble a chronic abscess or pyogranuloma. The purulent discharge usually contains distinct, small granules which are black-brown in color when associated with *Curvularia geniculata*, and cream-white when the organism is *Pseudoallescharia boydii*.

Diagnosis and treatment
- A diagnosis is based on clinical signs with a history of the chronicity and failure to respond to any normal treatment; it may be confirmed by culture and biopsy.
- Some cases can be successfully treated with surgical removal but recurrence is common.
- Oral potassium iodide (5–10 g q 12 h orally) for 3–6 weeks may also improve the condition.
- Oral antifungals can be used, but in most instances are prohibitively expensive.

Phaeohyphomycosis
This is a chronic subcutaneous and systemic infection caused by *Drechslera speciferum* in tropical countries. The condition often occurs as solitary, painless nodules on the face which exude pus.

Diagnosis and treatment
- Diagnosis is based on history, physical examination, biopsy and culture. It should be differentiated from infection with *Alternaria* spp. in temperate climates which occurs most commonly on the head and ears.
- Surgical removal is generally curative but topical antifungals may also be beneficial.
- Some cases resolve spontaneously.

Sporotrichosis (Fig. 9.71)
This is a chronic progressive infection of skin and subcutaneous tissues that occurs when skin wounds are contaminated by the soil saprophyte *Sporothrix schenckii*. It is generally regarded as a non-contagious disease but is zoonotic. Clinical signs include cording of the lymphatics and enlarged cutaneous nodules on the legs and body. Ulceration with crusting and discharge of a thick red/brown pus or serosanguineous fluid is common. Generalized body infection may show as similar crusted nodules and plaques.

Diagnosis
- Characteristic cording of lymphatics and nodular skin lesions are highly suggestive.
- Gram stain of exudates.
- Culture can be attempted but is difficult.
- Biopsies are rarely diagnostic.

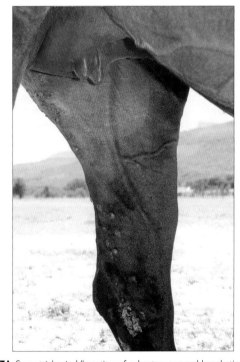

Figure 9.71 Sporotrichosis. Ulceration of subcutaneous and lymphatic nodules.
Differential diagnosis:
- Bacterial/fungal granulomatous dermatitis
- Cutaneous histoplasmosis
- Glanders.

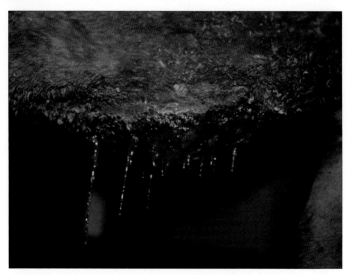

Figure 9.72 Pythiosis. Subcutaneous, ulcerative granulomatous lesions commonly are found in areas of the body that are in contact with infected water such as the ventral abdomen, limbs and face. Stringy, hemorrhagic, serum exudate forms hanging 'leeches'.

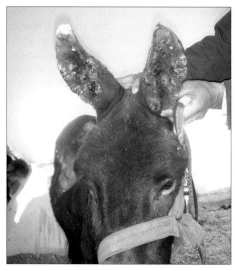

Figure 9.73 Nodular and ulcerated lesions of the pinnae in this donkey which are typical of cryptococcosis. The lips are the other site that is also frequently affected.

Treatment

- Iodine therapy. Sodium iodide 40 mg/kg as a 20% solution intravenously q 24 h for 3–5 days followed by 10 g potassium iodide daily until resolution is achieved.
- Treatment may be prolonged.
- Surgical removal of lesions is difficult but may help in limiting it.

Pythiosis (phycomycosis, bursatti, swamp cancer, Florida horse leeches, hyphomycosis) (Fig. 9.72)

This is a relatively common disorder of the skin caused by *Pythium insidiosum*, occurring in tropical and subtropical areas and particularly in the Gulf States of America, Australia and South America. It is usually associated with swampy conditions where horses either habitually graze in water, or are flood-bound, standing in water for long periods. The organism induces a severe pyogranulomatous reaction as it spreads throughout the tissues. The expansion of the lesion is extremely rapid due to the formation of granulation tissue and hemorrhage is a common feature of these lesions. Blood loss may be sufficient to cause significant anemia. Most lesions are found on the distal extremities and the ventral abdomen and chest, and are usually single. However, bilateral and multiple lesions may occasionally be encountered. Lesions are often initially relatively small and innocuous-looking, roughly circular, ulcerative granulomas, but they may arise explosively from an area which has previously only appeared to be mildly swollen. However, the lesions rapidly destroy surrounding tissue and may spread through lymphatic vessels to the regional lymph nodes, and sometimes even into the abdominal cavity. The cutaneous manifestation of the condition is characterized by the copious out-pouring of a stringy, mucopurulent, serosanguineous discharge. The presence of large 'kunkers' or 'leeches', which are found in the multiple draining tracts, represents cores of necrotic tissue containing the organism. Pruritus may be severe and result in extensive complicating self-inflicted trauma. Old lesions show chronic surrounding fibrosis and there may be long periods of time without the characteristic discharge. Lesions can occur on the lower limbs and frequently then involve tendons and joints or may occur at any other sites where the organism is introduced to wounds.

Diagnosis

- History of access to water and characteristic lesions and locations.

- Biopsy and culture on Sabourauds agar from early lesion are diagnostic.
- ELISA and PCR although these may not be readily available in all areas.

Treatment and prognosis

- Early treatment is essential as successful outcomes in chronic cases are more difficult to achieve.
- Complete surgical removal is required with a wide margin of excision required to help avoid recurrences.
- Intravenous sodium iodide may also be beneficial.
- Amphotericin B can be applied topically and administered systemically but some strains show resistance to the drug.
- Prognosis depends largely on the chronicity and location of the lesion. All cases with bone involvement have to date died.

Note: Differential diagnosis of all fungal diseases should include bacterial granuloma, habronemiasis, exuberant granulation tissue, foreign body reactions, sarcoid and various neoplasms. It is also possible to encounter mixed infections involving fungi, sarcoid and habronema larvae in a single lesion. A very careful clinical assessment and confirmatory biopsy and culture are then a necessity.

Systemic mycoses (Fig. 9.73)

Systemic mycoses which cause fungal infection of internal organs may have secondary skin manifestations. Typically most responsible fungi exist in soil and vegetation and are rare pathogens. Even where organisms occur endemically, exposed animals do not often develop clinical disease.

Infections with *Cryptococcus neoformans*, *Coccidioides immitis*, *Histoplasma capsulatum* var. *farciminosi* and *Blastomyces dermatitidis* have all been reported to cause skin disease in horses.

Cryptococcosis is unusual in distribution and is believed to be spread by pigeon droppings. The disease normally affects the respiratory and central nervous systems, bone and rarely the skin where it has been reported to cause granulomas on the lip.

Blastomycosis has also been recorded as causing multiple granuloma and abscesses around the mammary gland and perineum. Coccidiomycosis has been associated with severe dust storms, high environmental temperatures and inhalation of organisms. Cutaneous infection may follow skin abrasions, and appears as cutaneous ulceration, abscesses and multiple draining sinus tracts. Specimens for culture from suspected cases should be submitted to specialist laboratories dealing in fungal diseases, due to the risk of human infection.

Histoplasmosis (epizootic lymphangitis, pseudoglanders, African farcy)

This is a serious debilitating fungal infection caused by *Histoplasma capsulatum* var. *farciminosum*, which is endemic in Africa, Asia and the Far East. It occurs in horses, mules and very rarely donkeys. Biting insects can be vectors of the disease and trauma appears necessary for infection to occur. Clinical signs initially include nodules (15–25 mm diameter) on the skin of the face, head, neck and rarely on the limbs. The nodules soften and eventually rupture, discharging a light-green, blood-tinged exudate. Progressive ulceration occurs with ulcers reaching up to 10 cm in diameter. Some cases show nodules and ulceration along lymphatic chains. The lesions are almost indistinguishable from those of farcy (cutaneous glanders) except that respiratory tract involvement is not common. Ocular histoplasmosis involving the medial canthus of the eye and, in particular, the puncta and naso-lacrimal duct is relatively common in donkeys but is rare in horses. Infections may also involve one or more joints, leading to a purulent synovitis and severe disabling lameness.

Diagnosis, treatment and prognosis

- Diagnosis is based on direct smears from discharging lesions. Biopsy and culture from biopsy can help, but growth is very slow.
- The prognosis for affected animals is poor and there is no effective treatment known.

Ectoparasitic diseases

Dermatoses caused by ectoparasites form a large proportion of the common skin disorders of horses. As a group they are generally associated with pruritus and hair loss. Irritability, rubbing of the mane and tail in particular and, in some instances, severe self-mutilation may be present. Ectoparasites are also important vectors for the transmission of some very serious viral, bacterial, fungal, protozoal and helminth diseases. While the detection of parasites may simplify the diagnosis, a very careful and thorough examination may still fail to identify the causative agents involved and may necessitate the use of night-light traps, skin scrapings, culture of skin scrapings, biopsy and prolonged environmental studies. Many of the dermatoses due to ectoparasites are geographically restricted as well as seasonal, and this may help significantly in the diagnosis of clinical conditions which can be difficult to differentiate on clinical grounds only.

Pediculosis (louse infestation) (Figs. 9.74 & 9.75)

This is one of the more common causes of skin disease throughout the world. Both biting and sucking lice occur in horses and donkeys and the clinical effect of each is correspondingly different according to the lifestyle of the parasite. Louse infestation is probably the most common form of pruritus in foals. Even small numbers of the biting louse, *Damalinia equi*, cause severe pruritus, scurf and alopecia of the head, the neck (usually under the mane) and the dorso-lateral trunk.

Much greater numbers of sucking lice, *Haematopinus asini*, are usually present. They are most frequently found at the base of the mane and tail, and over the croup and lower limbs. In horses with long (winter) hair coats, the infestation may extend over the entire skin surface giving the animal a 'moth-eaten' appearance. Severe tail-rubbing with hair loss and skin damage are usually encountered. These signs are also common to *Oxyuris equi* infestation, culicoides hypersensitivity and tail mange due to *Psoroptes cuniculi* or *Chorioptes equi* parasites. All louse infestations may be transmitted by direct contact and groups of horses housed in close proximity are therefore likely to develop the condition. Debilitated, diseased and horses

suffering from immune suppression disorders, including pituitary adenoma, are particularly liable to harbor enormous populations of the parasites. Under these conditions both the physical demands of persistent pruritus and, in the case of the sucking lice, blood loss, may result in further dramatic deterioration in body condition and health status.

Diagnosis

- *Damalina equi*: Careful, prolonged examination of the horse is essential as the number of parasites involved is usually small, and skin scrapings from pruritic areas may be necessary to locate them or their eggs; a hand-lens may be a useful aid.
- *Haematopinus asini*: Both the eggs (nits) which attach to the hair and the adult lice are visible to the naked eye.

Treatment

- *Haematopinus asini*: Ivermectin at 200 μg/kg orally every 2 weeks for three treatments is effective.

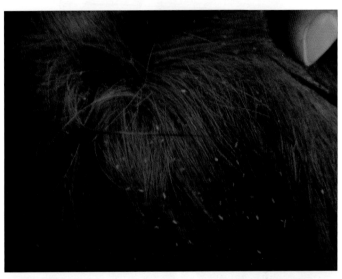

Figure 9.74 Pediculosis. Heavy infestation of lice in a thick winter coat. Mites are usually visible to the naked eye. Typical predilection sites shown include face, base of the mane and over the lateral thorax. Severe pruritus resulted in self-inflicted skin excoriation.

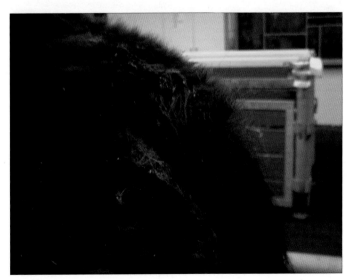

Figure 9.75 Pediculosis. Tail rubbing as a result of lice infestation.

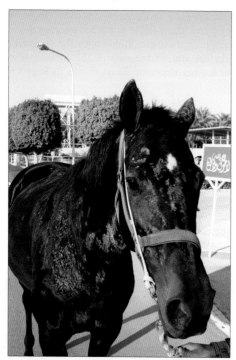

Figure 9.76 Psoroptic mange. Severe longstanding case of psoroptic mange. There was marked prurutis and hyperkeratinization of the affected areas. Numerous horses were affected in the same yard. Lesions were primarily based around the head and ears but longer-standing cases had lesions along the neck and ventral midline. All the cases involved resolved following treatment with body washes and ivermectin.

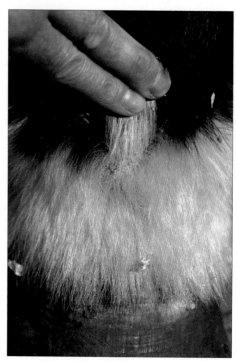

Figure 9.78 Typical scaling of the pastern region in a draft horse with chorioptic mange.

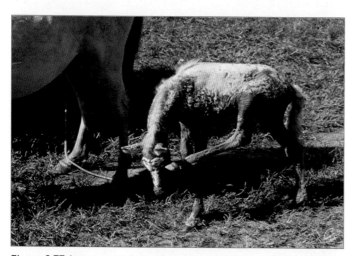

Figure 9.77 Intense pruritis has resulted in large areas of alopecia in this young foal with psoroptic mange.

- *Damalina equi*: Ivermectin is not effective and dips or powders should be used. Lime sulfur and pyrethrin dips have the fewest associated side effects but it is important to follow label instructions carefully.

Mange mites

Psoroptic mange (Figs. 9.76 & 9.77)

Although *Psoroptes* spp. only occasionally cause significant clinical problems, *Psoroptes cuniculi* is considered a possible cause of head-shaking. *Psoroptes equi* (which is reportable in the US) may cause intense pruritus, crusting and alopecia, especially of the head (ears),

mane and tail. It occurs in all ages of horses and particularly those in close contact or those which have common grooming and saddlery equipment. Once introduced into stables, it may infest most of the horses. In particular, yearlings being prepared for sales may display general body pruritus as well as tail rubbing. 'Lop ears' and pruritus with crustiness around the tail base are clinical indicators of this parasite.

Diagnosis and treatment

- Clinical signs are usually diagnostic, along with skin scrapings obtained from the affected areas which usually contain eggs or entire parasites.
- This condition can be treated with ivermectin at 200 µg/kg every 2 weeks for three doses.

Chorioptic mange (Figs. 9.78 & 9.79)

Horses with 'feathered' legs can become infected with chorioptic mange due to *Chorioptes equi*. The disease is particularly prevalent in winter months and is particularly common in the heavy draught breeds. The parasite burrows into the skin of the pastern, fetlock and cannon (and occasionally the tail head), causing severe pruritus, leg-stamping, self-mutilation and heavy scale and scab formation. Neglected cases of chorioptic mange in draught horses may eventually lead to a severe, proliferative and exudative dermatitis known as 'greasy heel'.

Diagnosis and treatment

- The diagnosis of the original instigating cause is often impossible in advanced cases due to heavy secondary bacterial infection, myiasis and the dense fibrous reaction in the underlying skin.
- This condition can be treated with ivermectin at 200 µg/kg every 2 weeks for three doses; this should be tried initially, but ivermectin-resistant mites have been reported. In such cases topical dips should

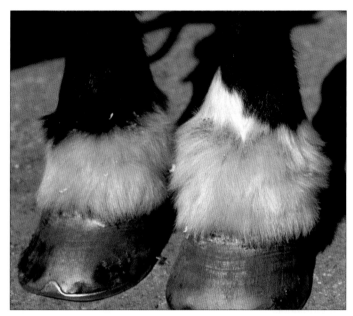

Figure 9.79 Chorioptic mange which is most commonly seen in horses with heavy "feathering".

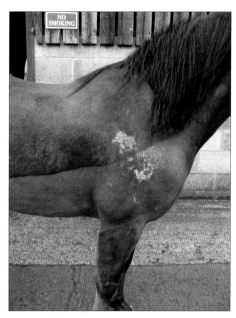

Figure 9.81 Poultry mites. Well-defined, circular alopecic lesions. ***Differential diagnosis:*** Dermatophytosis (*Trichophyton equinum* var. *equinum*).

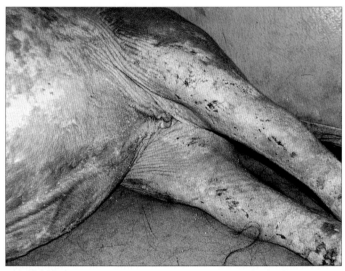

Figure 9.80 Sarcoptic. This mare had a severe generalized pruritis and *Sarcoptes scabiei* were identified in skin scrapings.

be used with the hair of the area first being clipped to improve penetration.

Sarcoptic mange (Fig. 9.80)

Infestations with *Sarcoptes scabiei* is uncommon but is a reportable disease in the US. It is contagious between horses and can also be transmitted to humans in contact with affected horses. Transmission by fomites is common as the parasite can survive off the host for 3 weeks. In early disease greatest concentrations are found around the head and neck with a particular predilection for the ears, thereafter the parasite spreads over the entire body. Intense pruritis is characteristic in horses as in other species and the itch–scratch reflex is normally easily induced in affected horses and while indicative of scabies is not diagnostic alone. Progression of the disease results in scaling and crusting with excoriations and lichenification.

Diagnosis and treatment

- As in other species, scabies is difficult to diagnose as skin scrapings are often negative. In many instances, diagnosis is based on ruling out other causes of pruritic dermatitis.
- This condition can be treated with ivermectin at 200 µg/kg every 2 weeks for three doses.

Demodectic mange

Demodex mites can sometimes be found in the skin of normal horses without the presence of any obvious clinical disease. On occasion, however, facial alopecia and scaling may be encountered. The most common location, even in normal horses, is in the eyelids and the neck. Clinical disease due to *Demodex caballi* or *Demodex equi* is only probably associated with a reduced immune capacity and this aspect should be seriously considered when a case of serious clinical demodicosis is encountered.

Diagnosis and treatment

- Deep skin scrapings from several locations are usually required to make a final diagnosis.
- As the condition is usually asymptomatic no treatment is given.
- If signs are present it is likely that there is immunosuppression as a result of a concurrent condition and this may require specific treatment.
- Treatment with avermectins or organophosphate washes may be curative if the condition is clinical.
- Amitraz which is used to treat canine demodecicosis should not be used as it is extremely toxic to horses.

Other mites (Fig. 9.81)

Free-living trombiculiform mites including *Trombicula* and *Neotrombicula* spp., forage mites (*Acarus* spp.) and occasionally poultry mites (*Dermanyssus gallinae*) can produce significant and sometimes alarming skin disease in horses. Trombiculid and acarine adults and nymphs are free-living; their larvae usually feed on small rodents but may attack horses. Infestations usually occur in late summer and autumn and are mainly seen in pastured animals although preserved hay and bedding straw may harbor significant numbers of parasites inducing clinical disease at other times. Clinical signs include restlessness and leg-stamping with the early skin lesions showing as papules or wheals. Extensive numbers of lesions may be present with small alopecic areas developing over the head, limbs and trunk after the mites fall off. The poultry mite *Dermanyssus gallinae* occasionally affects horses when stabled in or near poultry houses. Infestation occurs at night, causing severe pruritus with papules and crusts forming around the affected skin of the face and lower limb.

Diagnosis and treatment

- The mites, which may just be visible to the naked eye, are characteristically a yellow-orange color, but some species are colorless and very difficult to locate.
- Groomings, scrapings and microscopic examination are necessary to reach a definitive diagnosis.
- Diagnosis may be particularly difficult as the mites only feed briefly for 1 or 2 days and then fall off.
- Lime sulfur dip or pyrethrin dip is used as a one-time treatment combined with prednisolone or prednisone for 3–5 days.

Ticks (Fig. 9.82)

Ticks are important seasonal ectoparasites on horses in most tropical and subtropical regions. Skin injury is caused by the local effects of the bites and rarely through consequent self-mutilation. It is unusual for horses to harbor one or two ticks only and their identification usually presents few problems to the clinician. Their major importance lies more in their ability to transmit viral, bacterial and protozoal diseases. Significant blood loss with obvious anemia may be an important aspect of massive infestations. Some ticks, even in very small numbers, may induce a distinctive neurological disorder known as tick paralysis which may be fatal.

Two major families of ticks are known to cause specific clinical entities in horses. The *Argasidae* (soft ticks) includes *Otobius megnini* (the spinous ear tick) which affects a wide range of large animals including horses. Severe otitis externa accompanied by head-shaking, head tilt, behavioral problems and a waxy discharge are typical. The parasite can usually be readily seen in the depths of the external auditory tube.

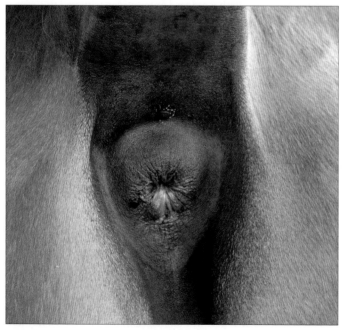

Figure 9.82 Ticks.

The *Ixodidae* family of hard ticks includes a number of individual species with the ability to transmit disease and induce specific skin disorders in various parts of the world. Tick-related dermatoses are seasonal and correspond with the periods of feeding behavior in the ticks concerned. Some ticks are slower to develop than others and some require more than one host during the life cycle. While most species will feed at any site, most have predilection sites such as the eyelids, ear, perineum, axillae and groin. The lesions resulting from the bite alone are usually localized swelling and edema but in many cases there is little local reaction, in spite of heavy infestations. Severe anemia and loss of blood proteins resulting in generalized debility and edema are possible in heavily parasitized animals. The complicating factors relating to the transmission of *Babesia* spp. parasites may exaggerate the clinical effects of these two signs. Any horse carrying ticks, even in low numbers, in areas where protozoal arthropod-borne infections are endemic should be carefully assessed for the possibility of these being of pathological significance. In Australia, hypersensitivity reactions have been recorded in individual horses to the larval stages of *Boophilus microplus*. Affected horses show a rapid onset (within 30 minutes) of multiple papules, principally of lower limbs and muzzle. Pruritus is intense with leg stamping, body rubbing and self-mutilation.

Diagnosis and treatment

- The ticks themselves can be found by careful examination and are normally most prevalent around the ears and in the tail.
- Manual removal may be necessary in some cases.
- Pyrethrin dips can be used but re-application may be required if reinfestation occurs. There is also much resistance and local resistance patterns and treatments should be sought.

Flies and other biting insects

A wide range of flies and other biting insects cause immense problems among horses both from local annoyance and the transmission of disease. Usually the presence of a small central scab or focus of inflammation is related to physical bite injury. In some cases there may be almost no superficial evidence of the bites but in most cases there is a surrounding area of edema and occasional animals show marked hypersensitivity reactions to the bites of flies, mosquitoes and midges. Eosinophilic keratitis is an important sequelae of fly molestation. *Stomoxys calcitrans*, the common stable fly, causes local irritation and hypersensitivity and is, furthermore, a potential vector for viral, fungal, protozoal and helminthic diseases. These, and other species of flies, are most prevalent in summer and autumn and are particularly active during warm humid periods. They induce severe irritation to horses causing restlessness, stamping, biting and self-mutilation. Clinically the flies cause pruritic, painful papules and wheals, often with a small central crust or depression.

Family tabanidae

Tabanus spp., *Chrysops* spp. and *Haematopota* spp., known together as 'horse flies', cause more severe bites, great annoyance and are often responsible for behavioral problems and significant irritation. Clinically, the bites are the most severe of the fly lesions, causing pruritic papules, wheals, ulceration and even hemorrhage from the bite site. Bites most commonly occur on legs, ventral body, neck and withers.

Family Muscidae

Haematobia spp. (horn flies, buffalo flies) also cause skin irritation, although the extent of the local lesion created by the bite is variable between individual horses. Clinically, the flies cause pruritus, painful papules and wheals with a central crust and in the United States of America appear to cause a well-recognized ventral midline dermatitis. Flies aggregate in huge numbers and may cause larger raised nodules and scabs. The bites of these flies usually involve some skin penetration and bleeding and in many cases this is an effective physical means for the transmission of viral, bacterial or protozoal (or other) disease.

Family Muscidae

Stomoxys calcitrans is the most important species of this fly worldwide. These 'stable flies' are known to transmit EIS and surra. Non-biting flies of the family may act as the intermediate host for *Habronema* and *Draschia* spp. helminths, which are the cause of non-healing wounds on the legs, face, lacrimal sac and elsewhere, known as 'summer sores' or 'swamp sores'.

Diagnosis and treatment

- Diagnosis of skin diseases related to fly damage relies heavily on observation, use of light-traps and careful assessment of the type of damage to the skin. Use of fly-masks is imperative in areas of dense populations of flies.
- There is no specific treatment but steps to reduce the number of flies in the environment, and use of repellent sprays are useful in many instances.

Family Ceratopogonidae

Culicoides spp. (gnats, sandflies, biting midges, 'punkies', 'no-see-ums') occur throughout the world, and cause severe irritation and hypersensitivity and are important vectors for diseases such as African horse sickness and equine viral arteritis. Different species have different preferred biting patterns and regional information, relating to the species and local climate, is useful in assessing their local significance. Adult *Culicoides* gnats are blood-sucking parasites and their bites are immediately painful and annoying for the horse. There is a characteristically rapid onset of pruritus, and the development of local papules and wheals at the site. Individual lesions last for several days, and frequent attacks cause almost continuous irritation. The majority of horses in a group are affected when the populations of *Culicoides* spp. are at their peak. In some enzootic areas in tropical and sub-tropical countries this can be continuous throughout the year. *Culicoides* spp. are most active at dusk and dawn, with little activity during the heat of the day and the cool of night. The preferred sites vary depending on the species, but the neck and back, the head, and ventral midline are commonly affected. They are also responsible for the development of a very common hypersensitivity disorder known as 'sweet itch' and for a ventral midline dermatitis.

Family Simulidae

Simulium spp. (black flies, sandflies, buffalo gnats) also cause severe irritation and tend to occur in vast numbers following rain in spring and early summer in northern parts of the USA, Canada and eastern Europe. The clinical signs associated with their presence are painful papules and wheals. With huge numbers of flies, lesions may become vesicular, hemorrhagic and necrotic. They may be vectors of the virus that cause pinnal acanthosis. Absorption of toxin from the bites has been recorded as causing cardiorespiratory dysfunction when depression, weakness, staggers, tachycardia, tachypnea, shock and death may be encountered.

Family Culicidae

Mosquitoes (*Aedes* spp., *Anopheles* spp., and *Culex* spp.) are locally annoying as well as being vectors for viral and protozoal disease. Multiple bites cause papules and small wheals. Contact scabs are difficult to see or may be absent. The presence of large numbers may cause irritation and weight loss in horses.

Family Glossinidae

Glossina spp. (tsetse flies) occur in sub-Saharan Africa and are aggressive blood feeders leaving large visible bite marks. Their chief significance however is in their ability to transmit trypanosome parasites.

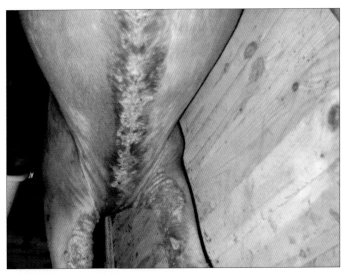

Figure 9.83 Equine ventral midline dermatitis. Distinctive small exudative, granulomatous papules associated with edema, alopecia and severe pruritus. The ventral midline is the predilection site for ventral biting species of *Culicoides* and for *Haematobia* spp. flies.

Equine ventral midline dermatitis (Fig. 9.83)

This is a dermatitis that is seasonally and geographically related to the presence of biting flies and particularly to *Haematobia irritans*, *Culicoides* spp., *Stomoxys calcitrans* and *Tabanus* spp. Usually the condition is caused by a mixture of insect species and in some cases a hypersensitivity may develop to one or more of the species involved.

The condition is more common in young horses (3–5 years of age). The dermatitis that develops along the ventral midline is highly pruritic and can result in severe self-trauma. Clearly demarcated areas with punctate ulcers, thickened skin, alopecia and in severe cases, an eczematous appearance, develop along the ventral midline of the abdomen, following even limited numbers of bites. Leukoderma occurs in longstanding cases.

Diagnosis and treatment

- Diagnosis is based on history, the presence of flies and the typical clinical appearance and distribution of the lesions.
- Skin biopsy shows variable degrees of superficial perivascular dermatitis with numerous eosinophils, indicative of a hypersensitivity reaction.
- Treatment is based on removal of the cause and relies heavily on management. Fly repellents, clothing, stabling and fans can all be used. Topical application of antibiotic/steroid creams may help provide relief during severe episodes.

Equine insect hypersensitivity (Figs. 9.84 & 9.85)

This is the most common skin hypersensitivity disorder of horses and is largely attributed to a reaction to the bites of *Culicoides* spp., although other biting insects may be involved in individual cases (*Stomoxys* spp., *Tabanus* spp. and mosquitoes). There is no sex or hair color predilection. Older horses are affected more commonly with lesions being rare in horses under 4–5 years of age. The condition is somewhat progressive with age. The condition is seasonal, related to increased activity of the insects.

Individual animals may have greater or lesser sensitivities to the individual species of flies but some are sensitive to more than one. Certain breeds, including the Icelandic Pony and the Welsh Pony, appear to be more likely to develop the condition, and there are strong familial associations within breeds, supporting the contention that the sensitivity is of genetic origin.

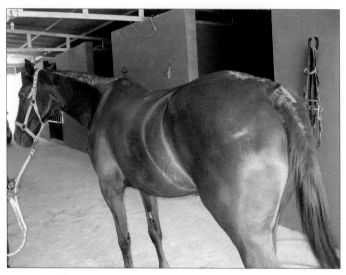

Figure 9.84 Hypersensitivity. Typical pattern of lesions due to dorsal-biting species of *Culicoides* over back, withers and dorsal neck with broken mane and tail hairs and localized alopecia and excoriation.

The mane and tail areas are most commonly affected. There is mild to severe pruritis which is worse in the early evening and morning corresponding to insect feeding times. Self-trauma as a result of the pruritis results in breakage of hairs, excoriation, exudation and skin thickening/lichenification with the development of rugae over time. Secondary bacterial infections can occur.

Diagnosis

- Diagnosis is usually based on classical clinical appearance. Response to specific avoidance measures such as application of clothing or stabling at times of increased insect activity is highly supportive.
- Skin testing and IgE/IgG estimation in blood are unreliable tests.

Treatment and control

- Control is the best approach but may be extremely difficult. Control measures include application of clothing to prevent access to the mane and tail area, stabling during the early evening and morning, application of insect repellents though these are rarely completely effective.
- Change of paddock to more open windy areas may also be beneficial.

Family Apidae (Apis mellifera, bee)

Horses attacked by bee swarms often have obvious stings in the skin and a surrounding area of edema and pain. The head and neck are most often attacked and show edema of the eyelids and muzzle. Papules with edema occur wherever stings have occurred. The identification of the sting lodged in the skin at the site of these lesions confirms the diagnosis but it may be particularly difficult to find them. An occasional horse suffers from an anaphylactoid reaction following even single (or few) bee stings. Severe respiratory embarrassment and gross urticaria with extensive edema are typical. Wasp stings are more often single but may be multiple from one or more wasps and the stings lead to the formation of painful papules and plaques over the body which closely resemble bee stings but which have no residual sting remnants. Edema of the head and muzzle, and anaphylactoid reactions may occur, however, and cases must be carefully assessed to eliminate the possibility of allergic diseases such as urticaria and angioedema.

Non-biting flies

Non-biting flies such as *Musca* spp. are surface feeders but often, due to high populations, can cause ulceration of moist skin, eyes, nostrils

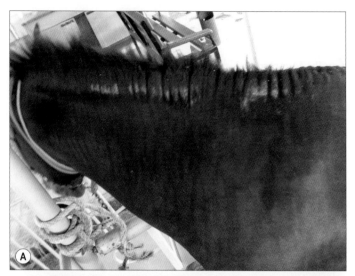

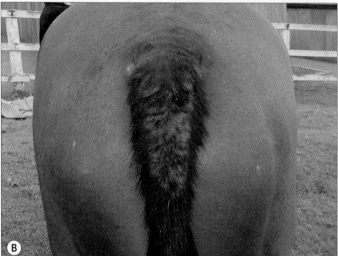

Figure 9.85 *Culicoides* hypersensitivity. (A) Chronic case showing lichenification and rugae formation with poor hair growth resulting from permanently damaged skin. (B) Chronic mild challenge by *Culicoides* spp. insects caused persistent tail rubbing with loss of hair and damage to the tail base and the formation of nodules of hyperkeratinized skin giving a 'rat-tail' effect.

and prepucial areas. *Musca autumnalis* (face fly of North America), *Musca domestica* (domestic house fly) and *Musca vetustissima* (bush fly of Australia) have a tendency to congregate around the eye and cause physical ulceration damage through sheer numbers in the periocular skin. These wounds are characteristically slow to heal and often become complicated by the presence of *Habronema* spp. larvae in the wounds, conjunctiva or in the nasolacrimal duct.

Myiasis flies (Fig. 9.86)

Flies of the genera *Calliphora*, *Chrysomyia*, *Lucilia*, *Phormia*, *Sarcophagi* and some other species may be involved with **fly strike (calliphorine myiasis)** in horses. This mostly occurs in contaminated, infected wounds, under badly managed plaster casts and occasionally in fresh surgical wounds such as castrations. The presence of the fly larvae is usually very obvious and the horse often bites or chews at the malodorous area. Bacterial cultures from wounds affected by myiasis are often surprisingly unrewarding and the wound is often remarkably free from tissue detritus. Removal of the larvae and normal wound management result in rapid healing in most cases although the tendency towards exuberant granulation tissue may still be a problem in some sites.

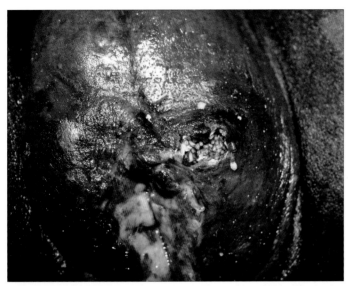

Figure 9.86 Fly strike. Opening of a caslick in this mare exposed an ideal surface for fly feeding and development of a fly strike.

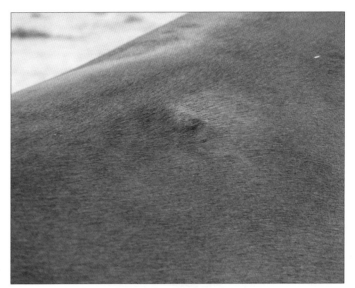

Figure 9.87 *Hypoderma bovis* larvae under the skin producing an inflamed painful nodule. The nodule failed to mature into a larva but was identifiable using an 18-MHz ultrasound scanner. Reproduced from Knottenbelt D, *Pascoe's Principles & Practice of Equine Dermatology*, second ed. (2009), with permission from Elsevier.

Differential diagnosis:
• Epidermoid/dermoid cysts
• Parafilariasis
• Infected granuloma (foreign body)
• Neoplasia (mast cell tumor, sarcoid)
• Eosinophilic granuloma.

Cochliomyia hominivorax (screw worm), and *Cochliomyia macellaria* in the Americas and *Chrysomyia bezziana* in Africa and Asia lay their eggs on open wounds, the umbilicus of neonates, body orifices and even onto moist intact skin. The larvae hatch within 12–24 hours and burrow into the underlying tissue causing intense pruritus and a severe malodor, which serves to attract more flies. The larvae leave the wound after 3–6 days but usually successive waves of maggots result in extensive tissue destruction.

Diagnosis and treatment
• The presence of the maggots is usually very obvious, but on occasion the extent of the invasion is not apparent until the area is clipped and examined closely.
• The wound should be thoroughly cleaned and debrided. All visible larvae should be removed.
• The wound should then be treated topically with either a small amount of injectable ivermectin mixed with petroleum jelly or conventional ivermectin paste applied directly.
• It may be necessary to repeat the treatment as more deeply embedded maggots become more obvious.

Hypoderma *spp. (warble flies)* (Fig. 9.87)
Hypodermiasis due to the tissue-migrating larval stages of *Hypoderma lineatum* and *Hypoderma bovis* occasionally affects horses, particularly those in contact with cattle over the warmer summer months. Younger horses in poor body condition are more likely to be affected. Small numbers of subcutaneous nodules and cysts appear in the skin along the dorsal midline between the withers and the tail head, in the early spring months in the year following infection. While most of these develop a breathing-pore in the overlying skin, some are more swollen and painful and produce no breathing aperture. Furthermore, anaphylactoid type reactions may occur following the rupture or death of third-stage larvae in the skin during accidental injury or attempts to squeeze the larvae out, or during their migration through the body tissues. A particularly serious complication may arise if the larvae penetrate the spinal cord and then die.

Diagnosis and treatment
• Clinical signs of typical lesions, history of contact with cattle and ultrasound examination of lesions demonstrating larvae are suggestive, but a diagnosis may be difficult to establish unless the larva can be identified after removal.

• Medical treatment with avermectin wormers is effective.
• The condition is now rare in most countries where the condition in cattle is largely under statutory control.

Gasterophilus *spp. (horse bots)* (Figs. 9.88 & 9.89)
There are various species of horse bots that occur worldwide while others are geographically restricted. Their main significance is distress and annoyance caused as they attempt to lay their eggs on the hairs of the legs and around the mouth. Many larvae may be found on the gastric mucosa during gastroscopic examination but they have not been found to be of any pathological significance.

Diagnosis and treatment
• Direct observation of eggs or larvae is usually diagnostic.
• Treatment is susceptible to avermectin wormers.

Nematode parasites causing skin disease
Habronema *spp.* (Figs. 9.90–9.92)
Cutaneous habronemiasis causes chronic ulcerative granulomata which are known variously as 'summer sores', 'bursautee', 'bursatti', 'swamp sore', 'kunkers', 'esponja', 'granular dermatitis'. The condition occurs commonly, particularly in the tropics and sub-tropics. The adult nematodes inhabit horses stomachs, eggs or larvae being passed in feces. The resultant larvae are ingested by the larvae of the intermediate host *Musca domestica* (the house/domestic fly) or *Stomoxys calcitrans* (the stable fly). These larvae are released from the adult flies while they feed on exudates or body secretions (such as in open wounds, facial skin moistened by lacrimation, the urethral process and the conjunctiva). The larvae penetrate intact skin or infest the surface of wounds or, if they are deposited near the mouth, they are swallowed to continue their lifecycle in the horse's stomach. It is believed that hypersensitivity by some horses to the larvae causes the appearance of clinical disease. The disease has a strong seasonal nature with spontaneous remission over the winter. Although horses

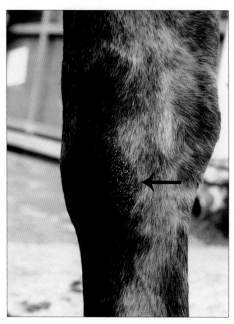

Figure 9.88 Bot eggs clearly visible attached to hairs on the forelegs (arrow).

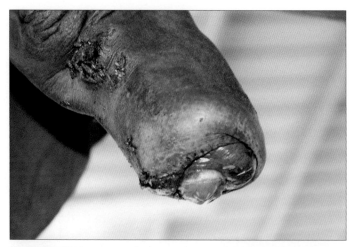

Figure 9.90 Habronemiasis of the penis. Note the multiple lesions of the penile shaft in addition to the proliferative lesion of the urethral process. These lesions are frequently markedly pruritic and lesions of the urethral process may also interfere with urination and ejaculation.

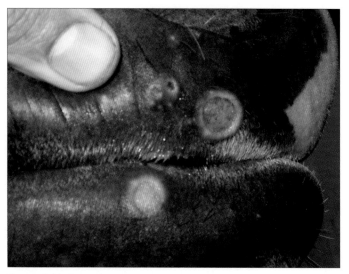

Figure 9.89 Gastrophilus ulcers.

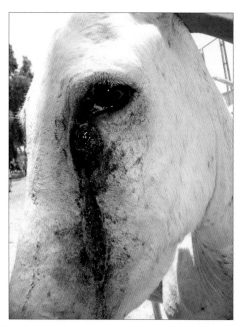

Figure 9.91 Habronemiasis of the facial skin below the medial canthus of the eye. Note also the dermatitis as a result of constant bathing of the skin in the exudative fluids.

may be congregated, single individuals may be affected. Often, the same horse is reinfected in the succeeding summers, indicating that there is little or no immunological or cellular resistance. Lesions commonly occur around the medial canthus of the eyes, face, urethral process, prepuce, ventral abdomen and legs. In the absence of an open skin wound progress of the disease is usually rapid with small papules on intact skin quickly enlarging and ulcerating. This is particularly obvious on the face, especially around the medial canthus, where the lesion can progress to large granulomatous sores within 4 weeks. Wounds which become infected with *Habronema* larvae develop granulation tissue particularly rapidly, and often show a saucer-like configuration and heal extremely slowly unless treated specifically for the habronemiasis. Untreated habronema lesions on the urethral process cause great enlargement which can lead to bleeding during coitus, thus causing a lowered fertility and reduced libido.

Diagnosis and treatment

- The diagnosis is usually easily made in endemic areas based on clinical signs. It can be confirmed by low-power microscopic examination of washings taken from the surface of an infected site.
- Treatment of skin lesions involves the application of topical ivermectin, with a second treatment being required in some cases 3–4 weeks later. This may be followed in some cases by topical corticosteroid creams.
- The ophthalmic form should be treated with oral ivermectin +/– topical corticosteroids (see also Chapter 10, p. 361). Lesions on the third eyelid should be curetted and then treated with topical corticosteroid eye drops and a solution of 50% injectable ivermectin in artificial tears.

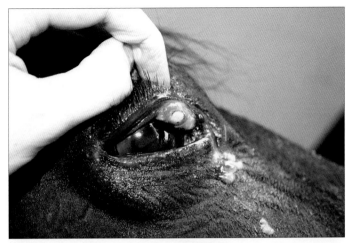

Figure 9.92 Habronemiasis of the upper eyelid showing typical yellow 'granule'.

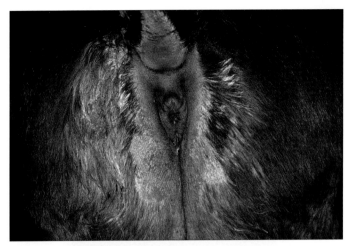

Figure 9.94 Oxyuriasis. Pruritis has resulted in local alopecia and skin excoriation.

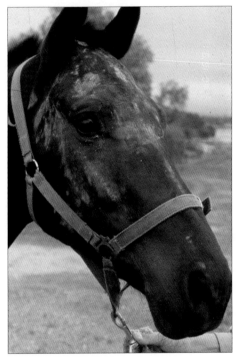

Figure 9.93 Onchocerciasis.Typical alopecic, hyperkeratotic roughly circular facile lesions of *Onchocerca cervicalis* infection.

Onchocerca cervicalis (Fig. 9.93)

Cutaneous onchocerciasis occurs as an unusual clinical syndrome and many horses may harbor larvae (microfilaria) without any clinical signs, with some parasites being regarded as a normal occurrence. Many horses (25–100%) are infected with *Onchocerca cervicalis*, but only a very few show clinical signs. The cutaneous form of the disease is thought to represent a hypersensitivity reaction. Affected horses are commonly older than 4 years, with horses under 2 years of age being particularly rarely affected. Clinical lesions may appear during any time of the year, but are usually more severe in warmer weather. This may also be related to increased activity of the insect vectors, such as *Culicoides* spp. The lesions, which are commonly located on the head, neck, ventral midline and palmar/plantar aspects of the limbs, are initially localized, poorly demarcated and intensely pruritic. Rubbing

and biting at the sites abates after some days and the lesions develop into circular patches of scaling and crusting. Longstanding *Onchocerca* lesions show leukotrichia and leukoderma which are usually irreversible.

Diagnosis and treatment

- Diagnosis is aided by biopsy and examination of minced skin for microfilaria. It is important to realize that microfilaria may be present in normal blood and in normal skin without any pathological effect.
- The use of ivermectin as an anthelmintic has resulted in a dramatic reduction in the incidence of this parasite in some parts of the world but the initial use of this drug may cause severe localized allergic-type reactions when the microfilaria are killed in the capillary beds of the skin.

Parafilariasis

This is a seasonal hemorrhagic nodular skin disease of horses which occurs in Eastern Europe and Great Britain. *Parafilaria multipapillosa* adult worms live coiled up in subcutaneous nodules which open to the skin surface, discharging a bloody exudate. *Haematobia atripalpis* serve as a vector for the parasite. The clinical disease appears in spring and summer with papules and nodules suddenly appearing, principally on the neck, shoulders and trunk. Lesions are not usually painful or pruritic. New lesions develop as the old regress.

Diagnosis

- The diagnosis may be confirmed by direct smears from the bloody exudate when larvae, rectangular embryonated eggs and numerous eosinophils will be visible, and by biopsy when nodular to diffuse dermatitis with coiled nematodes is present.
- ***Differential diagnosis:*** Fungal, bacterial and other parasitic granuloma and hypodermiasis.

Oxyuris equi (pinworm) (Figs. 9.94 & 9.95)

Oxyuriasis may cause pruritus of the anus and rubbing of the tail. The adult female worms deposit their eggs in a gelatinous mass around the perianal area. Clinical signs include tail-rubbing and a rat-tail appearance develops with increasing self-depilation.

Diagnosis and treatment

- Diagnosis is confirmed by finding characteristic triangular eggs around the perineum. A strip of adhesive cellulose tape is a useful way of harvesting the eggs for examination.
- This parasite is susceptible to avermectins.

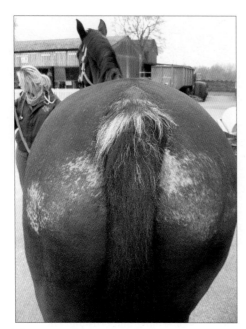

Figure 9.95 Oxyuriasis. Tail rubbing causing breakage of hairs and localized alopecia.

Neoplastic disorders

Equine sarcoid (Figs. 9.96–9.100)

Equine sarcoid is the commonest skin tumor of horses and can be seen in horses of all ages, colors and breeds, although Thoroughbreds are under-represented. There is some evidence of transmission between horses and across an individual horse suggesting an infectious etiology and possible vector involvement. Genetic predisposition occurs in a large number of horses and familial tendencies are also recognized. There are six different types of sarcoid recognized, each with its own prognosis, differentials and therapeutics. A number of different types can occur on the same horse, although non-metastatic equine sarcoid can be very locally invasive.

Note: Individual lesions are likely to be exacerbated over time. There is also a tendency to exacerbation following biopsy, surgery or accidental injury. Additional sarcoids are likely to develop in the same horse over time. Treatment is always difficult and new sarcoids may occur in horses that have had previous successful treatments. Prognosis is always guarded as all treatment methods have failures and new lesions are likely to develop.

Occult sarcoid

Clinically, these are recognized as a well-defined alopecic area. With time, the area of alopecia may increase or it may remain static for months or years, without any tendency to return to normal. The lesion involves only the most superficial layers of the dermis and alopecic areas may have a flaky surface and are often mistaken for ringworm lesions (dermatophytosis). It is quite common for these to develop areas of more warty, gray, hyperkeratinized tissue or obvious single or multiple nodules (nodular sarcoid) in and under the skin. Many of these lesions are not progressive and unless traumatized, do not clinically change over long periods. Some, however, gradually develop increased numbers of nodules or hyperkeratinized areas which may become more verrucous (warty), but still remain relatively sessile. These hyperkeratotic nodules may further increase in size and if abraded, may result in the development of a more aggressive fibroblastic form of the tumor. Predilection sites include the head and neck and medial aspect of the forelimb and thigh.

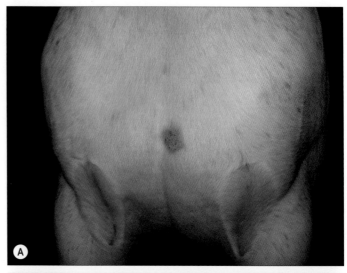

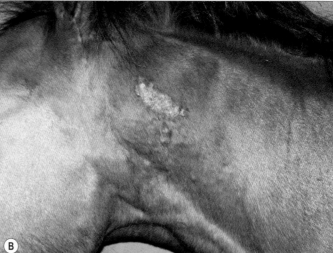

Figure 9.96 (A, B) Occult sarcoid. Discrete area of alopecia.
Differential diagnosis:
• Dermatophytosis
• Traumatic/rubbing injury.

Note: Due to the frequently benign nature of these lesions, they are often left untreated.

Verrucose (warty) sarcoid

An increased dermal involvement results in the appearance of obvious, irregular flat areas of hyperkeratosis with marked skin thickening. The extent of hyperkeratosis is very variable with those occurring in the periorbital skin often being almost smooth and hairless. They may be sessile, with a broad base or pedunculated. Extensive verrucous sarcoids are sometimes present on the medial thigh and in the axiliary region. Typically, this type is slow-growing and seldom become more aggressive until abrasion, injury or surgical interference occurs. They may then become granulomatous and commonly adopt a more aggressive, fibroblastic appearance.

Predilection sites include the face (particularly eyelids), body, axillae and groin areas. This form is rare on the limbs. The treatment chosen frequently depends on number, severity and location of lesions.

Nodular sarcoid

This form of sarcoid is entirely subcutaneous, although occasionally they may erupt through the overlying skin and then have a similar

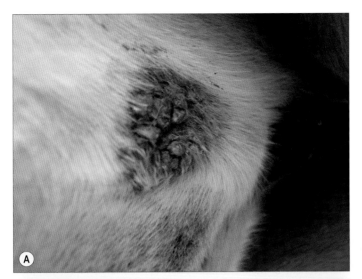

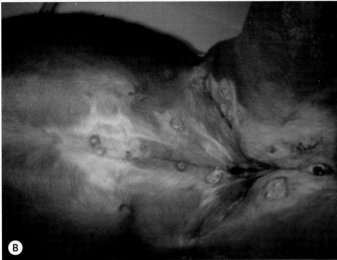

Figure 9.97 Typical warty appearance of verrucose sarcoid.

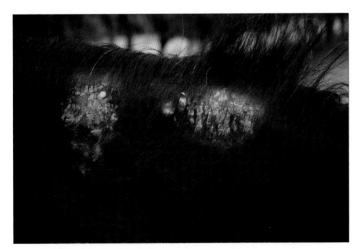

Figure 9.98 Multiple nodular sarcoids of the ventral abdomen and inner thigh.

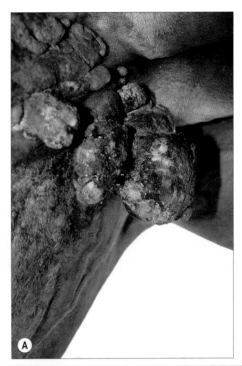

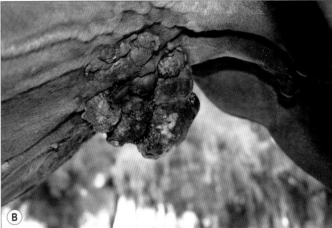

Figure 9.99 (A, B) Fibroblastic sarcoids of the ventral abdomen in this mare. Many variations of fibroblastic sarcoids can be seen. They may be pedunculated or sessile and frequently resemble fleshy granulation tissue especially on the distal limbs.

appearance to the fibroblastic form. The more usual appearance is of one or many, dense, often spherical nodules lying below the skin. Typical sites for the development of this type of lesion are the thin-skinned areas of the inguinal region, the sheath, medial thigh and the eyelids. Nodules are divided into two distinct categories based on the involvement of the overlying skin. These groups are further subdivided based on the relationships to surrounding tissue (see Table 9.2).

Fibroblastic sarcoid

These have a characteristic aggressive, fleshy, ulcerated appearance frequently with a fibrocellular 'scab' and secondary infection. Fibroblastic sarcoids are divided into two broad, clinically recognizable groups (see Table 9.3). They may enlarge rapidly, especially those occurring on the lower limbs, and may attain considerable size within weeks or months and then may remain static for years, showing variable periods of apparent improvement and deterioration. They

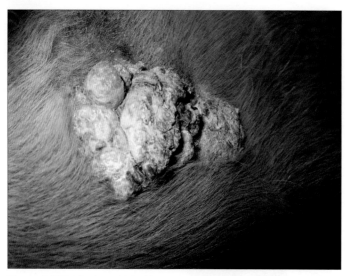

Figure 9.100 Mixed sarcoid. In this case nodular and verrucose forms are visible. This type of sarcoid is probably a progressive state.

Table 9.2 Nodular sarcoid classification

Type	Subtype	Clinical and gross pathological features
A No cutaneous involvement Single or multiple Individual or multilobular No occult changes directly associated with nodules	I	No deep tissue involvement Loose fibrocellular capsule Defined margins
	2	Deep tissue involvement Invasive 'bound down' character Ill-defined margins
B Cutaneous involvement Single or multiple Individual or multilobular Possible occult and occasionally verrucose margin on skin	I	No deep tissue involvement Loose fibrocellular capsule Defined margins
	2	Deep tissue involvement 'Bound down' nature Ill-defined margins

Table 9.3 Fibroblastic sarcoid classification

Fibroblastic type	Subtype	Features
I Pedunculated	a	Distinct pedicle No deep tissue involvement
	b	Distinct pedicle Wide/palpable root Invasive 'Bound down' character Ill-defined margins of root
2 Sessile/broad based		Bound down character Ill-defined margins

are highly vascular and many bleed significantly following minimal trauma. Some of the largest fibroblastic lesions develop when the other, more superficial, types have been traumatized and others can be associated with wound scars. Lesions occurring on the distal limbs are frequently mistaken for granulation tissue. A particularly aggressive fibroblastic sarcoid (malevolent form), which spreads along lymphatic vessels creating extensive nodules and multiple, ulcerating fibroblastic masses, is occasionally encountered and represents an advanced stage with a very poor prognosis. Occasional fibroblastic forms on the lips may erode through to give ulceration on the buccal mucosa. The superficial appearance of fibroblastic sarcoids may belie the extent of dermal and subdermal involvement and surgical excision is often followed by rapid regrowth of an increasingly aggressive fibroblastic tumor-like mass. Multiple lesions are also common at sites of attempted excision or cryosurgery.

Mixed (verrucose, fibroblastic and nodular) sarcoids

A wide variety of mixed sarcoids occurs, having areas which are characteristic of the other more easily defined single types, and they may merely represent a transition from the occult, verrucose or nodular sarcoids to the more aggressive fibroblastic type.

Interference with any of the individual types may result in marked increase in the fibroblastic component of the mass and it is likely then that the mixed forms are the result of minor or major, localized or generalized insults applied to otherwise less aggressive lesions. It is unusual for the verrucose, nodular or occult forms to develop into anything other than the fibroblastic form following interference (including biopsy or accidental damage).

Diagnosis

- History and clinical features are usually highly suggestive but a definitive diagnosis is not always straightforward, unless any one of the differential diagnosis also occur simultaneously.
- **Differential diagnosis:** squamous cell carcinoma (usually localized with definitive histology); lymphangitis (also accompanied by diffuse swelling and edema); glanders and epizootic lymphangitis should be considered in geographical areas where these conditions occur; scarring/granulation tissue (frequently occurs simultaneously on the distal limbs with history of wound or trauma); lymphoma/lymphosarcoma is usually accompanied by systemic involvement.
- Partial or excisional biopsy is generally diagnostic (exception occurs when a sarcoid is diffusely mixed with granulation tissue), but there is a large risk of exacerbation. Therefore a therapeutic plan should be in place before the biopsy is performed.
- Note: It is preferable to take a total excisional biopsy rather than a simple biopsy if a sarcoid is suspected. Superficial swabs from surface lesions can be PCR tested for the bovine papilloma genome (believed to be part of the etiology) but a deeper swab may be required if the skin is intact or hyperkeratotic as the genome is not found in keratinocytes.

Treatment

Table 9.4 outlines the relative value of treatment methods. The choice of treatment method is not only dictated by the relative value of the method but also by many other factors:

- *Patient variation*: each horse responds individually to treatment and horses with similar lesions may respond differently to the same treatment
- *Location*: certain anatomical locations have restrictions on therapy related to the serious side effects or consequences of certain treatments. This would most notably include periorbital lesions, lesions of the penis or prepuce, coronary band, over limb joints and around the mouth and ears

Table 9.4 Relative value of treatment methods for the various forms of equine sarcoid

Treatment	Type of sarcoid				
	Occult	Verrucose	Nodular	Fibroblastic	Mixed
Surgical					
Ligation	N/A	N/A	***	#	#
Excision	***	*	***	*	*
Cryosurgery	**	**	N/A	*	*
Hyperthermia	**	*	N/A	*	N/A
Electrocautery	**	**	***	*	*
CO$_2$-YAG laser	***	**	***	*	*
Photodynamic	**	**	NA	*	*
Topical					
(AW4-LUDES)	****	***	**	***	**
Podophyllin	*	#	N/A	#	#
5-Fluorouracil	***	***	*	*	N/A
Tazarotene	***	**	N/A	N/A	N/A
Imiquimod	**	**	N/A	*	*
Sanguinaria/ZnCl[a]	**	**	N/A	*	*
Intralesional injection/cytotoxic/antimitotic					
5-Fluorouracil	N/A	N/A	**	**	*
Cisplatin	N/A	N/A	***	***	N/A
Immune methods					
Autogenous vaccines	#	#	#	#	#
BCG	N/A	N/A	****[b]	*** #	#
Radiation					
Brachytherapy	N/A	N/A	*****	*****	***
Teletherapy	*****	*****	*****	*****	*****

N/A, not appropriate modality.

*****, Expected results over 80–90% success; ****, expected 60–80% success; ***, 40–60% success; **, 20–40% success; *, 20% success.

#, liable to be worse.

[a]Sanguinaria canadensis and zinc chloride marketed as XXTERRA an345d SARC-OFF.

[b]BCG therapy has a good reputation in the treatment of nodular lesions around the eye but a poor one elsewhere. The results are particularly poor on limb or body lesions.

Reproduced from Knottenbelt D, *Pascoe's Principles & Practice of Equine Dermatology*, second ed. (2009), with permission from Elsevier.

- *Type of sarcoid.*
- *Previous treatments*: the likelihood of success is much less if there have been previous unsuccessful treatments. Complications such as co-existence of other factors such as granulation tissue infection, myiasis or other neoplasia
- *Facilities and practicality of the treatment*: not all treatments are available in all areas. The best treatment for a given lesion may not be economically viable if the lesions are extensive. Consequences such as severe scarring may be intolerable to the owner
- *Owner compliance*: predicting the length of some therapies may be difficult and regular/continuing veterinary care combined with other care (fly control, housing) may result in poor owner compliance
- *Patient compliance*: the age and temperament of the horse may influence treatment choices, e.g. daily topical treatments may not be tolerated by previously unhandled or fractious horses
- *The possibility of a contagious nature*: this can be a large stimulus to treatment of a horse in a grazing group.

Squamous cell carcinoma (Figs. 9.101 & 9.102)

This is the second most common skin tumor of horses, with a predilection for non-pigmented skin and mucocutaneous junctions. The most

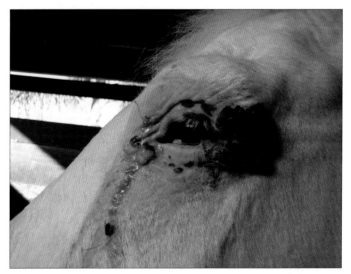

Figure 9.101 Advanced eyelid squamous cell carcinoma. In this case it has a raised cauliflower-like appearance with a broad base of attachment. These lesions bleed easily and are frequently locally invasive in addition to having a high metastatic rate to regional lymph nodes.

Table 9.5 The main forms of squamous cell carcinoma in the horse and their common features

Form	Location	Features	Assumed carcinogen	Type of horse affected	Age (years)	Progression	Clinical behavior	Features / Notes
Ocular	Palpebral	Proliferative	UV light	Pale skin/colored/cremello/albino/vitiligo	All	Slow	Benign/locally aggressive	Can be slow at first and become destructive
		Destructive						
	Caruncular			All				
	Nictitans	Proliferative		Pale exposed mucosa (no pigmented margin)			Benign but can be aggressive if on inner conjunctiva	Usually localized
		Destructive						
	Conjunctival	Proliferative		Pale non-pigmented limbal conjunctiva			Benign	Can invade cornea
	Corneal[a]	Proliferative Superficial spread mostly remaining intra-epithelial	Not known	All			Benign	Can be deeper and involve calcium deposition
Cutaneous	Skin Hoof	Invasive/destructive	UV light/uncertain	Non-pigmented skin	>10	Slow	Usually highly destructive	Hoof forms are very rare
	Preputial		Not known	All	>7	Rapid	Malignant	Can be very benign in appearance but this form is very dangerous
Penile		Proliferative	Smegma Pale skin/mucosa	Geldings All colors/breeds	10+	Slow	Benign in older horses Younger horses have more aggressive/malignant forms	Very common Precarcinomatous changes are common Older horses tend to have more proliferative forms
		Destructive			5+	Rapid		
Vulval	Labial	Destructive	Unknown	Pigmented skin can be affected	>8	Slow	Benign	Locally destructive
	Clitoral	Proliferative/destructive	Smegma			Slow	Benign	Converts to destructive
	Vaginal	Proliferative	Not known	All		Slow	Benign	Can be invasive
Oral	Mouth/tongue, pharynx	Destructive	Not known	All	>12	Rapid	Malignant	
Respiratory/nasal	Sinus/nasal cavity/pharynx	Proliferative, invasive, destructive	Not known	All	>6	Slow		Space-occupying mass or destruction
Gastric	Squamous epithelium/margo plicatus	Invasive	Not known, possible bacteria/parasites	All	>12	Rapid	Highly malignant	

Although there are some typical characteristics, as with all neoplastic diseases, the clinician should not be surprised to find different clinical appearances and behavior.
[a]Intra-epithelial carcinoma (in-situ carcinoma).
Reproduced from Knottenbelt D, *Pascoe's Principles & Practice of Equine Dermatology*, second ed. (2009), with permission from Elsevier.

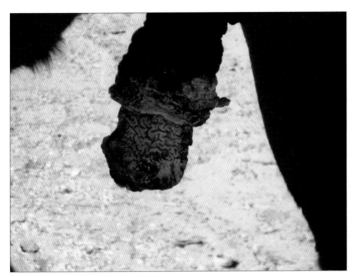

Figure 9.102 Precancerous changes of squamous cell carcinoma evident on the penis of this aged stallion. Note the thickening of the penile skin and single small cauliflower-type lesion.

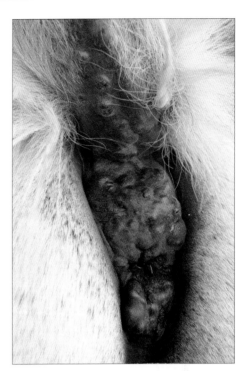

Figure 9.103 Typical location and presentation of perineal melanomas.

common forms occur at mucocutaneous junctions. Horses of all ages can be affected and lesions at different anatomical locations may have differing etiologies. Most are malignant, locally invasive and some metastasize. Some are highly active and require immediate aggressive treatment and carry a poor or guarded prognosis, while others are less aggressive and surgical removal has a good prognosis.

Table 9.5 outlines the main forms of SCC in the horse, the assumed etiology and clinical features.

Diagnosis and treatment
- While clinical appearance may be suggestive a definitive diagnosis is generally required. Scrape cytology or surgical biopsy is useful. Impression smears may be sufficient for periorbital lesions.
- *Differential diagnosis:* Sarcoids (variable forms are usually present and are rarely destructive); melanoma (highly pigmented and in typical sites of gray horses); papilloma (may be benign or a precursor of carcinoma); mast cell tumor (isolated single nodular lesions with little destructive nature); lymphosarcoma (definitive histological features); granulation tissue (history of wound); Botryomycosis/pyogranuloma (history of wound or local inflamed pustule); habronemiasis (geographical and seasonal restriction); phycomycosis (geographical restriction).
- Treatment consists of total excisional biopsy where possible, which can confirm the diagnosis and degree of differentiation.
- Table 9.6 outlines the treatment options and relative values of each.

Melanoma and melanosarcoma (Figs. 9.103–9.106)
These may occur in any age of horse and are most commonly recognized in gray or color-diluted horses. Table 9.7 outlines the different clinical syndromes, their pathological features and treatments. Over 80% of gray horses greater than 1 year of age will have one or more melanoma. Over 95% of cases are benign at the time of diagnosis but up to 30% can become malignant and may metastasize.

Diagnosis
- Clinical appearance and history are usually characteristic. Fine-needle aspirate yields black pigmented material. Biopsy.
- *Differential diagnosis:* Nodular sarcoid (other forms do not appear black in color); parotid salivary gland pathology; most other conditions and tumors can be ruled out due to the lack of pigmentation.

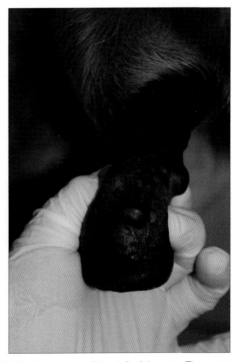

Figure 9.104 Small melanomas of the shaft of the penis. They were not associated with any clinical signs.

Neurofibroma (schwannoma, neurilemoma, neurinoma) (Fig. 9.107)
Neurofibroma and the less common neurofibrosarcoma arise from dermal or subcutaneous Schwann (nerve sheath) cells, without any known predisposing factor. They can occur in horses of any age and at any site but are most commonly seen in the upper eyelid and

Table 9.6 Relative value of treatment modalities for treatment of common forms of cutaneous squamous cell carcinoma

	Surgical ablation	Cytotoxic/antimitotic	Cryosurgery	Immunomodulation	Radiation
Cutaneous	**	**	*	**	**** (β) (γ)
Labial	*	**	N/A	***	**** (γ)
Clitoral	***	**	N/A	**	**** (γ)
Penile					
<8–10 years	*	N/A	N/A	N/A	N/A
>10 years	****	N/A	N/A	N/A	N/A
Palpebral	N/A	**	*	*	**** (γ)
Nictitans	****	***	*	N/A	N/A
Corneolimbal	**	**	N/A	N/A	**** (β)
Carcinoma in situ	**	*	N/A	N/A	**** (β)

N/A, not applicable or invariably fails to help.

*, Unlikely to be effective; **, effective in some cases or partially effective; ***, effective or partially effective in most cases; ****, likely to be effective in almost all cases (the best approach).

Reproduced from Knottenbelt D, *Pascoe's Principles & Practice of Equine Dermatology*, second ed. (2009), with permission from Elsevier.

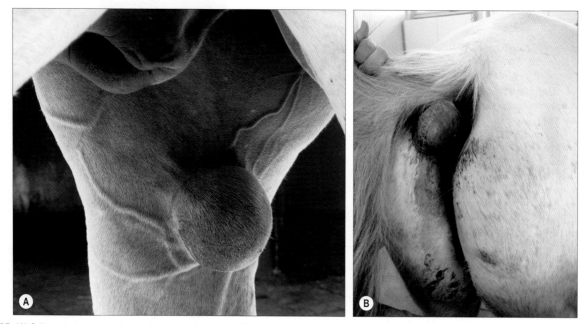

Figure 9.105 (A) Solitary melanoma on the medial aspect of the thigh. (B) Solitary melanoma on the tail.

periorbital subcutaneous tissue. The tumors are frequently hard, shot-size nodules (2–3 mm) in the upper eyelids which gradually enlarge and finally, if untreated, erode through the epidermis.

Diagnosis and treatment

- Biopsy or excisional histopathology is required for diagnosis. Fine-needle aspirates are not usually sufficient as the tumors are very dense with little intercellular matrix.
- Complete surgical removal is the treatment of choice but is frequently difficult to achieve due to the location.
- Intralesional injections of BCG over an extended period can be effective but results are not as good as surgical removal.
- Intralesional injection of cisplatin or 5-fluorouracil can also be effective but resolution takes a long time.
- Another possible alternative is gamma radiation brachytherapy.

Table 9.7 Melanoma: features and treatment

Melanoma	Clinical features	Pathological features	Treatment
Melanocytic nevus/ melanocytoma	Young horses (mean 5 years) Gray and non-gray horses Solitary/few Localized/non-encapsulated Legs/trunk/neck (not perineum) Commonly ulcerated Benign	Superficial dermis Epithelial involvement Distinct sheets or nests of melanocytes Mixture of epithelioid and spindle cells with large euchromatic nuclei Low mitotic activity Moderate to heavy melanin pigmentation	Surgical excision curative Partial excision results in recurrence
Dermal melanoma/ melanomatosis	>10 years Gray horses Multiple Perineum, lips, eyelids and prepuce High metastatic rate overall but may take years Progressive	Pleomorphic/atypical melanocytes in sheets and cords Little involvement of junctional region between dermis and epidermis Variable mitotic index Malignant formas may be less pigmented/amelanotic	Total surgical excision Cryonecrosis for smaller lesions Intralesional cisplatin has variable reports of success/ failure/recurrence with larger lesions requiring debulking first Cimetidine (lack of convincing evidence of benefit) BCG immunostimulation (not proven successful) Autogenous vaccine: successful in one case, other results not as convincing
Malignant (anaplastic) melanoma	7–20 years Gray and non-gray horses Rapid extensive metastasis	Aggressive metastatic dissemination High mitotic index Amelanotic forms occur	Usually there is extensive metastasis by the time of diagnosis

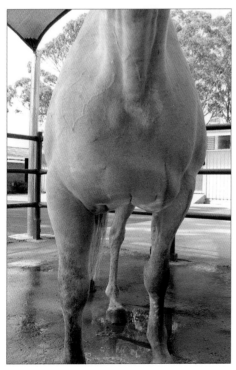

Figure 9.106 Sternal edema and edema of the right forelimb associated with thoracic metastasis of melanoma.

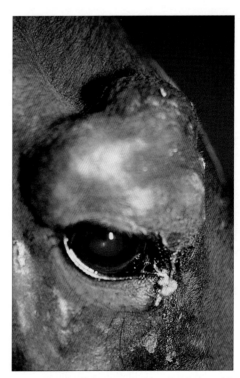

Figure 9.107 Neurofibroma of the upper eyelid with multiple nodules of varying size. Eyelid distortion resulted in a purulent ocular discharge and intermittent corneal ulceration. Reproduced from Knottenbelt D, *Pascoe's Principles & Practice of Equine Dermatology*, second ed. (2009), with permission from Elsevier.

Differential diagnosis:
• Sarcoid
• Equine cutaneous mastocytoma
• Cutaneous lymphosarcoma
• Cutaneous nodules caused by insect bites.

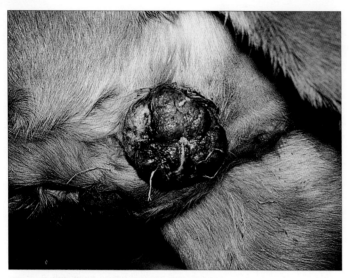

Figure 9.108 Fibrosarcoma in the girth region with a typical ulcerated cauliflower appearance. Reproduced from Knottenbelt D, *Pascoe's Principles & Practice of Equine Dermatology*, second ed. (2009), with permission from Elsevier.

Differential diagnosis:
• Sarcoid
• Exuberant granulation tissue
• Foreign body reaction
• Lymphoma/lymphosarcoma
• Other tumors (depending on location).

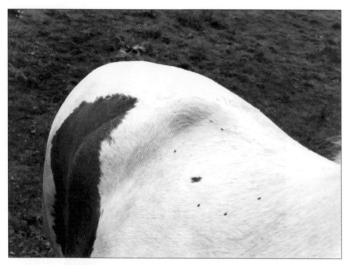

Figure 9.109 Subcutaneous lipomas over the dorsal flank area in this aged pony.

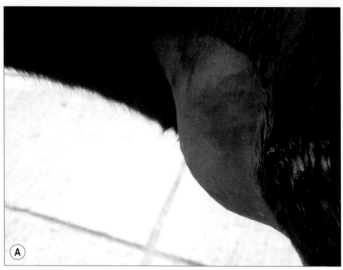

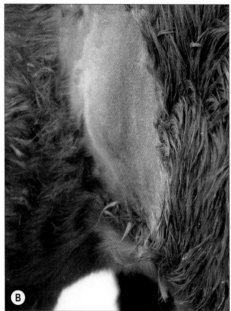

Figure 9.110 (A, B) Discrete cutaneous nodules of cutaneous lymphosarcoma. It is infrequently seen as a skin-only neoplasm.

Fibromas and fibrosarcomas (Fig. 9.108)

These are uncommon tumors of dermal or subcutaneous origin. They are reported to occur in older horses, usually as a solitary tumor. Fibromas may be firm (*fibroma durum*) or soft (*fibroma molle*), well-circumscribed nodules in dermis or subcutaneous tissue. Fibromas in the foot also occur as firm fleshy growths of the frog and like the more usual dermal lesions, surgical ablation is usually successful. Fibrosarcomas tend to be poorly demarcated, firm infiltrating subcutaneous tumors. The surface of the tumors may ulcerate, but more commonly, fibrosarcomas may clinically resemble the fibroblastic form of the equine sarcoid.

Diagnosis, treatment and prognosis

• Histopathological examination is required to confirm the diagnosis.

• Fibromas can be effectively treated with surgical excision or cryotherapy. Fibrosarcomas are more difficult to treat with both surgical excision and cryotherapy yielding poor results.
• Fibromas are benign and remain localized, but fibrosarcomas may be multiple and locally invasive but rarely metastasize.

Lipomas (Fig. 9.109)

Lipomas are benign tumors arising from subcutaneous fat. They are soft to flabby, well-circumscribed, and occur about the neck, lower chest, abdomen and, occasionally, the limbs. These grow slowly and may fluctuate in size somewhat depending on body condition.

Diagnosis and treatment

• Ultrasound examination is useful and reveals a typical pattern.
• Histopathology of biopsy or needle aspiration is diagnostic.
• Surgical removal is effective.

Cutaneous lymphosarcoma (Fig. 9.110)

See p. 194.

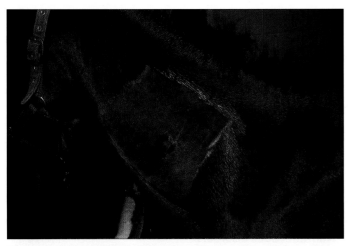

Figure 9.111 Solitary subcutaneous mastocytoma in the mid neck region of this horse. Mastocytomas most commonly occur on the head and are frequently ulcerated but they can be found in other regions and be entirely subcutaneous as in this case. The differentials for mastocytomas depend on the location and type.

Differential diagnosis (subcutaneous):
• Sarcoid
• Dermoid
• Deep dermal mycosis
• Insect bite/sting
• Eosinophilic/allergic granuloma
• Cutaneous amyloidosis.

Differential diagnosis (ulcerated/head): All of the above plus squamous cell carcinoma and habronemiasis.

Mastocytomas (mast cell tumors) (Fig. 9.111)

These are rare and there is some debate as to whether or not they are actually tumors. They are found most frequently in middle-aged male horses. Three forms are recognized:

1) ***Nodular cutaneous mastocytosis.*** They have a variable clinical appearance, but are usually nodular. The head, neck and limbs are the predilection sites for these solitary tumors which may vary from 2–20 cm in diameter. They may be firm or fluctuant, and the overlying skin may or may not be alopecic, ulcerated or hyperpigmented. A few cases are reported to be pruritic but rarely are they painful.

2) ***Malignant equine mastocytosis.*** In the few reported cases there has been pruritis at the site or generalized pruritis with lameness or pain. There have also been elevated circulating eosinophil counts and hyperfibrinogenemia with metastasis to local lymph nodes also reported.

3) ***Congenital equine mastocytosis.*** This form is detected at or soon after birth and consists of widespread nodules along the back and trunk from 2–3 mm to 3–4 cm in diameter. There may be ulceration of the overlying skin. Some cases have resolved spontaneously.

Diagnosis and treatment

• Diagnosis may be achieved by biopsy but the definitive description is not well described as cases are so rare. It should also be borne in mind that mast cells are attracted to an eosinophilic focus and, in some cases, the masses may be merely reactive tissue rather than true neoplasms.

• Surgical excision is the most common form of treatment and is normally curative but location of the lesion may prevent excision in some cases.

Reference and further reading

Knottenbelt, D.C., 2009. Pascoe's Principles and Practice of Equine Dermatology, second ed. Saunders, Oxford, UK.

CHAPTER 10

Disorders of the eye

CHAPTER CONTENTS

Part 1 Orbit and globe

Congenital/developmental conditions

Microphthalmos/anophthalmos

(Figs. 10.1–10.4)

Microphthalmos is a developmental anomaly that presents as a congenital defect in foals. Thoroughbreds are most commonly affected, although the heritability of the condition is unknown. One or both eyes are affected, and the globe is smaller in size than a normal globe. The small size of the globe may be the only defect, or there may be a wide range of accompanying abnormalities within the eye, such as colobomas within the eye or heavy pigmentation of the globe itself. The palpebral fissure is usually small also. Vision may be normal if small size is the only ocular abnormality, however accompanying defects or very small globes may result in blindness.

Anophthalmos is diagnosed if no eye tissue can be located. It is an extreme form of microphthalmos and is actually very rare. The main differential diagnosis for microphthalmos is non-congenital phthisis bulbi (see below). The microphthalmic eye should be examined carefully to assess whether there is vision present, using the menace response. The dazzle reflex and pupillary light reflex should also be tested. The globe is carefully evaluated for additional abnormalities such as lens coloboma or cataract.

Diagnosis and treatment

- Diagnosis is made by direct observation of a small globe. The third eyelid normally protrudes, which may obscure the globe. If the eye is very small, it may not be visible.

- Treatment is not usually possible. If a cataract is the only abnormality found and the other reflexes are normal, the cataract could be surgically removed.

- Very small globes may lead to chronic ocular discharge and entropion. In this situation, enucleation is recommended if there is no vision. Removing a globe from a young foal may lead to poor orbital development and therefore an orbital prosthesis might be considered.

- Repeating the same sire/dam breeding should be avoided in Thoroughbreds.

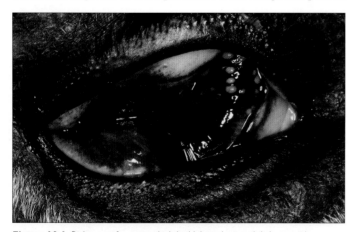

Figure 10.1 Right eye of a pony which had bilateral microphthalmos, with thickened and pigmented conjunctiva and pink lymphoid nodules.

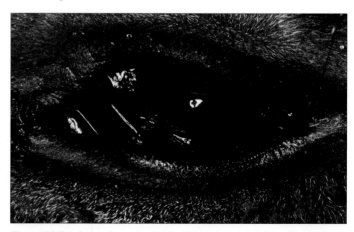

Figure 10.2 Left eye of a pony which had bilateral microphthalmos. The third eyelid is protruding, and the visible conjunctiva and cornea are densely pigmented.

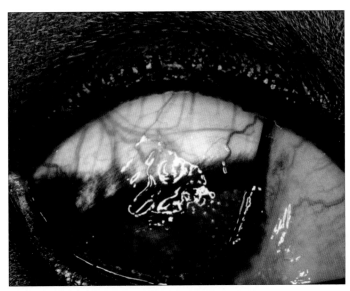

Figure 10.3 Right eye of a Thoroughbred foal which had bilateral microphthalmos. The third eyelid is protruding and the globe is visibly small. The cornea is thickened, pigmented and nodular.

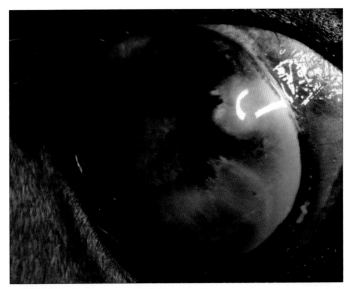

Figure 10.5 Multiple ocular anomalies in a foal with anterior segment dysgenesis. There is opacity of the peripheral cornea due to corneal endothelial abnormalities, fine strands of persistent pupillary membranes and some lens opacity.

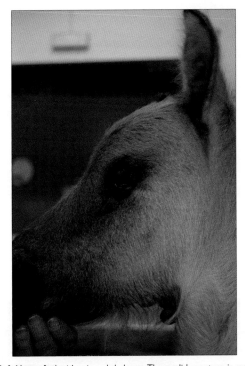

Figure 10.4 Young foal with microphthalmos. The eyelid aperture is small and the globe cannot be seen. There is mucoid ocular discharge. Courtesy of Kim Hughes.

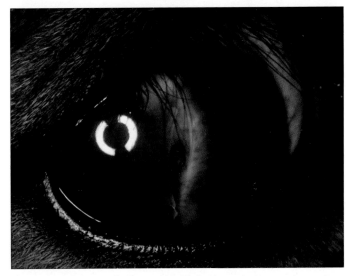

Figure 10.6 Right eye of a Thoroughbred foal with anterior segment dysgenesis. The lateral globe was relatively normal but there is a vertical corneal opacity and the medial iris is thickened and contacting the medial cornea.

Anterior segment dysgenesis (Figs. 10.5 & 10.6)

Anterior segment dysgenesis is failure in the normal development of the tissues of the anterior segment of the eye. It leads to abnormalities in the structure of the adult anterior segment, which can result in corneal opacity, visible intraocular abnormalities and an increased risk of glaucoma. Multiple congenital ocular abnormalities can occur as a congenital condition in Rocky Mountain horses. These usually feature megalocornea (an abnormally large cornea) along with a syndrome of ocular abnormalities including cysts of the iris, ciliary body and retina, iris hypoplasia, cataracts and retinal dysplasia. The condition is likely to be inherited, and therefore affected animals should not be used for breeding. However, any breed of horse can be affected with congenital anterior segment dysgenesis and multiple ocular abnormalities.

Diagnosis and treatment

- Diagnosis is made by observing congenital abnormalities in an eye which can include a range of symptoms, such as corneal opacity due to stromal, Descemet's membrane or corneal endothelium abnormalities, megalocornea, adhesions of the iris to other structures in the eye (the cornea or the anterior lens capsule), cataract, lens coloboma or microphakia.
- Treatment is not usually possible. If a cataract is present but the cornea is clear and the other reflexes are normal, the cataract could be surgically removed.

Non-infectious conditions

Phthisis bulbi (Figs. 10.7–10.9)

Phthisis bulbi is a shrunken, atrophic globe as a result of injury or inflammation. The affected eye is always permanently blind. The third eyelid usually protrudes due to the reduction in orbital volume. Entropion may occur. Ocular discharge often builds up due to incomplete blinking.

Diagnosis and treatment

- Diagnosis is made by combining the history of ocular trauma or inflammation with the appearance of a shrunken globe, usually with a vascularized and fibrosed cornea. The eye should be assessed for discomfort, observing blepharospasm or ocular discomfort. The eyelids should be assessed for entropion.
- If the eye appears uncomfortable, it should be enucleated and the orbit should be closed.

Orbital fat prolapse (Fig. 10.10)

The extraorbital fat pad is positioned around the base of the third eyelid. Occasionally, this fat may herniate through weak fibrous connective tissue. This appears as a smooth conjunctival swelling arising from behind the third eyelid. The cause is not known, and one or both eyes might be affected.

Diagnosis and treatment

- Diagnosis is usually made on the characteristic clinical appearance. However, if the diagnosis is not clear from the clinical appearance alone, a fine-needle aspirate or biopsy would confirm the presence of fat.
- **Differential diagnosis:** nictitans gland cyst, inflammation, granuloma and neoplasia.
- In most instances, this is a cosmetic condition that does not cause any problem to the affected horse.

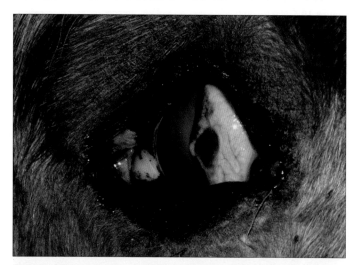

Figure 10.7 Mucoid ocular discharge, third eyelid protrusion, thickening of the conjunctiva, edema of the cornea and a small globe in an eye with phthisis bulbi after blunt ocular trauma.

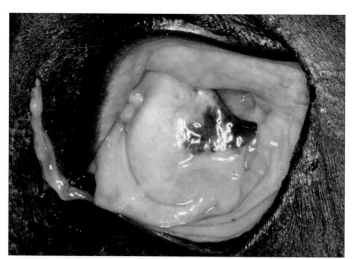

Figure 10.9 Close view of the left phthitic eye in Fig. 10.8. The globe was tiny and barely visible, there is mucoid ocular discharge, a protruding third eyelid and proliferation of conjunctiva.

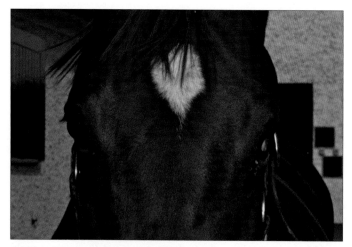

Figure 10.8 Enophthalmos of the left eye of a Thoroughbred yearling with third eyelid protrusion, due to phthisis bulbi.

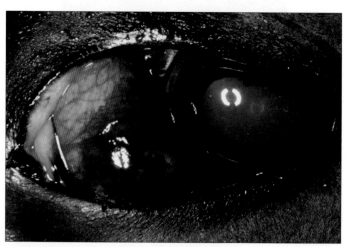

Figure 10.10 There is a smooth swelling protruding between the globe and the third eyelid, which is protrusion of the ocular fat pad covered with conjunctiva.

- Occasionally it leads to epiphora and the herniation may be extensive. In the latter cases, it may be surgically resected subconjunctivally, along with suturing the conjunctiva to prevent recurrence. The prognosis is very good.

Orbital neoplasia (Figs. 10.11–10.15)

The presence of neoplasia within the orbit can affect the eye, and the owner may be first alerted to the problem because of an abnormal eye. Types of orbital neoplasms include neuroendocrine tumors, extra-adrenal paraganglioma, anaplastic sarcoma, lymphosarcoma and squamous cell carcinoma. Orbital neoplasia can arise in adjacent structures such as the sinus or nasal cavity.

Diagnosis

- Signs that may be noticed include exophthalmos (forward displacement of the globe due to a retrobulbar space-occupying lesion), prominent third eyelid, deviation of gaze (strabismus), asymmetry of the eyelash angle and distension of the supraorbital fossa.
- The affected globe should be retropulsed, there is normally resistance to retropulsion but no pain (compared with a retrobulbar

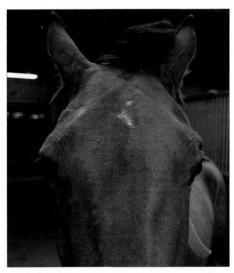

Figure 10.13 Exophthalmos of the right eye with forward and upward displacement of the globe. The cause was extensive retrobulbar lymphoma. Courtesy of Kim Hughes.

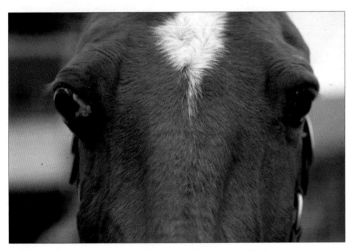

Figure 10.11 Pronounced exophthalmos in the right eye with forward displacement of the globe and protrusion of the third eyelid. This was due to a neuroendocrine tumor (paraganglioma).

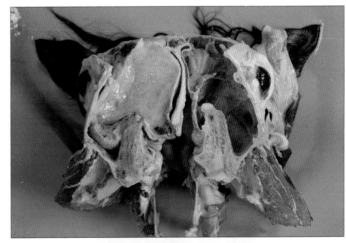

Figure 10.14 Gross pathology photograph of the horse featured in Fig. 10.13. The mass occupies the maxillary sinus, also invading the frontal sinus, and was pushing the eye outwards. Courtesy of Kim Hughes.

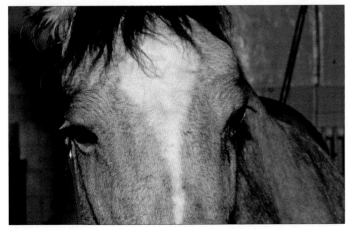

Figure 10.12 Exophthalmos of the left eye of a pony with marked distension of the supraorbital fossa due to orbital lymphoma.

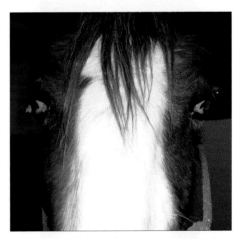

Figure 10.15 Bilateral exophthalmos which was caused by lymphosarcoma which was affecting the retrobulbar region and had infiltrated the conjunctiva and eyelids.

abscess, which is painful), local lymph nodes should be examined and a neurological assessment performed.

- Orbital ultrasound might be useful in order to take a guided biopsy of the area. Ideally, further diagnostic imaging such as radiography, CT or MRI is undertaken.

Treatment

- This involves surgical removal of the neoplasm, if there is no evidence of metastasis. Surgical treatment may involve enucleation or exenteration (removal of eye, adnexa and part of bony orbit).
- Chemotherapy or radiotherapy might be appropriate, depending on the type of tumor present.
- Otherwise, palliative care might be provided if removal of the neoplasm is not an option.

Orbital trauma (Fig. 10.16)

Orbital and periorbital trauma may be caused by kicks or collisions. The periorbital bones which might be fractured include the zygomatic arch, orbital rim and supraorbital process. Globe rupture might also occur. The eyelids may not be able to blink completely due to nerve damage or because of the malaligned bones. Diagnosis is made by visualizing and then palpating the deformity of the periorbital bones. This can be confirmed with radiology. Bony fragments may rub against the globe, causing irritation and threatening penetration. Treatment depends on the extent of the injury and on the level of cosmesis required. It may be possible to manually reposition displaced fragments, or surgically remove them. Surgical repair is possible, and preferred soon after the injury.

Sinusitis and sinus neoplasia

See Chapter 3, p. 142 & 153.

Part 2 Eyelids, third eyelids, conjunctiva and nasolacrimal diseases

Congenital/developmental disorders

Entropion (Figs. 10.17 & 10.18)

Entropion occurs when the eyelid margin is inverted, causing the eyelid to roll inwards. The lower eyelid is affected most commonly. This allows for the facial hairs to contact the globe (trichiasis), leading to ocular discharge, conjunctivitis, keratitis and potentially corneal ulceration. It is the most common ocular abnormality in foals. The

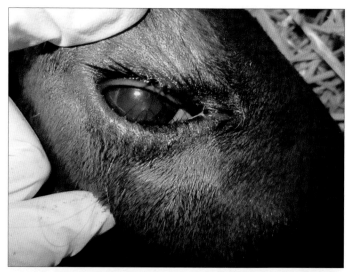

Figure 10.17 Entropion of the lower eyelid of a neonatal Thoroughbred foal. Facial hairs are contacting the cornea because the eyelid is inverted, and the cornea is cloudy due to keratitis.

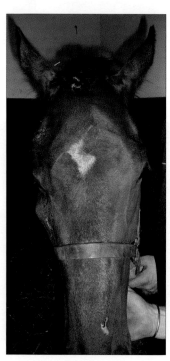

Figure 10.16 Dyssymmetry of the periorbital region after orbital rim and zygomatic arch fracture due to collision with a gate.

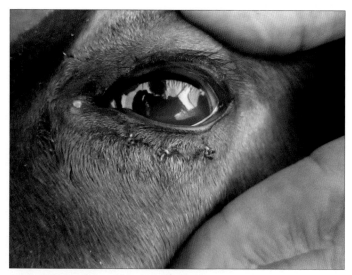

Figure 10.18 Entropion of the lower eyelid post repair with three temporary tacking sutures, which are visible below the lower eyelid. The eyelid is slightly de-pigmented due to the chronic moisture.

cause can be a primary anatomical problem, but also can be secondary to dehydration or cachexia in the neonatal foal. It may arise as a result of loss of orbital volume such as with microphthalmos or phthisis bulbi. At any age, eyelid trauma, eyelid scarring (cicatricial entropion) or blepharitis might result in entropion.

Diagnosis

* Direct observation of the eyelid margin rolling inwards allowing hairs to contact the globe.
* Fluorescein dye should be applied to the cornea to assess for corneal ulceration.

Treatment

* In young foals this normally involves placing three to four temporary tacking vertical mattress sutures to evert the eyelid margin, relieving the anatomical and spastic components of the condition. Usually this allows sufficient time for the underlying problem, such as dehydration, to be rectified.
* Topical lubricating ophthalmic ointment should be used during this time. A topical antibiotic should be used if the cornea is ulcerated.
* If entropion persists despite several temporary tacking procedures, permanent surgical repair is required. The Hotz-Celsus procedure involves removing a section of adjacent eyelid skin, everting the affected eyelid.
* Cicatricial entropion requires surgery to remove the scarred eyelid.

Cilia disorders (Fig. 10.19)

Cilia disorders are uncommon in horses. Distichia are hairs that arise from meibomian gland orifices. These may contact the globe and result in frictional irritation, manifested as blepharospasm, ocular discharge and keratitis, occasionally becoming ulcerative. Ectopic cilia are cilia that arise from the palpebral conjunctiva and contact the globe. A cases series of seven cases has been published (Hurn et al. 2005), and ophthalmic examination revealed a single translucent cilium in the upper eyelid palpebral conjunctiva, emerging approximately 5 mm from the eyelid margin. Post-traumatic trichiasis might occur as a result of inappropriately healed eyelid trauma.

Diagnosis

* Diagnosis is achieved by direct observation of aberrant cilia, and magnification greatly facilitates this.
* An assessment of the degree of irritation caused by the hairs should be made, and the cornea should be stained with fluorescein to check for corneal ulceration.

Treatment

* Application of topical ocular lubrication is sufficient if the irritation is mild. However, permanent destruction of the hair follicles is preferable, and this might be achieved with electrolysis or cryotherapy.
* Treatment of ectopic cilia is with transconjunctival surgical excision.
* Treatment of trichiasis as a result of eyelid scarring involves corrective blepharoplasty. Prognosis is very good with appropriate treatment.

Nasolacrimal duct atresia (Figs. 10.20 & 10.21)

Lacrimal punctum agenesis and lacrimal duct atresia are congenital conditions in the foal. They may occur unilaterally or bilaterally. Typically the condition is not noticed in the very young foal, but when the animal is several months old it develops a chronic copious mucopurulent ocular discharge.

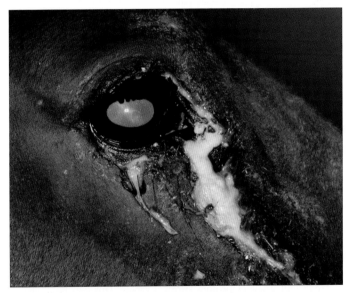

Figure 10.20 Profuse purulent ocular discharge in a yearling which was unresponsive to antibiotics. There was no passage of fluorescein down the nares due to congenital nasolacrimal duct atresia.

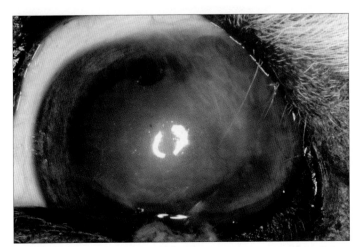

Figure 10.19 Hairs are emerging from the lateral aspect of the upper eyelid. The distichia have caused chronic frictional irritation on the cornea, resulting in keratitis and mucoid ocular discharge.

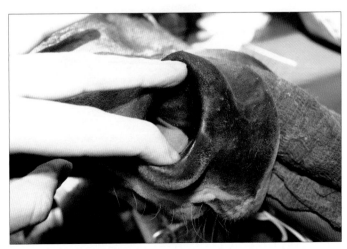

Figure 10.21 No opening for the nasolacrimal duct was present in the nasal meatus.

Diagnosis

- Diagnosis is made by observing the absence of a distal nasolacrimal duct punctum in the nares. It is normally positioned on the floor of the nostril in the ventral nasal meatus. Fluorescein is applied to the lacrimal sac, and there is no passage of the dye to the nares because of the lack of normal drainage.

- Contrast radiography may be used to locate the level of the obstruction, but it is most commonly present at the distal region.

Treatment

- Surgical recreation of a patent nasolacrimal system is required. This usually involves cannulating the nasolacrimal duct from the proximal aspect, through either the upper or lower nasolacrimal punctum. A No. 5 French urinary catheter or polyethylene tubing may be used. The catheter is advanced towards the nose and a quantity of fluid is instilled.

- This usually causes a distension over the mucosa in the nares, and an incision can be made at this site, allowing advancement of the catheter. If no distension is seen, the tip of the catheter might be palpated at the expected site, and the incision made over this. The catheter or tubing is passed through the false nostril and sutured to the side of the face, and it is left in position for several weeks.

Non-infectious disorders

Eyelid injury (Figs. 10.22–10.25)

Traumatic injury of the eyelids is a relatively common occurrence in horses, often resulting in eyelid laceration. The severity of injury varies, but all full-thickness lacerations require surgical repair. The eyelid has an excellent blood supply, and therefore heals very well and repair is normally successful.

Diagnosis, treatment and prognosis

- Diagnosis is usually obvious but the orbit should be carefully assessed for fractures by gently palpating the orbital rim. The conjunctiva and cornea should also be assessed for injury. If the wound is near the medial canthus, the nasolacrimal puncta and canaliculi should be carefully assessed for injury.

- ***Differential diagnosis (of a chronic laceration):*** ulcerated mass such as squamous cell carcinoma or severe solar blepharitis.

- Treatment involves prompt surgical repair. This can be achieved with topical and regional anesthesia, with sedation. The eyelid

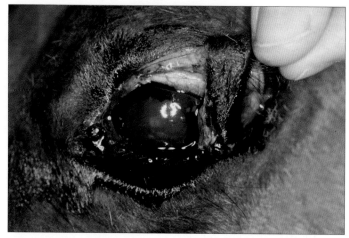

Figure 10.23 Laceration of the upper eyelid resulting in a pedicle of upper eyelid. Surgical repair is indicated.

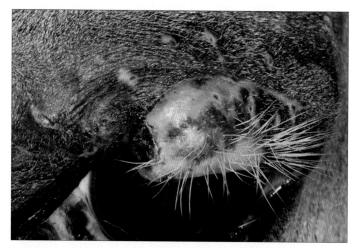

Figure 10.24 Laceration of the upper eyelid was repaired in an imprecise manner 10 days previously, resulting in a large irregularity in the upper eyelid margin.

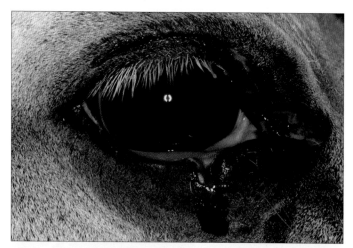

Figure 10.22 Full-thickness laceration of the lower eyelid will require surgical repair.

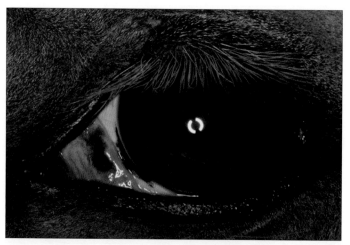

Figure 10.25 The eyelid featured in Fig. 10.24 was repaired again resulting in good eyelid apposition, which was possible because the initial surgery preserved the eyelid tissue.

should be cleansed with a dilute disinfectant which is not harmful to the eye, such as 10% povidone iodine solution, at a 1 : 50 dilution. Minimal debridement is required, and hanging eyelid pedicles should be replaced rather than amputated.

- Full-thickness laceration may require two-layer closure, and a deep conjunctival layer should first be gently apposed using a continuous pattern with an absorbable suture (for example 6-0 polyglactin 910).
- The eyelid margin should be carefully re-aligned using a figure-of-eight suture. The external skin is then repaired with simple interrupted sutures. Poor realignment or second intention healing can result in incomplete eyelid closure which can lead to drying to the exposed cornea and subsequent ulceration.
- The prognosis is normally very good with meticulous and timely surgical repair.

Acquired nasolacrimal duct obstruction
(Figs. 10.26–10.29)
Nasolacrimal duct occlusion or stenosis may be acquired due to dacryocystitis (inflammation of the duct), trauma, foreign body, parasite obstruction, tooth root disease or sinusitis. Clinical signs are chronic epiphora, which occurs if there is no infection, or mucopurulent to purulent ocular discharge if infection occurs.

Diagnosis
- A complete ocular examination is indicated, along with the Jones test for fluorescein dye passage. Absence of fluorescein dye at the ipsilateral nares 5–10 minutes after application indicates an obstruction of normal tear drainage down the nasolacrimal duct.
- If the discharge is purulent, an aerobic and anaerobic bacterial culture and sensitivity test is indicated.
- The adnexa and head should be examined for possible causes of nasolacrimal duct obstruction.
- Contrast radiography might be employed to ascertain the location of the blockage.

Treatment
- Careful flushing of the nasolacrimal duct, which may be cannulated at either the proximal end and flushed towards the nose, or at the nasal ostium and flushed towards the eye. If the blockage is successfully alleviated, the duct should be carefully but copiously flushed.

- An indwelling catheter or tubing might be sutured in place for 2–3 weeks to retain patency.
- An ophthalmic eye drop containing an antibiotic and a steroid is prescribed for application up to four times daily until the inflammation has fully settled and then at reduced frequency for several days.
- Systemic antibiotics may also be required.
- If an underlying cause such as a sinus or tooth root problem is identified, this is treated appropriately.

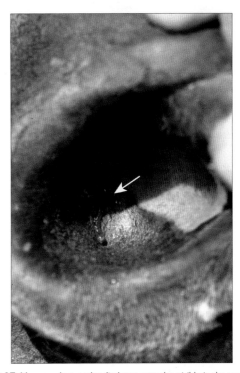

Figure 10.27 Mucopurulent ocular discharge was also visible in the nasolacrimal opening in the nasal meatus (arrow).

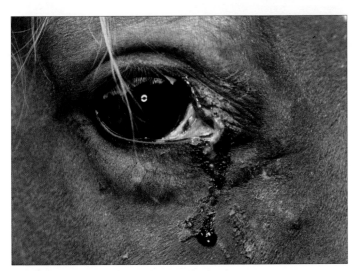

Figure 10.26 Acquired nasolacrimal duct obstruction in an older horse. Mucopurulent ocular discharge was emerging from the nasolacrimal duct.

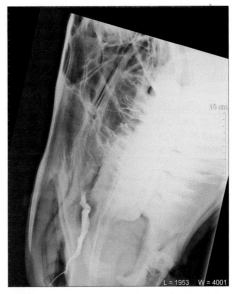

Figure 10.28 A dacryocystorhinogram with contrast material injected through the ventral nasolacrimal opening. The level of the obstruction is visible corresponding with PM2 and is due to inflammation around the first cheek tooth.

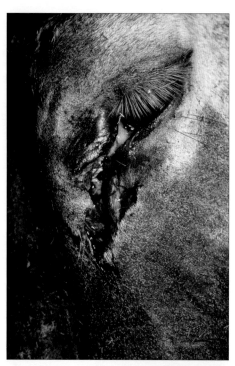

Figure 10.29 Extensive injury to the skin at the medial canthus, overlying the nasolacrimal duct. The duct is identified and preserved during surgical repair.

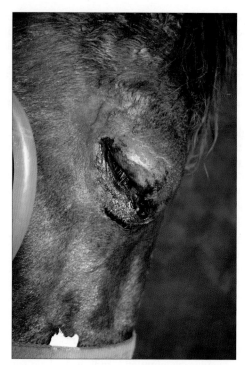

Figure 10.30 Trauma to the head has resulted in blepharoedema and ulceration of the upper eyelid.

- Surgical correction is occasionally required if repeated flushing cannot alleviate the obstruction, establishing drainage with a more invasive procedure such as a conjunctivorhinostomy or a conjunctivosinusotomy.

Non-infectious/infectious disorders

Blepharitis (Figs. 10.30–10.34)

Blepharitis involves inflammation of the eyelids. The main types of blepharitis that occur in the horse are infectious, traumatic, allergic, immune-mediated, actinic and parasitic blepharitis.

- *Infectious blepharitis* may be due to bacterial infection with *Moraxella equi*, *Listeria monocytogenes* or opportunistic bacteria. Fungal blepharitis might be caused by many organisms, depending on geographical exposure, and include *Trichophyton*, *Microsporum* and *Histoplasmafarciminosus*.
- *Traumatic blepharitis* is also a common cause of inflammation.
- *Allergic blepharitis* might arise as a result of a local or a systemic allergy, and blepharoedema may be the most striking sign. The allergen might be environmental, e.g. mold, dust, pollen, or it could be due to topical or systemic medication or shampoos, or a food allergy.
- *Immune-mediated blepharitis* is uncommon, but might arise as part of the pemphigus foliaceus or bullous pemphigoid complexes, which will also affect other mucocutaneous junctions.
- *Solar blepharitis* affects eyelids with little or no protective pigment which are exposed to UV light. Actinic blepharitis could be a precursor for later development of squamous cell carcinoma.
- *Parasitic infestation* can result in blepharitis, and those that might affect the eye include *Onchocerca cervicalis*, *Habronema muscae*, *Habronema microstoma* and *Draschia megastoma* and *Thelazia lacrymalis*. *Onchocerca* principally affects the conjunctiva,

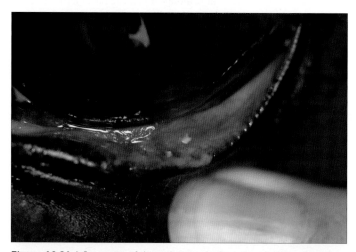

Figure 10.31 Inflammation of the meibomian glands on the palpebral conjunctiva, the eyelid has been gently pressed and yellow material has expressed from the meibomian glands. Bacterial meibomianitis.

with focal conjunctivitis present as nodules lateral to the limbus or as regions of de-pigmentation. Habronema causes mainly blepharitis, with thickened ulcerative caseous nodules on the eyelid margin or palpebral conjunctiva. *Thelazia* infestation might cause dacryocystitis but is often asymptomatic.

Blepharitis symptoms vary depending on the underlying cause but include some of the following: blepharoedema, hyperemia of the palpebral conjunctiva, eyelid hyperemia, pruritis and focal swellings on the eyelid margins or palpebral conjunctiva.

Diagnosis

- The conjunctival fornices and region behind the third eyelid should be examined carefully for the presence of a foreign body.

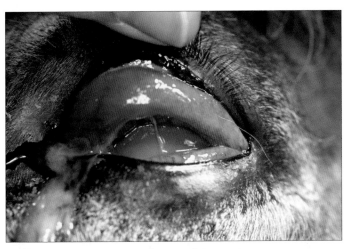

Figure 10.32 Dramatic chemosis due to an allergic reaction.

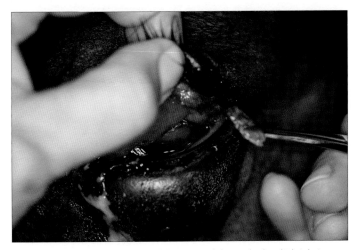

Figure 10.33 Inflamed upper eyelid due to a stick foreign body, which is being gently removed.

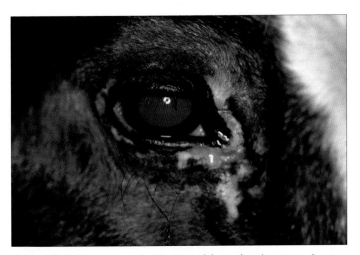

Figure 10.34 The depigmented regions around the eye have become sun-burnt. Solar blepharitis is a risk for progression to squamous cell carcinoma.

- A swab should be submitted for bacterial and fungal culture and sensitivity.
- Cytology of the affected region with scraping may allow more rapid diagnosis of the condition. If the cause is not evident, biopsy of the area may allow for an accurate histopathological diagnosis.

Treatment

- Infectious blepharitis should be treated as appropriate, based on culture and sensitivity. Systemic anti-inflammatory treatment might be required for allergic blepharitis, along with exclusion from the underlying trigger factor.
- It is recommended that horses with solar blepharitis are shielded from the sun with UV-protecting eye wear, the provision of shade and with the application of sun block.
- Habronema is effectively controlled with ivermectin (0.2 mg/kg) but the lesions may also need to be treated with topical compresses, de-bulking, topical antibiotics or lubricants and systemic anti-inflammatories if severe.
- Systemic ivermectin at the same dose is effective at controlling *Onchocerca* microfilaria, and this treatment will need to be repeated, as it is not effective against adult worms. *Thelazia* might be treated with topical irrigation with 0.5% iodine solution and 0.75% potassium iodide. Topical application of 0.03% echothiophate iodide or 0.025% isoflurophate has also been reported to be successful.

Horner's syndrome and facial nerve paralysis

See Chapter 11.

Neoplasia

Eyelid sarcoids (Figs. 10.35–10.37)

Equine sarcoids are benign fibroblastic cutaneous tumors which are very common in horses. Metastasis of sarcoids is rare but recurrence is common. They can affect the skin of the eyelid and periocular region, where they may affect the eye by direct contact with the globe. Location next to the eye can make surgical removal challenging. Retrovirus or palpillomavirus may be involved in the etiology.

Diagnosis

- Diagnosis is normally made based on the characteristic clinical appearance. Any of the five broad categories of sarcoid (occult, nodular, verrucose, fibroblastic or mixed) may affect the periocular region (see p. 342).

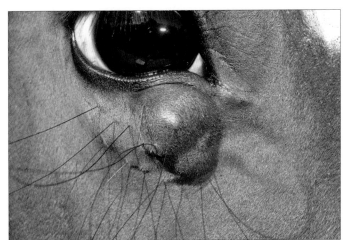

Figure 10.35 Focal subcutaneous nodular thickening under the lower eyelid in a yearling, representing a nodular type A sarcoid.

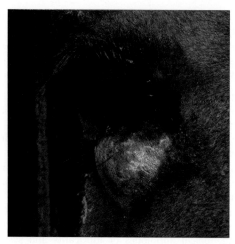

Figure 10.36 A nodular type B sarcoid (also involving the epidermis) on the lower eyelid of a 6-year-old Thoroughbred.

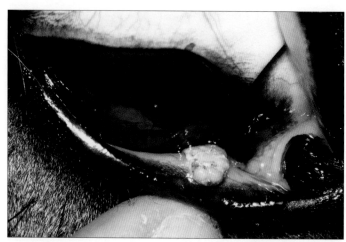

Figure 10.38 Squamous papilloma arising from the palpebral conjunctiva. A viral papilloma needs to be distinguished from a squamous cell carcinoma by biopsy.

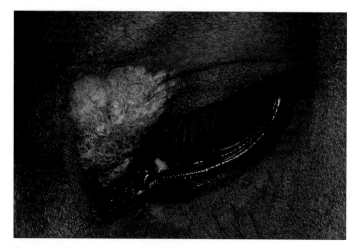

Figure 10.37 A verrucose sarcoid on the upper eyelid with thickened hyperkeratotic skin.

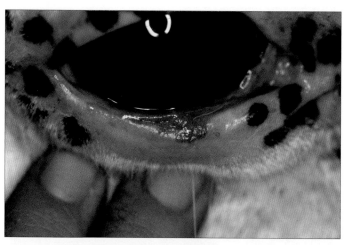

Figure 10.39 Lower eyelid ulcerative squamous cell carcinoma on a depigmented eyelid margin.

- Biopsy and histopathology provide definitive diagnosis. This also helps distinguish the lesion from granulation tissue, *Habronema* infestation, blepharitis, squamous cell carcinoma, papilloma or melanoma.

Treatment

- Periocular sarcoids present a therapeutic challenge as some of the treatment modalities, which are amenable to other parts of the body, are contraindicated around the eye because of the possibility of damaging the globe.
- Historically, sarcoids were treated with topical irritants, such as engine grease, tea tree oil, and oil of rosemary, which served to stimulate the local immune system to mount a response against them. However they would cause a severe keratitis if they were allowed to come into contact with the cornea.
- Surgical excision is usually difficult because of the size of the mass and the lack of available tissue for blepharoplasty procedures. It has also been suggested that sarcoids that recur after surgery are less amenable to further adjunctive treatments.
- Immunotherapy using BCG injections at fortnightly intervals has been very successful at treating periocular sarcoids, although local

and systemic anaphylaxis is a risk and should be anticipated with pre-treatment with systemic NSAIDs.

- Chemotherapy with intralesional cisplatin or topical 5-fluorouracil has been reported to be successful, although 5-fluorouracil is irritant to the globe.
- Cryotherapy and hyperthermia have both been reported with some success. Brachytherapy is reported to be very successful although facilities for radiation treatment must be available.
- The prognosis is poorer when recurrence develops, therefore the initial treatment should be well thought out and thorough.

Squamous cell carcinoma of the eyelid and third eyelid (Figs. 10.38–10.42)

Squamous cell carcinoma (SCC) is the most common neoplasm to affect the eye and adnexa of the horse. An increased incidence has been observed in draft breeds and the Appaloosa. The average age at diagnosis is about 11 years. Horses with light-colored coats are more susceptible than those with darker pigmentation. Actinic solar blepharitis may transform into a squamous cell carcinoma. UV light may mutate the tumor suppressor gene *p53*, allowing the neoplasm to develop.

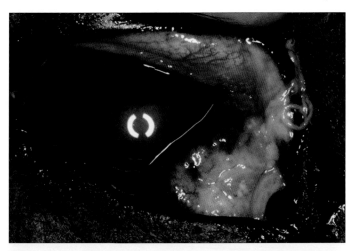

Figure 10.40 White necrotic ocular discharge on an irregular depigmented lobulated third eyelid with squamous cell carcinoma.

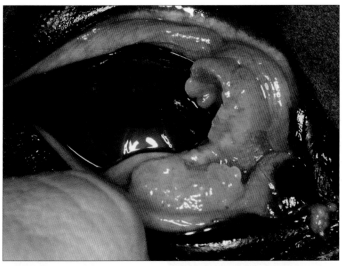

Figure 10.41 More advanced third-eyelid squamous cell carcinoma is visible on manual protrusion of the third eyelid, with lobulated pink tissue on the anterior surface of the third eyelid.

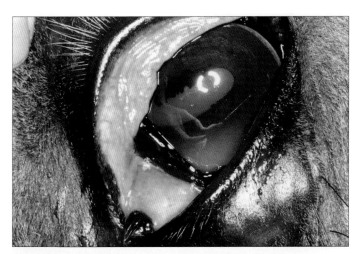

Figure 10.42 Squamous cell carcinoma initially affected the lower eyelid as a subcutaneous nodule, but rapidly invaded the conjunctiva, the cornea and was also intraocular. Orbital exenteration was performed.

Diagnosis

- SCC may be suspected on the clinical appearance of the lesion. Eyelid SCC typically presents as an erosive, erythematous thickening of the eyelid. Third-eyelid SCC typically presents as a lobulated, irregular pink cobblestone-like mass on the third eyelid.
- Definitive diagnosis requires biopsy and histopathology. Histopathology will also distinguish between plaque (carcinoma in situ), papillomatous, non-invasive or invasive SCC.
- Gentle palpation of the orbital rim should be undertaken to assess for extension of the tumor.
- A metastasis assessment should be made before treatment is considered, assessing the regional lymph nodes and salivary glands, the thorax, and the orbit and sinus for evidence of local extension.

Treatment

- Treatment of periocular SCC is challenging. While complete surgical resection is the treatment of choice, extensive eyelid re-construction is often not possible.
- Removal of the entire third eyelid, over-sewing the remaining conjunctiva to prevent fat prolapse, may be curative for third-eyelid SCC.
- Eyelid SCC may require surgical debulking with adjunctive treatment, or adjunctive treatment alone. Methods successfully employed include immunotherapy (BCG injections), chemotherapy (e.g. intralesional cisplatin, 5-fluorouracil), cryotherapy (double or triple freeze–thaw cycle to −25°C), brachytherapy (radioactive isotopes gold, iridium, radon, etc.) or hyperthermia (41–50°C).
- The most recently reported treatment with a favorable outcome is photodynamic therapy (Giuliano et al 2008) although it is still undergoing further investigation as a suitable treatment modality.
- There is a poor prognosis for eyelid SCC compared with third-eyelid SCC, and reported metastasis rates vary from 6% to 15%.

Other adnexal tumors (Figs. 10.43–10.51)

Other adnexal neoplasms arise occasionally. In all cases, the diagnosis might be suspected from the clinical appearance but can only be confirmed by fine-needle aspirate, biopsy or excisional biopsy. Other non-neoplastic swellings can occur in the area, such as *Habronema* granulomas or orbital fat prolapse.

Eyelid and subconjunctival melanomas are most common in gray horses. They may cause frictional irritation on the globe. They present as firm pigmented nodules on the eyelid margin or beneath

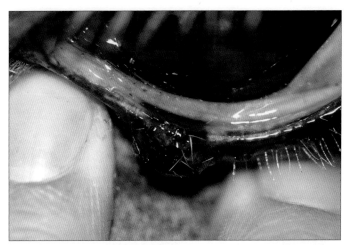

Figure 10.43 Melanoma affecting the lower eyelid and palpebral conjunctiva in a gray horse.

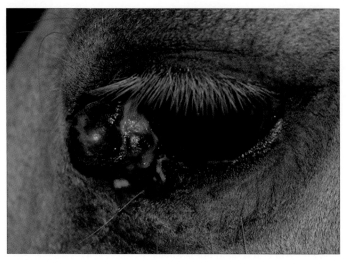

Figure 10.44 A larger melanoma affecting the lower eyelid, medial canthus and lacrimal caruncle.

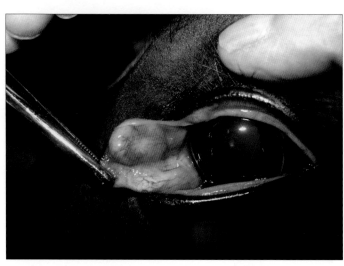

Figure 10.47 Nodular thickening underneath the conjunctiva was removed by excisional biopsy and the diagnosis was a nodular lymphoma.

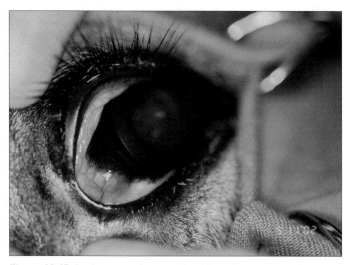

Figure 10.45 A subconjunctival pigmented nodular melanoma in a gray horse.

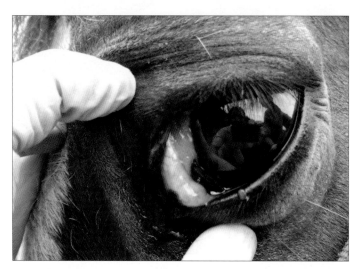

Figure 10.48 More generalized thickening of the conjunctiva due to conjunctival infiltration with lymphoma, diagnosed with a fine-needle aspirate.

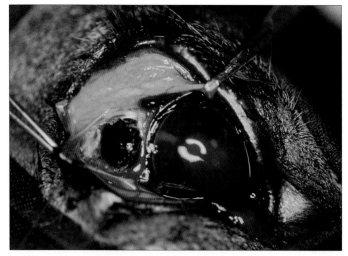

Figure 10.46 During surgical removal, the overlying conjunctiva is reflected to reveal the melanoma underneath.

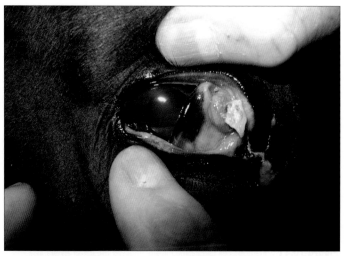

Figure 10.49 Nodular lesion on the anterior surface of the third eyelid with a caseous exudate, diagnosed on excisional biopsy as a mast cell tumor.

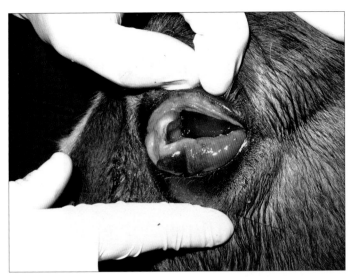

Figure 10.50 Extensive conjunctival reddening and thickening due to a hemangioma.

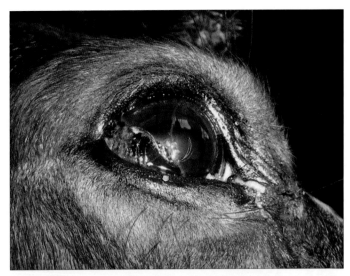

Figure 10.52 Haired and pigmented skin on the ventral aspect of the cornea (dermoid), giving rise to purulent ocular discharge, in a 5-year-old pony.

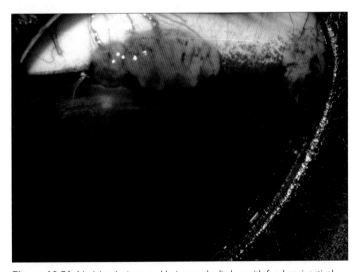

Figure 10.51 Nodular depigmented lesion on the limbus with focal conjunctival pigmentation also.

Part 3 Cornea

Congenital/developmental conditions

Dermoids (Fig. 10.52)

A dermoid is normal skin that is present in an abnormal location (a choristoma). They are congenital but may become more obvious as the animal gets older, and the hair grows a little longer. They may be located on the conjunctiva, cornea or eyelid, and may be unilateral or bilateral. Associated clinical signs include the physical presence of haired skin on the eye or adnexa. They most commonly occur on the dorsal limbus but may be located elsewhere. The skin may be pigmented, making their presence more obvious. The consequences of its presence are also visible as irritation results in epiphora or mucopurulent ocular discharge, and occasionally blepharospasm.

Diagnosis, treatment and prognosis

- Diagnosis is made based on clinical signs and examination.
- Treatment is by surgical resection, which is usually a superficial keratectomy.
- The prognosis is excellent as surgical removal is curative.

Linear keratopathy (Fig. 10.53)

Paired parallel well-defined corneal striae in a linear pattern occasionally present in an apparently normal eye. These linear opacities occur at the level of Descemet's membrane, and there is no associated corneal edema. It may travel in any direction, but most often extends from limbus to limbus across the center of the cornea, and may branch one or more times. The cause is unknown, but they are thought to arise due to a transient increase in intraocular pressure during parturition. Identical opacities are found in some horses with glaucoma, and in others that have suffered blunt ocular trauma.

Diagnosis and treatment

- A careful ocular examination to attempt to identify other signs of glaucoma is indicated. These would include visual deficits, mydriasis, reduced pupillary light responses, corneal edema, mild iridocyclitis, retinal degeneration and optic nerve cupping.
- Tonometry to measure the intraocular pressure is indicated.
- If linear keratopathy is the only abnormality present, the condition is considered incidental and no treatment is required.

the conjunctiva. The adjacent area should be carefully examined to determine the full extent of the mass. Surgical resection is the preferred treatment, and cryotherapy might also be considered. Oral cimetidine has been used to treat cutaneous melanomas but there are no reports of using it for periocular melanomas.

Lymphosarcoma is an uncommon tumor of the adnexal region. It has a variety of presentations. There may be infiltration of the conjunctiva and eyelids. Orbital involvement may result in exophthalmos. Nodular swellings of the conjunctiva may occur occasionally, and have been referred to as pseudotumors. A full systemic examination is indicated. Most cases represent multicentric lymphosarcoma which makes the prognosis very poor. Treatment with systemic dexamethasone 30 mg every second day has been reported.

Mast cell tumors are not common. They are associated with eosinophilic infiltration and may resemble a *Habronema* granuloma. They may result in a diffuse thickening of the affected eyelid. Surgical resection is indicated if this is possible.

Other less common adnexal tumors include hemangioma, hemangiosarcoma, basal cell carcinoma, lacrimal gland carcinoma, fibroma and fibrosarcoma.

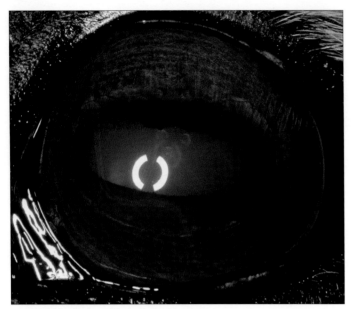

Figure 10.53 Well-defined linear refractile opacity (linear keratopathy) traversing the cornea in a horse with a normal intraocular pressure. Incidentally three round posterior subcapsular cataracts are also present.

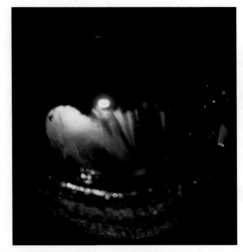

Figure 10.55 Hemorrhage in the vitreous and fibrin in the anterior chamber after ocular blunt trauma.

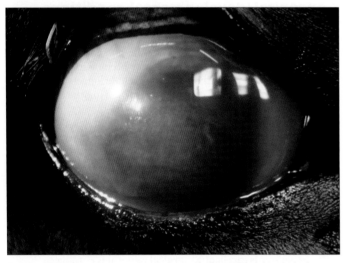

Figure 10.54 Blunt trauma to the eye has resulted in peripheral corneal edema and hemorrhage (hyphema) in the anterior chamber. Courtesy of Kim Hughes.

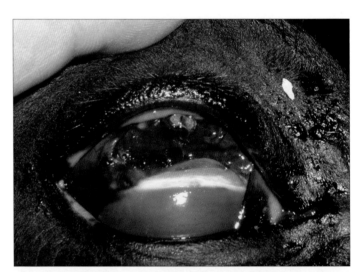

Figure 10.56 Severe blunt trauma has resulted in rupture of the globe at the superior limbus, with dark uveal tissue visible outside the eye. Courtesy of Kim Hughes.

Non-infectious disorders

Corneal trauma (Figs. 10.54–10.60)

Horses are very vulnerable to both blunt and sharp penetrating ocular trauma, and this can have a variety of effects on the globe. Sharp penetrating corneal trauma will cause laceration. If the wound is full thickness, there may also be damage to the iris or lens. Blunt force energy is transmitted throughout the globe. Corneal perforation may also occur but it is more likely that there will be more serious structural damage, worsening the prognosis. The traumatized eye presents with ocular pain, manifested as blepharospasm, alteration in the angle of the eyelashes and epiphora. The eye is usually cloudy, due to corneal edema and/or aqueous flare, and red due to inflammation or hyphema. Corneal trauma invariably results in secondary iridocyclitis, with miosis, iritis, aqueous flare and possibly hypopyon. Full-thickness corneal laceration may be associated with a shallow

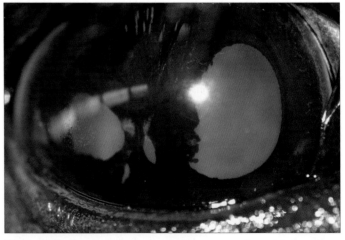

Figure 10.57 As a sequel to blunt trauma, there is a central synechia where the dorsal and ventral iris are adhered centrally in the pupil.

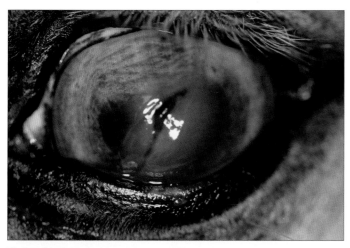

Figure 10.58 Corneal laceration injury with corneal edema, dark uveal tissue within the laceration and miosis.

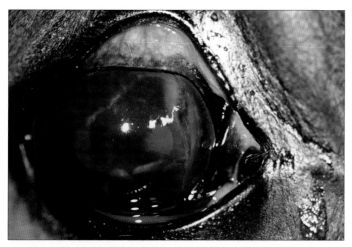

Figure 10.59 Full-thickness corneal laceration medially, with iris tissue visible within the laceration along with hyphema and aqueous flare.

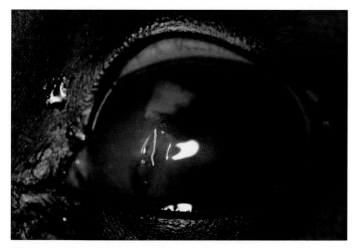

Figure 10.60 Full-thickness corneal laceration injury with protrusion of iris covered with an aqueous clot, along with hyphema and miosis.

anterior chamber, hyphema and iris prolapse. If the corneal laceration is peripheral, it should be carefully checked if it traverses the limbus as the sclera may also be ruptured. Scleral rupture is more difficult to see clinically because of the posterior location and because it is covered by conjunctiva which will be inflamed and swollen.

Diagnosis

- Diagnosis is made with the history of trauma and by careful examination of the eye. As the eye will be painful, sedation, regional nerve blocks and topical anesthesia will be required for a thorough examination.
- The cornea should be examined with magnification to determine if any foreign body is still present.
- Fluorescein stain is applied to assess the presence of corneal ulceration. The Seidel's test is carried out simultaneously as follows. The corneal wound is examined carefully after liberal application of fluorescein dye. If the wound is leaking, a small stream of clear aqueous will flow through the concentrated fluorescein, appearing brighter green as it is diluted. This is a positive Seidel's test.
- If the cornea is stable and the eye cannot be examined thoroughly due to opacity in the ocular media, B-mode ultrasound is a useful method to look for lens luxation, lens capsule rupture, hemorrhage or inflammatory membranes in the vitreous and retinal detachment.

Treatment and prognosis

- Treatment depends on the extent of the injury. Small corneal lacerations, which are not full thickness, can be treated medically as for corneal ulcers. This involves topical antibiotics and mydriatics, along with systemic NSAIDs.
- If the edges of the corneal wound are edematous and therefore everted or irregular, or if the corneal wound is full-thickness, the wound should be surgically repaired. Direct simple interrupted corneal sutures are normally sufficient, but occasionally a conjunctival graft might be necessary to support healing. Systemic antibiotics and NSAIDs will be required as well as topical antibiotics and mydriatics.
- Iris prolapse requires surgical repair. Ocular survival has been reported to be 80% after surgery with vision in 33% of horses with iris prolapse due to corneal lacerations.
- The prognosis is best for corneal lacerations that do not involve any other ocular structures, and that are presented promptly for treatment. Corneal lacerations could potentially become complicated by bacterial or fungal infection, corneal melting, anterior synechiae, glaucoma, or uncontrolled uveitis due to lens capsule disruption causing lens-induced uveitis. Intraocular bacterial inoculation might result in endophthalmitis.

Corneal foreign bodies (Figs. 10.61–10.67)

Corneal foreign bodies are not unusual in the horse. Regions of the north-eastern USA have a plant burdock pappus with sharp bristles that can lodge in the conjunctiva and damage the cornea. They result in ocular pain and chronic non-healing ulcers. The eye needs to be examined with magnification to determine whether any bristles are retained. If there are, they are gently removed with a forceps after application of topical anesthesia, and both motor and sensory nerve blocks. Treatment as for a corneal ulcer is then given, with topical antibiotics and atropine, with systemic NSAIDs until the eye is comfortable and the cornea is negative for fluorescein uptake.

Small bedding, pasture or feed foreign bodies can adhere to the cornea. They typically present with acute-onset ocular discomfort. Plant material can sometimes penetrate the cornea and perforate the globe. This results in severe iridocyclitis and it may introduce infection into the eye, resulting in endophthalmitis.

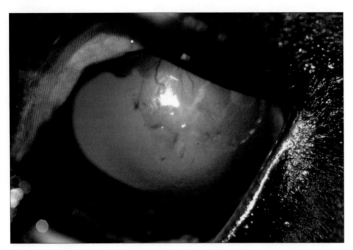

Figure 10.61 Cactus prickle keratopathy with multifocal linear corneal ulcers, corneal edema and neovascularization. The prickles did not remain in the cornea but the ulcerative keratitis is still present.

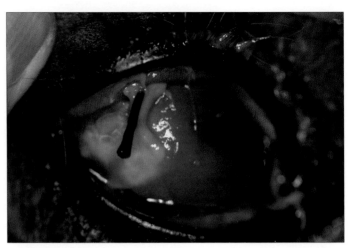

Figure 10.64 Thorn impailed through the cornea with severe intraocular and corneal inflammation.

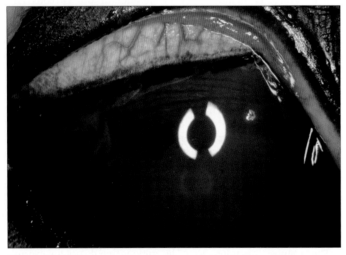

Figure 10.62 Common presentation of a corneal foreign body which has adhered to the cornea at the one o'clock position.

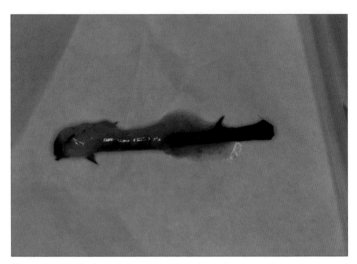

Figure 10.65 The barbed thorn was removed, purulent material remains adhered to it.

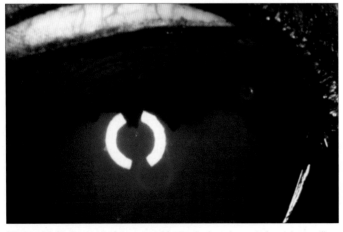

Figure 10.63 Removal of the corneal foreign body under topical anesthesia will leave a small stromal corneal ulcer.

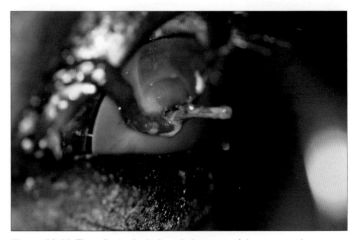

Figure 10.66 Thorn foreign body through the center of the cornea with hemorrhage, corneal edema and a surrounding corneal ulcer.

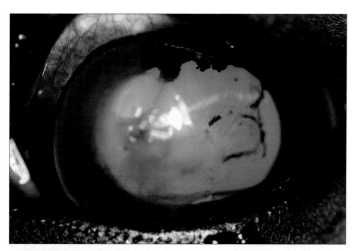

Figure 10.67 The thorn was removed. Keratitis, hyphema, fibrin in the anterior chamber and pigment on the anterior lens capsule remain, but the eye is responding well to treatment.

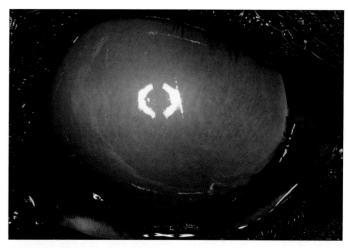

Figure 10.68 Pan-corneal edema following blunt ocular trauma. Corneal ulceration is not evident.

Diagnosis, treatment and prognosis

- Careful examination of the eye, aided with magnification, reveals the foreign body on the surface of the cornea. After application of topical anesthesia, the foreign body is gently dislodged either by flushing with sterile saline or with a needle. This leaves a superficial ulcer, which is treated as for a routine superficial corneal ulcer.
- In cases where the foreign body has penetrated the cornea, an assessment is made as to whether the penetration extends full thickness through the cornea, and if deeper structures such as the lens have been damaged.
- Perforation of the lens carries a guarded prognosis due to severe phacoclastic uveitis. A general anesthetic is indicated. The corneal foreign body is removed and the cornea is repaired. Systemic antibiotics will be required as well as topical antibiotics. Systemic NSAIDs are necessary. Topical atropine is given for the iridocyclitis.
- The prognosis depends on the extent of intraocular damage and if infection is introduced.

Non-infectious/infectious disorders

Ulcerative keratitis

Corneal ulceration is a very common occurrence in horses. It is potentially a vision- and eye-threatening condition; therefore it is imperative that timely and appropriate treatment is given. Corneal ulcers range from superficial through to deep. Corneal healing can be complicated by a number of factors, such as bacterial or fungal infection, collagenolysis (corneal melting), uveitis, eyelid dysfunction, distichiasis and the presence of a foreign body. Careful examination for such complicating factors is imperative in order to create the most appropriate treatment plan. Laboratory tests such as corneal scraping and bacterial/fungal culture and sensitivity are commonly used. Treatment needs to be provided without delay to prevent potentially serious outcomes such as progression to corneal perforation, endophthalmitis, phthisis bulbi and blindness.

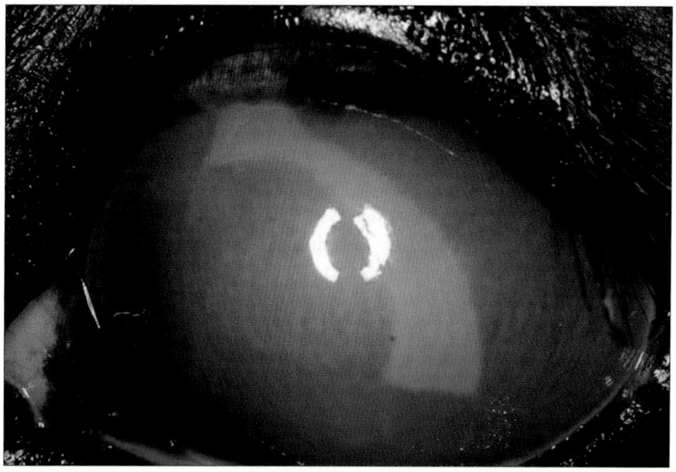

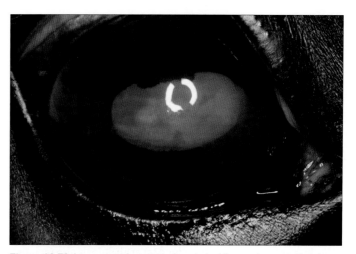

Figure 10.69 The same eye stained with fluorescein, the superficial corneal ulcer can be clearly seen highlighted with fluorescein dye. All corneal opacities should be stained with fluorescein.

Superficial corneal ulceration (Figs. 10.68–10.71)

A superficial corneal ulcer involves focal loss of the epithelium, which represents about 10% of the corneal thickness. Many are assumed to be traumatic in origin, but in reality we often do not ascertain the cause. Because the cornea is densely innervated, the eye is usually very uncomfortable, and the horse presents with blepharospasm and

Figure 10.70 Linear corneal opacity in the palpebral fissure, due to accidental contact with alcohol during surgical preparation of the throat and resulting in iatrogenic superficial corneal erosion.

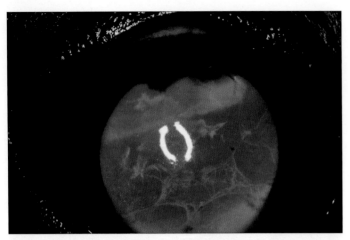

Figure 10.71 A superficial fluorescein-positive ulcer at the one o'clock position on the cornea has caused reflex uveitis with fibrin in the anterior chamber. The pupil has been dilated with atropine.

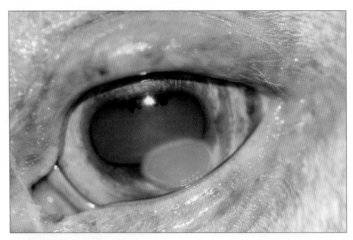

Figure 10.72 Superficial indolent corneal ulcer with retention of fluorescein dye and seepage of the dye underneath the epithelium at the edge of the lesion as it is non-adherent.

epiphora. There is usually conjunctival hyperemia. There may be focal corneal edema within the ulcerated area, but there may be no signs of neovascularization or cellular infiltrate at the early stages. Reflex uveitis is often a secondary result, with miosis, aqueous flare and reduced intraocular pressure. These ulcers are generally not infected.

Treatment

In the absence of complicating factors, these ulcers are expected to heal at the rate of 0.6 mm/day, and are supported with topical broad-spectrum prophylactic antibiotics and topical mydriatics to control the secondary reflex uveitis, along with systemic NSAIDs, while healing occurs.

Non-healing superficial corneal ulceration
(Figs. 10.72 & 10.73)

Superficial ulcers may fail to heal, despite the absence of complicating factors. These are termed 'indolent' or non-healing corneal ulcers. Older horses are more likely to be affected than younger horses. These ulcers are characterized by chronicity (at least a week), and a non-adherent rim of epithelium at the edge of the ulcer. There are likely to be defects in the anterior stroma and extracellular matrix, as occurs in dogs affected by a similar non-healing superficial corneal ulcerative condition.

Diagnosis

- Diagnosis of a superficial ulcer is made on uptake of fluorescein stain by the exposed corneal stroma, and this fluorescence is highlighted with a cobalt-blue light source. The eye needs to be carefully assessed for predisposing causes or complicating factors, such as eyelid dysfunction, tear film quantitative deficiency (keratoconjunctivitis sicca), tear film qualitative deficiency (e.g. premature evaporation of the tears due to inadequate blinking) and the presence of a corneal foreign body.
- A non-healing superficial ulcer is diagnosed based on the chronicity of the problem, and on the characteristic spreading of fluorescein underneath the edge of the loose epithelium at the periphery of the ulcer.

Treatment

- Treatment of non-healing ulcers requires the same medical support as is provided with superficial ulcers. However, in order to induce healing, debridement of the redundant epithelium is also required. This is carried out after application of topical anesthesia (e.g. proxymetacaine/proparacaine 1%). Sterile dry cotton-tipped

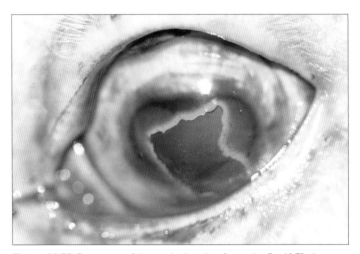

Figure 10.73 Progression of the non-healing ulcer featured in Fig. 10.72, the ulcer is more extensive. Both fluorescein and Rose Bengal dye have been applied.

applicators are gently but firmly rubbed radially outwards, starting at the center of the ulcer.
- Additional therapy might also be required to alter the anterior stroma, allowing the epithelium to adhere to it during the healing process. This might involve a grid or punctate keratotomy, and the use of thermal cautery has also been reported.
- A soft therapeutic bandage contact lens will provide instant comfort and is thought to aid healing.
- Cases that do not heal after the methods outlined often benefit from a surgical superficial keratectomy, as it removes the abnormal anterior corneal stroma.
- The use of topical steroids is contraindicated.

Stromal and deep corneal ulceration
(Figs. 10.74–10.77)

Corneal ulceration that extends deeper into the stroma is a more serious condition than superficial ulceration. This might occur because the initial injury caused a deep ulcer, or with progression of a superficial corneal ulcer due to infection or collagenolysis. Once the normal epithelial barrier is removed, the stroma is exposed to the commensal ocular organisms along with environmental pathogens

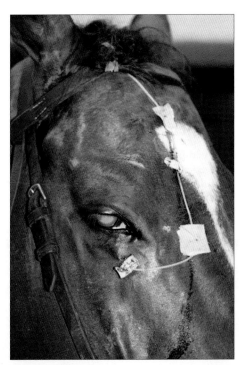

Figure 10.74 A subpalpebral lavage catheter can be inserted through the lower or upper eyelid and secured to the mane, to increase compliance and effectiveness of drug delivery.

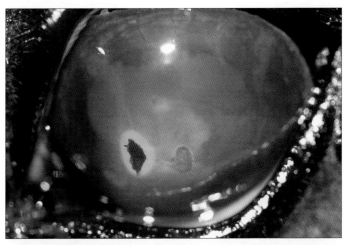

Figure 10.75 Stromal corneal ulceration after application of both fluorescein, staining the limits of the ulcer, and Rose Bengal staining the center. An adjacent corneal facet has epithelialized so is not uptaking either dye.

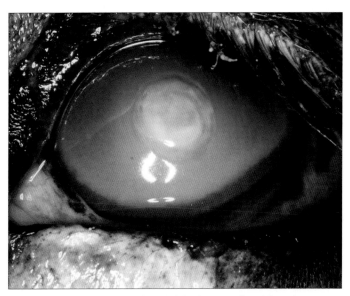

Figure 10.76 Stromal corneal ulcer which has become infected. It is white in color due to cellular infiltration, necrosis and infection. There is corneal edema and deep neovascularization.

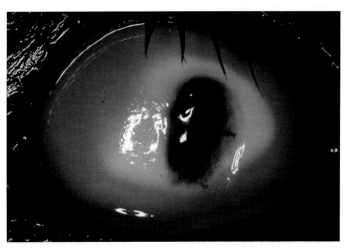

Figure 10.77 Deep corneal ulceration has progressed to globe rupture, with iris prolapse. There is deep corneal vascularization, edema and cellular infiltration.

and particles. Pathogens can overwhelm the natural ocular defense system and result in progressive corneal stromal infection and destruction. They usually induce a local inflammatory response. This results in excessive production of proteases by the invading microorganism, as well as by host neutrophils, fibroblasts and epithelial cells. This leads to progression of the corneal ulcer through collagenolysis, and can lead to corneal 'melting' (see below). The eye is painful and there may be a mucopurulent or purulent ocular discharge. Conjunctival hyperemia is expected and there is often chemosis. Corneal edema is always present within the defect but often involves the entire corneal stroma to a lesser degree. Vascularization is very variable, depending on the pathogenesis and chronicity of the

ulcer. There may be cellular infiltrate, visible as yellow to white stromal opacity.

Diagnosis

- Diagnosis of stromal and deep corneal ulceration is made on the basis of characteristic clinical signs.
- The ulcer is expected to take up fluorescein stain. The depth of the ulcer might be ascertained using the slit lamp biomicroscope. Ulcers to a depth of Descemet's membrane lack any stroma, and therefore there is no fluorescein uptake at the base of the lesion. However, with a descemetocele, fluorescein uptake can normally be seen in the 'walls' of the ulcer, but it is missing from the base.
- Secondary reflex uveitis is invariably present, and is recognized as miosis, aqueous flare, and occasionally hypopyon.
- Laboratory testing is strongly recommended in all cases of deep stromal ulceration. Cytology provided by corneal scraping at the edge of the lesion provides a rapid and low-cost evaluation of the cells and pathogens present.

- Bacteria and fungi can be rapidly identified. Bacterial and fungal culture and sensitivity are also recommended, but treatment will have to commence before these results are available. However, they provide very useful information should the ulcer fail to heal.

Treatment

- The use of a subpalpebral lavage catheter is highly recommended because the eye is usually very painful and treatment depends on frequent and reliable delivery of medication to the eye.
- Topical antibiotics are always indicated. Gentamycin or fluoroquinolones are chosen if Gram-negative bacterial infection is suspected, whereas chloramphenicol or cefazolin are better choices if Gram-positive infection is present.
- Use of a topical anticollagenase to prevent corneal melting is recommended (see below).
- Topical antifungals are required if fungal organisms are present (see fungal keratitis below).
- Topical mydriatics and systemic NSAIDs are essential to control the inevitable uveitis.
- Surgical repair might be indicated for deeper ulcers. This allows the corneal ulcer to be surgically debrided, thus reducing the bacterial or fungal burden. Conjunctival pedicle grafts provide a blood supply and a strong epithelium to the vulnerable region. Amniotic grafts and penetrating keratoplasties have been performed successfully on appropriate cases. Third-eyelid flaps are generally contraindicated as they prevent visual appraisal of the ulcer, trap infection and are a barrier to penetration of medication.
- The use of topical steroids is contraindicated.

Melting corneal ulcer (Figs. 10.78–10.81)

Tear film proteinases are enzymes that provide an essential maintenance role for the health and repair of the corneal epithelium and stroma. The enzymes operate in a delicate balance with inhibitory factors, which act to control the action of these enzymes and therefore prevent excessive destruction of the healthy cornea. In the presence of corneal ulcers, tear film matrix metalloproteinase-2 (MMP-2), MMP-9 and neutrophil elastase (NE) levels are increased. These destructive collagenases and proteinases are produced by the invading micro-organism, as well as by host tear film neutrophils, epithelial cells and fibroblasts. Excessive destruction of the corneal stroma results in liquifactive necrosis that clinically appears like gelatinous soft cornea, which is called a 'melting' cornea because of the appearance. The use of topical corticosteroids on an ulcerated cornea can induce corneal melting. An untreated melting corneal ulcer will invariably progress to globe perforation.

Diagnosis

- Diagnosis is made on the classical presentation of white or gray (due to edema +/– inflammatory cell infiltration) malacic corneal stroma that appears to be sloughing ventrally from a corneal ulcer.
- The contour of the globe is normally disrupted with the cornea appearing flat within the ulcerated region because the stroma is so thin. As for deep stromal ulcers, corneal scraping and swabs for pathogen culture and sensitivity are indicated. Sometimes no microbial agent is identified and the melt is considered sterile.

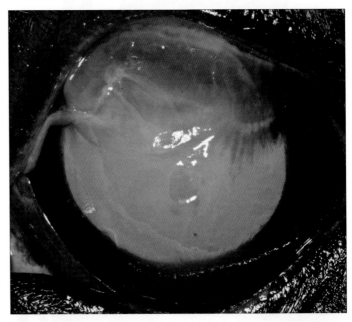

Figure 10.79 Chronic deep corneal ulcer with deep corneal neovascularization, progressed to melting with soft gelatinous cornea exuding from the superior aspect of the ulcer.

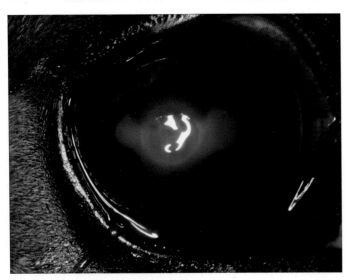

Figure 10.78 A focal central corneal ulcer with white malacic gelatinous 'melt' extending onto the lower eyelid.

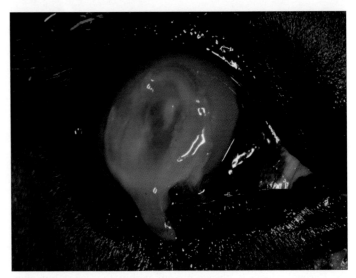

Figure 10.80 Severe melting ulcer with soft malacic cornea extending onto the lower eyelid. The rest of the cornea is opaque due to edema and cellular infiltration.

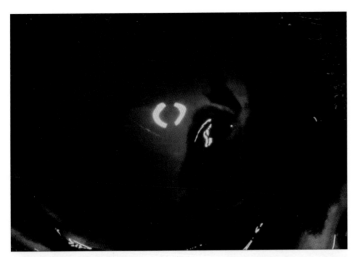

Figure 10.81 Four weeks after surgical repair of the eye in Fig. 10.80 with a 360 degree conjunctival graft. Pigmented conjunctiva has adhered to the ulcerated site but reasonable vision is present.

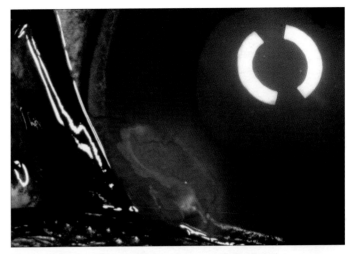

Figure 10.82 Superficial corneal ulceration next to the limbus with neovascularization and white coloration. Corneal scraping revealed eosinophils as well as other inflammatory cells.

Treatment

- It is imperative that treatment is commenced as soon as possible. A subpalpebral lavage catheter is strongly advised.
- Topical anticollagenase treatment is essential to counteract the destructive enzymes. This might be provided by topical serum, acetylcysteine, EDTA, heparin, tetanus antitoxin or ilomastat. Serum reduces proteolytic activity because it contains inhibitory substances such as alpha-2 macroglobulin, along with platelet-derived growth factor and epidermal growth factor. It is obtained from clotted blood, stored in the fridge, and applied topically frequently (every 2–3 hours). The other topical anticollagenase agents work by chelating calcium and zinc, thereby reducing the activity of the MMPs. Prolonged use of acetylcysteine may retard epithelial repair by degrading tear film mucins. In addition to anticollagenase medication, treatment as for a deep stromal corneal ulcer is prescribed.
- Surgical treatment to provide vascular supply and structural support may be indicated as well as medical treatment, such as a conjunctival graft or amniotic membrane graft.

Eosinophilic keratitis (Figs. 10.82–10.84)

Eosinophilic keratitis occurs more commonly in the USA, compared with Europe. It arises more frequently in the spring and summer months. The cause has not yet been determined, although parasites and environmental allergens have been considered. Horses which are turned out appear to be affected more frequently than stabled horses, possibly connected to increased contact with flies. Eosinophilic keratitis is a chronic inflammatory condition of the cornea, which may affect one or both eyes. It presents with mild blepharospasm, mucoid ocular discharge and conjunctival hyperemia. There is a white necrotic plaque within the surface of the cornea, usually at the periphery although it can extend axially with time.

Diagnosis and treatment

- Diagnosis is reached based on the clinical signs and on the cytology findings on a corneal scraping specimen. Typical cytology reveals numerous eosinophils, along with a few other inflammatory cells such as mast cells, lymphocytes and plasma cells.
- Treatment with topical anti-inflammatories is indicated. Topical steroids (e.g. dexamethasone 0.1% or prednisolone acetate 1%) are often used although the horse must be monitored carefully as many

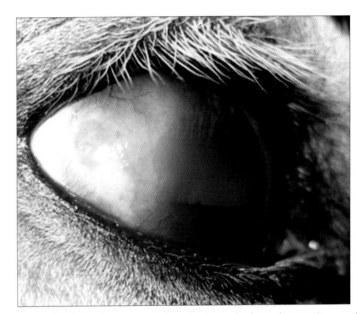

Figure 10.83 The lateral cornea is infiltrated with a whitish vascular necrotic plaque, typical of eosinophilic keratitis. Courtesy of Ida Gilbert.

have superficial corneal ulceration. For this reason, topical antibiotics are often used concurrently.
- In a recent study in the US, systemic corticosteroid treatment was found to decrease therapy duration. Also, treatment with cetirizine was associated with a decreased risk of recurrence (Lassaline-Utter et al, 2013).
- If the horse is uncomfortable, surgical superficial keratectomy will speed the resolution of the condition.
- Anthelmintics should be administered if they are due. Turn-out time should be reduced and the use of a fly mask is advised.

Immune-mediated keratitis (Figs. 10.85–10.91)

Non-ulcerative immune-mediated keratitis is a very common presentation in equine practice. It was succinctly described by Matthews and Gilger in 2009, reviewing the different presentations in the UK and

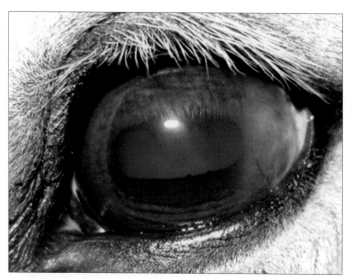

Figure 10.84 The left eye of the same horse as in Fig. 10.83 is also affected, but less severely. Courtesy of Ida Gilbert.

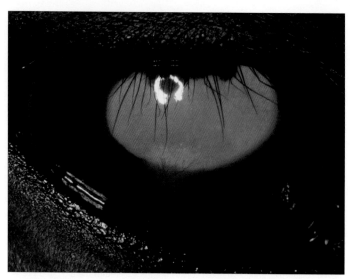

Figure 10.86 Early superficial immune-mediated keratitis, with superficial branching corneal neovascularization and subtle stromal cellular infiltrate.

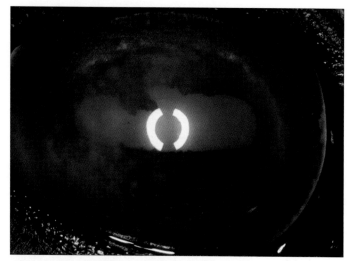

Figure 10.85 Epithelial immune-mediated keratitis. There was conjunctival hyperemia, no corneal vascularization and multifocal subepithelial opacities which responded to topical steroids.

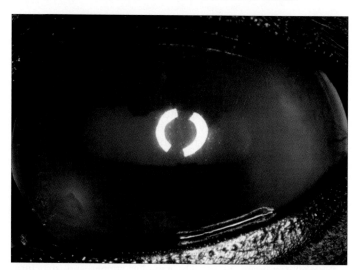

Figure 10.87 More advanced superficial immune-mediated keratitis with much yellow stromal cellular infiltrate laterally with superficial neovascularization, and there is a paralimbal ulcer medially.

the USA. This group of inflammatory keratopathies is thought to be the result of upregulated immunoreactivity within the cornea, a structure that is normally immunologically passive. Local auto- or heteroantigens are thought to disrupt the normal immunoregulatory microenvironment, triggering and then perpetuating the inflammation. Histopathology has revealed lymphocytic–plasmacytic stromal infiltrate along with migration of histiocytes and polymorphonuclear cells. No infectious agents were observed in histopathology studies. The clinical presentations may be divided into four main groups, and differ in presentation in the UK and USA (Matthews et al 2010).

1) Epithelial immune-mediated keratitis in the UK presents with a diffuse, central, superficial, non-vascularized corneal opacity, with conjunctival hyperemia and some blepharospasm. In the USA, a similar condition presents with multifocal punctate opacities in the ventral and ventral-paracentral non-vascularized corneal epithelium, with conjunctival hyperemia but usually without blepharospasm.

2) Superficial immune-mediated keratitis in the UK is described as chronic superficial keratitis, with prominent subepithelial arborizing vascularization involving corneal edema and stromal cell

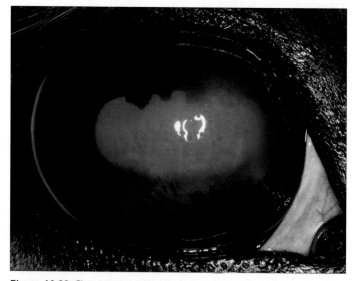

Figure 10.88 Chronic recurrent keratitis with mid-stromal lacunae and a fibrovascular response.

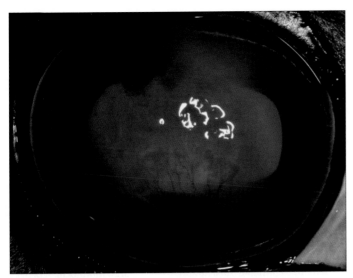

Figure 10.89 Chronic recurrent keratitis with mid-stromal greenish lacunae and a fibrovascular response.

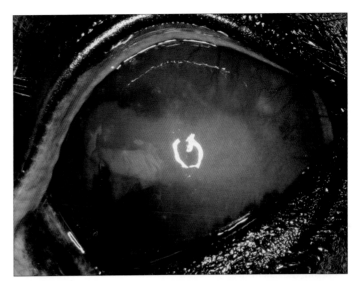

Figure 10.91 Chronic active recurrent immune-mediated keratitis with cellular infiltrate and fibrovascular reaction.

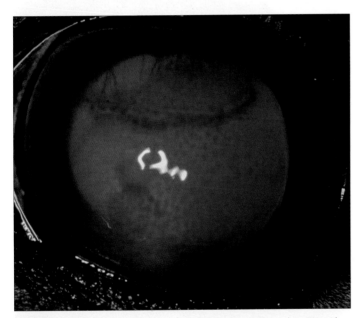

Figure 10.90 Endotheliitis with features of chronic deep recurrent keratitis, with edema and hydrops of the cornea as well as greenish lacunae and deep stromal neovascularization.

infiltrate, which occurs usually underneath the upper eyelid and occasionally underneath the third eyelid. There is moderate discomfort and the other eye may become affected in time. In the USA, there is an area of subepithelial yellow stromal infiltrate with superficial vascularization in the ventral paracentral cornea, occasionally in the ventral paralimbal region or centrally. There is no associated discomfort, and the condition typically waxes and wanes.

3) Midstromal immune-mediated keratitis in the UK is described as chronic recurrent keratitis, with a region of extensive mid to deep stromal edema and fibrovascular response. There is no discomfort unless subepithelial bullae form and result in superficial erosions. The condition recurs episodically. In the USA, a similar condition there is vascularization and cellular infiltrate present in the mid-stroma in the lateral paracentral, ventral or central cornea.

4) Endothelial immune-mediated keratitis presents similarly in the UK and the USA. It presents as diffuse opacity due to corneal edema and fibrocellular opacity of the ventral or ventrolateral cornea. It is non-painful but is slowly progressive. Bullous keratopathy may develop later with associated superficial corneal ulceration.

Diagnosis

- Diagnosis is made on the basis of the clinical signs, as described. The corneal opacity is present for several weeks, featuring cellular infiltrate, corneal vascularization and edema. There may be no or moderate discomfort. There is no uptake of fluorescein stain because the condition is non-ulcerative. There is no secondary uveitis.
- Corneal surface cytology and microbial culture and sensitivity are not carried out in every case, but when they are, no pathogen is identified.
- In more severe cases, a corneal biopsy might be indicated.
- One commonly employed diagnostic test is the response to treatment.

Treatment

- Treatment involves topical local immunosuppression and anti-inflammatory therapy. Epithelial keratopathy and endotheliitis are treated with topical steroids in the UK, and the response to treatment is usually very good. It is suggested that chronic superficial keratitis is treated with topical cyclosporine, while chronic deep keratitis is treated with a combination therapy of both topical cyclosporine and dexamethasone. These conditions should respond to treatment but will improve slowly, and recurrence is possible.
- In the USA, it is recommended that epithelial, superficial stromal and mid-stromal keratopathies are treated with topical neomycin, polymyxin and dexamethasone four times daily along with topical cyclosporine twice daily, gradually weaning first off the topical steroid and then reducing to once daily cyclosporine. Endotheliitis is considered difficult to treat in the USA with a poor prognosis, and similar treatment is used but a poorer prognosis is given. Topical bromfenac (a NSAID) has been used with some anecdotal reports of success in the USA.

Calcific keratopathy (Figs. 10.92 & 10.93)

Calcific keratopathy is also referred to as calcific band keratopathy because sometimes the opacity appears as a band due to its location in the interpalpebral fissure. It is a degenerative condition in which deposits of dystrophic calcium are laid down beneath the corneal epithelium. The condition may occur as a complication of severe and chronic equine recurrent uveitis. However there is a possibility that chronic topical steroid use, which might be prescribed because of chronic uveitis, may potentiate the condition.

Diagnosis

- Diagnosis is made based on direct observation of dense white gritty subepithelial corneal deposits.
- There may be variable multifocal regions of fluorescein uptake around these lesions as the calcium can disrupt the overlying epithelium, resulting in corneal ulceration. This can be quite painful, resulting in blepharospasm and epiphora.

Treatment

- Treatment involves manual debridement of any loose epithelium with a sterile cotton bud under topical anesthesia. Topical 1% sodium EDTA is applied in an attempt to reduce the tear film pH and chelate the calcium.

- The underlying uveitis should be controlled with systemic NSAIDs, along with topical NSAIDs and mydriatics.
- Topical antibiotics are indicated if there is corneal ulceration.
- Some cases benefit from surgical superficial keratectomy to shorten the course of disease. This removes the painful calcium deposits, which allows healing of the corneal ulceration.

Infectious disorders

Multifocal punctate keratopathy (viral keratitis) (Figs. 10.94–10.96)

Multifocal punctate keratopathy is not uncommon. In many cases, the cause is thought to be equine herpesvirus-2 (EHV-2). However it may be difficult to definitively identify an etiological agent, as there is a high seropositivity rate for EHV-2 among horses (90%). Affected horses present with varying degrees of ocular pain, and there is usually conjunctivitis. There is a variable degree of corneal edema, caused by epithelial disruption. There are multifocal corneal

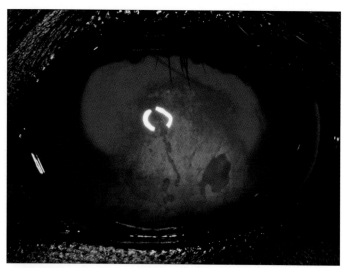

Figure 10.92 White subepithelial calcium deposits causing ulceration and ventral vascularization representing calcific keratopathy in a horse with equine recurrent uveitis (ERU).

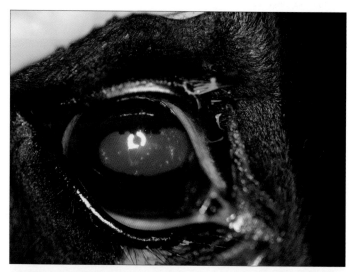

Figure 10.94 Superficial punctate keratitis with scattered multiple white fine linear opacities, presumed to be viral keratitis type I.

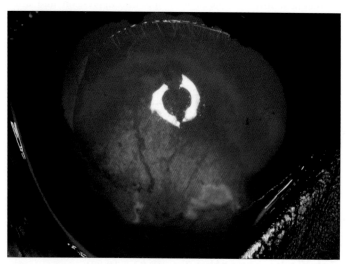

Figure 10.93 Fluorescein staining of calcific keratopathy shows irregular fluorescein uptake.

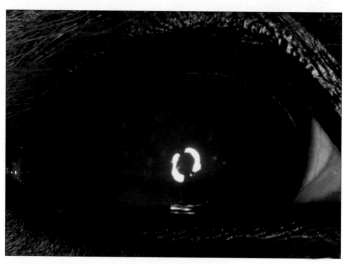

Figure 10.95 Superficial punctate keratitis with the pattern of viral keratitis type II, with multiple focal white superficial opacities and mild edema.

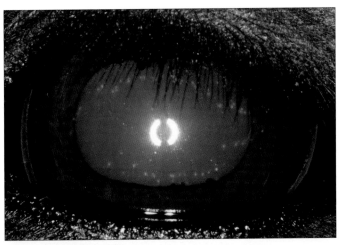

Figure 10.96 Superficial punctate keratitis with the pattern of viral keratitis type II, with multifocal white non-ulcerative superficial corneal opacities.

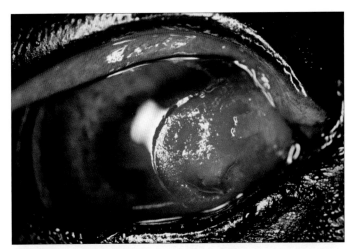

Figure 10.97 Corneal ulceration with a white irregular stippled appearance due to fungal keratitis. The differential diagnosis of eosinophilic keratitis can be distinguished with corneal cytology.

opacities, which are usually very superficial. Two forms of superficial keratopathy have been identified. Type I lesions are scattered white fine linear opacities. There may be fluorescein-positive fissures, which can coalesce to appear dendritic in shape. This form of the condition is not associated with corneal neovascularization. Type II lesions are multiple round fluorescein-positive pinpoint corneal opacities with surrounding focal corneal edema, and there may be corneal neovascularization.

Diagnosis

- Diagnosis is made based on clinical signs and examination. It also involves ruling out differential diagnosis.
- Fluorescein retention implies a full-thickness epithelial defect, which is ulceration.
- Rose Bengal dye can highlight even more superficial corneal epithelial damage as it can penetrate the ocular surface in regions where there are disruptions in the tear-film integrity or dysfunction in the production of tear-film components.
- **Differential diagnosis:** early keratomycosis (which might present with multifocal Rose Bengal uptake), immune-mediated keratitis, other causes of corneal ulceration, such as keratoconjunctivitis sicca, and corneal degeneration.
- Virus isolation and PCR have been used to try to identify the virus, but more commonly a rapid response to antiviral treatment is used as a confirmatory diagnostic test.

Treatment

- Topical antiviral medication is used as treatment; 1% idoxuridine or 1% trifluorothymidine are used but need to be applied frequently (4–6 times daily) because they are virostatic rather than virucidal.
- Topical NSAIDs are used also if the eye is painful. Topical antibiotics are used if there is fluorescein uptake until the epithelium heals. Recurrence is possible, and therefore the owners should be educated to monitor for the early signs of the condition so that prompt treatment can be implemented.

Fungal keratitis (keratomycosis)

(Figs. 10.97–10.103)

Fungal keratitis is much more common in temperate climates, but has also been diagnosed worldwide. The fungal organisms which most

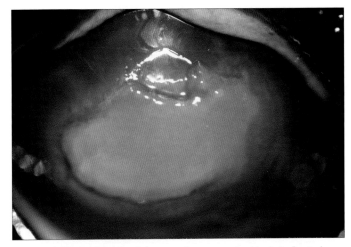

Figure 10.98 A defined fungal plaque on the cornea resembles 'cake frosting' with a granular appearance, surrounded by a furrowed rim.

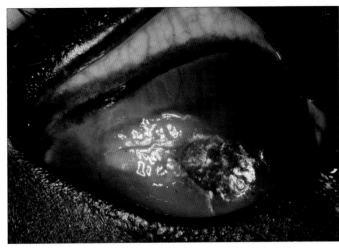

Figure 10.99 Deep corneal ulceration with neovascularization and a yellow necrotic plaque. Corneal scraping revealed fungal hyphae.

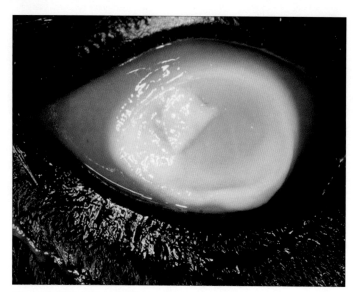

Figure 10.100 Deep stromal corneal ulceration with stromal cellular infiltration. The eye had been inappropriately treated with topical steroids.

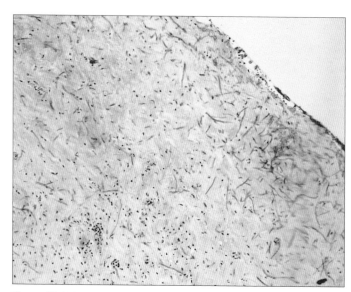

Figure 10.102 H&E section of a keratectomy sample shows a dense infiltration with fungal organisms, along with inflammatory cellular infiltration.

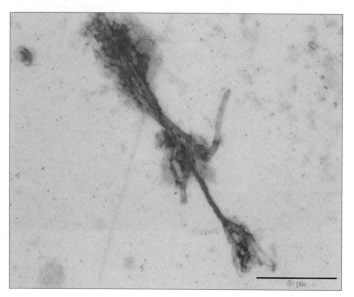

Figure 10.101 Corneal scraping from the previous eye, showing branching septate fungal hyphae.

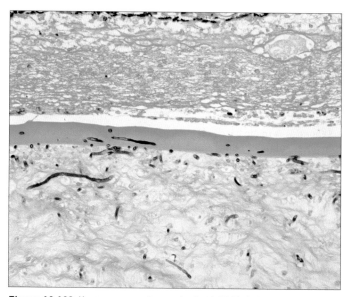

Figure 10.103 Keratectomy specimen stained with GMS which shows a tropism of the darkly stained fungal organisms for Descemet's membrane.

commonly affect the eye are *Fusarium* spp. and *Aspergillus* spp. There are various clinical manifestations and the clinical signs vary between those categories.

Superficial keratomycosis presents with punctate lesions of the epithelium and subepithelial stroma, likely as a result of microerosion, and this can result in superficial ulceration. More severe stromal keratomycosis presents with a plaque or deep stromal infiltration with ulceration, sometimes with a surrounding furrow. Stromal abscessation occurs when fungal or bacterial organisms get trapped beneath an intact epithelium (see below). Multiple superficial microerosions can progress to superficial corneal ulceration and this is very painful, with epiphora, blepharospasm and secondary uveitis. Within the superficial ulcer, a granular stippled white 'cake-frosting' appearance is considered a sign of fungal keratitis. Stromal fungal infection may result in a superficial or deeper plaque on the cornea. A trough or furrow may develop around the plaque, and this indicates that the surrounding stroma is being digested and is a negative prognostic

sign. Plaques surrounded by a furrow are best treated surgically with a conjunctival, corneal or amniotic membrane graft. The infected stroma may be a yellow color and the ulcer may progress to perforation and iris prolapse.

Accompanying uveitis is severe and the eye is normally very painful. Use of topical corticosteroids or over-use of topical antibiotics may predispose the eye towards keratomycosis.

Diagnosis

- Diagnosis is made on the characteristic clinical appearance, along with laboratory confirmation.
- The quickest and simplest diagnostic test is a corneal scrape from the edge of the lesion, and cytology with a Diff-Quik stain will show easily identifiable fungal hyphae if present.
- Fungal culture and PCR are useful also but the time required is prohibitive in most cases. A corneal biopsy or keratectomy sample may be evaluated, and the organisms have an affinity for Descemet's

membrane and are often found in greater numbers in the deeper corneal stroma.

Treatment and prognosis

- Treatment should be prompt and aggressive. It is directed at the fungal organisms but also at the uveitis.
- Topical antifungals used include natamycin, miconazole, itraconazole with DMSO, fluconazole, voriconazole, povidone iodine solution or silver sulfadiazine. These are administered every 2–4 hours but the initial fungal death will exacerbate the uveitis. Systemic NSAIDs are very important in the early stages.
- Topical mydriatics such as atropine are important to control the uveitis and to act as a cycloplegic.
- Broad-spectrum topical antibiotics are also required in most cases.
- Surgical treatment may be required to reduce the fungal burden, to repair a stromal deficit and to provide a blood supply.
- Severe cases may benefit from systemic antifungal treatment also, such as voriconazole, itraconazole or fluconazole.
- Treatment needs to be prolonged for several weeks.
- The prognosis depends on the stage of presentation and diagnosis and the use of appropriate treatment.

Stromal abscess (Figs. 10.104–10.106)

A corneal stromal abscess is a focus of inflammatory cells located within the corneal stroma, usually underneath an intact corneal epithelium. It is thought that focal trauma to the epithelium allows the introduction of microbes or foreign agents through micropunctures. The epithelium subsequently heals over the area, trapping the organism within the stroma. Due to the avascular and immune-privileged nature of the cornea, an infection can flourish. Abscesses may be bacterial (for example due to *Staphylococcus* spp. or *Streptococcus* spp.), fungal (for example *Aspergillus* spp. or *Fusarium* spp.) or sterile, with no infectious agent identifiable. There is an increased incidence of stromal abscessation in horses with keratomycosis.

Diagnosis

- The abscess is normally recognizable as a dense yellow to white stromal opacity, often with a feathery appearance at the edge of the opacity. There is variable corneal vascularization towards the lesion, and some fungi have antiangiogenic properties. The eye is usually very painful, with blepharospasm and epiphora. Anterior uveitis might be present, manifested as hypopyon, aqueous flare and miosis.
- There is commonly no fluorescein uptake over the lesion.

- Confirmation of the diagnosis with a corneal scraping and culture may be hampered by the deep location within the corneal stroma underneath an intact corneal epithelium.

Treatment and prognosis

- Aggressive medical treatment is indicated and involves the use of topical and systemic antibiotics, topical mydriatics and systemic NSAIDs. Treatment is facilitated by the placement of a subpalpebral ocular lavage catheter.
- Topical antifungal medications are indicated in regions where mycotic infection is common. Topical medications that can penetrate an intact epithelium are necessary, and chloramphenicol and some fluoroquinolones have superior biphasic solubility.
- Debridement of the overlying epithelium will aid penetration of the medications to reach the target area.
- Surgical treatment may be necessary if the lesion does not improve with medical treatment. Ideally the diseased area is targeted and only this area is surgically removed, being replaced with healthy corneal tissue or a substitute. This may be achieved with a targeted

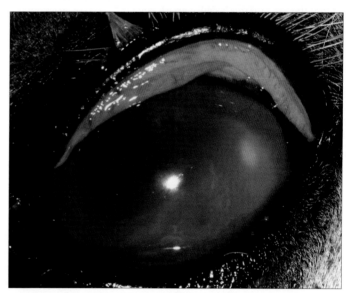

Figure 10.105 A small yellow corneal stromal abscess present laterally has caused vascular keratitis along with corneal edema, fibrin in the anterior chamber and miosis.

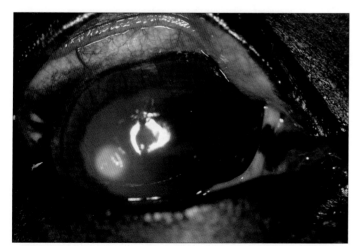

Figure 10.104 A focal yellow stromal abscess with corneal neovascularization not reaching the region, likely due to antiangiogenic factors released by the fungal organisms. Conjunctivitis and miosis are present.

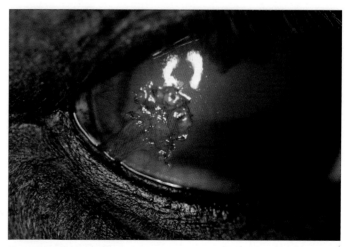

Figure 10.106 A conjunctival pedicle graft has been placed after a keratectomy for a corneal stromal abscess.

lamellar keratoplasty; either a posterior lamellar keratoplasty or a deep lamellar endothelial keratoplasty. The surgical techniques are reviewed in detail elsewhere (Brooks 2010).

- At the time of surgery, culture specimens and biopsy samples for histopathology are obtained. On histopathology, fungal hyphae are often found next to Descemet's membrane, and they seem to display a tropism towards this location.
- Depending on the stage at presentation and the treatment approach used, the prognosis for vision is guarded, and in a few cases, enucleation is required.

Part 4 Uvea

Congenital/developmental conditions

Iris coloboma (Figs. 10.107 & 10.108)

Aniridia is the congenital complete absence of the iris, and it is very rare. It has been reported in the Quarterhorse and in the Belgian horse. Slightly more commonly, a focal full-thickness hole occurs within the iris, and this is called an iris coloboma. A typical coloboma is one that arises in the area of the embryonic optic fissure, which is ventral or slightly ventro-nasal, whereas an atypical coloboma occurs in any other position. One or both eyes may be affected.

Diagnosis, treatment and prognosis

- Diagnosis is made through visual observation.
- They have no pathological significance, although technically the affected animal may be more photophobic because of the increased passage of light to the retina.
- No treatment is required.

Iris hypoplasia ('iris stromal cysts')
(Figs. 10.109–10.111)

Congenital thinning of the iris may be most easily observed in eyes with a blue iris. It is commonly observed in the Welsh pony in the UK. They are most commonly located within the dorsal iris, which appears to bulge forwards towards the cornea. The curvature changes when the pupil dilates, and the area appears more wrinkled. They used to be referred to as anterior uveal cysts but are now more correctly termed regional iris hypoplasia. The tapetal reflection might be observed through the thin iris. The area may otherwise appear dark, making iris melanoma an important differential diagnosis. The condition has no pathological consequences and no treatment is needed.

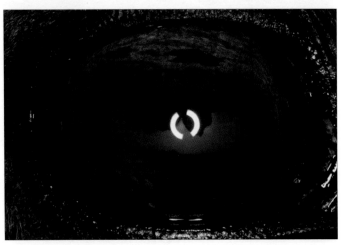

Figure 10.107 Congenital iris coloboma at the seven o'clock position with a full-thickness hole through the iris tissue.

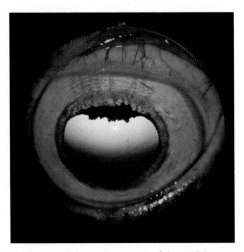

Figure 10.109 Thinning of the pupillary margin of the pupil due to iris hypoplasia in a subalbinotic eye; the tapetal reflection can be seen through the thin region.

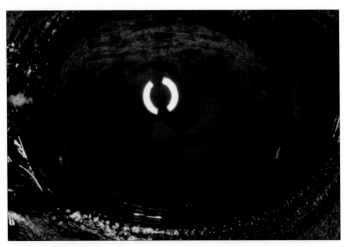

Figure 10.108 Left eye of the same pony as in Fig. 10.107 with a similar iris coloboma.

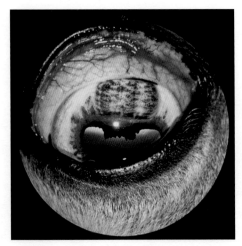

Figure 10.110 The dorsal iris appears focally darker and is bulging forward due to iris hypoplasia in a typical position.

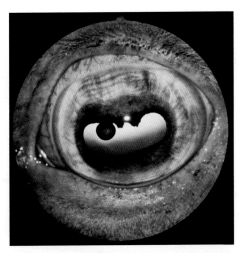

Figure 10.111 The pupillary margin of the iris is thin and the dorsal aspect appears darker because it is bulging forwards due to iris hypoplasia. There is also uveal cyst associated with the superior granulairidica.

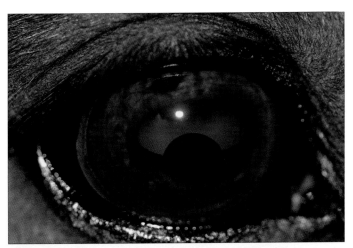

Figure 10.112 A dark iris cyst associated with the granulairidica remains attached at the ventral pupillary margin.

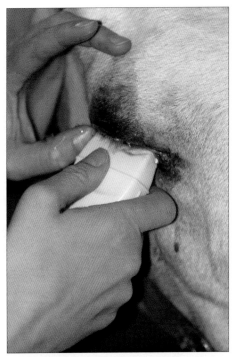

Figure 10.113 The ultrasound transducer is placed directly on the cornea after application of topical anesthesia, or the eye may be scanned through closed eyelids.

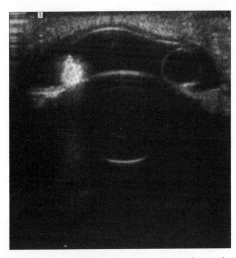

Figure 10.114 With B-mode ultasound, iris cysts show as hyperechoic circular lesions with a dark fluid-filled center, as on the right of this photo. The dense granula iridica shows up as a dense white hyperechoic lesion on this image, to the left. Courtesy of Kim Hughes.

Anterior uveal cysts/cystic corpora nigra
(Figs. 10.112–10.114)

Anterior uveal cysts may involve hyperplastic corpora nigra, or arise from the posterior iris epithelium and appear at the pupil margin or be free-floating in the anterior chamber. There is no known cause for the condition. Anterior uveal cysts may also occur as part of the multiple congenital ocular anomaly syndrome which can occur in the Rocky Mountain horse. They are dark, smooth-edged, spherical masses, often remaining attached at the pupil margin. The number and size of cysts varies greatly.

Diagnosis and treatment
- Diagnosis is normally easily made on the characteristic clinical appearance alone.
- *Differential diagnosis:* melanoma or inflammatory masses. If the distinction is not clear, ocular B-mode ultrasound will clearly show whether the mass is fluid-filled, as expected with a cyst, or a solid structure.
- Small cysts are of no consequence. However, if the cysts are large and obscure the visual axis, they may cause significant visual disturbance manifesting in head shaking or spooking.

- The use of semiconductor diode laser for deflation and coagulation of anterior uveal cysts in horses has been reported (Gemensky-Metzler et al 2004, Gilger et al 1997).

Non-infectious/infectious disorders

Equine recurrent uveitis (Figs. 10.115–10.121)

Equine recurrent uveitis (ERU) is also known as moon blindness, periodic ophthalmia and iridocyclitis. It is reported to be the most common cause of equine blindness worldwide. It is a more common condition in the USA (prevalence 2–25%) and in Europe (prevalence 8–10%)

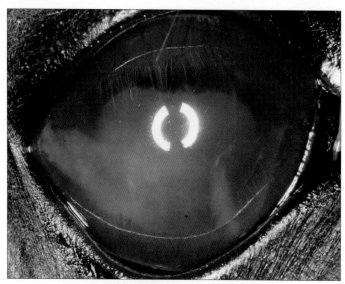

Figure 10.115 A draft horse with bilateral ERU presents with a flare up of uveitis, with corneal neovascularization, fibrin in the ventral anterior chamber and aqueous flare.

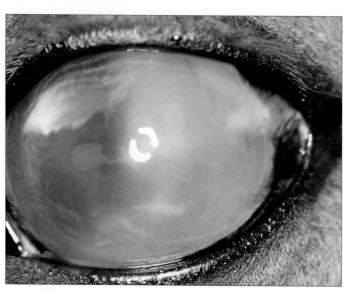

Figure 10.118 Chronic ERU has led to corneal opacity due to fibrosis and miosis is present.

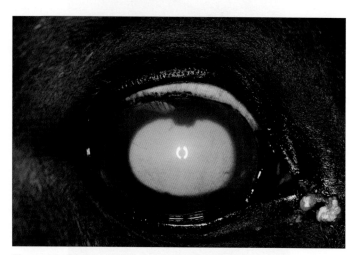

Figure 10.116 Chronic ERU with corneal edema and cellular deposits on the corneal endothelium, along with atrophy of the corpora nigra.

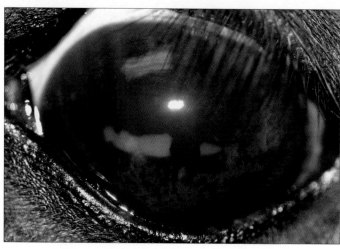

Figure 10.119 Subepithelial calcification may occur with ERU, and miosis is also present.

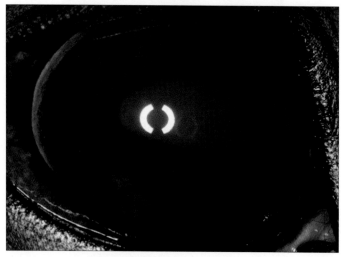

Figure 10.117 Atrophy of the granulairidica in a horse in a quiescent stage between bouts of ERU.

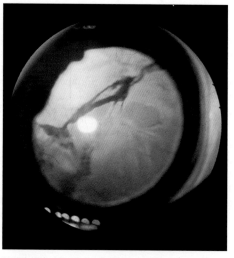

Figure 10.120 Chronic inflammatory debris in the vitreous is common in horses with ERU.

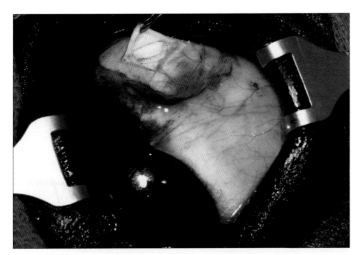

Figure 10.121 Insertion of a suprachoroidal cyclosporine implant in a case of ERU.

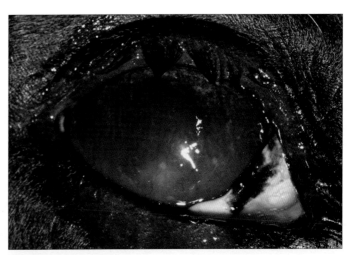

Figure 10.122 Sore eye with epiphora, corneal vascularization and intense miosis due to uveitis.

than it is in the UK (prevalence <1%). This regional variation is likely to be due to both genetic factors and environmental factors such as the presence of causative infectious organisms. ERU is characterized by recurrent episodic bouts of intraocular inflammation, with intervening apparent periods of remission. This is in contrast to an acute, single bout of inflammation as occurs with acute anterior uveitis.

ERU has multiple etiologies, which include infectious and immune-mediated causes. *Leptospira* spp. and all of the causes of anterior uveitis listed above have been implicated as inciting causes. After the initial inflammation, immune mechanisms can trigger future inflammation. The role that *Leptospira* plays in perpetuating inflammation is poorly understood. *Leptospira* microbial peptides have been shown to have antigenic homology with potentially uveitogenic intraocular autoantigens and MHC Class I peptides. The initial inflammation may cause loss of local ocular immune tolerance, allowing for cross-reaction between the leptospiral organism and autoantigens. A genetic predisposition has been demonstrated, with German Warmblood horses expressing the MHC haplotype ELA-A9 shown to be more susceptible to developing ERU. Appaloosa horses are more susceptible to developing ERU, and are affected with a severe type of ERU, which is poorly responsive to treatment.

Diagnosis

- Clinical signs need to have been present at least once in the past for the condition to be classified as recurrent. It is unilateral in approximately 50% of horses, although it is bilateral in up to 80% of Appaloosa horses.
- In the active phase there are similar clinical signs to acute anterior uveitis outlined above. The eye might not be obviously painful. There may be conjunctival hyperemia, corneal edema and peripheral vascularization, aqueous flare, miosis, a dark iris, posterior synechia, atrophy of the corpora nigra, iris pigment on the anterior lens capsule, cortical cataracts, yellowing of the vitreous, chorioretinitis and exudative retinal detachments.
- Fundus changes visible in the quiescent phases can include peripapillary retinal degeneration in a butterfly pattern and single or multiple chorioretinal 'bullet-hole' lesions. However these retinal changes can be present in eyes with no evidence of previous inflammation, and they are not pathognomonic for ERU.
- Depending on the geographical location and other systemic clinical signs, it may be appropriate to undertake diagnostic tests including complete blood count, biochemistry, urinalysis and serology for

local prevalent serovars of *Leptospira* along with *Brucella* and *Toxoplasma*. A veterinary ophthalmologist may elect to take a sample of aqueous for testing to compare the systemic levels with those within the eye to further support the etiology of inflammation.

Treatment

- Symptomatic medical therapy is given to control the inflammation with systemic and topical corticosteroids or NSAIDs. Topical mydriatics are often used. Systemic antibiotics are administered if an infectious cause is found or suspected.
- It is very important to treat the eye until all signs have abated, and to continue treatment at a reduced level for several weeks afterwards.
- Surgical treatment may be appropriate. Pars plana vitrectomy has been shown to reduce the recurrence of inflammation in horses with vitreal opacity and those that have positive leptospiral titers in the vitreous. The technique involves surgically removing the visibly turbid vitreous by aspiration through a small scleral incision, while simultaneous irrigation through a separate scleral incision keeps the fluid volume constant. The highest success rates have been reported in Europe with this treatment.
- A sustained-release cyclosporine implant has been developed and studies have concluded that it is beneficial at controlling the signs of ERU in many horses. The implant is surgically inserted under the sclera onto the choroid, and therapeutic levels can be absorbed by the eye for up to 3 years. This has resulted in a decreased frequency of recurring bouts of inflammation, and a decreased amount of medication required to manage the inflammation.

Anterior uveitis (Figs. 10.122–10.130)

Anterior uveitis is inflammation of the iris (iritis), or of the iris and ciliary body (iridocyclitis). Acute anterior uveitis must be distinguished from chronic recurring uveitis (ERU). While the clinical signs may be similar, the prognosis is very different for the two conditions. Uveitis is due to damage to the anterior uvea, which results in a breakdown of the blood–ocular barrier. Induced inflammatory mediators increase vascular permeability and attract inflammatory cells to the region. This allows for leakage of the inflammatory cells, protein and fibrin into the aqueous humor.

Acute anterior uveitis may arise due to a number of causes. These include systemic infections and non-infectious causes such as trauma, neoplasia, lens-induced uveitis or idiopathic disease.

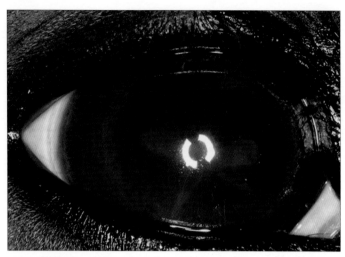

Figure 10.123 Fibrin and hemorrhage in the anterior chamber with miosis and yellowing of the vitreous due to uveitis.

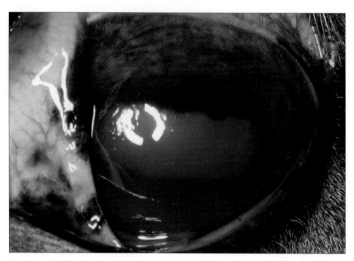

Figure 10.126 Conjunctival hyperemia, aqueous flare, hypopyon and miosis in an eye with uveitis.

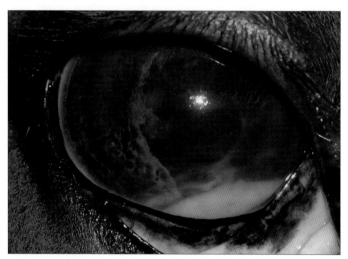

Figure 10.124 White inflammatory cells in the ventral aspect of the anterior chamber representing hypopyon, along with miosis in an eye with uveitis.

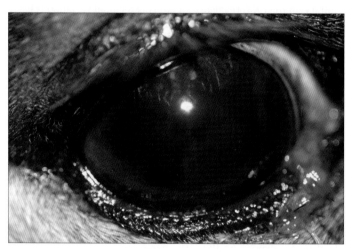

Figure 10.127 Hemorrhage in the anterior chamber (hyphema) and miosis in an eye with uveitis.

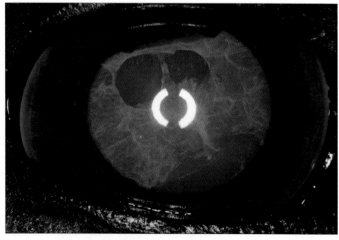

Figure 10.125 A meshwork of fibrin spans the pupil in an eye with uveitis. The pupil has been pharmacologically dilated.

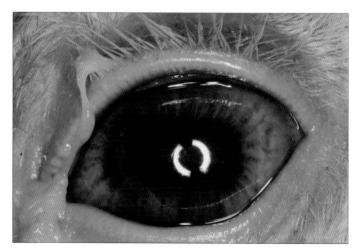

Figure 10.128 Mucoid ocular discharge, yellowing of the iris and hyperemia of the iris in a foal with uveitis which had a blue iris prior to inflammation.

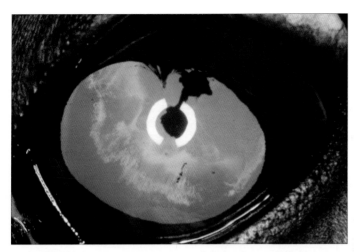

Figure 10.129 Sequels to traumatic uveitis include detachment of the corpora nigra and inflammatory material in the vitreous, in this case resting on the posterior lens capsule.

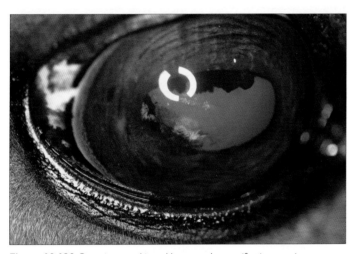

Figure 10.130 Posterior synechia and lens capsular opacification remain permanently after uveitis due to corneal trauma in this horse.

Bacterial causes include infection with *Rhodococcus equi*, *Streptococcus* spp., *Leptospiras* spp., *Escherichia coli* and *Brucella* spp. Viral causes include EHV-1, equine influenza virus, equine viral arteritis and equine infectious anemia virus. Other implicated agents include *Borrelia*, *Onchocerca*, *Toxoplasma* and strongyles.

Clinical signs of anterior uveitis can vary with the degree of inflammation present. The eye is usually uncomfortable, with blepharospasm and epiphora. There is conjunctival hyperemia. The cornea is usually mildly edematous and may have some peripheral deep neovascularization. The anterior chamber may appear cloudy due to aqueous flare (leakage of protein) or due to a cellular infiltrate, which can settle at the bottom of the anterior chamber as hypopyon. The anterior chamber may also contain fibrin or blood (hyphema). The pupil may be very constricted to a horizontal slit. It may be difficult to view the posterior segment because of this and because of the corneal and anterior chamber opacity.

Diagnosis

- Clinical signs and ocular examination are diagnostic.
- Tonometry reveals a low intraocular pressure typically, although uncontrolled uveitis can lead to a raised intraocular pressure and glaucoma. Fluorescein staining of the cornea is recommended to

determine whether topical corticosteroids can be safely used for treatment. A range of diagnostic tests may be indicated, including complete blood count, biochemistry, urinalysis and serology for specific infectious agents. At the later stages, there may be posterior synechia, pigment on the anterior lens capsule, a darkening of the iris and cortical cataracts. Uncontrolled uveitis can lead to secondary glaucoma or phthisis bulbi.

Treatment

- Symptomatic medical treatment is indicated to control the inflammation associated with uveitis. This includes prescribing both topical and systemic corticosteroids or NSAIDs.
- Topical mydriatics are indicated to stabilize the blood–ocular barrier, reduce the painful spasm of the iridal musculature, and dilate the pupil, reducing the risk of synechia. Atropine 1% is commonly used, and may be available as a drop or an ointment. The effect of atropine lasts up to 14 days in a non-inflamed eye, but in an eye with uveitis, it may need to be applied up to four times daily.
- Topical atropine may be absorbed systemically, especially when the eye is inflamed. It can reduce intestinal motility, and therefore the owner should be warned to monitor for signs of colic.
- A horse with a pharmacologically dilated pupil should be protected from bright light, as they will be unable to constrict the pupil to protect the retina. Once pupil dilation is achieved, the frequency is reduced to effect, which may be once daily or once every second day.
- Tropicamide 1% is an alternative mydriatic; it is shorter-acting and it is most often used to dilate the pupil of a normal eye for examination purposes, and is not as powerful as atropine when uveitis is present. Topical phenylephrine 10% will not cause pupil dilation when used alone, but it may improve the mydriatic effect of atropine when used in combination.
- If a specific cause of the uveitis can be found, for example *Rhodococcus equi* infection in a foal, the appropriate systemic medication is also administered. Treatment needs to be intensive and the animal needs frequent examinations until the inflammation is under control. Undesirable sequelae of poorly controlled inflammation include cataract formation, posterior synechia, glaucoma, endophthalmitis, phthisis bulbi or relapse of inflammation after apparent initial resolution, which may represent ERU.
- Cases with fibrin in the anterior chamber may benefit from an intracameral injection of 25 µg of tissue plasminogen activator, which can dissolve the fibrin. This procedure is usually carried out by an ophthalmologist.

Prognosis

- The prognosis is good for cases in which the inciting cause can be identified and treated but is guarded for cases in which the cause cannot be identified and there is a poor response to therapy.
- Undesirable sequelae of poorly controlled inflammation include cataract formation, posterior synechia, glaucoma, endophthalmitis, phthisis bulbi or relapse of inflammation after apparent initial resolution, which may represent ERU.

Neoplasia

Intraocular melanoma (Figs. 10.131–10.137)

Tumors of the uveal tract are not common, but the most common intraocular tumor is a melanoma of the iris. They may arise in horses of any age, whereas cutaneous melanomas tend to occur in older horses. They are more common in gray horses. They are most commonly benign, but are slow-growing and can lead to glaucoma. The main differential is iris nevi, which are benign foci of pigmentation. It is possible that iris nevi could change with time and give rise to melanomas. Metastasis is very uncommon.

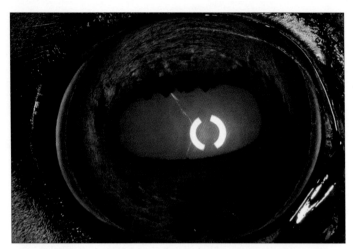

Figure 10.131 Melanosis of the iris is very common, where focal or multifocal regions appear more darkly pigmented. The iris surface is regular and not thickened.

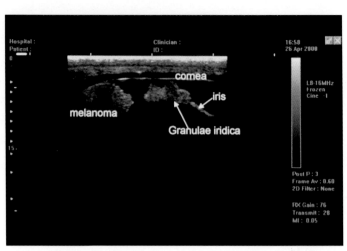

Figure 10.134 B-mode ultrasonography is useful to determine the extent of the mass and to distinguish from iris cysts. The white hyperechoic melanoma is visible to the left of the picture.

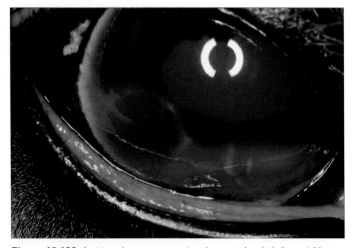

Figure 10.132 An iris melanoma rests against the corneal endothelium, visible as a dark opacity. There is also keratitis.

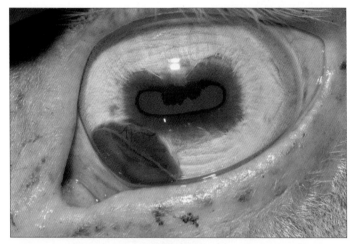

Figure 10.135 A liver-colored melanoma with surface vascularization arises from the iris and occupies the anterior chamber. Courtesy of Prof Sheila Crispin.

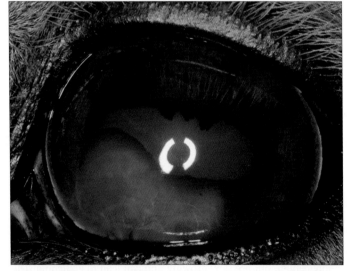

Figure 10.133 There are three iris melanomas in this eye; a darkly pigmented lesion at the 10–11 o'clock position on the iris, a discolored lesion at the 1–2 o'clock position on the iris, and ventrally a third melanoma rests against the corneal endothelium causing a white opacity.

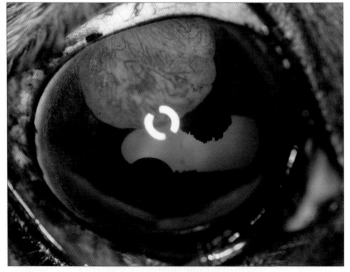

Figure 10.136 A pink vascularized mass occupies the superior anterior chamber. An incidental iris cyst is present. Retinoblastoma was diagnosed on histopathology.

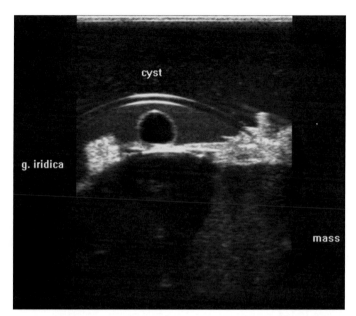

Figure 10.137 The extent of the mass featured in Fig. 10.136 was apparent on B-mode ultrasonography, where it was seen to occupy a significant portion of the vitreous chamber.

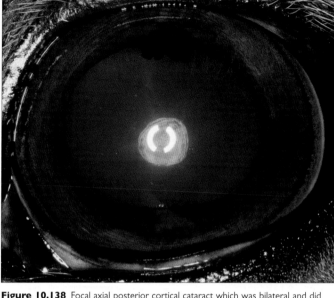

Figure 10.138 Focal axial posterior cortical cataract which was bilateral and did not progress.

Diagnosis

- The diagnosis is made by observing the presence of the melanoma in the eye. The affected eye is most often comfortable and visual. The melanoma appears as a dark swelling on the iris, occupying the anterior chamber. There may be corneal edema on the overlying cornea if there is physical contact of the mass with the corneal endothelium. More than one melanoma may be present.
- As the mass slowly enlarges, it may lead to secondary glaucoma with ocular discomfort, more diffuse corneal edema, distortion of the iris and aqueous flare.
- An ocular ultrasound is indicated as the mass may also involve the ciliary body and extend posteriorly into the vitreous.
- The intraocular pressure should be measured with tonometry, and monitored periodically.

Treatment

- Most often, no treatment is given but the mass is kept under surveillance. In some circumstances where there is a discrete well-defined melanoma affecting the iris, it might be surgically removed with a sector iridectomy.
- Laser treatment has been used to reduce the size of the mass.
- If there is secondary glaucoma, enucleation is advisable.

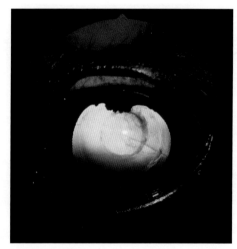

Figure 10.139 Nuclear cataract with a perinuclear halo.

Part 5 Lens and glaucoma

Congenital/developmental conditions

Cataracts (Figs. 10.138–10.153)

A cataract is an opacity of the lens or its capsule. They may be congenital or acquired. Eyes with congenital cataracts may have a range of other accompanying abnormalities, including microphthalmia (see above), persistent pupillary membranes, persistent hyaloid vasculature, microphakia (a congenitally small lens), lens coloboma (a mis-shapen lens with a peripheral section 'missing') and lenticonus (a bulging of the lens capsule and the underlying cortex). Most commonly, cataracts are associated with uveitis or trauma in horses, but they could also be hereditary, senile or due to metabolic disease or

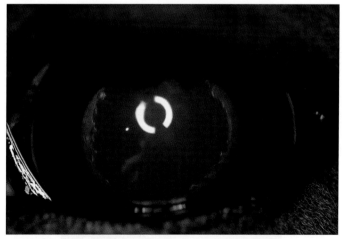

Figure 10.140 Peripheral equatorial cataract, which could easily be missed without mydriasis.

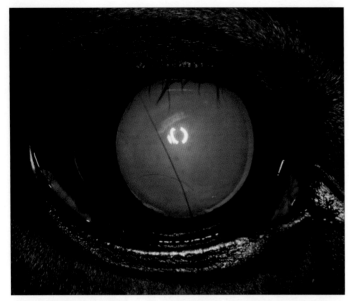

Figure 10.141 Congenital mature cataract which was present bilaterally in a Clydesdale foal. Note the clear periequatorial cortex.

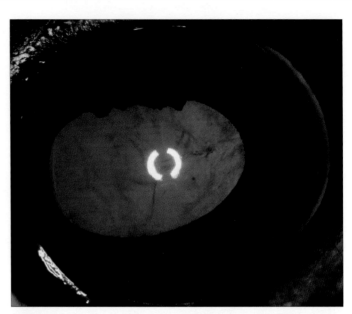

Figure 10.144 Immature cataract with opacity of the cortex and nucleus; the anterior suture lines are visible.

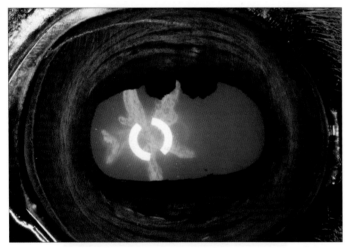

Figure 10.142 Floriform developmental cataract in the posterior perinuclear cortex.

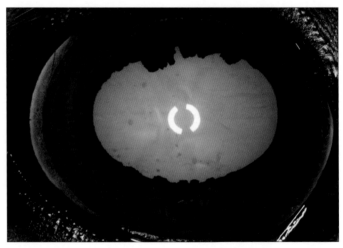

Figure 10.145 Mature cataract involving the lens cortex and nucleus.

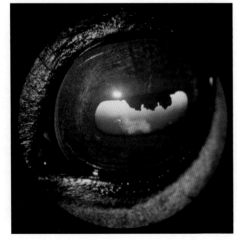

Figure 10.143 Focal anterior cortical cataract (these may be progressive).

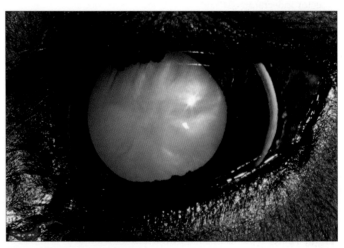

Figure 10.146 Chronic mature cataract.

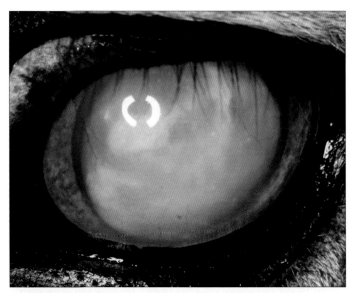

Figure 10.147 Hypermature cataract, which is beginning to luxate anteriorly, with keratitis.

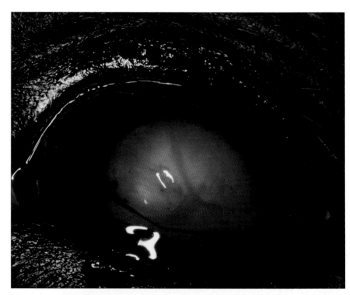

Figure 10.150 Severe blunt ocular trauma has resulted in rupture of the anteior lens capsule in a foal, with iris pigmentation on the ruptured lens capsule.

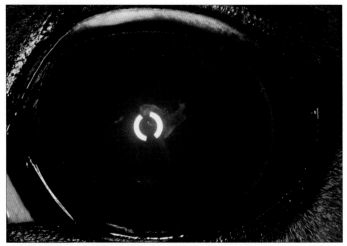

Figure 10.148 Whip-lash type opacity with trauma resulting in opacity of the posterior lens sutures, appearing Y-shaped.

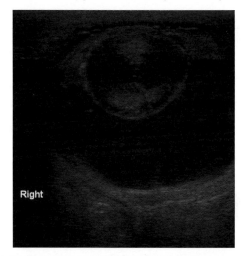

Figure 10.151 The lens is very amenable to ultrasound. There is a smaller anterior cortical opacity and a larger posterior capsular opacity.

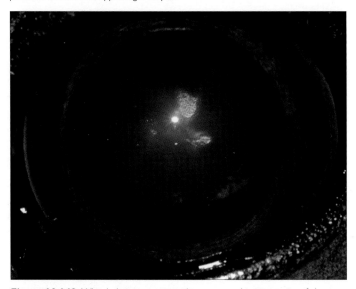

Figure 10.149 Whip-lash type opacity with trauma resulting in opacity of the posterior lens sutures, appearing tri-radiate.

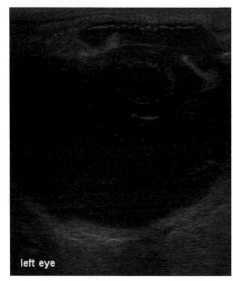

Figure 10.152 A perinuclear opacity is visible on B-mode ultrasound.

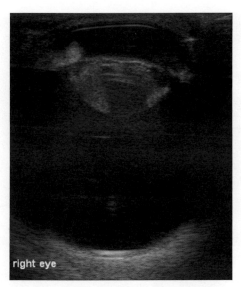

Figure 10.153 A mature cataract is seen on B-mode ultrasound.

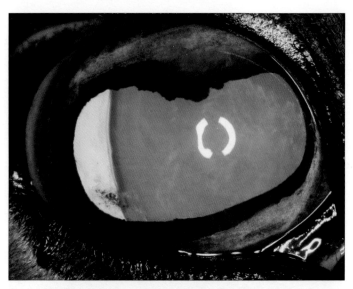

Figure 10.154 Lens luxation with a total cataract. The dorsal edge of the lens is visible through the pupil along with a tapetal reflection above the lens.

systemic toxins. Cataracts may remain static and not change with time (commonly nuclear and posterior cataracts) or may progress (commonly cataracts associated with uveitis or anterior cortical cataracts).

Diagnosis

- The diagnosis of a cataract is made on the observation of an opacity of or within the lens. A useful technique is distant direct ophthalmoscopy, when the tapetal reflection is used to highlight opacities in the visual pathway, and they appear as a dark shadow. Direct observation with illumination and magnification is also used. To observe the entire lens, the pupil should be pharmacologically dilated with tropicamide, and observed 20–30 minutes later.
- Cataracts are classified a number of ways, including by the degree of opacity (incipient, immature, mature or hypermature), the age of onset (congenital, juvenile, senile), location (anterior, posterior, perinuclear, nuclear or equatorial, and capsular, subcapsular or cortical) and cause (traumatic, inflammatory, toxic, metabolic).
- Depending on the location (central or peripheral) and extent of opacity, cataracts may have little effect on vision or may cause blindness.

Treatment

- Not all cataracts require treatment, and continued observation is recommended. However, if there is visual impairment or progression, treatment is indicated. If inflammation is present, this is controlled with topical and systemic steroids or NSAIDs. However, the only method of improving or restoring vision is by the surgical removal of the cataract. This is achieved with phacoemulsification.
- Not every cataract is suitable for this procedure, and the horse should be referred to a veterinary ophthalmologist for assessment, which will include an ocular ultrasound and electroretinography. Other pre-existing accompanying ocular disorders, such as retinal detachment or congenital stationary night blindness, would imply that there would be insufficient improvement in vision despite successful cataract removal. Surgery is avoided in such cases.
- Foals may be considered for surgery once they are halter broken. Surgery is not delayed as the cataracts may not be suitable for surgery at a later age due to the development of complications such as lens-induced uveitis. Some surgeons will operate on both eyes of a foal during one surgery.

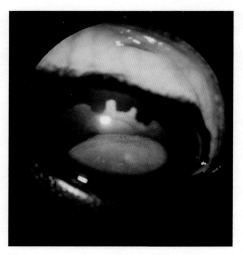

Figure 10.155 Lens luxation with a total cataract. The dorsal edge of the lens is visible through the pupil along with the fundus; there is retinal detachment around the optic nerve.

- A smaller intraocular lens is available for foals. If the eye is found to be otherwise suitable, but a vitreal opacity is present, a vitrectomy will need to be planned during the surgical procedure. Intraocular lenses have now been developed for horses, and allow for improved quality of vision after surgery.
- There are several complications that can arise after surgery, including hyphema, glaucoma, uveitis, retinal detachment, corneal ulceration and intraocular infection.
- Expert surgery along with prolonged post-operative medication and regular monitoring reduce the likelihood of these undesirable complications.

Non-infectious disorders

Lens luxation (Figs. 10.154–10.157)

Lens luxation and lens subluxation occur when the lens dislocates from its normal position within the patellar fossa. It might arise because of congenital abnormalities of the supporting lens zonules, or more commonly secondary to chronic uveitis, glaucoma or blunt ocular trauma. Lens subluxation presents with the dorsal equator of

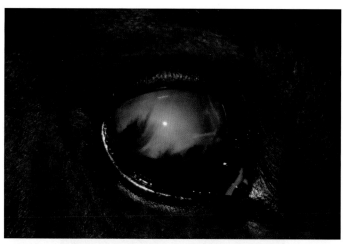

Figure 10.156 Corneal fibrosis and pigmentation with mydriasis. The diagnosis is not clear due to the corneal opacity and ocular ultrasound is indicated. Courtesy of Kim Hughes.

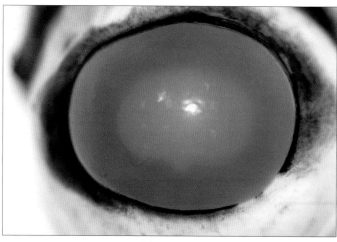

Figure 10.158 Corneal edema and mid-range mydriasis were the only obvious clinical signs of glaucoma in this eye. The intraocular pressure was high.

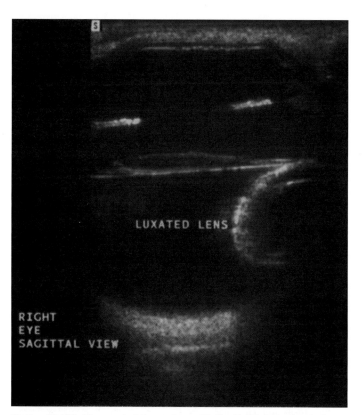

Figure 10.157 Ultrasound of the eye featured in Fig. 10.156 shows that the lens is completely luxated and situated eccentrically in the vitreous chamber. Courtesy of Kim Hughes.

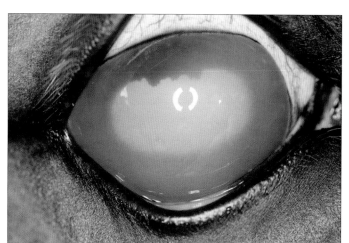

Figure 10.159 Pancorneal edema, some multifocal endothelial depositis and mid-range mydriasis in an eye with a high intraocular pressure and glaucoma.

the lens visible as the lens has slipped ventrally, exposing some stretched lens zonules. An aphakic crescent is visible where a crescent-shaped bright tapetal reflection is seen between the iris margin and a subluxated lens. Total lens luxation involves dislocation of the entire lens into the vitreous chamber. Anterior lens luxation into the anterior chamber is less common. Initially the lens is clear but invariably a total cataract develops. There may be ocular discomfort manifested as blepharospasm and epiphora, and there may be conjunctival hyperemia or corneal edema. The intraocular pressure should be measured, as lens luxation can be a cause or effect of glaucoma. The main differential diagnosis for lens subluxation is sector lens coloboma, where a peripheral portion of the lens is congenitally missing and the lens zonules may be seen within the aphakic crescent.

Treatment

If glaucoma or uveitis is present and causing the lens luxation, these underlying conditions should be medically controlled. Lens luxation surgery is a challenging undertaking. However, despite previous reports of poor success, with careful surgical technique and the increasing availability of phacoemulsification and vitrectomy, some cases without glaucoma or uveitis are now considered suitable for surgery. The prognosis however is guarded.

Glaucoma (Figs. 10.158–10.161)

Glaucoma is a group of ocular diseases that result in the increase of intraocular pressure (IOP) above a threshold in which the retinal ganglion cells and optic nerve can function normally. Normal intraocular pressure in a horse is 15–30 mmHg, and this is measured using tonometry. There are several causes of glaucoma, and it can be congenital, primary or secondary. Secondary glaucoma is by far the most common type. Possible causes include uveitis, ERU, hyphema, lens luxation, neoplasia of the iris or ciliary body, or intraocular surgery.

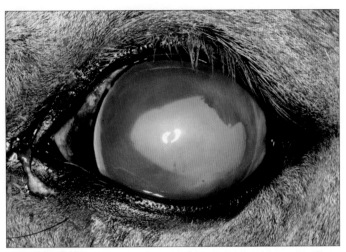

Figure 10.160 Chronic glaucoma with corneal edema and a dilated and distorted pupil.

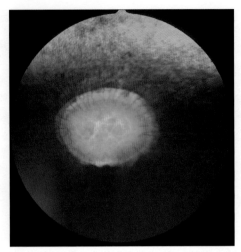

Figure 10.162 Fundus photo of a normal horse. Courtesy of Andy Matthews.

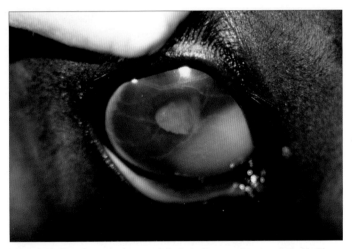

Figure 10.161 Corneal edema medially, linear keratopathy representing Haab's striae and a cataractous luxated lens in an eye with chronic glaucoma secondary to ERU.

Risk factors that have been found include the Appaloosa breed, increasing age, and the presence of current or previous uveitis.

Diagnosis
- Diagnosis is made by observing clinical signs of glaucoma, and is confirmed by tonometry.
- Typical clinical signs include moderate ocular discomfort, reduced vision, afferent PLR deficits, generalized corneal edema, corneal linear band opacities, slight mydriasis, iridocyclitis and optic nerve atrophy or cupping.
- The clinical signs depend on the length of time the pressure has been raised and on the degree of elevated pressure.
- Corneal edema may be the most consistent clinical sign associated with glaucoma.

Treatment and prognosis
- Both medical and surgical treatments are available for glaucoma in horses. Medical treatment is undertaken most commonly. If uveitis is present, every attempt is made to control the inflammation, which may in turn reduce the IOP.

- Anti-inflammatory therapy includes the use of both topical and systemic steroids or NSAIDs.
- Topical atropine is useful for the control of uveitis, and has been found in many cases to reduce IOP. However, it does occasionally cause IOP spikes, so the eye needs to be monitored carefully if atropine is prescribed.
- Topical glaucoma drops are also used. However, many of them have not been studied in horses with glaucoma. The topical β-adrenergic blocker timolol maleate 0.5% has been shown to reduce the IOP of normal horses when administered twice daily. Topical carbonic anhydrase inhibitors dorzolamide 2% and brinzolamide 1% have been shown to reduce the IOP of normal horses when administered twice daily.
- Combination therapy of timolol maleate and dorzolamide ('Cosopt', Merck) is often used.
- Topical prostaglandin analogs are very effective at reducing the IOP of humans with glaucoma, but because the horse often has an inflammatory aspect to the glaucoma, it may exacerbate uveitis and actually cause increased IOP along with ocular discomfort. For this reason, the topical prostaglandin analogs are best avoided in horses.
- Surgical treatment might be considered in combination with medical treatment. Destruction of the ciliary body, which makes the aqueous humor, reduces the IOP by reducing the volume of aqueous produced. Contact trans-scleral laser cyclophotocoagulation using Nd:YAG or diode laser has been shown to cause a decrease in IOP which can be sustained and can therefore result in preservation of vision. Medical treatment is continued after treatment and gradually withdrawn. On-going monitoring is required.
- The prognosis remains guarded, especially in the Appaloosa breed. If the IOP cannot be controlled, enucleation is indicated.

Part 6 Posterior segment

Normal ocular fundus and variations of normal

The fundus of the horse (Figs. 10.162 & 10.163) is very amenable to examination using direct or indirect ophthalmoscopy. Examination of the fundus is required in horses with eye problems, but is also an essential part of the pre-purchase examination. Pharmacological

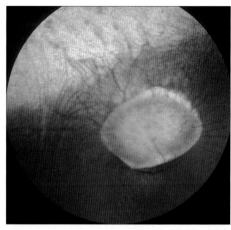

Figure 10.163 Fundus photo of a normal color dilute horse. There is no tapetum and little pigment in the retinal pigment epithelium. Larger choroidal blood vessels are visible as well as the fine retinal vessels arising from the optic disc. Courtesy of Andy Matthews.

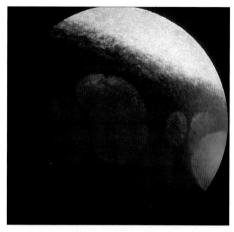

Figure 10.164 Multiple circumscribed focal regions of depigmentation in the lateral fundus representing atypical colobomas. Courtesy of Andy Matthews.

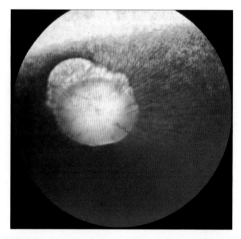

Figure 10.165 A focal depigmented region of peripapillary depigmentation represents an atypical coloboma. Courtesy of Andy Matthews.

dilation of the pupil with 1% tropicamide, which takes 20–30 minutes to achieve dilation, greatly facilitates the examination procedure. The fundus is composed of the transparent neurosensory retina, with its visible vasculature, the retinal pigment epithelium, the underlying choroid, which contains the tapetum, and the optic nerve head (optic disc or papilla). The tapetal fundus is the roughly triangular region above the optic nerve, which has a reflective tapetum in the choroidal layer. The color of the tapetum can vary from shades of yellow, green and blue. Within the tapetum there are multifocal dark dots, and these represent an end-on view of blood vessels in the choriocapillaris. These are called the 'stars of Winslow'. In the non-tapetal fundus, the pigment of the retinal pigment epithelium is visible. The degree of pigmentation usually depends on the coat color of the horse. Horses with lighter coat colors may have less pigment in this layer, allowing for the underlying choroidal blood vessels to be seen. This may occur in a focal region or may occur diffusely throughout the non-tapetal fundus, and may be referred to as 'partial albinism'. The optic nerve is ovoid in shape although this can vary slightly. It is normally pink in color with a white reticulate pattern on the surface due to the lamina cribosa. Thirty to 60 blood vessels extend from within the edge of the disc to approximately two optic disc diameters beyond the disc radially. There is an absence of blood vessels at the central ventral aspect of the disc, where there is usually a notch. There are several anatomical variations of normal. Familiarity with the normal fundus allows the clinician to appreciate when an abnormality is present, and this can only be achieved through examination of hundreds or thousands of animals.

Congenital/developmental conditions

Colobomas of the retinal pigment epithelium
(Figs. 10.164 & 10.165)
A coloboma is an absence of tissue. In the eye they are called 'typical' if they occur in the anatomical location of the optic fissure at 6 o'clock, and atypical if they occur elsewhere. Usually they have no affect on vision and they do not progress, but they may be easily seen on examination of the fundus so it is important to be able to identify them as they are a common incidental finding. They may be more common in the Quarterhorse, and may affect one or both eyes. The lesion is very variable in appearance but is a single or multiple well-circumscribed focal region of decreased pigmentation, which may be white or pink in color. The underlying choroidal vasculature, and the overlying and adjacent retinal vasculature, are normal. No treatment is required.

Congenital stationary nightblindness
Congenital stationary night blindness (CSNB) is an inherited, congenital, non-progressive visually impairing condition, which occurs due to a defect in neurotransmission through the ON-bipolar cells in the rod pathway. The Appaloosa breed is most frequently affected, but it may also affect the Thoroughbred, Paso Fino, Thoroughbred and Standardbred. In the Appaloosa and the Miniature Horse, it is associated with homozygosity for the *Leopard Complex* spotting allele, which has a white-spotting coat pattern. Vision is very poor in dark conditions, but may appear normal in bright conditions. The fundus usually appears normal on examination, and there may be a dorso-medial strabismus, microphthalmia or 'star-gazing'.

Diagnosis and treatment
- Diagnosis is confirmed with electroretinography, which has a normal a-wave but a decreased photopic b-wave and an absent scotopic b-wave (Sandmeyer et al 2007).
- There is no treatment for the condition, and affected animals should not be used for breeding.

Retinal hemorrhages

Occasionally, multifocal intraretinal and subretinal hemorrhages are observed in both eyes of neonatal foals. They are thought to arise due to temporary vascular hypertension during parturition. These hemorrhages occasionally appear more numerous in foals with neonatal maladjustment syndrome. They do not cause any notable visual impairment, and they resolve over a few weeks. No treatment is required.

Non-infectious disorders

Asteroid hyalosis (Figs. 10.166 & 10.167)

Asteroid hyalosis is a normal aging change in the vitreous, but it is not commonly seen. Multifocal refractile calcium-phosphate crystals develop and are suspended within the vitreous. They are easily seen on distant direct ophthalmoscopy as multifocal black dots behind the lens against the tapetal reflection. They are an incidental finding and are not considered pathological. They are not thought to be associated with significant vision problems.

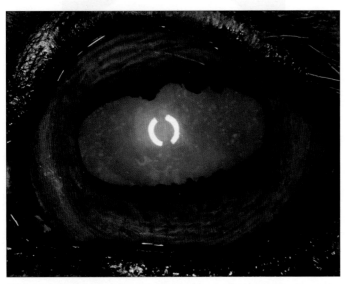

Figure 10.166 Multiple refractile inclusions suspended in the vitreous of an aged pony representing asteroid hyalosis.

Retinal detachment (Figs. 10.168–10.170)

Retinal detachment occurs when there is separation of the neurosensory retina from the underlying retinal pigment epithelium. It may be congenital or acquired, and it may affect one or both eyes. There are several different types of retinal detachment. The most common type is post-uveitis retinal detachment, where an accumulation of transudates and exudates from the choroid enter the subretinal space. This may be focal or complete, and may occur as a flat detachment with no demarcation or as a bullous detachment with a dark line of demarcation. Cyclitic membranes and organized vitreal hemorrhage can lead to vitreal traction bands, which also lead to retinal detachments. A complete retinal detachment occurs when the retina is torn from its firm attachment at the peripheral ora ciliaris retinae, but remains attached at the optic nerve. This is visible as a free-floating gray or pink veil in the vitreous overlying the optic disc. In this situation, the tapetum is hyper-reflective, because of the absence of overlying retina. Apart from uveitis, other possible causes of retinal detachment include congenital non-attachment, trauma, neoplasia, perforating wounds of the globe, after intraocular surgery or idiopathic. If it is not possible to visualize the fundus due to opacity of the ocular media, B-mode ultrasound can be employed which may clearly show the retina floating in the vitreous, sometimes showing the classic seagull sign.

Treatment

- Treatment involves controlling underlying inflammation, if it is present. This may allow bullous retinal detachments to re-attach.
- Transpupillary retinopexy is indicated occasionally for retinal tears, to attempt to prevent progression of the tear. The prognosis for vision after complete retinal detachment is hopeless.

Equine motor neuron disease

(Figs. 10.171 & 10.172)

Chronic deficiency in oral vitamin E leads to degeneration of motor neurones in the ventral horn of the spinal cord and some brain stem nuclei. A lipid retinopathy also occurs in the majority of cases that manifests as a retinal pigment epithelium dystrophy due to accumulation of ceroid lipofuscin. This appears as a mosaic of irregular reticulated pigment deposits on the upper aspect of the non-tapetal fundus, later extending into the lower tapetal area and involving more of the fundus as time goes on. Both eyes are affected, but vision is normally unaffected. The ocular signs may be present before the musculoskeletal symptoms develop.

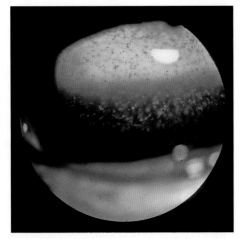

Figure 10.167 A closer view of the refractile vitreal inclusions of asteroid hyalosis.

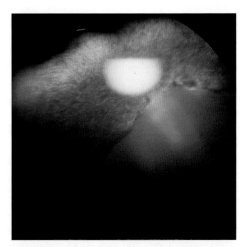

Figure 10.168 Rhegmatogenous retinal detachment which is a giant retinal tear, or disinsertion of the retina at the peripheral ora ciliaris retinae while it remains attached around the optic disc. The detached retina is overlying the optic disc. Courtesy of H.S. Donaldson.

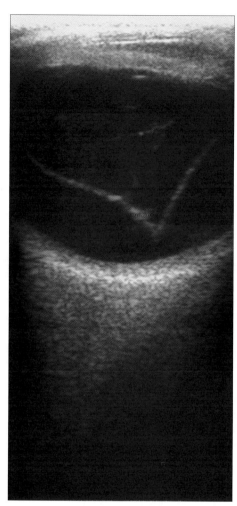

Figure 10.169 Ultrasound image showing the classic 'seagull' sign of a retinal detachment.

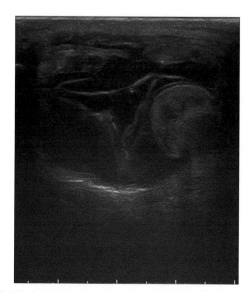

Figure 10.170 Corneal opacity made it impossible to clinically assess this eye after a penetrating injury. Ultrasound shows both lens luxation and retinal detachment. Courtesy of Kim Hughes.

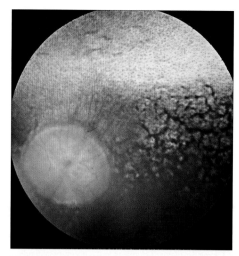

Figure 10.171 Honeycomb pattern of pigment deposits in the non-tapetal fundus and extending upwards into the tapetal fundus in an aged Shetland pony. Equine motor neurone disease was confirmed after serology. Courtesy of Andy Matthews.

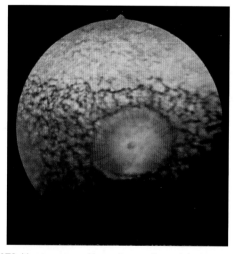

Figure 10.172 Mosaic pattern of hyperpigmentation and depigmentation due to equine motor neurone disease.

Diagnosis and treatment

Diagnosis is confirmed by measurement of plasma vitamin E concentration (see Chapter 11, p. 427).

Treatment

- Treatment involves supplementation with vitamin E orally, along with foods rich in vitamin E such as fresh forage.
- Treatment aids with the musculo-skeletal symptoms but the fundus changes are irreversible.

Senile retinopathy (Figs. 10.173–10.175)

Signs of aging may commonly manifest as a bilateral senile retinopathy in horses over the age of 15 years. This appears as an irregular linear depletion of pigment in the non-tapetal fundus below the optic disc. The retinal vasculature usually appears normal. The tapetal fundus is not normally affected. Vision is not noticeably affected. The cause is not known and therefore treatment is not given.

Optic nerve atrophy (Fig. 10.176)

Optic nerve atrophy occurs as an end result of several different disease processes. These might include trauma, inflammation, ischemia

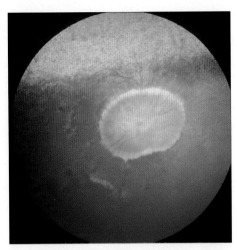

Figure 10.173 Irregular pigment clumping in the non-tapetal fundus and notable retinal blood vessel attenuation due to senile retinopathy. Courtesy of Andy Matthews.

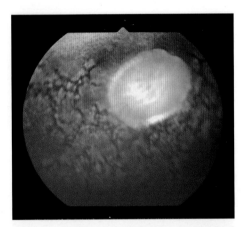

Figure 10.174 Mosaic of pigmentation and depigmentation confined to the non-tapetal fundus along with retinal blood vessel attenuation, due to senile retinopathy.

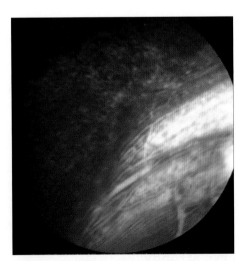

Figure 10.175 Degeneration of the retina and choroid is resulting in white scleral exposure, which was chorioretinal degeneration in an old pony. Courtesy of Andy Matthews.

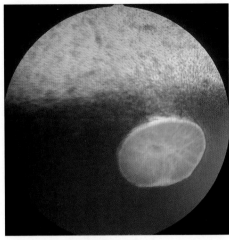

Figure 10.176 Atrophy of the optic disc with attenuation of the retinal blood vessels. Courtesy of Andy Matthews.

(acute blood loss), glaucoma, sphenopalatine sinusitis and neoplasia. Tumors along the visual pathway, or compression from inflammatory lesions or space-occupying lesions adjacent to the visual pathway, can compress the optic nerve and result in wallerian degeneration and atrophy.

Diagnosis

- Diagnosis is made on the characteristic clinical signs. There is a negative menace response, dazzle reflex and pupillary light response, both direct and consensual. The optic disc is pale, and there is granular-appearing texture due to visualization of the lamina cribosa. The surrounding retinal blood vessels will be severely attenuated or not visible at all.
- History taking is very important, given the wide range of possible causes.
- The eye is examined for other signs such as hemorrhage or inflammation. The intraocular pressure is measured if glaucoma is suspected. Orbital masses might cause exophthalmos, or intracranial masses might cause other neurological signs.
- In appropriate cases, further diagnostic imaging such as MRI may be indicated.

Treatment and prognosis

- There is no treatment and the prognosis for return of vision is hopeless.
- Caution might be expressed regarding the future of the unaffected eye if the cause is not known.
- An orbital tumor can affect the optic chiasm at a later date, which could cause blindness.

Ischemic optic neuropathy

Ischemic optic neuropathy occurs when there is a sudden and severe reduction of blood volume to the optic nerve. It occurs due to surgical treatment for guttural pouch mycosis, severe systemic blood loss, after a severe head trauma or as a result of thromboembolic disease. Guttural pouch mycosis can result in chronic epistaxis. One treatment used for this condition is arterial occlusion of the internal carotid, external carotid and greater palatine arteries. This can lead to profound ischemia of the optic nerve on the same side, resulting in sudden-onset blindness. The affected optic nerve initially appears pale but within 1–2 days becomes edematous and congested, with some multifocal hemorrhages and exudative white lesions around the optic disc. The pupil is dilated and visual responses and pupillary light reflexes are absent. Several weeks later, optic nerve atrophy develops. Sudden-onset bilateral blindness has been reported after severe blood loss that occurred after castration. There is no treatment for this condition, and the affected eye will remain permanently blind.

Traumatic optic neuropathy (Figs. 10.177 & 10.178)

Severe head trauma is caused by blunt trauma to the head or when a rearing horse falls backwards. Damage to the basisphenoid bone can cause compression, contusion or hemorrhage in one or both optic nerves. The blunt trauma can also result in the tearing of the dural sheath of the optic nerve.

Diagnosis

- Diagnosis is based on a history of cranial trauma. One or both eyes might be affected. The affected pupil is dilated, and there is an absence of visual responses and pupillary light responses.
- Initially the optic nerve may appear normal, although it may also become edematous and congested, with some multifocal hemorrhages and exudative white lesions around the optic disc. Several weeks later, optic nerve atrophy develops.

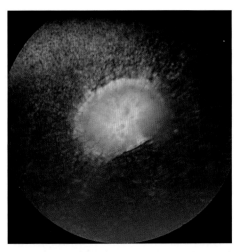

Figure 10.177 Fundus image taken shortly after traumatic blunt ocular injury showing optic disc congestion, retinal blood vessel attenuation and depigmentation of the non-tapetal fundus, as a precursor for optic atrophy. Courtesy of McNeill Lugton.

Treatment and prognosis

- Immediate aggressive treatment is instigated. Systemic anti-inflammatory agents such as corticosteroids or NSAIDs along with dimethyl sulfoxide may restore some vision in a few cases.
- The prognosis is poor and most do not regain any vision.

Proliferative and exudative optic neuropathy (Fig. 10.179)

Proliferative optic neuropathy may be an incidental finding in otherwise normal older horses. They are sometimes called benign exudative neuropathy. Vision is not normally affected. The clinical appearance is of a white lesion arising from the optic disc, usually in one eye. It may be difficult to distinguish this condition from a tumor of the optic nerve, such as an astrocytoma (see below). No treatment is needed and the prognosis is very good.

Exudative optic neuropathy has been described as a bilateral condition that occurs in older horses that present with sudden-onset blindness. On examination of the posterior segment, there are hemorrhages associated with the optic discs and retina, along with swollen optic discs. There are white exudates present over the optic disc. The cause of the condition is not always apparent, but might be associated with head trauma or significant systemic hemorrhage. There is no treatment available. The prognosis is hopeless for vision, and the optic discs are likely to develop optic nerve atrophy with time.

Non-infectious/infectious disorders

Chorioretinitis (Figs. 10.180–10.182)

Chorioretinitis refers to inflammation of the choroid and retina, which are in close contact. The condition may occur as part of equine recurrent uveitis, or may be an ocular manifestation of a systemic disease. Recent and current pathology are termed 'active' chorioretinitis, while older stationary lesions are termed 'inactive' chorioretinitis.

Diagnosis

- Diagnosis is made on the clinical signs observed on funduscopic examination. The lesions may be focal or diffuse, and most commonly affect the non-tapetal region of the fundus. Active lesions may appear as focal or multifocal white or gray areas with edema and cellular infiltrate. Inactive lesions may be more circular, well-demarcated depigmented or hyper-reflective lesions, sometimes with a pigmented clumping centrally. Large areas of depigmentation may be present lateral and medial to the optic disc, in some cases appearing as the classic 'butterfly' lesion.

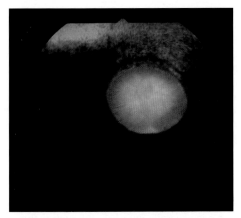

Figure 10.178 The optic disc has some pallor and the retinal blood vessels are attenuated a few days after blunt ocular trauma. Optic disc atrophy developed over the following fortnight.

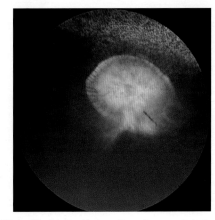

Figure 10.179 A white lobulated lesion with surface vascularization is present on the dorsal border of the optic disc and represents proliferative optic neuropathy. Courtesy of Andy Matthews.

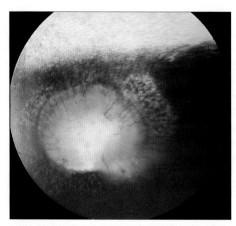

Figure 10.180 Peripapillary chorioretinitis with depigmentation exposing choroidal vessels lateral and medial to the optic disc. There is also a region of active inflammation visible on the 4–6 o'clock sector over the optic disc and extending into the retina. Courtesy of Andy Matthews.

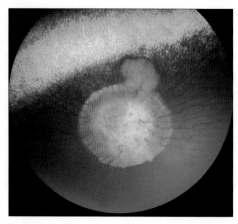

Figure 10.183 The optic disc is fluffy and irregular in the 6–9 o'clock position due to inflammation with both neovascularization and blood vessel attenuation, representing optic neuritis and retinitis. Courtesy of Andy Matthews.

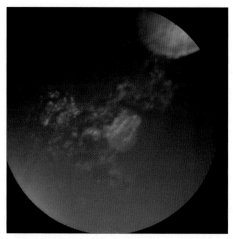

Figure 10.181 Chorioretinal degeneration with depigmentation exposing the choroidal vasculature. Courtesy of Andy Matthews.

- The significance of this condition is that the lesion has been reported to be present in up to 5% of adult normal horses, as well as in horses with previous equine recurrent uveitis.
- The history, retinal vasculature and other signs of previous uveitis such as atrophic corpora nigra should be carefully assessed.
- Focal chorioretinopathy may have one, or more usually several, so-called 'bullet-hole' lesions. These are small round well-demarcated depigmented regions that represent focal atrophy of the retinal pigment epithelium and choroid. A few bullet-hole lesions present usually does not imply any visual impairment or on-going inflammation. However, if they are widespread, they may be part of a general retinal degeneration, which is more likely to impact on vision.

Treatment

- Inactive chorioretinitis does not require any treatment. Active chorioretinitis requires investigation as to an underlying cause by an infectious agent such as *Leptospira*, EHV-1 *Toxoplasma* or *Onchocerca*, with treatment as appropriate.
- More generally, active chorioretinitis is treated with systemic NSAIDs.

Optic neuritis (Fig. 10.183)

Optic neuritis is not a common condition. As the optic nerve is part of the central nervous system (CNS), any inflammatory condition of the CNS may present with optic neuritis. Reported causes of optic neuritis include septicemia, bacterial infection with *Streptococcus equi* or *Borrelia burgdorferi*, viral infection with EHV-1, EHV-4, Borna disease or togavirus, fungal infection such as *Cryptococcus*, protozoal encephalitis and immune-mediated disease. The ocular clinical signs are bilateral blindness and mydriasis. There may be no other obvious ocular clinical signs, except for those found on funduscopy. The optic disc appears hyperemic, hemorrhagic, congested, swollen and therefore out of focus. There may be some exudates on and at the periphery of the disc.

Treatment and prognosis

- Treatment involves investigating the underlying cause, and specifically treating the etiological agent if it can be identified.
- The prognosis is generally guarded, although if the cause can be identified and treated, vision could return. The disc may develop atrophy over time.

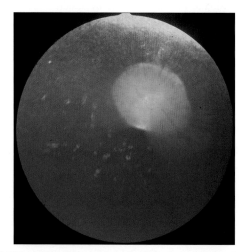

Figure 10.182 Multifocal chorioretinal white 'bullet-hole' lesions in the non-tapetal fundus with some active inflammation visible over the optic disc at the 3–6 o'clock region. Courtesy of Andy Matthews.

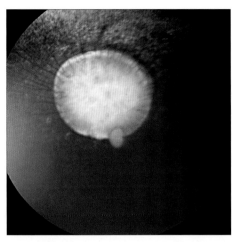

Figure 10.184 A small white lesion is arising from the periphery of the optic disc at the 6 o'clock position without any surface neovascularization, representing an astrocystoma. Courtesy of Andy Matthews.

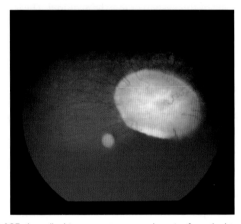

Figure 10.185 A small white astrocytoma can also arise from the lateral fundus.

Neoplasia of the retina and optic disc

Tumors arising from the retina and optic disc are uncommon (Figs. 10.184 & 10.185). The glial cells are most likely to be affected. Medulloepitheliomas have been reported in young horses, appearing as a white mass visible through the pupil (leukocoria). Astrocytomas, gliomas and schwannomas have been described, and occasionally confirmed histologically. Secondary neoplasia could also occur, most commonly due to lymphoma.

Diagnosis

• Diagnosis is made on the observation of a well-demarcated, round to oval raised nodular lesion, which may be white or pale pink. They are commonly located at the periphery of the optic disc, but may also arise in the peri-papillary fundus.

• The diagnosis can only be definitively confirmed with histopathology. However, as the eye is typically comfortable and visual, and the tumor is often benign and very slow-growing, usually histopathology would not arise.

• **Differential diagnosis:** proliferative optic neuropathy (the clinical appearance can be very similar).

Prognosis

• The prognosis is usually good, but it is advisable to be cautious and continually monitor the lesions for progression.

• Lymphoma normally has a more varied appearance, with accompanying uveitis, hyphema and retinal detachment possible.

• The prognosis is poor for metastatic tumors.

References and further reading

Barnett, K.C., Crispin, S.M., Lavach, J.D., Matthews, A.G., 2004. Equine Ophthalmology: An Atlas and Text, second ed. Elsevier Saunders, Edinburgh.

Brooks, D.E., 2010. Ophthalmology for the Equine Practitioner, second ed. Teton New Media, Jackson, Wyoming.

Brooks, D.E., 2010. Targeted lamellar keratoplasty in the horse: A paradigm shift in equine corneal transplantation. Equine Vet J Suppl 37, 24–30.

Cutler, T.J., 2004. Updates in ophthalmology. Vet Clin North Am: Equine Pract 20 (2), 285–506.

Gelatt, K.N., Gilger, B.C., Kern, T.J., 2013. Veterinary Ophthalmology, vol. 2, fifth ed. Wiley-Blackwell, Iowa.

Gemensky-Metzler, A.J., Wilkie, D.A., Cook, C.S., 2004. The use of semiconductor diode laser for deflation and coagulation of anterior uveal cysts in dogs, cats and horses: a report of 20 cases. Vet Ophthalmol 7, 360–368.

Gilger, B.C., 2011. Equine Ophthalmology, second ed. Elsevier Saunders, Maryland Heights, MO, USA.

Gilger, B.C., Davidson, M.G., Nadelstein, B., Nasisse, M., 1997. Neodymium:yttrium-aluminium-garnet laser treatment of cystic granulairidica in horses: eight cases (1988–1996). JAVMA 211, 341–343.

Giuliano, E.A., MacDonald, I., McCaw, D.L., et al., 2008. Photodynamic therapy for the treatment of periocular squamous cell carcinoma in horses: a pilot study. Vet Ophthalmol 11, 27–34.

Hurn, S., Turner, A., McCowan, C., 2005. Ectopic cilium in seven horses. Vet Ophthalmol 8, 199–202.

Lassaline-Utter, M., Miller, C., Wotman, K.L., 2013. Eosinophilic keratitis in 46 eyes of 27 horses in Mid-Atlantic United States (2008-2012). Vet Ophthalmol [Epub ahead of print].

Matthews, A., Gilger, B., Hughes, K., 2010. Reviews in memory of Keith Barnett. Equine Vet J Suppl 37 Equine Ophthalmology III.

Matthews, A., Gilger, B.C., 2009. Equine immune-mediated keratopathies. Vet Ophthalmol 12, 10–16.

Matthews, A., Gilger, B.C., 2010. Equine immune-mediated keratopathies. Equine Vet J Suppl 37, 31–37.

Sandmeyer, L.S., Breaux, C.B., Archer, S., Grahn, B.H., 2007. Clinical and electroretinographic characteristics of congenital stationary night blindness in the Appaloosa and the association with the leopard complex. Vet Ophthalmol 10, 368–375.

CHAPTER 11

Disorders of the nervous system

CHAPTER CONTENTS

Abnormal behavior patterns, alterations in mental status, seizures and weakness are commonly encountered in horses. Such clinical signs may be referable to the nervous system or may be secondary to disorders of other body systems. Definitive diagnosis of a neurological disorder may be challenging and localization of the neurological lesion even more challenging.

Developmental disorders

Developmental disorders of the nervous system of the horse are usually manifested by disturbances of function evident at, or shortly after, birth. Most of these are the result of genetic defects or insults which have affected the foal during gestation. These include a variety of virus or toxemic disorders affecting the mare. The clinical manifestations depend largely upon the stage of development at which the insult is applied and the extent of the consequent deficit. Thus, virus infections affecting a pregnant mare at the time of neurological development (early in gestation) might produce severe effects on the neurological development of the foal. In many cases the effects are life-threatening to the fetus and intrauterine death is common.

In some cases the clinical effects of minor neurological problems in foals may be dramatic. In others, even apparently gross abnormalities might have surprisingly little effect.

Hydrocephalus (Figs. 11.1–11.3)

Hydrocephalus is usually an easily recognized, isolated, developmental abnormality which is not consistent with life long term. Affected foals are usually born dead or die during parturition, as a result of massive increases in intracranial pressure. They are often premature, with an obvious cranial deformity. However, cranial deformity is not invariably present in hydrocephalic foals and in such cases a diagnosis may be difficult without diagnostic imaging. Conversely, some foals born with apparently domed skulls may not be suffering from hydrocephalus. A sagittal section of the head of an affected foal shows the gross distension of the lateral ventricles with generalized compression of the cerebral hemispheres.

Hydrocephalus can also be acquired following conditions such as meningitis or following hemorrhage. Hydrocephalus can be further classified as normotensive or hypertensive. Normotensive hydrocephalus usually is incidental to hypoplasia or loss of brain parenchyma after destructive prenatal or postnatal infection or injury. The CSF volume passively expands to fill the space that is normally occupied by the brain tissue. Hypertensive hydrocephalus is a result of obstruction of the CSF conduit between the sites of production, in the third and lateral ventricles, and the sites of absorption by the arachnoid villi

in the subarachnoid space. Blockage may be due to hypoplasia or aplasia of a part of this system or may be acquired. The increased CSF pressure results in dilation of the third and lateral ventricles with resulting tissue damage. The clinical signs seen include abnormal behavior patterns such as lack of recognition of dam, compulsive walking, bizarre postures and apparent blindness.

Diagnosis and treatment

- Diagnostic imaging techniques such as computed tomography or magnetic resonance imaging allow for ante-mortem diagnosis.
- Post-mortem examination confirms the diagnosis. In either case the etiology usually cannot be determined.
- There is no treatment at present.

Myelodysplasias (Figs. 11.4 & 11.5)

Failure of the cranium and overlying skin to close during development, with prolapse of either the meninges (**meningocele**) or the meninges with parts of the brain (**encephalocele**) is occasionally seen in neonatal foals. The condition which is almost exclusively in the midline may be very small, or involve almost the entire cranium, and may be accompanied by other developmental disturbances including spina bifida. Affected foals are usually either aborted or are born dead or die soon after birth.

Myelodysplasias may be clinically evident at birth or manifested soon after as stable neurological abnormalities such as paraparesis. A bunny-hopping gait and bilaterally active reflexes in the limbs at the level of the defect are prominent features.

Progressive neurological defects resulting from spinal cord compression are associated with severe vertebral anomalies.

Diagnosis and treatment

- Diagnosis by visual and clinical examination with no differentials.
- Affected foals that are born alive should be euthanized as the condition is incompatible with life.

Cerebral hypoplasia

Cerebral hypoplasia is not a common clinical disorder of the horse. Affected foals are recumbent and convulsive from birth, and other defects such as cataracts, limb deformities, hydrocephalus and myopathy, are usually present. Unilateral hypoplasia of one cerebral hemisphere may be responsible for unilateral central blindness, epileptiform convulsions and ataxia but may also be asymptomatic.

Diagnosis and treatment

- Diagnosis is normally made at necropsy.
- There is no treatment at present.

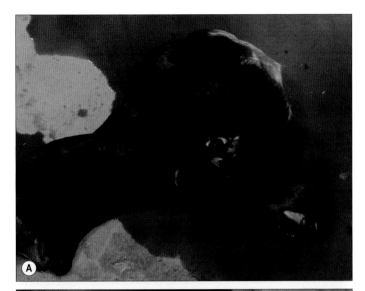

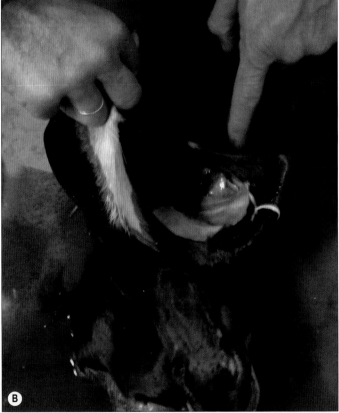

Figure 11.1 (A, B) Hydrocephalus in an aborted fetus. Note the marked fluid distension of the cranium which results in compression of other cerebral tissue.

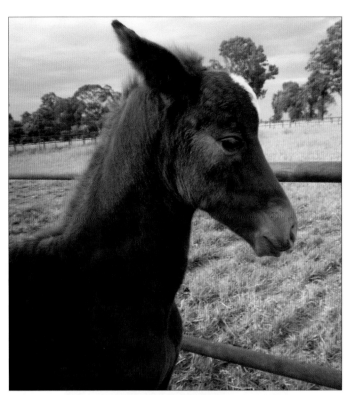

Figure 11.2 Hydrocephalus in a young foal. Note the marked doming of the skull. This foal had abnormal behavior patterns present from birth. ***Differential diagnosis:*** Any condition capable of producing abnormal behavior patterns including HIE, electrolyte imbalances/hypoglycemia, meningitis/septicemia and prematurity.

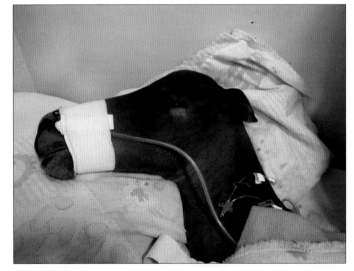

Figure 11.3 Domed skull in a newborn premature foal. This foal did not have a hydrocephalus.

Cerebellar hypoplasia (Fig. 11.6)

Cerebellar syndromes and degenerative lesions are seen in Thoroughbred and Paso Fino foals. Unlike ruminants no toxin or virus has been linked with abnormalities of cerebellar development in foals and congenital malformation or hypoplasia of the cerebellum appears to be rare. Signs including dysmetria and ataxia are evident as soon as the foal attempts to stand and walk.

Diagnosis and treatment

- Ataxia at birth makes this distinguishable from other conditions such as cerebellar abiotrophy that develop later. Definitive diagnosis is only possible at post-mortem. The cerebellum is grossly and histopathologically abnormal.
- No treatment is possible but less severely affected animals may survive with a satisfactory quality of life.
- As it has not been shown to be an inherited condition continuing to breed from the parents is unlikely to result in the birth of another similarly affected foal.

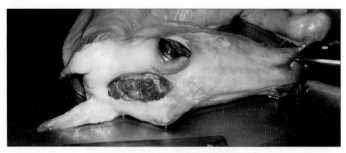

Figure 11.4 Encephalocele in an aborted fetus. Courtesy of Irish Equine Centre, Ireland.

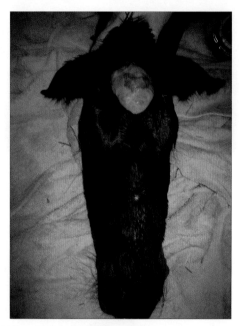

Figure 11.5 Encephalocele in a newborn foal.

Cerebellar abiotrophy

'Abiotrophy' means 'premature (postnatal) degeneration', and in the case of cerebellar abiotrophy refers to degeneration of neurons, particularly Purkinje cells, in the cerebellum. Cerebellar abiotrophy is a familial disease that occurs in purebred Arabian or Arabian crossbred horses in addition to Oldenburg, Gotland and Eriskay ponies. While it is rare, there is strong evidence to suggest that it is an inherited abnormality. Foals of either sex may be affected and the foal is usually of normal size and is bright and alert.

Foals are usually normal at birth with onset of signs normally developing at a few weeks of age. Ataxia with jerky head movements, an intention tremor and an abnormal menace response are the most common signs. Comparison with age-matched controls may be useful as the gait of young foals is naturally somewhat ataxic with jerky head movements.

Diagnosis and treatment

- The condition may be suspected on the basis of clinical signs and suitable breed but currently can only be confirmed at post-mortem examination. A cerebellum to whole brain weight ratio of less than 10% confirms relative smallness of the cerebellum. In some cases transverse cerebellar sections show an obvious loss of white matter.
- Newer imaging modalities, where available, may be useful for ante-mortem diagnosis but to date there are no reports of their use.
- Histopathology shows degeneration of Purkinje cells, atrophy of cerebellar folia and loss of the external granular layer.
- ***Differential diagnosis:*** Cerebellar abiotrophy (must be differentiated from other rare congenital tremor syndromes such as *in utero* exposure to organophosphates or Arnold-Chiari malformation although these may also have other neurological signs); acquired diseases (abscessation and migrating parasites).
- There are no treatment options and clinical signs can be expected to progress.

Occipitoatlantoaxial malformation (OAAM)
(Fig. 11.7)

OAAM is reported in Arabians, Morgans, Standardbreds and rarely in other breeds and includes fusion of the atlanto-occipital joint, atlantalization of the axis and hypoplasia of atlantal wings. Foals can be born dead, be ataxic at birth or show progressive ataxia as yearling

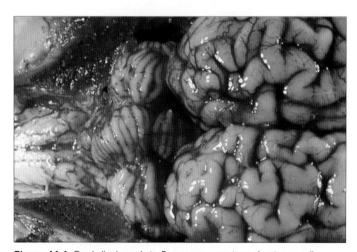

Figure 11.6 Cerebellar hypoplasia. Post-mortem specimen showing a smaller than normal cerebellum. Reproduced from McAuliffe SB, Slovis NM (eds), *Color Atlas of Diseases and Disorders of the Foal* (2008), with permission from Elsevier.

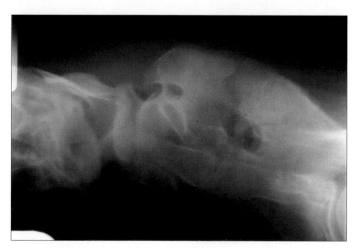

Figure 11.7 Occipitoatlantoaxial malformation. This radiograph shows atlantalization of the axis and fusion of C1 and C2.

Differential diagnosis: Cervical fractures and cervical vertebral malformation should be ruled out.

animals. Occasionally restricted neck movements are the only clinical signs.

In spite of severe (physical and radiographic) malformations some cases show little or no neurological deficit until a gross displacement occurs, when a severe compromise of the neurological function will be evident immediately.

Animals often have extended neck posture with reduced flexion of the atlanto-occipital junction. A malformation of C1 and C2 may be palpated. Usually there are varying degrees of cervical spinal cord signs (tetraparesis and ataxia in all four limbs).

Diagnosis and treatment

- The disease can be confirmed by plain radiography. Malformations of the occiput, C1 and C2 are present including atlanto-occipital fusion and hypoplasia of the dens. Healed atlanto-axial fractures can mimic OAAM.
- No treatment is indicated in most cases and since the disease is most likely inherited in the Arabian, the owners should be counseled not to breed close family lines.
- Laminectomy has been used to alleviate spinal cord compression and clinical signs.

Juvenile epilepsy (Fig. 11.8)

Juvenile epilepsy occurs mainly in Egyptian Arabs or Arabian crosses. The disorder results in seizures in foals that are otherwise normal from several days to several months of age and unlike true epilepsy is usually outgrown.

Clinical signs

- Single or multiple epileptiform seizures. Frequently, these seizures are not seen and all that is noticed is evidence of self-trauma. If seen these seizures usually follow a consistent pattern which is individual for each foal.
- Prodromal signs and postictic signs are also usually consistent for a given animal. Amaurosis (central blindness) is common before and after seizures and is frequently noted by owners.

Treatment

- Although this disorder is outgrown, anticonvulsant therapy (phenobarbital) should be initiated at the first signs and maintained for several weeks to months.

It is administered at a dose rate of 12 mg/kg PO/IV loading dose and then 6 mg/kg PO/IV q 12 h. Note: Phenobarbital induces microsomal enzymes, which may alter the metabolism of the drug with repeated administration. Serum phenobarbitol concentrations should be monitored and maintained between 10–30 µg/ml.

- Failure to treat these animals may result in neuronal death and further possibly permanent seizure foci.
- Underlying problems such as fever that may initiate further seizures should be corrected.

Lavender foal syndrome/coat color dilution lethal (Fig. 11.9)

This is a rare, genetic disease of Arabian foals inherited as an autosomal recessive. It is most commonly encountered in Egyptian Arabians but has also been seen in some Crabbet lines. The condition gets its name as the most striking feature of some of these foals is the dilute or 'bleached-out' hair coat color. In a few cases, the color is a very striking iridescent silver to pale lavender hue, hence the name 'lavender foal syndrome'. Coat color dilution lethal is a more appropriate name, as many affected foals do not exhibit the striking lavender color. Other dilute coat colors observed are pewter (pale slate gray) and pale chestnut (pink). Foals with LFS are unable to stand, and sometimes cannot even attain sternal recumbency (to roll from their side to lie upright, resting on the sternum, a precursor position to standing). They may lay with their necks arched back, make paddling motions with their legs, and often have seizures.

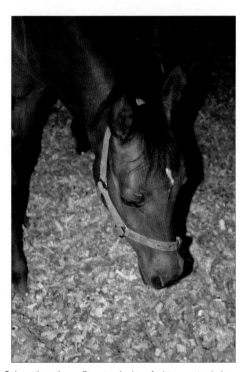

Figure 11.8 Juvenile epilepsy. Egyptian Arabian foal in post-ictal phase of a seizure. These seizures started spontaneously at 3 months of age. He was treated with oral phenobarbital with a total treatment time of 6 months. Thereafter he did not experience any further seizures. Reproduced from McAuliffe SB, Slovis NM (eds), *Color Atlas of Diseases and Disorders of the Foal* (2008), with permission from Elsevier.

Differential diagnosis: (any condition capable of producing seizure activity)
- Meningitis
- Other infectious agents such as strangles, viral encephalitis
- Trauma
- Metabolic disorders
- Disorders of the cardiovascular system
- Liver failure
- Heat stroke
- Fever resulting from infectious process elsewhere.

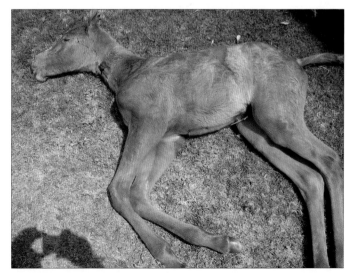

Figure 11.9 Lavender foal. Diluted coat color.

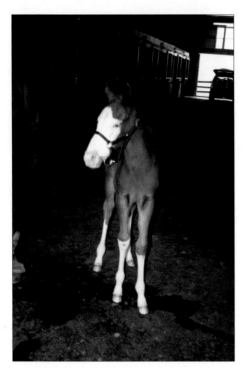

Figure 11.10 Deaf foal. This Thoroughbred foal had two blue eyes and was noted to be deaf when he did not respond as expected to environmental noise. Deafnesss has been associated with the presence of blue eyes in other species and overo horses.

Diagnosis and treatment
- The condition should be suspected in any Arabian foal showing coat color dilution with appropriate clinical signs. It may be somewhat more difficult in foals without obvious coat color dilution.
- There is genetic testing available in the US and Australia at present.
- There is no effective treatment and affected foals are usually euthanized within a few days of birth.

Deafness (Fig. 11.10)
This is poorly documented in the horse but is thought to occur in some overo-colored horses with blue eyes.

Diagnosis and treatment
- The brainstem auditory-evoked response (BAER) test measures responses in brain waves that are stimulated by clicks in the ear to check the auditory pathways of the brainstem.
- Normal values have not been established for foals, however marked delays can be predicted from normal adult horse values.
- There is no treatment available.

Hypoxic ischemic encephalopathy (neonatal maladjustment syndrome) (Fig. 11.11)
Hypoxic ischemic encephalopathy (HIE) is a specific syndrome characterized by alterations in behavior, neurological signs and ischemic and/or hemorrhagic CNS lesions associated with perinatal asphyxia. Foals are often normal for the first few minutes to hours after birth and then may be unable to locate the udder or suck properly and lose affinity for the dam.

Clinical presentation is dependent on the degree of hypoxia. Signs are variable and may include somnolence, lethargy and hypotonia. There may also be a loss of suckle reflex, dysphagia, odontoprisis, central blindness, mydriasis, anisocoria, nystagmus and head tilting. Foals that have been exposed to more moderate hypoxia/ischemia are

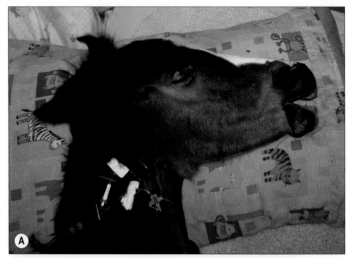

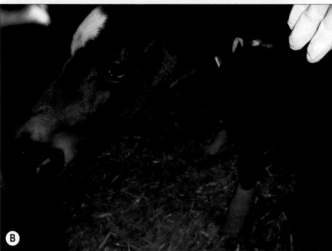

Figure 11.11 (A, B) Hypoxic ischemic encephalopathy. (A) Seizure activity including abnormal mouth and lip movements in this foal. (B) Milder seizure behavior noted as abnormal behavior patterns in this foal. He would have repeated 'chewing' seizures and adopt abnormal positions. Both foals were treated symptomatically and made good recoveries.

Differential diagnosis:
- Metabolic disorders (e.g. hyponatremia)
- Hyperosmolality (hyperlipemia, hyperglycemia)
- Hepatoencephalopathy
- Infectious conditions
- Bacterial meningitis
- Bacteremia
- EHV-1 meningitis
- Cranial trauma
- Development conditions
- Hydrocephalus
- Cerebellar abiotrophy.

more likely to experience seizures characterized by eye blinking, eye deviation, nystagmus, paddling movements and a variety of oral-buccal-lingual movements.

Diagnosis
- HIE is principally a diagnosis of exclusion. Foals typically present within 24–36 hours of birth.
- The condition should be expected in any foal which has a history of abnormal placentation of the mare, premature placental separation, delivery by cesarian section, prolonged dystocia, premature

delivery or in foals that have required resuscitation for any reason after delivery.

Treatment and prognosis

Treatment of HIE has been described extensively and the success rates have improved significantly, however many commonly used treatments are still quite controversial. The goals of treatment are listed below with many of the recommended treatments.

- *Treatment of the mare.* Prevention of intrauterine asphyxia by early treatment of placentitis in mares may help to decrease intrauterine asphyxia (see Chapter 12, p. 471).
- *Treatment of the foal*:
  - Maintaining adequate ventilation
  - Maintaining adequate perfusion
  - Maintaining adequate glucose levels
  - Controlling seizures
  - Control of brain swelling (see Treatment of CNS trauma in p. 410)
  - Other treatments:
    1. *Free radical scavengers*: Allopurinol (xanthine oxidase inhibitor)
    2. *NMDA* (N-methyl-D-asparate) receptor blockers such as magnesium
    3. *Ascorbic acid* (vitamin C)
    4. *Thiamine*: 1 gram IV in 1L of fluids SID. Thiamine increases the activity of the ATP-dependent sodium pump, thus regulating ion uptake and decreasing cellular water
    5. *Hypothermia* has been shown to be neuroprotective. However the exact level of hypothermia has not been established for equine patients but currently it is advisable to stay below rather than above normal temperature. Thus avoid overheating by the judicious use of heating lamps, blankets, etc.
    6. *Good nursing care* is vital.
- Survival rates have been reported as high as 90% but the prognosis is poorer for premature foals, foals with concurrent sepsis and foals showing clinical signs immediately after birth.

Narcolepsy/cataplexy

Narcolepsy is a disorder of rapid eye movement (REM) sleep and is usually accompanied by cataplexy (profound loss of muscle tone). It is occasionally reported in foals and is familiar in miniature horses and Suffolk horses. The syndrome can be present from birth or can be precipitated after an intervention such as surgery.

The underlying etiology is unknown but may involve a defect in function of receptors of the neurotransmitter hypocretin (known to be involved in arousal and food intake in other species).

Clinical signs including episodes of collapse that may occur spontaneously or be precipitated by a stimulus such as manipulation or, most commonly, feeding. An attack may progress from buckling at the knees to sudden collapse with rapid eye movement, loss of skeletal muscle tone and absence of reflexes (e.g. patellar reflexes). Foals can be aroused with varying degrees of difficulties.

There are no abnormalities between episodes and cardiovascular function is normal.

Diagnosis and treatment

- The diagnosis is made on clinical signs. Electroencephalography is used in other species, but interpretation in foals requires considerable experience.
- **Differential diagnosis:** Epilepsy and cardiovascular causes of collapse (these however are not associated with rapid eye movement or loss of reflexes).
- There is no treatment but it resolves in some foals.

Non-infectious disorders

Cervical vertebral malformation/cervical vertebral stenotic myelopathy (Figs. 11.12–11.15)

Cervical vertebral malformation (CVM) is a common cause of ataxia in horses and tends to affect young adults. Compression of the cervical spinal cord results in lesions to proprioceptive and motor tracts to the thoracic and pelvic limbs. This results in ataxia (resulting in inconsistent foot placement and excessive circumduction of the pelvic limbs when turning) and paresis (shown by weakness when pulling on the tail while the horse is walking in a straight line). Table 11.1 outlines a system for grading neurological deficits that is useful in the evaluation of horses with suspected CVM as it allows for accurate

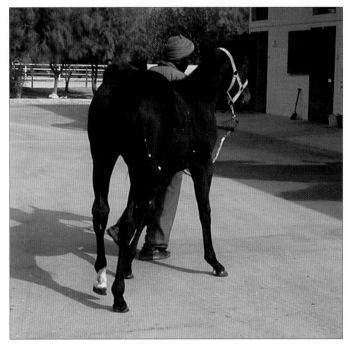

Figure 11.12 Wobbler. Circumduction and truncal sway in this yearling with cervical vertebral malformation.

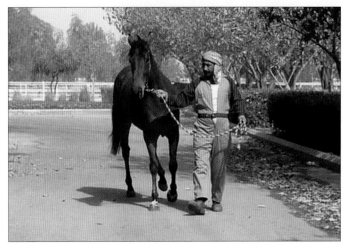

Figure 11.13 Wobbler. Note again in this image the circumduction of the hindlimb on the turn and the truncal sway.

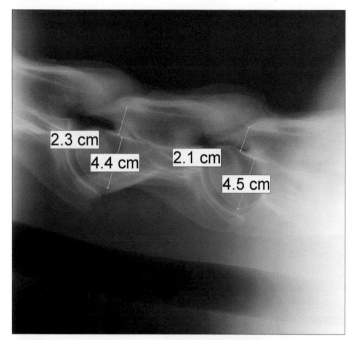

Figure 11.14 Minimum sagittal diameter measurements of the vertebral foramina. The vertebral foramen of C6 is small. There is a mild subluxation at C5–C6 with non-displaced osteochondral fragments of the articular processes and caudal epiphyseal flaring. The intravertebral sagittal ratio is A : B, thus at C5 is 52% and at C6 is 46%. Reproduced from McAuliffe SB, Slovis NM (eds), *Color Atlas of Diseases and Disorders of the Foal* (2008), with permission from Elsevier.

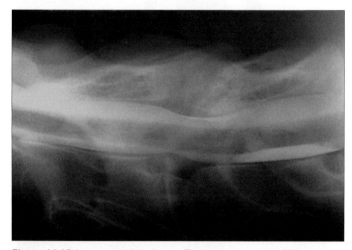

Figure 11.15 Lower cervical myelogram. There is approximately a 50% narrowing of the dorsal contrast column at C6–C7. Reproduced from McAuliffe SB, Slovis NM (eds), *Color Atlas of Diseases and Disorders of the Foal* (2008), with permission from Elsevier.

Table 11.1 System for grading of neurological gait deficits

Grade	Description
0	No gait deficit
1	Deficit barely detectable at walk or trot, but present with special tests
2	Deficit detected during walk and trot, exaggerated by special tests
3	Deficit prominent at walk or trot, may fall during special tests
4	Stumbling, tripping or falling spontaneously at normal gait
5	Down, cannot rise

Box 11.1

Two forms of CVM/CVSM are recognized: dynamic and static.

- In horses with **dynamic stenosis**, compression of the spinal cord occurs only during movement of the neck, particularly flexion. Dynamic compression occurs most commonly at C3–C4 and C4–C5 and primarily affects horses from 8–18 months of age. Compression may not be evident on neutral radiographic views.
- **Cervical static stenosis** is narrowing of the vertebral canal with subsequent compression of the spinal cord regardless of the position of the neck. Compression is evident on neutral radiographic views but in many cases is also exacerbated by extension of the neck indicating coexisting dynamic compression. Static stenosis is most frequently seen at C5–C6 and C6–C7 and is usually seen in older animals, 1–4 years.

recording and monitoring of progression. There are two different types of CVM/CVSM that are recognized and are outlined in Box 11.1.

Due to the peripheral location of pelvic limb tracts in the spinal cord they are affected more severely, resulting in paresis and ataxia, which is more notable in the pelvic limbs. In mild cases the thoracic limbs will not appear to be affected even though the lesion is in the cervical cord. It can sometimes have a history of acute onset ataxia.

Diagnosis

- Neurological examination usually reveals symmetrical ataxia, paresis, dysmetria and spasticity in all four limbs, though usually more noticeable in the pelvic limbs. Asymmetry of clinical signs can be seen in horses with significant degenerative joint disease of the articular processes. At a walk signs of ataxia and paresis such as truncal sway, circumduction of the hindlimbs, toe-dragging and stumbling can be seen. These signs can be exacerbated by walking the horse up or down a slight slope, walking over obstacles (e.g. kerb), turning in circles or elevating the horse's head. Evidence of hypermetria such as exaggerated limb movements or hypometria such as stiff-legged movements are also frequently seen.
- The diagnosis can be made from good-quality cervical radiographs. Subjective assessment reveals enlarged physeal growth plates, caudal extension of the dorsal border of the orifice of the vertebral canal, angular fixation, delayed ossification of bone and degenerative joint disease.
- Stenosis of the vertebral canal corrected for radiographic magnification can be determined by measurement of the intravertebral ratio. A ratio of less than 50% at C4, C5 or C6 or less than 52% at C7 is associated with a high likelihood of having CVSM.
- Myelography can be used to confirm stenosis of the vertebral canal but should only be used when the results will alter the treatment of the case.
- Contrast-enhanced computed tomography has been used in a few cases. Currently the indications are presurgical evaluation and assessment of lateral compressive lesions in horses without myelographic evidence of compression that are strongly suspected of having lesions based on clinical signs. Availability, cost and patient size are limiting factors for the use of this technique at present.

Treatment

- Early diagnosis of CVM in young Thoroughbred horses has been successfully treated using a restricted, paced diet and confinement. Treatment with anti-inflammatory drugs is also common. The use of corticosteroids is controversial due to lack of evidence regarding efficacy, potential negative side effects and the fact that corticosteroids are contraindicated in EPM. Without definitive diagnostic techniques differentiation between CVM and EPM in endemic areas may be difficult.

- Although fusion of cervical vertebrae can result in resolution of clinical signs in selected adult cases of CVM, it would be hard to justify in a foal.

Traumatic injuries

Traumatic injuries to the nervous system of the horse are a frequent occurrence and affect the central nervous system as well as the peripheral nerves.

Cerebral trauma (Figs. 11.16–11.20)

Cerebral trauma does not always have to be severe enough to cause outward evidence of damage, although this is common. Fractures of the forehead are often compound (open) and involve direct cerebral laceration and hemorrhage. These injuries are most commonly the result of kicks from other horses or from impact with solid objects. In some cases rearing or pulling back from a firmly fastened head collar or halter may be responsible for significant trauma, particularly in young horses.

Closed head injuries (those in which there are no skull fractures) often result in brainstem damage with localized bleeding and, often quite extensive subarachnoid bleeding. The signs that are seen are the result of mechanical injury to the brain, cerebral edema, parenchymal hemorrage and ischemia produced by brain swelling and intravascular clotting. The neurological signs are very variable depending on the site of the trauma and its relationship to underlying structures, and the extent of any intracranial bleeding and/or physical disruption.

There may be an initial period of unconsciousness, which can be of variable length, followed by fluctuating neurological signs which are

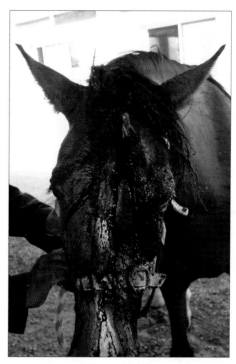

Figure 11.16 Cerebral trauma. Open head injury following impalment on a metal spike.

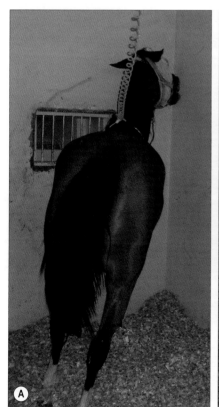
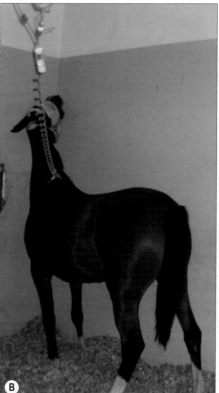
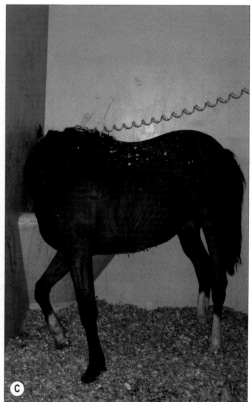

Figure 11.17 Cerebral trauma (same mare as Fig. 11.16), 24 hours later demonstrating neurological signs. (A) Ataxia and proprioceptive deficits, note positioning of hindlimbs. (B) Seizures and abnormal behavior; repeated prolonged and frantic episodes of wall licking and chewing. (C) Compulsive circling. The mare was euthanized shortly after these images were taken.

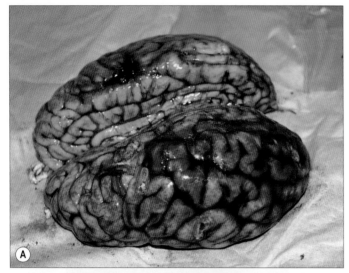

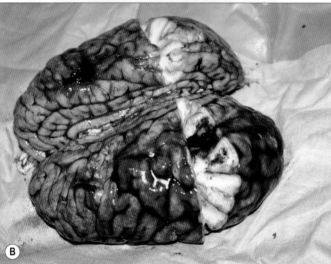

Figure 11.18 (A, B) Brain from the mare in Figs. 11.16 and 11.17. Marked edema and hemorrhage are evident. Cut surface indicates marked hemorrhage at the site of injury. Paint from the railing was found within this area.

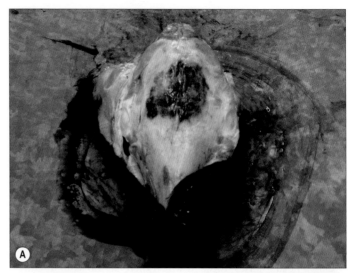

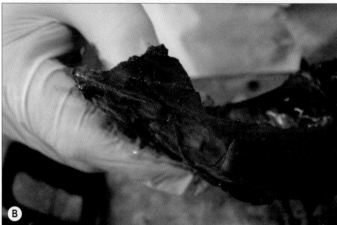

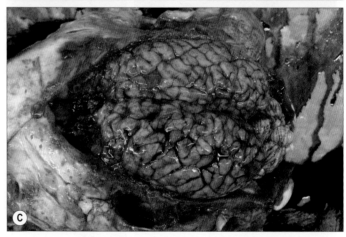

Figure 11.19 Head trauma in a foal. (A) Marked subcutaneous hemorrhage in the area of injury. (B) Skull fracture associated with the trauma. (C) Cerebral hemorrhage associated with the site of trauma and skull fracture.

dependent on the degree of intracranial hypertension associated with cerebral edema and hemorrhage.

Wandering toward the side of the lesion and depression are commonly seen but ataxia is not usually seen unless there is progressive involvement of other parts of the brain.

Pupillary light responses are usually brisk in the early stages but may become more delayed as cerebral edema worsens. There may be some asymmetry of the pupils and miosis and characteristically there is central blindness and depressed menace responses.

The development of a midbrain syndrome (dilated unresponsive pupils and tetraparesis), associated with swelling of the cerebral hemispheres and herniation caudally against the midbrain, warrants a poor prognosis, whereas an uncomplicated cerebral syndrome usually has a good prognosis as response to treatment for brain swelling can be good.

Basioccipital and basisphenoid fractures
(Figs. 11.21 & 11.22)

These fractures most commonly occur after rearing accidents or head collar injuries. Typically, the neurological signs associated with this type of trauma are very variable. Individual cases may be comatose

but others may show subtle neurological deficits, which may be limited to the individual cranial nerves in the region of the fracture; in which case the signs may be unilateral.

Petrous temporal bone fractures
(Figs. 11.23–11.30)

Bleeding from the ear following head trauma is indicative of damage to the petrous temporal bone and the vestibular nerve and/or its

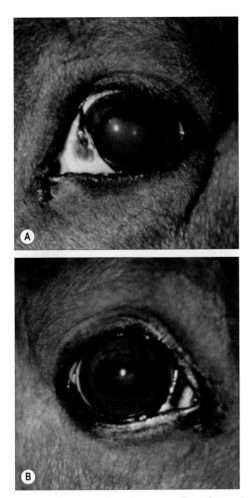

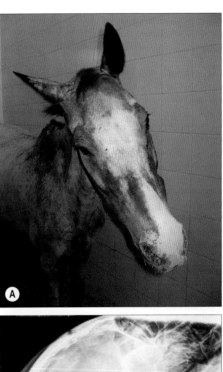

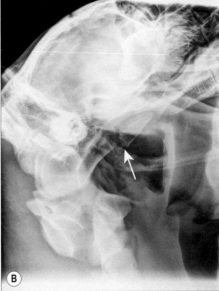

Figure 11.20 Anisocoria or asymmetry of the pupils. This is frequently found with fractures that involve the optic or vestibulo-cochlear nerves.

nucleus. Affected horses have a marked head tilt towards the affected side, and are obviously disoriented with circling and nystagmus in which the fast phase is away from the affected side. Usually there is complicating concurrent damage in the base of the brain and weakness, depression and ataxia, amongst other signs.

Fractures involving the base of the cranium

These will frequently involve one or more of the cranial nerves, and the clinical signs of this damage may be difficult to identify in conjunction with the more severe effects of cerebral, cerebellar or brainstem disruption. Commonly, however, the signs include depression and/or dementia.

Fractures which affect the optic or vestibulo-cochlear nerves

These fractures or their central nuclei will have dramatic and easily recognized signs (see Fig. 11.20). In the former, blindness and pupil-light-reflex deficiencies or discrepancies between the two eyes will be present. Concurrent retinal damage (including detachment) and/or lens dislocation may be found.

Diagnosis

- In many cases the diagnosis of trauma is an obvious diagnosis but diagnostic imaging techniques can be useful to help identify the exact site and thus allow for a more informed assessment of involved structures. Advanced imaging techniques such as CT and MRI can provide additional information such as enlargement of cerebral hemispheres.

Figure 11.21 (A) Fracture of basisphenoid with head tilt towards the side of the lesion. (B) Radiograph of the head showing a fracture of the basisphenoid (arrow) and soft issue opacity of the guttural pouch consistent with blood within the pouch.

Differential diagnosis:
- Otitis media/interna
- Petrous temporal bone fracture/vestibular injury
- Cerebral trauma.

- Basioccipital and basisphenoid fractures may be difficult to appreciate radiographically, but endoscopic examination of the roof of the medial compartment of the guttural pouches will often identify either bruising or even the presence of a hematoma over the site of the fracture.
- Fractures of the hyoid bone may possibly be detected radiographically and by endoscopic examination of the guttural pouch(es).
- Ultrasound examination of the atlanto-occipital space can be used in some cases to determine the presence of intracranial hemorrhage.
- Cisternal puncture and aspiration of blood-stained cerebrospinal fluid confirms intracranial hemorrhage but in many cases may be contraindicated due to increased risk of mid brain herniation.

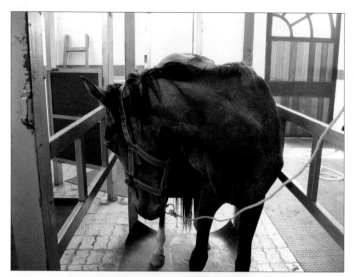

Figure 11.22 Head trauma with head and neck turning to the side of the lesion. For differentials see Fig. 11.21.

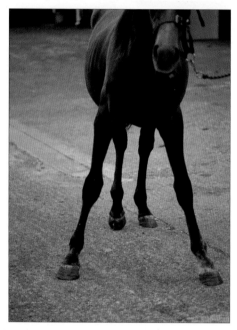

Figure 11.23 Cerebellar injury with typical wide-based stance.

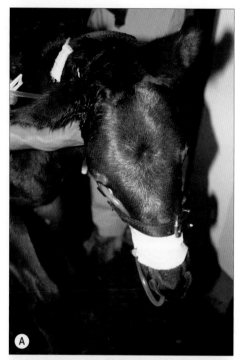

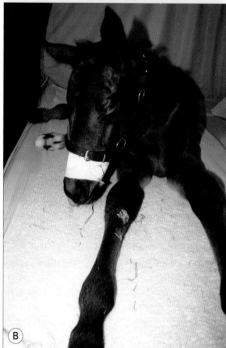

Figure 11.24 (A) Vestibular head tilt. (B) Vestibular injury resulted in whole body turning towards side of lesion.

Treatment

- The general principles for treatment of CNS trauma are administration of osmotic diuretics, nutritional and fluid support and protection from self-inflicted trauma and the effects of prolonged recumbency.
- Seizures or excessive, difficult-to-manage thrashing may require sedation or short-term anesthesia. Diazepam 5 mg (foal) up to 100 mg (adult) can be repeated as necessary to control seizures. Phenobarbital or pentobarbital may also be used to control seizures. The alpha 2 agonists should be avoided for the treatment of seizures in the acute stages as they can cause transient hypertension, exacerbating CNS hemorrhage and they also suppress ventilation.
- Horses with CNS signs following cranial trauma should probably receive dexamethasone (0.1–0.25 mg/kg q 4–6 h) for 1–4 days. However, the benefits should be weighed against the possible complications of steroid administration in the horse (laminitis).

- Intravenous administration of 20% mannitol (0.25–1 g/kg) has been used for the treatment of increased intracranial pressure. Its use however is contraindicated in cases of ongoing cerebral hemorrhage. Response to mannitol is usually noted within 1 hour and if a response is noted, mannitol administration should be repeated every 4–6 hours for the first day.
- DMSO, is frequently given slowly at 1 g/kg as a 10% solution in isotonic fluids. DMSO has several beneficial pharmacological effects including diuresis, free-radical scavenging, inhibition of platelet

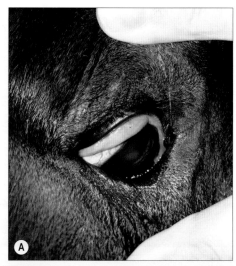

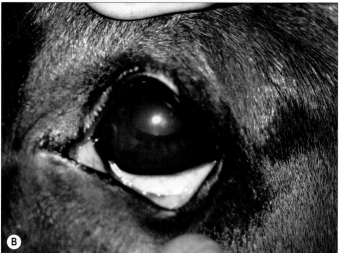

Figure 11.25 (A, B) Vestibular injury (same foal as Fig. 11.24). Note the difference in positioning of the eyes. Nystagmus was present bilaterally but more obvious in the eye on the side of the lesion with the fast phase away from the side of the lesion.

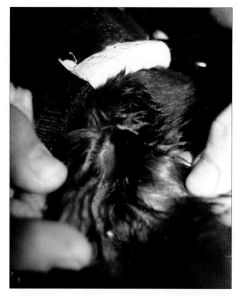

Figure 11.26 Serosanguinous discharge from the right ear was present in this foal (same foal as Figs. 11.24 and 11.25). This type of discharge is typically seen with fractures of the petrous temporal bone.

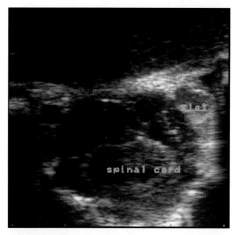

Figure 11.27 Ultrasound examination of the atlanto-occipital space (same foal as Figs. 11.24–11.26) revealed the presence of a blood clot. Concurrent injuries to the base of the brain are common with petrous temporal bone fractures.

aggregation, vasodilation and increased penetrance of steroids and antibiotics into the brain. There are many anecdotal reports of successful treatment with DMSO but clinical trials in other species have not shown a clear benefit in treating CNS trauma. Adverse effects include intravascular hemolysis which has been associated with too rapid administration or administration of a more concentrated solution. DMSO administration can be repeated every 12 hours for 3–4 days if clinical improvement is seen.

- Hypoxemia and hypercapnia should be avoided as hypoxia exacerbates brain swelling and hypercapnia increases intracranial blood volume and pressure. Recumbent horses should be rolled every 4–6 hours to minimize pulmonary arteriovenous shunting and ventilation perfusion mismatching. Ideally the head should also be maintained at heartbase level or higher to avoid hypostatic intracranial congestion. Maintenance of hydration is important but overhydration should be avoided as it can exacerbate brain edema.
- Close monitoring and good nursing care are essential. If an improvement is noted in 6–8 hours, treatment should be repeated. If no improvement is seen more aggressive treatment may be warranted, including exploratory craniotomy.

Prognosis

- Complicated combinations of neurological deficits can arise from even relatively minor trauma and may take some hours or days to produce their full neurological effect. Many consequences of cranial trauma such as hemorrhage, laceration necrosis, secondary ischemia and midbrain injury are inaccessible to therapy and the presence of some of these lesions is difficult to diagnose with failure to improve or deterioration in neurological condition being the only clue to their existence.
- The most accurate prognosis is based on repeated detailed neurological examinations with assessment of the rate of progression or resolution and the responses to specific therapeutic measures.
- Cerebral and cerebellar lesions usually carry a better prognosis than brainstem lesions and therefore those injuries which are accompanied by bleeding from the ear but few other outward signs are possibly more serious than the more dramatic injuries to the frontal and facial bones.

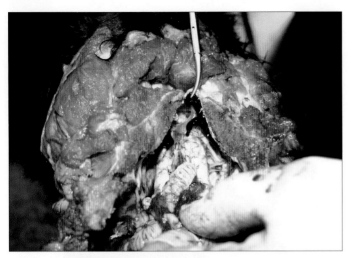

Figure 11.28 Clot within the spinal canal found at necropsy (same foal as Figs. 11.24–11.27).

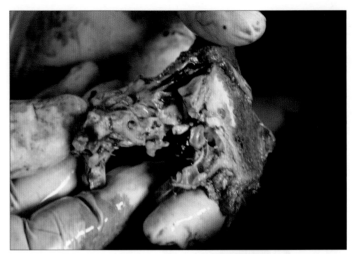

Figure 11.30 Fractured petrous temporal bone.

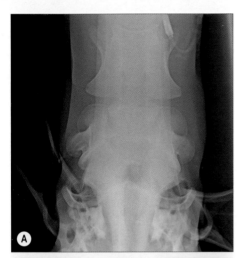

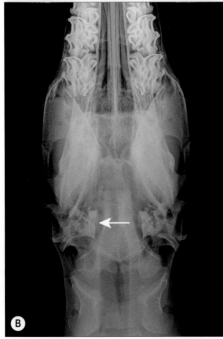

Figure 11.29 (A) Dorsoventral radiograph of skull from a normal foal. (B) Dorsoventral radiograph of skull from foal in Fig. 11.24 with a fracture of the petrous temporal bone (arrow).

- If no improvement is seen or deterioration is noted in a comatose patient 36 hours after surgery or anesthesia, euthanasia may be indicated.

Cord trauma

Suspected spinal cord trauma is one of the most common neurological disorders presented to equine practitioners. Spinal cord trauma typically occurs following a traumatic incident such as a fall and may or may not be associated with vertebral trauma. Fractures rarely occur secondary to other pathology such as neoplasia. The cervical vertebrae are a common site for vertebral fractures, especially the occipitoatlantoaxial region in foals. The lower cervical and cranial thoracic sites are the most common areas for vertebral fractures in the adult horse. Fractures of the thoracic dorsal spinous process are not usually associated with neurological signs, whereas fractures of the vertebral body, arch or articular processes are usually associated with neurological signs.

Clinical signs

The signs seen depend heavily upon the location of the injury and the extent of damage to the cord or to the meninges and/or to the peripheral nerves as they pass through the intervertebral foramina.

Gross displacement of adjacent vertebrae which results in severance of the cord is accompanied by immediate loss of all conscious proprioception and voluntary motor function distal to the site of the lesion. In some cases, however, the extent of the apparent bony damage may not necessarily correspond to the extent of the neurological deficits.

Many cases of vertebral trauma with or without neurological signs have been reported.

Cervical spine (Figs. 11.31–11.34)

A recumbent horse with a lesion at C1–C3 has difficulty raising its head off the ground; whereas, a recumbent horse with a lesion at C4–T2 should be able to lift its head and cranial neck. C1–T2 lesions may result in tetraplegia, but may also present as tetraparesis and ataxia. Spinal cord lesions above the C6 segment will result in normal to increased muscular tone and spinal reflexes (panniculus, triceps and biceps) in all limbs. If the lesion is located at the sixth to eighth cervical spinal cord segments, the forelimb reflexes are diminished or absent and those of the hindlimbs are normal or increased.

Thoracic spine (Figs. 11.35–11.38)

Lesions of T3–T6 may cause paraplegia or paraparesis and ataxia. A paraplegic horse that 'dog-sits' usually has a lesion caudal to T2. Most

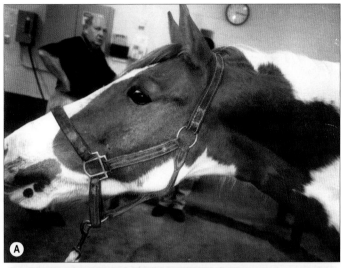

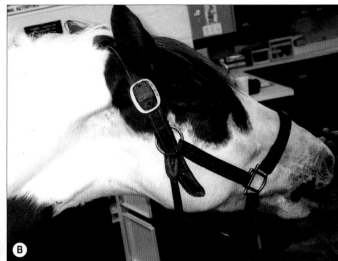

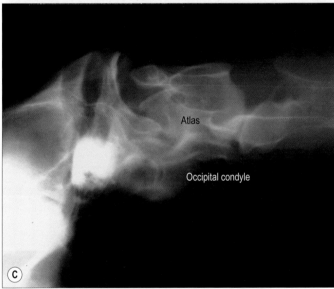

Atlas

Occipital condyle

Figure 11.31 Cervical trauma. This horse was left tied to a post and on return the owner noted that the horse had become hung up in his tie rope and had marked swelling of the head of the neck. The horse was presented 6 weeks after the initial incident for abnormal head carriage. (A, B) A fixed extended neck position was noted with a marked disparity in the position of the wings of the atlas between the left and right side of the neck. (C) Radiographs revealed a healed fracture of C1 with occipitoatlantal dislocation. The atlas is seen to be clearly separated from the dens. Due to the chronic nature of the condition with minimal clinical signs and the possibility of worsening the condition with surgical intervention no specific treatment was given. The horse remained stable over the following 10 years.

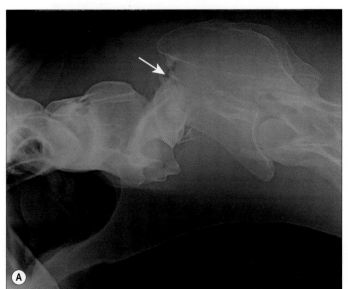

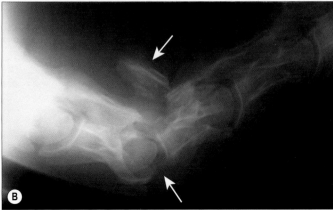

Figure 11.32 (A) Fractured dens (arrow). There was a gross deformity of the neck but no neurological signs associated with this lesion. (B) Multiple fractures of a cervical vertebrae (arrows) which resulted in obvious external ventral deviation of the neck.

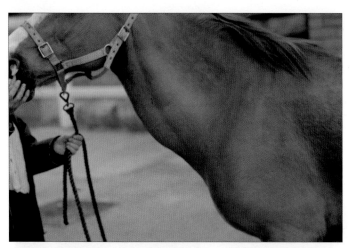

Figure 11.33 Deviation of neck in sagittal plane associated with cervical vertebral fracture.

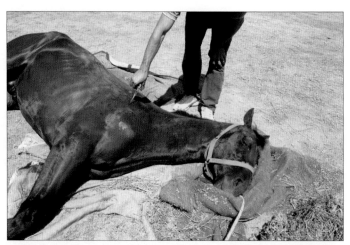

Figure 11.35 Thoracic vertebral fracture. This horse presented with acute-onset recumbency. There was no obvious external lesions. Hypalgesia was present at the level of T2–T4. Post-mortem examination revealed a fracture of the vertebral body of T3.

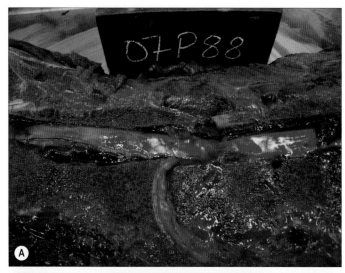

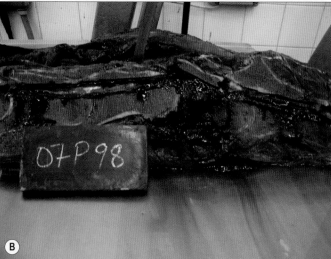

Figure 11.34 (A) Fracture of dorsal spinous process of a cervical vertebrae. (B) Fracture of body and dorsal process of a cervical vertebrae. Courtesy of Irish Equine Centre, Ireland.

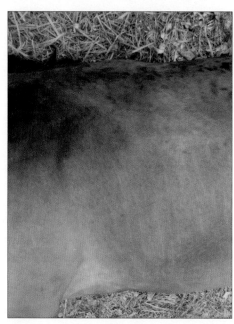

Figure 11.36 Thoracic vertebral fracture. Obvious step defect in thoracic spine. This yearling was seen to have fallen over a gate during an electrical storm. A fracture of a thoracic vertebrae could be imaged radiographically.

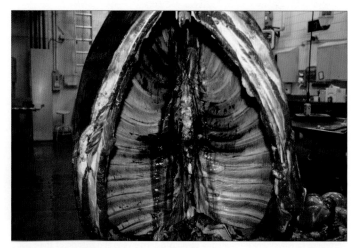

Figure 11.37 Hemorrhage in the thoracic wall associated with fracture of the thoracic vertebrae (same horse as Fig. 11.36).

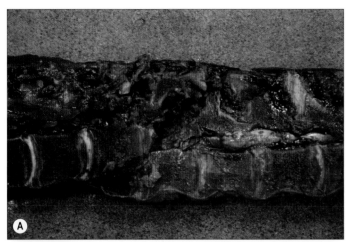

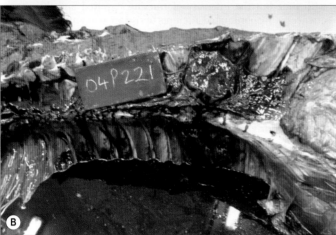

Figure 11.38 Thoracic vertebral fractures. (A) Complete fracture of the thoracic vertebrae (same horse as Fig. 11.37). Note the extensive local hemorrhage. (B) Marked hemothorax as a result of a thoracic vertebral fracture (Courtesy of Irish Equine Centre, Ireland).

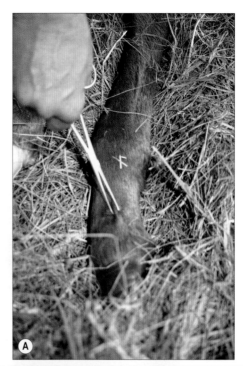

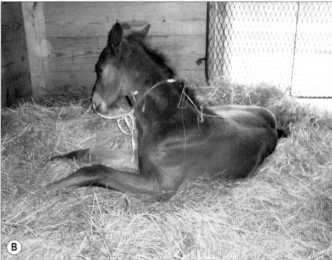

Figure 11.39 Lumbar vertebral fracture. (A) Lack of spinal reflexes in the hindlimbs of this foal with an L6 fracture. The foal had been found down in the field and was unable to stand. (B) The foal retained good reflexes in the forelimbs and was able to put itself in a sternal position.

animals with thoracic spinal cord injury have normal to exaggerated spinal reflexes and hypertonia of the rear limbs. Some degree of asymmetry may be present with spinal cord trauma, but signs are almost always bilateral. The level of hypalgesia on the neck or back indicates the cranial extent of the lesion. In the early post-trauma phase, a region of hyperesthesia may be detected just cranial to the lesion. Strip patches of sweating may occur when thoracolumbar spinal nerve roots are damaged. Whole-body sweating, seen frequently in horses with a broken neck or back, may be due to involvement of pain pathways and sympathetic spinal cord pathways.

Lumbar spine (Figs. 11.39–11.41)

Lesions at L1–L3 spinal cord segments result in normal or hypertonic and hyper-reflexic hindlimbs. Lesions at L4–S2 may result in hypotonia and hyporeflexia of the hindlimbs. The bladder is distended, but sphincter tone is normal. Tail and anal tone are normal.

Thoraco-lumbar lesions which are associated with posterior paralysis and forelimb extensor rigidity (Schiff-Sherrington reaction) and which gradually ascend are most serious.

Sacrococcygeal spine

Lesions of spinal cord segments S1–S2 result in decreased conscious proprioceptive responses of the hindlimbs and diminished flexor reflexes of those limbs. Anal tone is diminished to absent and the bladder is distended and hypotonic. Atony of the urethral sphincter results in incontinence and urine scalding. The tail is flaccid and paralyzed.

Clinical pathology and radiographic findings

- Plain radiography is the most helpful aid in confirming vertebral trauma, but does not directly evaluate the presence or extent of spinal cord damage. Abnormalities that are seen that indicate injury are displacements of vertebral components, shortened or abnormally shaped vertebrae, slipped physeal plates and fractures.
- Fracture-induced changes in the CSF may be useful for ancillary diagnosis. These changes can be classified as acute (<24 hours) or chronic (>24 hours). The acute changes include diffuse blood contamination, a high red blood cell (RBC) count, a normal to high white blood cell (WBC) count, and a high protein concentration.

Chronic CSF changes include a normal to slightly increased WBC count, normal to increased RBC count, increased protein concentration and xanthochromia.

Treatment
- Pain should be managed with non-steroidal anti-inflammatories and other medication recommendations are similar to those for cerebral injury. Good nursing care is essential, especially for recumbent patients and should include bladder and rectal evacuation if necessary.

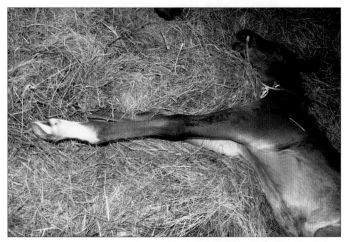

Figure 11.40 Same foal as Fig. 11.39, 24 hours later showing a Sciff-Sherrington response in the forelimbs. This is seen with severe injuries of the thoracic or lumbar spinal cord.

- If the spinal fracture appears stable and the animal can stand with assistance, it may be placed in a water tank and supported for long periods. Other methods of support include slings, but these should not be used for animals that cannot support themselves as severe respiratory compromise or myositis may result. Slinging of animals with mild neurological signs may help minimize secondary complications, improve extensor tone and hasten recovery.
- Horses which suffer from spinal pain and/or posterior paralysis often show extremes of panic and their management is most difficult and frequently dangerous for the handlers involved. Priority should be given to human safety at all times.

Prognosis
- The prognosis is best judged on the basis of repeated neurological examinations. The longer a patient remains recumbent and neurologically impaired the poorer the prognosis. In general the prognosis for horses suffering from spinal trauma is poor. Some may recover with time but the intensity of nursing required and the consequences of incoordinated attempts to rise are often most distressing for the horse, the owner and the attendants.
- Healing of fractures frequently results in vertebral malalignment. Delayed callus formation and degenerative changes in adjacent articulations can result in permanent spinal cord compression even after apparent healing and resolution of clinical signs.

Other cranial nerve disorders
The trigeminal nerve (CN-V) (Fig. 11.42)
This is the largest cranial nerve and has both motor and sensory functions. Motor functions include aspects of prehension, mastication and swallowing, while the sensory components control mouth and eye sensation and sensation in the skin of the head.

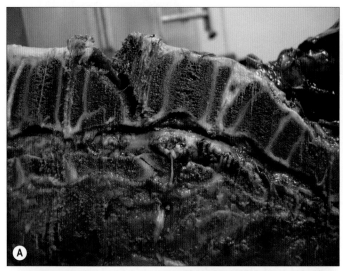
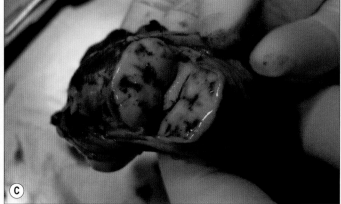
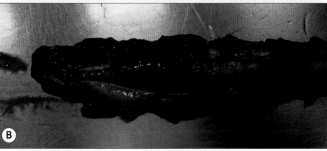

Figure 11.41 (A, B) Necropsy specimen from the foal in Fig. 11.39 showing a fracture through L6 and marked hemorrhage associated with the spinal cord. (C) Cross-section of the spinal cord shows extensive hemorrhages throughout the cord.

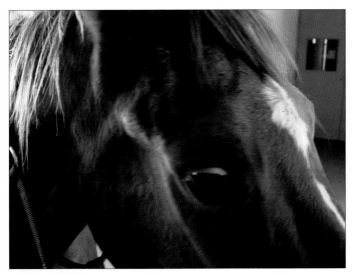

Figure 11.42 Trigeminal nerve disruption resulting in masseter atrophy. Damage to the trigeminal nerve can be peripheral or central and can be unilateral or bilateral.

Differential diagnosis:
• Hyoid fractures (peripheral)
• Equine protozoal myeloencephalitis (central or peripheral)
• Central multifocal disorders
• Botulism (central effect of neurotoxin on nerve nucleus)
• Degenerative disorder of the peripheral nerve fiber
• Cauda equina neuritis (equine polyneuritis syndrome)
• Idiopathic trigeminal neuritis.

Clinical signs

• Bilateral loss of motor activity results in a dropped jaw, inability to chew and tongue protrusion. Repeated, unconscious biting of the cheeks and tongue during mastication may result in severe damage which may be unilateral or bilateral, and is most often indicative of a trigeminal sensory deficit. Prehension may be possible in some cases where the sensory function is maintained and where the facial nerve (CN-VII) is unaffected, but chewing is almost always severely affected.
• Atrophy of the temporal, masseter and the distal part of the digastricus muscles develops over the following 2–3 weeks. Atrophy may be unilateral or bilateral depending on whether the lesion is unilateral or bilateral.

Diagnosis

• The diagnosis of trigeminal nerve disorders is difficult and relies heavily upon a detailed assessment of motor and sensory functions and unilateral disorders are particularly difficult to assess in the early stages.
• Loss of sensation in the muzzle and medial wall of the nasal cavity are supportive findings but central lesions often only affect the motor function.
• Once atrophy of individual and definable muscle blocks occurs the diagnosis becomes simpler but determining an actual etiology may remain difficult.

Facial nerve (VII) (Fig. 11.43)

Perhaps the most common cranial nerve injury in the horse occurs to the **facial nerve (CN-VII)**. The nerve is liable to be traumatized in

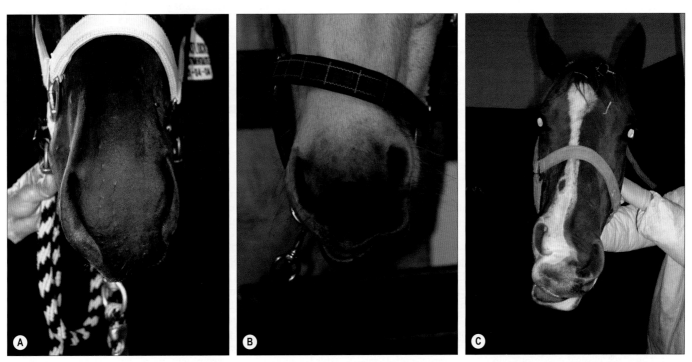

Figure 11.43 Facial nerve paralysis. (A) Right side, affecting upper lip only. Lesion probably on side of face in one or more localized branches. (B) Right side, peripheral lesion. Both upper and lower lip affected. Ear and eyelid were not affected. Lesion probably at vertical ramus of mandible. (C) Facial paralysis (neurapraxia) (Right side, central or root lesion). Note: Paralysis of left lip (upper and lower), drooping left ear and paralysis of upper eyelid. Corneal ulcer was also present as a result of poor blink-efficiency and a consequent area of keratoconjunctivitis sicca (dry eye).

Differential diagnosis:
• Equine protozoal myeloencephalopathy
• Cauda equina neuritis (*polyneuritis equi*) syndrome
• Guttural pouch mycosis
• Fracture of basisphenoid or hyoid bone (or both)
• Central neoplasia.

view of its very superficial path. The nerve is closely related at its root to the styloid process of the hyoid bone and to the guttural pouches. The most superficial portions of the nerve pass round the caudal border of the vertical ramus of the mandible and cross the side of the face, lying subcutaneously. It may be damaged at any point along its length from the cranial outflow to the more distal branches. As the nerve is responsible for the motor activity of the muscles of facial expression, the consequence of damage (whether mild and temporary or more permanent) is an abnormality of facial expression.

Lesions occurring at the base of the brain, including **fractures of the hyoid bone, fractures of the cranial floor** and **guttural pouch mycosis** and **diverticulitis**, would probably affect all three major branches of the nerve (i.e. the auricular, palpebral and buccal branches), exerting a more extensive effect than more peripheral lesions. Central, facial nerve lesions are unusual, but may be a sign of generalized degenerative disorders such as cauda equina neuritis syndrome (polyneuritis equi). The most common sites for damage to the nerve coincide with the location of the metal buckles on head collars and halters. Sudden snatching of the head against the head collar, or direct trauma, particularly when the animal falls onto the side of the face (such as sometimes occurs during the induction of anesthesia) might result in damage at, or beyond, the caudal edge of the vertical ramus of the mandible.

Clinical signs

- Cases in which all three branches are affected present with paralysis of the ipsilateral upper and lower lips, a drooping of the ipsilateral ear and often a ptosis of the upper eyelid. The more distal the lesion, the more limited will be the effect on facial expression. Damage occurring over the side of the face rostral to the end of the facial crest will result in limited deviation of the upper lip only.
- Bilateral lesions involving the peripheral (or central) pathway of the nerve result in a symmetrical drooping of the upper and lower lips with profound effects on prehension and obvious saliva drooling may be present. Jaw tone and mastication are normal however, in contrast to trigeminal nerve lesions. Secondary consequences of facial nerve paralysis include an inability to prehend effectively, epiphora and corneal ulceration.

Treatment and prognosis

- In most cases treatment is aimed at treating secondary effects.
- Most cases of traumatically induced facial nerve damage are temporary and mild, but irreparable damage (**neurotmesis**) results in a permanent distortion of facial expression.
- Some return of function may occur gradually over many years, even in severed nerves where the damage occurred more distally.

Horner's syndrome (Figs. 11.44 & 11.45)

The clinical signs of Horner's syndrome include ptosis of the upper eyelid, enophthalmus resulting in prolapse of the third eyelid, miosis of the pupil and sweating along the affected side of the face. Any condition which results in inflammation or damage of the cranial sympathetic trunk or ganglion can result in Horner's syndrome. Additionally, damage to the internal carotid nerve which contains postganglionic sympathetic fibers can also result in Horner's syndrome. Therefore, clinical conditions which may present with Horner's syndrome include: inflammation within the guttural pouch such as in guttural pouch mycosis or extravascular injection of irritant substances in the jugular groove, lacerations at the base of the neck (or higher), injury or infarction of the cranial thoracic spinal cord, avulsion of the brachial plexus, space-occupying lesions in the thoracic inlet such as abscesses, hematomas or mediastinal and thymic lymphosarcoma and multiple/extensive, thoracic melanoma or carcinoma.

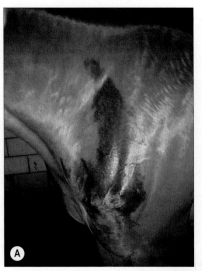

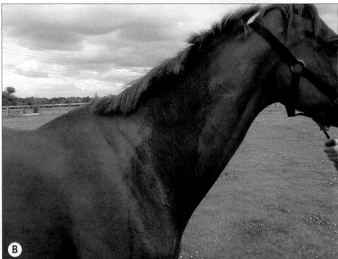

Figure 11.44 (A, B) Focal sweating associated with local damage to the sympathetic trunk.

The consequences of loss of sympathetic tone include cutaneous vasodilatation with localized hyperthermia and consequent sweating. Thus, damage to the trunk in the lower or mid-cervical region results in sweating over the side of the neck and, in Horner's syndrome, on the ipsilateral side. The characteristic feature of this clinical sign is the sharp cut-off of the sweating down the midline of the face. Where the lesion responsible for the damage is situated in the guttural pouch and damage to the trunk is beyond the cranial sympathetic ganglion, the area of sweating is usually limited to a small area just under the ear. Loss of sympathetic control of the upper eyelid and pupillary diameter results in a ptosis, miosis (which may not be very obvious) and enophthalmos on the affected side. The nictitating membrane (third eyelid) may be prominent as a secondary consequence of enophthalmos. Damage to the sympathetic fibers within the spinal cord results in sweating down the whole side of the horse, as well as Horner's syndrome, which may then be bilateral. Equine protozoal myeloencephalitis (EPM) is one of the few generalized disorders which may produce signs of central-origin Horner's syndrome and the condition may be attributed, in these cases, to extensive brainstem disruption and specific damage within the tectotegmental tract of the spinal cord.

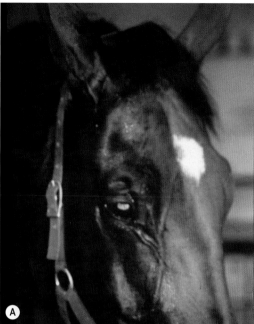

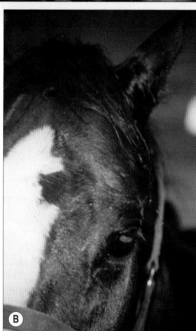

Figure 11.45 (A, B) Horner's syndrome. Sweating restricted to one side of the face with ptosis (drooping of the ipsilateral eyelid).

Diagnosis and treatment

- Diagnosis of Horner's syndrome itself is obvious on the basis of clinical signs but diagnosis of the cause of the Horner's syndrome may be somewhat more difficult and requires eliminating all possible causes.
- Treatment is aimed at the primary disorder.

Peripheral nerve damage

Damage to peripheral nerves occurs relatively frequently as a result of direct trauma to superficial nerves or as a result of excessive distraction of nerve roots and plexuses. The damage may be mild and result in a temporary or partial loss of function (neurapraxia) or more severe, causing permanent loss of function (neurotmesis). The extent

of the damage is important when assessing the prognosis of peripheral nerve lesions; although some regeneration of peripheral nerve is possible, this is extremely slow. Damage involving the sensory nerves is often accompanied by no detectable clinical effect (such as those in the distal limb), but loss of sensation in other areas, such as the face, may cause severe distress, and result in self-trauma.

Damage to individual peripheral motor nerves of visible muscles results in a very obvious and rapidly developing atrophy. The extent of the atrophy depends largely on the location of nerve disruption. Denervation atrophy is usually rapid and particularly well-defined when compared to secondary atrophy following physical muscle damage or interference with blood supply.

Suprascapular nerve 'Sweeney' (Fig. 11.46)

Fractures of the neck of the scapula, the scapular tuberosity, or blows to the shoulder, or extremes of movement (particularly caudal extension of the shoulder) may result in clinically significant damage to the **suprascapular nerve**. The path of the suprascapular nerve around the neck of the scapula makes it liable to stretching and bruising trauma, even in the absence of any obvious fractures. Damage to this nerve is often complicated by concurrent damage in the brachial plexus.

Damage to the nerve results in neurogenic atrophy of the infraspinatus and supraspinatus muscles resulting in prominence of the scapular spine.

Consequent loss of lateral support for the shoulder joint normally maintained by these muscles results in a characteristic outward bowing of the joint when the animal is weight-bearing.

The sudden outward excursion of the shoulder joint itself may be responsible for continued stretching (and, therefore, dysfunction of the nerve), even in the event that the damage is slight initially.

Diagnosis, treatment and prognosis

- In most cases the diagnosis is retrospective when muscle atrophy becomes apparent but can be suspected early on the basis of history of trauma and characteristic movement of shoulder joint.
- In most cases any trauma would have been treated at the time of injury. There is no specific treatment and recovery is usually prolonged due to the slow regeneration of nerve fibers. Stall confinement (at least initially) may help limit ongoing damage.
- Prognosis is dependent on whether there is brachial plexus involvement, which unfortunately may be impossible to diagnose without other more obvious signs of brachial plexus involvement.

Radial nerve paralysis (Figs. 11.47 & 11.48)

The radial nerve is the largest outflow from the brachial plexus and innervates the extensors of the elbow, carpus and digit. It also has a sensory component to the front of the antebrachium (forearm). Trauma involving **brachial plexus disruption**, from simultaneous over-extension and adduction of the shoulder causing overstretching of the plexus, or damage to the shaft or overlying muscles of the humerus, may affect the function of the radial nerve. The clinical signs depend upon the severity and location of the damage. True **radial paralysis** is not common; usually some brachial plexus involvement occurs simultaneously. However, recognition of the differences is important with respect to prognosis and the nursing requirements.

Damage to the radial nerve distal to the brachial plexus results only in loss of elbow extension and limited skin hypoalgesia. Damage involving only the radial nerve is not common but is encountered both from relatively minor trauma and is associated with humeral shaft fractures. Characteristically the limb cannot be voluntarily extended and, unless placed in its natural position by an attendant, is unable to bear weight. However, once the limb is placed appropriately, the horse may bear weight relatively normally, until a

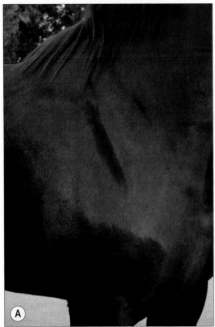

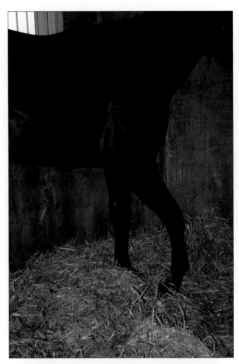

Figure 11.47 Radial nerve paralysis. Note the dropped elbow. The radial paralysis in this case was temporary following anesthesia.

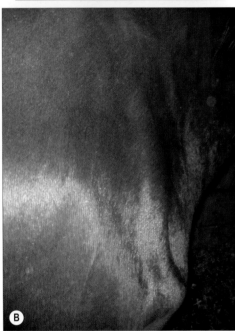

Figure 11.46 Sweeney. (A) Atrophy of infraspinatus and supraspinatus muscles. This image was taken 1 week after known injury had occurred indicating the speed at which neurogenic muscle atrophy occurs. This horse never recovered fully, indicating the possible presence of concurrent brachial plexus injury. (B) Severe atrophy of the infraspinatus and supraspinatus muscles with prominence of the scapular spine. This image was taken some months after the initial injury. This horse in contrast made a full recovery over 12 months and raced successfully.

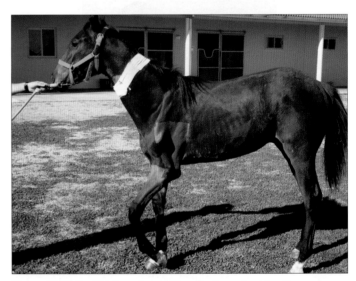

Figure 11.48 Brachial plexus damage. Note the dropped and flaccid appearance of the limb and regional muscle wastage.

step is required. In most cases the branch of the nerve to the triceps muscle is most severely involved and the elbow therefore has a dropped appearance while the distal limb is flexed. The limb typically rests with the dorsum of the pastern on the ground and voluntary movement is undertaken by thrusting the limb forward from the shoulder. Mild, partial damage to the radial nerve may only produce a tendency to stumble when the affected foot encounters a slight obstacle. Long-standing damage results in atrophy of the muscles innervated by the

nerve including, most obviously, the triceps brachialis, extensor carpi radialis, ulnarislateralis and the digital extensor muscles. The loss of triceps function does not always result in a severe handicap with some horses adapting very well.

Brachial plexus damage involves both extensors and flexors of the forelimb and the limb is completely unable to bear weight even when placed in its natural position. The limb has a flaccid appearance with a dropped shoulder, in addition to the signs of more distal radial nerve paralysis. The limb appears to be too long for the horse. Brachial plexus disruption is accompanied in most cases by suprascapular paralysis.

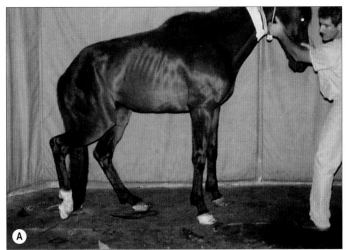

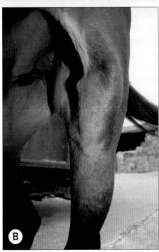

Figure 11.49 (A) Femoral nerve paralysis. (B) Quadriceps wasting associated with chronic femoral nerve paralysis.

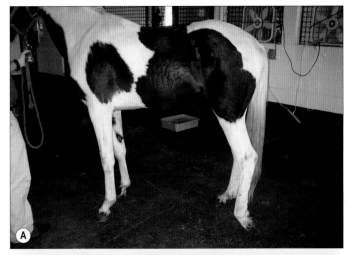

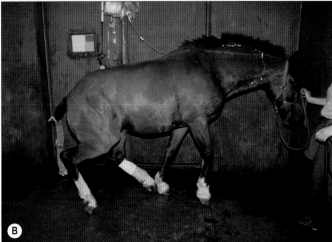

Figure 11.50 Sciatic nerve paralysis. (A) Unilateral, note the extension of the stifle and hock. (B) Bilateral, note inability to bear weight adequately with knuckling over onto dorsum of hoof with attempts to move.

Femoral nerve (Fig. 11.49)

The femoral nerve, which innervates the quadriceps femoris group of muscles on the dorsal and lateral aspects of the thigh, is prone to damage from direct trauma or from over-stretching as a result of over-extension of the limb. Affected horses are unable to bear weight, with all the joints of the limb flexed. Hypoalgesia of the medial thigh may be detectable. Ultimately, atrophy of the quadriceps femoris and vastus muscle masses results in the formation of dense fibrous metaplasia, which may feel like tendons rather than muscle masses. Femoral and/or sciatic nerve neurapraxia sometimes occurs in newborn foals after assisted deliveries, particularly where there has been considerable force applied as the hips are delivered through the pelvic canal in either anterior or posterior presentations.

Sciatic nerve (Fig. 11.50)

Damage to the sciatic nerve is a result of either direct trauma associated with coxo-femoral luxations, fractures of the acetabulum, pelvic fractures or sacral/pelvic osteomyelitis. The most common cause is misdirected injections of irritant drugs in the caudal buttock, which results in loss of both tibial and peroneal nerve function. While the loss of sensory functions results in hypoalgesia of the distal limb (from the stifle down), the loss of motor function results in poor limb flexion with the stifle and hock extended (i.e. virtually straight) and the fetlock flexed; possibly even standing on the dorsum of the

pastern. Weight can be born on the limb if it is placed into its normal position, but if the animal moves the weight is supported by the dorsum of the hoof.

Obturator nerve (Fig. 11.51)

Damage to the obturator nerve occurs much less frequently in the horse than in the bovine, but fetal oversize and dystocia may nevertheless cause obturator neurapraxia. The loss of adductor ability affecting the muscles of the medial upper thigh is characteristic. The affected limb may not support weight effectively, particularly when sudden movement or turning is attempted. There is a persistent danger in these cases of serious adductor muscle rupture or coxo-femoral dislocations and femoral, pelvic or sacral fractures.

Stringhalt (Figs. 11.52 & 11.53)

Stringhalt is an involuntary hyperflexion of one or both hindlimbs during movement. In most parts of the world it occurs as an isolated disorder in individual horses, but in Australasia it sometimes occurs in epidemics associated with the ingestion of flatweed (*Hypochaeris radicata*), dandelion (*Taraxacum officinale*), or sweet pea (*Lathyrus* spp.) plants. The clinical features of both forms of the disorder are similar with respect to the appearance of the involuntary flexion, but in the Australian form both hindlimbs are usually affected and, occasionally, the forelimbs and neck may also be involved.

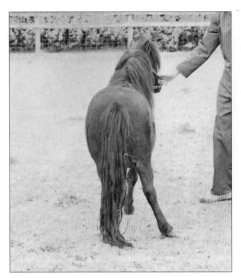

Figure 11.51 Obturator paralysis. Assisted parturition 6 hours previously. Loss of adductor ability in both hindlimbs with the right worse affected.

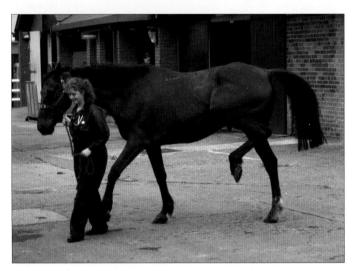

Figure 11.52 Stringhalt, unilateral. Note the marked hyperflexion of the affected limb.

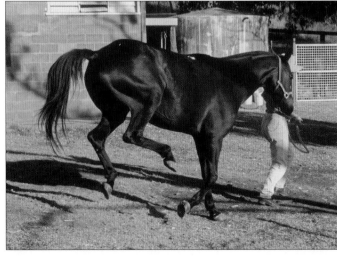

Figure 11.53 Bilateral stringhalt.

The two conditions differ clinically only in degree, with the sporadic form usually being milder, sometimes unilateral and possibly permanent. Individual horses affected by the sporadic form show a sudden jerking of the hind leg during walking of variable severity, which may be occasional or occur with every step. Less severe cases may show only a slight spasm of the leg without marked lifting of the foot. In more severe cases, however, the dorsal aspect of the fetlock may even hit the abdominal wall with considerable force and this will obviously have a marked effect upon gait. It can often be made more obvious by turning or backing the horse. Progression is sometimes ungainly, but the animal appears unconcerned, and any pace faster than a walk is usually normal or nearly normal. Although the etiology of the sporadic form is uncertain, it is considered to be a neurogenic disorder.

In **Australian stringhalt**, both hindlimbs are generally, equally and severely affected, and the signs may be severe enough to prevent forward movement, with extreme spasms of both flexor and extensor muscle groups resulting in a state of tetanus. The extensor and flexor muscles of the hindlimbs below the stifle, in severe cases, frequently become atrophied giving a 'peg-leg' appearance. Affected horses may develop concurrent laryngeal paralysis (usually restricted to the left side but occasionally right-sided or bilateral).

Diagnosis and treatment

- The characteristic gait is usually diagnostic.
- Traditionally sporadic cases of stringhalt were thought to have a poor chance of recovery or improvement without surgical intervention. Tenotomy or tenectomy of the lateral digital extensor tendon has been the surgical treatment of choice. Conservative management techniques of gradually increasing exercise, anti-inflammatories or corticosteroids have resulted in favorable responses in some individual cases and one report showed no difference between horses treated surgically and those treated conservatively.
- Some cases of Australian stringhalt may resolve spontaneously over weeks or months, provided that no further ingestion of the offending plants is allowed. In some cases, however, obvious neurological deficits including laryngeal paralysis remain.

Polyneuritis equi (cauda equina neuritis)
(Fig. 11.54)

Horses of all ages and types are occasionally affected by a granulomatous polyneuritis known as the cauda equina neuritis syndrome (polyneuritis equi). While the clinical signs of the disorder are classically

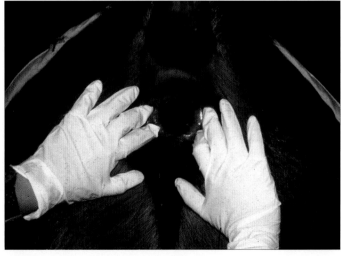

Figure 11.54 Cauda equina neuritis poor tail tone

associated with neurological deficits within the cauda equina, the disorder has a number of alternative features. Most cases are presented with some degree of urinary and fecal incontinence, with anal flaccidity, accompanied by a well-defined area of hypalgesia or analgesia in the perineal area. Bladder sphincter atony results in urine dribbling from a flaccidly distended bladder; squirts of urine appearing during vocalization or when the horse moves or, particularly, when it rises from recumbency. Tail paralysis is a common finding. The loss of rectal, anal and bladder reflexes and perineal sensation results in a dramatic accumulation of progressively drier food material and progressively more bladder distension, often to the point where the horse develops colic symptoms associated with primary impaction of the small colon and/or chronic cystitis. In some cases subtle alterations in hindlimb gait are noticeable and, in these, or occasionally independently of this sign, there may be profound unilateral muscle atrophy of the gluteal muscles.

Involvement of nerve roots including cranial nerves and individual spinal nerves may be present. Subtle or sometimes obvious cranial nerve deficits including facial paralysis, trigeminal deficits and vestibular disturbances may be present at the same time or, indeed, without concurrent cauda equina symptoms. The **cranial nerve syndromes** are often subtle and may easily be overshadowed by the more dramatic perineal and pelvic deficits or may be missed completely when, as may rarely occur, they exist on their own. Their distribution may be very localized, even to the point of affecting only one branch of the facial nerve.

The rate of progression of this untreatable disease may be very variable with some cases deteriorating rapidly while others appear to maintain a static state for months or years.

Diagnosis, treatment and prognosis
- The detection of circulating antibodies to myelin sheath (P2) proteins is a useful means of confirming the diagnosis.
- The prognosis is, at best, poor but the progression may be slow or almost inapparent.
- At post-mortem examination a moderate to severe granulomatous polyneuritis with discoloration and hemorrhage of the cauda equina can usually be found. In some cases, however, there may be little obvious pathology and histopathological examination may be required.
- Cases involving cranial nerves, or specific spinal nerves without cauda equina involvement, may show only histological evidence of the progressive neuropathy characteristic of the disorder.

Shivers (Fig. 11.55)
Shivering is a condition of unknown etiology with a suspected genetic origin that has been long recognized in draft breeds. It is characterized by spasmodic muscle tremors affecting the hindlimbs and tail and is most commonly observed if the horse is asked to back, turn or lift a hindlimb. Typically, one limb is held in a flexed and abducted position with muscle trembling for a few moments and is then slowly lowered to a normal position. Elevation and tremor of the tail are also commonly observed. Forced flexion of the hock, such as during farrier work, may produce signs in an otherwise normal-appearing animal.

Diagnosis, treatment and prognosis
- Diagnosis is based on clinical signs but these may be subtle.
- This condition is slowly progressive, although in some cases the signs may plateau. Hence there is a guarded long-term prognosis with no effective treatment.

Gomen disease
Gomen disease is a progressive degenerative cerebellar disease recognized in the northwest part of New Caledonia, which causes mild to severe ataxia. The pathogenesis is unknown but is thought to involve

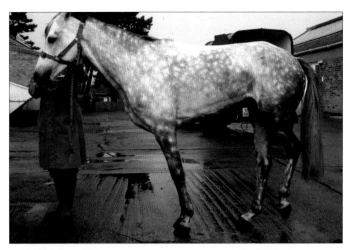

Figure 11.55 Shivers. Note the abduction of the hindlimb and raised tail.

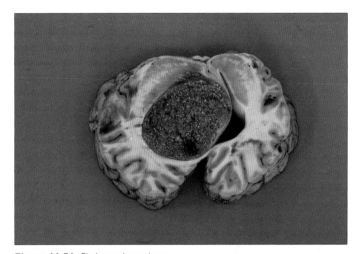

Figure 11.56 Cholesterol granuloma.

a metabolic disorder, perhaps resulting from toxicity. It occurs in indigenous and introduced horses that are allowed to roam free with confined horses generally unaffected. Signs may take 1–2 years to develop following introduction to an endemic area. Prominent signs include ataxia and a wide-based stance referable to cerebellar involvement and weakness likely due to brainstem or spinal cord involvement. The condition is progressive with most horses dying or being euthanized within 3–4 years.

Diagnosis
- Diagnosis can be suspected on the basis of clinical signs but confirmed at necropsy where gross examination of the brain reveals cerebellar atrophy, with severe depletion of Purkinje neurons visible histologically.
- There is moderate to severe lipofuscin pigmentation of neuron cell bodies throughout the brain and spinal cord that is considered greater than what would normally be expected in horses of a similar age.

Cholesterol granuloma (Fig. 11.56)
Cholesterol granulomas are found incidentally in the choroid plexuses of up to 20% of older horses. They occur more commonly in the fourth ventricle but usually reach a larger size in the lateral ventricles and are thus more likely to cause clinical signs. They appear as

brownish nodular thickenings and microscopically consist of abundant cholesterol crystals interspersed with hemosiderin, empty clefts and an inflammatory reaction consisting of giant cells and macrophages. Compression of brain tissue or an obstructive hydrocephalus may result. Clinical signs are insidious in onset and include altered behavior, depression, somnolence, seizures ataxia, weakness and unconsciousness.

Diagnosis and treatment

- Diagnosis is difficult although advanced imaging techniques may now result in increased ante-mortem diagnosis.
- There is no specific treatment and relief of clinical signs is usually attained symptomatically.

Nutritional and metabolic conditions resulting in neurological disease

Nutritional and metabolic derangements may exert powerful and profound effects upon nerve function. While few of these diseases present illustratable clinical features, they are of importance with respect to differential diagnosis.

Hypoglycemia

Blood glucose levels of less than 40-50 mg/dl may result in weakness, depression and ataxia, and can progress to loss of consciousness. Hypoglycemia is not normally associated with seizure activity except in neonates. If untreated, hypoglycemia may result in irreversible brain damage. The principal lesion of hypoglycemia is ischemic neuronal cell change, similar to that of cerebral hypoxia, with neurons of the cerebral cortex most severely affected.

Hyponatremia (Fig. 11.57)

Hyponatremia is most commonly associated with conditions such as diarrhea, excessive sweat loss and adrenal insufficiency, which cause sodium depletion. The neurologic signs that are seen are a result of the rapidly developing hypotonic hyponatremia and include depression, convulsions and coma. Progressively, severe disturbances can be seen as the serum sodium concentration falls below 115 mg/dl, and then below 100mg/dl. The severity of signs depends not only on the degree of hyponatremia, but also on how quickly it develops.

Hypernatremia

Hypernatremia may occur in the initial stages of diarrhea, vomiting or renal disease if water loss exceeds electrolyte loss. The

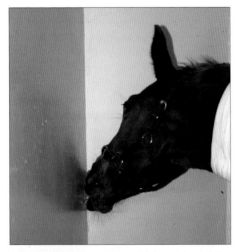

Figure 11.57 Hyponatremia. Compulsive wall licking in this foal that presented for enterocolitis and had severe hyponatremia. The clinical signs disappeared when the sodium levels were returned to normal.

hypernatremia that is observed in salt poisoning of ruminants and swine is associated with water restriction in animals that have been maintained on a high salt diet. Salt poisoning is associated with severe gastrointestinal and neurological signs, including head-neck extension, blindness, aggressiveness, hyperexcitability, ataxia, proprioceptive deficits and head pressing. The pathophysiology involves deposition of sodium ions in the CNS which, when followed by access to ion-free water, results in cerebral edema and death occurring by respiratory failure.

Hypocalcemia

See Chapter 6, p. 220.

Thiamine deficiency

Deficiency of thiamine either in absolute dietary terms (which is very unusual) or through the repeated ingestion of thiaminase enzymes also has significant effects upon neurological function. The bracken fern (*Pteridium aquilinum*) is very poisonous to horses when ingested over periods of 30–60 days or more, but is not usually palatable unless food is scarce. The entire plant contains a thiaminase which is not destroyed by drying and which results in a clinical thiamine deficiency syndrome. Nervous tissue is the first to suffer the effects of thiamine deficiency and the earliest signs affect the peripheral motor nerves. Gradual myelin degeneration in peripheral nerves causes a progressive weakness and incoordination (bracken staggers). Muscle weakness is initially only apparent during exercise, but progresses to recumbency and opisthotonus. Arching of the back, a base-wide, hindlimb stance and crossing of the front legs, followed by advancing weakness and recumbency are typical. Cardiac tachydysrhythmias and hemolytic crises are also encountered. The affected horse is dull and weak and there is often a concurrent pharyngeal paralysis.

Diagnosis and treatment

- A curative response to thiamine therapy is diagnostic in horses with an appropriate contact history.
- Poisoning with *Equisetum arvense* (Marestail) is clinically and physiologically identical.

Toxic plants (Fig. 11.58)

Many plants from all areas of the world are known to have serious toxic effects characterized by neurological signs. In some cases the clinical signs may appear to be related to the nervous system although the plant toxins actually have their major effects upon the liver (in particular) or other organs.

Some plants, however, are known to have marked direct toxic effects upon the central nervous system. In most cases they cause a diffuse encephalopathy with a wide range of signs including blindness, depression, dementia, seizures and in some cases subtle behavioral changes. *Astragalus* spp., *Oxytropis* spp., and crotalaria spp. plants, known as 'locoweeds' in North America, and *Swainsonia* spp. in Australia, contain the alkaloid locoine, and are perhaps the best identified plants producing notable clinical signs including aggression, dementia, ataxia, posterior paralysis and weight loss. The same group of plants accumulates selenium and repeated ingestion over a long period may produce clinical signs typical of selenium poisoning, including laminitis and hair loss.

Sorghum toxicity (see Chapter 5, p. 205) (Fig. 11.59)

A small proportion of horses ingesting large amounts of *Sorghum* spp. grasses (including Sudan and Milo grass) over prolonged periods may develop a paralysis of the bladder with persistent urine dribbling and, often, some degree of hindlimb ataxia. In some cases the condition may be indistinguishable from the cauda equina neuritis syndrome except that hindquarter ataxia and paralysis are more prominent features of sorghum toxicity. Diagnosis is based on history of access to sorghum-containing pasture and ruling out similar conditions.

Nigropallidal encephalomalacia

Sustained ingestion of significant amounts of the Yellow Star Thistle (*Centaurea solstitialis*) (and other members of this species such as Yellow Burr, Russian Knapweed and creeping knapweed), over some weeks, causes a specific equine neurological disorder characterized by difficulty with prehension, mastication and swallowing. The plant is found widely in the Western United States of America and in Australia and affected animals may obtain the plant directly from pastures or, more commonly, in preserved feeds. While the plant is not usually palatable to horses, some appear to become addicted to it and this represents the most dangerous situation. The disorder is associated with a progressive and profound malacic degeneration of the substantia nigra and the globus pallidus and is known as nigropallidal encephalomalacia.

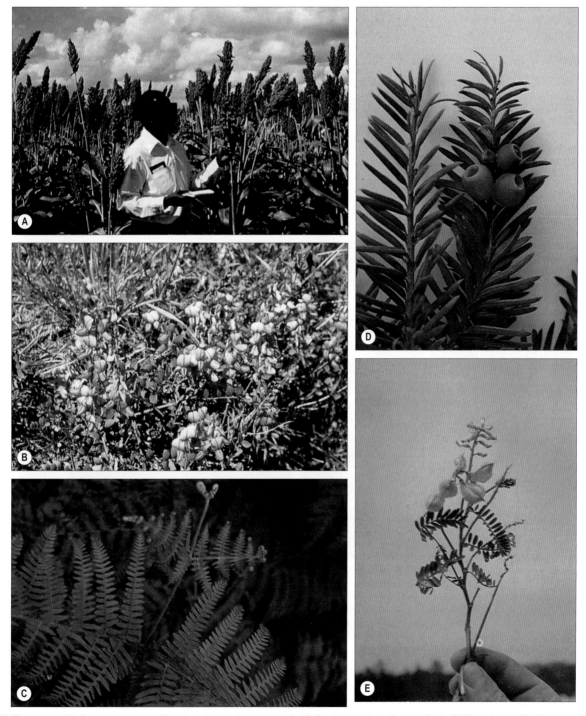

Figure 11.58 Toxic plants. (A) *Sorghum* spp. grass. (B) *Lathyrus hirsuitis* (singletary pea). (C) *Pterdium aquilinum* (bracken fern). (D) *Taxus baccata* (English yew). (E) *Astralagus* spp.

Continued

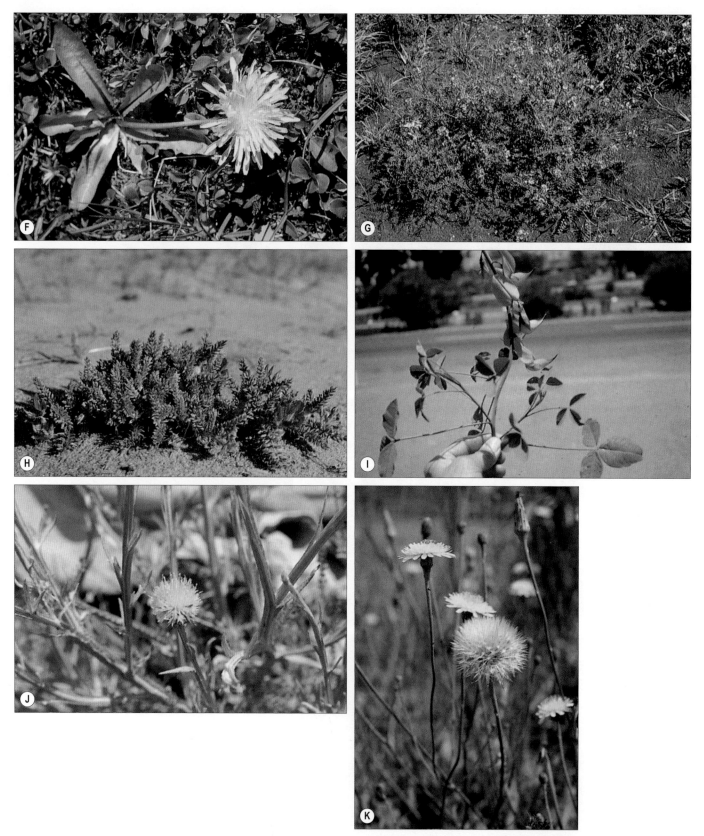

Figure 11.58, cont'd (F) *Taraxacum officinale* (dandelion). (G) *Swainsonia galegifolia*. (H) *Oxytropis* spp. (I) *Crotalaria* spp. (loco weed). (J) *Centauriasol stitialis* (yellow star thistle). (K) *Hypochaeris radicata* (flatweed).

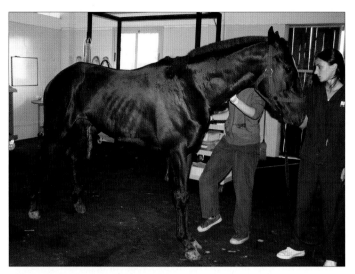

Figure 11.59 Sorghum toxicity. Paraphimosis and bladder paralysis. This horse had also loss of anal tone and hindlimb ataxia.

Differential diagnosis:
- Cauda equina neuritis (polyneuritis equi)
- Epidural anesthesia
- Equine herpes-1 virus infection (neurological syndrome)
- Sacrococcygeal fracture/luxation
- Cord neoplasia (melanoma, squamous cell carcinoma, lymphosarcoma).

There is a sudden onset of an obvious masticatory difficulty and affected horses are seen to prehend and then make ineffective chewing movements. Hay may be seen protruding from the mouth for prolonged periods, during which futile chewing movements continue. Mastication and swallowing are not effective and food material and water are apparently unable to be moved into the caudal parts of the oral cavity. The tongue may be seen to move back and forth from the mouth. Attempts to drink are often frustrated, with head dipping (often up to the eyes), and some horses resort to tipping the head back to allow water to run passively into the pharynx. Persistent unrewarding feeding attempts may result in a severe edema of the muzzle and nose. Wandering, ataxia and fasciculation of the masticatory muscles and dramatic weight loss occur in almost all cases.

More generalized central nervous signs such as head pressing, semi-conclusive seizures and incoordination are sometimes present but may reflect other aspects of the metabolic consequences of starvation and water deprivation. The condition has a very high mortality once clinical signs are present.

The donkey and mule are much less susceptible to the poisoning and, in spite of ingesting large amounts over long periods, seldom show any clinical effects.

Diagnosis and treatment
- Ante-mortem diagnosis relies largely on history of access to the plants and clinical signs. Where available magnetic resonance imaging can be used to demonstrate typical lesions.
- At post-mortem examination a pathognomonic liquefactive necrosis of the nigropallidal regions of the brain which may be extensive and obvious or subtle, with only microscopic evidence of the problem, are identified.
- There is no effective treatment and control by limiting exposure to the plants is the best policy.

Mycotoxicosis

Central nervous signs are also a feature of mycotoxicosis and the best defined form of this group of disorders is due to toxins produced by molds such as *Fusarium moniliforme* in corn. Sustained ingestion of the toxin over 4 weeks or more induces a progressive liquefactive necrosis of the cerebral cortex (leukoencephalomalecia, see also Chapter 2, p. 91). Characteristically this causes sudden and unexpected death in one or more animals under the same managemental regime. Dementia, blindness, convulsions and ataxia may be seen prior to death. Death is virtually certain within 24 hours of the development of any of the clinical signs, although some horses suspected of being affected have survived with longstanding/permanent neurological (cerebral) deficits. Cranial nerve signs include dysphagia and laryngeal paralysis, and facial and trigeminal disorders occur in some cases.

Diagnosis
- Post-mortem examination usually shows definite areas of liquefactive necrosis of the subcortical white matter in the cerebral hemispheres.
- In some cases hepatic pathology is also present and may produce obvious icterus, hemorrhagic diatheses and signs of hepatoencephalopathy.

Yew poisoning

Ingestion of leaves and berries of the ornamental yew tree (*Taxus baccata* and *Taxus caspicata*) results in sudden death related to the alkaloid, taxine. The horse is one of the most sensitive species to the effects of the alkaloid and a single mouthful may be lethal. The leaves remain poisonous in a dry state.

Diagnosis

Death is abrupt and post-mortem examination shows no pathognomonic features. Fortunately the needles are distinctive and masticated pieces of them can usually be found in the mouth or stomach of affected horses. However, the small amounts required to cause death may make their detection very difficult.

Equine motor neuron disease (EMND)
(Figs. 11.60 & 11.61)
Motor neuron disease is a degenerative disorder of the somatic lower motor neurons of horses. The disease was first described in the 1990s with results of epidemiological, laboratory and experimental studies

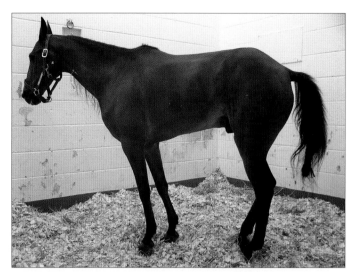

Figure 11.60 EMND. Shifting weight between the hindlimbs and raised tail.

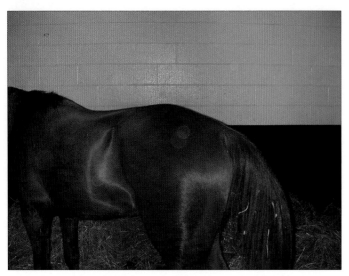

Figure 11.61 EMND. Muscle tremors of the upper limbs and tail were present.

supporting vitamin E deficiency as the primary risk factor for EMND. Most affected horses have a history of limited or no access to pasture which accounts for the vitamin E deficiency seen. However, there is a smaller group of affected horses that have had access to pasture but in these there has also been low serum vitamin E levels. Oxidative damage (as a result of this deficiency) to somatic neurons and the retina account for the clinical signs seen.

Affected horses frequently have a hyperalert, worried facial expression and extensive muscle fasciculations, which are most apparent in the muscles of the head and the upper limbs. Weight shifting from one leg to another, a stance with the hindlegs tucked under the abdomen and diffuse sweating are encountered and are associated with the increased muscular effort associated with maintaining a standing posture. The animal usually takes every available opportunity to rest and lies down with difficulty, resting the head either by propping itself up by the muzzle or by profound relaxation in full lateral recumbency.

Diagnosis
- Clinical signs and history are suggestive in many cases.
- Plasma vitamin E concentrations are consistently <1 µg/ml, selenium concentration is normal, vitamin A concentration is low to normal and serum ferritin concentration is frequently high. Slight increases in muscle enzymes are commonly seen. Glucose absorption tests show low serum glucose concentrations, which are thought to result from increased glucose utilization.
- Biopsy of the sacrocaudalis dorsalismedialis muscle or spinal accessory nerve has a sensitivity of 90% for confirming the diagnosis.
- *Differential diagnosis:* other neuromuscular disorders, chronic myopathies and equine dysautonomia (which may have similar clinical signs).

Treatment
- Treatment consists of supplementing vitamin E. This is usually done with a combination of oral supplementation and moving the horse to lush pasture. Affected horses should be rested for 2–3 months after which controlled exercise may be started provided the clinical condition of the horse allows.
- Other drugs with antioxidant potential have been used but their efficacy has not been evaluated.

Prognosis and prevention
- Forty percent showed a marked improvement and response to therapy; 20% will have permanent muscle atrophy; 40% will continue to deteriorate, ultimately requiring euthanasia.
- Wherever possible horses should have access to green forage. If this is not possible supplementation with vitamin E is required. This can be done through feeds with a high content or supplements; 10 000 IU/day/horse is commonly used.

Equine degenerative myeloencephalopathy

Equine degenerative myeloencephalopathy (EDM) is a diffuse degenerative disease of the spinal cord and brainstem. The disease has been shown to have a familial hereditary basis in some breeds including Morgans, Appaloosa, Standardbreds and Paso Finos and is suspected in a number of other breeds. Vitamin E deficiency early in life has been implicated as a causative factor; although the exact pathogenesis is not known. By the time that clinical signs become apparent the vitamin E levels may be normal. The disease usually occurs in foals of either sex but may affect horses up to 3 years of age.

The disease may occur in an individual or may affect groups of young horses (usually related). The onset of signs may be abrupt or insidious. Symmetric ataxia, paresis and dysmetria are seen with pelvic limb signs worse than thoracic limb signs. Clinical signs may stabilize for several months or may progress to causing recumbency. Other signs that are reported include marked hyporeflexia over the neck and trunk, including absent slap test, cutaneous trunci reflex and cervicofacial reflex.

Diagnosis, treatment and prognosis
- It is difficult to differentiate this disease from other differential diagnosis, especially cervical stenotic myelopathy (CSM) (see p. 408). A definitive diagnosis can only be made by histopathological evaluation of the spinal cord which demonstrates diffuse axonal degeneration, myelin digestion and astrocytosis.
- Treatment should include oral supplementation of vitamin E (2–3 000 IU/day) in addition to ample green forage.
- No remission or recovery has ever been reported and treatment is aimed at stabilizing clinical signs. Affected animals and their parents should not be bred because of the heritable nature of the disease.

Neuroses

Neuroses (vices) are a common problem in horses, particularly those which are under-exercised and stabled. There is good evidence that these habits are quickly learned from other horses.

Crib-biting and wind-sucking

The most common vices are crib-biting and wind-sucking. Many animals are afflicted by both vices at the same time. Crib-biting is the habit of forceable grabbing of a fixed object between the incisor teeth and biting hard. Those which simultaneously wind-suck, then arch their necks and suck in air. The bolus of air is then swallowed and may create secondary disorders of gastrointestinal function including colic and weight loss. The appearance of the cribbing behavior is characteristic, and the wear pattern created on the incisor teeth as a result of the persistent misuse results in a typical appearance of wear on the buccal margin of the upper incisors which in early or mild cases, may be subtle. Some cases may wind-suck without crib-biting, and while most of these have a characteristic arching of the neck, others may extend the neck. Some may show no neck muscle involvement but still make obvious swallowing movements. The accompanying noise made by this swallowing is characteristic. In almost all cases there is a concurrent hypertrophy of the muscles of the ventral neck and the sternocephalicus in particular. Horses can be treated for this condition by the application of a cribbing strap or metal cribbing bar but some manage to wind-suck or crib with these in place. The condition is virtually impossible to treat effectively without recourse to surgical myectomy and neurectomy but even this has a high rate of failure.

Self-mutilation syndrome

Mature lightweight stallions, in particular, are prone to the self-mutilation syndrome (see Chapter 9, p. 312). Horses with a nervous disposition whose circumstances change dramatically may develop the disorder. Dramatic self-mutilation, with biting and chewing at particular sites on the body, is evident. Most cases show a variety of associated nervous signs including squealing and spinning round, and seem to pick on a particular site, usually one stifle or shoulder, biting and chewing at it incessantly. The odor of seminal fluid seems to act as a particular trigger for the behavior, which may result in alopecia, leukotrichia and localized scarring. As it occurs in horses which are bored and which have recently changed environment, it may be that the condition is a neurosis. Most cases can be temporarily and easily distracted.

Head shaking (Fig. 11.62)

Head shaking is a widely recognized disorder characterized by persistent or intermittent, spontaneous and repetitive vertical, horizontal or rotary movements of the head and neck. Other signs seen with this disorder are snorting, sneezing, nose rubbing, flipping the upper lip, striking at the face, corner seeking and nostril clamping. The signs seen can be mild or can be severe enough to lead to the horse being dangerous and unusable.

There are many possible cited etiologies, a combination of which may be present in any given case. The two that have received most attention are photophobia and trigeminal neuralgia. Other causes are rider or bit resentment, dental, ophthalmic or guttural pouch disease; cranial nerve abnormalities, cervical injury, ear mites or allergic rhinitis.

The majority of horses are affected seasonally in the spring and summer but many are affected year round. Many features of head shaking in horses are similar to trigeminal neuralgia in humans with certain trigger factors inducing sudden sharp pain.

Diagnosis and treatment

- A complete clinical examination should be performed to rule out as many causes as possible.
- Diagnostic blockade of the trigeminal nerve branches (infraorbital nerve or posterior ethmoidal nerve), may help in identifying trigger points in affected horses. Early indications showed that neurectomy may be a possible treatment but the results of neural blockade and neurectomy do not always correlate and because of complications such as neuroma formation, neurectomy is no longer recommended.
- Therapies aimed at decreasing the response to trigger factors can be effective in up to 70% of horses. These include tinted contact lenses, face masks or hoods and nose nets.
- Cyroheptadine (0.3 mg/kg orally q 12 h) has been used with reported success in a large number of cases. A combination of cyproheptadine with carbamazepine (4–8 mg/kg PO q 6–8 h) has been reported to be effective in horses that have failed to respond to cyproheptadine alone.

Infectious disorders

Otitis media-interna/temporohyoid osteoarthropathy (Figs. 11.63–11.65)

Otitis media-interna is uncommon in horses compared to other species. It is assumed that infection of the middle ear arises as a result of hematogenous spread or a direct extension of infectious processes in the pharynx, guttural pouch or external ear. Clinical signs that are seen are normally those of a peripheral vestibular syndrome, with head tilt, circling and ataxia. Concurrent ipsilateral facial paralysis is common and usually results from extension of the suppurative process from the middle ear into the adjacent facial canal or internal acoustic meatus containing cranial nerve VII. Signs of facial nerve damage

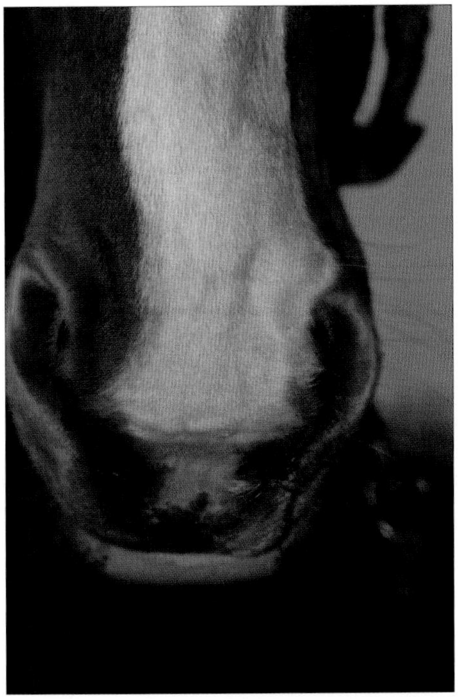

Figure 11.62 Nostril clamping which is a frequently encountered feature of headshaking.

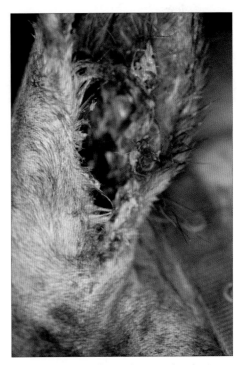

Figure 11.63 Otitis externa most frequently occurs alone but in rare cases there may be extension of the infection to the middle ear resulting in otitis media. Such outwards signs of disease make diagnosis a lot easier.

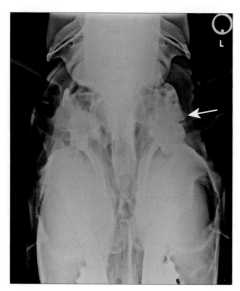

Figure 11.64 Otitis media. Radiograph showing sclerosis and thickening of the affected tympanic bulla (arrow).

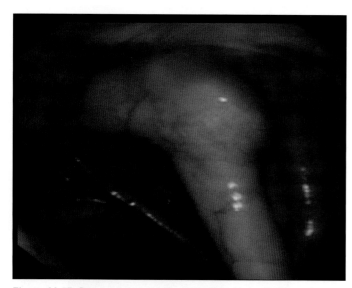

Figure 11.65 Otitis media interna endoscopic image showing thickening of the proximal portion of the stylohyoid bone.

such as exposure keratitis may precede the vestibular signs. Discharge from the external ear following rupture of the tympanic membrane is rarely seen. Head shaking has been reported as another rare clinical sign in cases of primary otitis media (Blythe 1997).

Diagnosis is based on clinical signs, endoscopy and radiography with or without isolation and culture of an infectious organism. Endoscopy may demonstrate pharyngitis, guttural pouch disease or proliferative lesions involving the petrous temporal bone and proximal portion of the stylohyoid bone. Radiographs show sclerosis of the affected tympanic bulla even in acute cases, thickening and sclerosis of the stylohyoid and petrous temporal bones. Exudates from the ear, guttural pouch or pharynx should be cultured in addition to any abnormal CSF (uncommon). Flushing sterile fluid through the middle ear via tympanocentesis can confirm the presence of sepsis. *Streptococcus* sp., *Staphylococcus* sp., *Actinobacillus* sp. and *Aspergillus* sp. have been cultured, but frequently the presence of infection or a causative agent cannot be determined. Many cases that are diagnosed

as otitis media or otitis interna are in fact secondary manifestations of temporohyoid joint disease without middle ear infection. However, antibiotic treatment is justified in all suspected cases of middle ear infection. Prolonged courses of antibiotic treatment are usually required in addition to short-term corticosteroid treatment (12–48 hours) and treatment of signs of facial nerve paralysis. Similar to cases of temporohyoid osteopathy removal of a section of the affected stylohyoid bone may minimize mechanical stresses resulting from ankylosis of the temporohyoid joint. Facial nerve and compensated vestibular function may remain following functional recovery.

Otitis media is rare in horses but ascending infections from guttural pouch infections and foreign bodies in the external auditory meatus (with concurrent otitis externa) are encountered occasionally. The clinical signs are usually somewhat less dramatic than in traumatic disruption of the vestibular nerve pathways. Aural discharges and systemic illness are often present.

Borna disease (Near Eastern encephalitis)

Borna disease (Flaviviridae) is an encephalitis of mammals with natural infections encountered commonly in horses, sheep, goats, cattle and rabbits. Outbreaks have been reported in countries across Europe and the Middle East. The viruses of borna disease and Near Eastern encephalitis are indistinguishable. The virus is transmitted between birds by the tick *Hyalomma anatolicum*. The borna disease virus is shed through nasal secretions and urine from infected animals. It is resistant to drying and adverse environmental conditions. Clinical signs are similar to those seen with other viral encephalitides; ataxia, head pressing, head tilt, compulsive movements and muscular tremors.

Diagnosis and treatment

- Identification of antibodies in the serum and CSF of infected horses.
- Gross pathology is usually unremarkable. Histologically, the characteristic lesion is the Joest-Degen inclusion body in the neuronal nucleus.
- Affected animals are usually euthanized, as the mortality rate is high and the virus can cause latent and persistent infections.

Alphavirus (Togaviridae) encephalitis of horses (Figs. 11.66–11.69)

- *Eastern equine encephalitis* (EEE). There is one EEE virus with two antigenic variants, North American and South American. EEE is recognized primarily in southeastern Canada and most of the United States east of the Mississippi river, although it has been recognized in the Carribean and Central and South America. Enzootic cycles in North America involve a mosquito vector, and passerine birds as an amplifying host. There is a seasonal variation in disease with peak incidence in late summer or early fall. Infected horses and humans are regarded as dead end hosts as the level of viremia that develops is insufficient to infect epizootic hosts.

- *Western equine encephalitis* (WEE). The WEE complex has seven virus species. WEE occurs throughout most of the Americas and Canada with extensive epizootics in Argentina. The principal enzootic vector is *Culextarsalis* and the epizootic mosquito vector is an *Aedes* species. At intervals of 5–10 years the level of viral transmission within the maintenance cycle is more intense with epidemics and epizootics occurring in horses and humans. Equine cases usually precede human cases by several weeks and thus act as a sentinel for humans. Similar to EEE, humans and horses are regarded as dead-end hosts for WEE infection.

- *Venezuelan equine encephalitis* (VEE). The VEE complex is one virus with six antigenic subtypes (I through VI). The geographic range is primarily South America with extension into Central

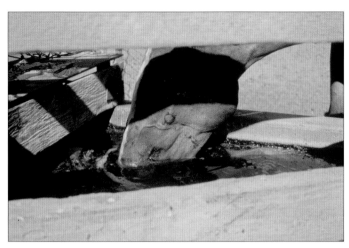

Figure 11.66 EEE. Due to pharyngeal and tongue paralysis affected horses frequently have difficulty drinking and may be seen to submerge a large proportion of the face in an attempt to obtain water.
Differential diagnosis: Nigropallidal encephalomalacia

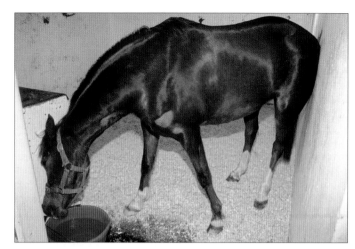

Figure 11.68 Abnormal behavior patterns and seizures can be seen in many encephalitis cases.

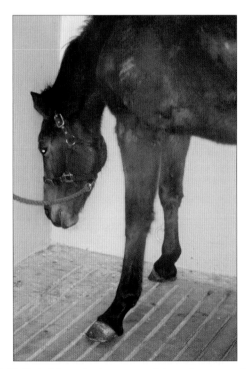

Figure 11.67 Marked depression is a common feature of many encephalitis cases.

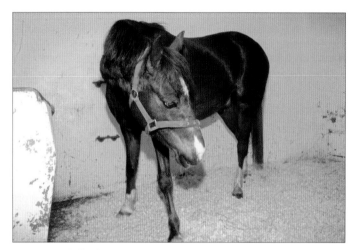

Figure 11.69 This horse experienced episodes of self-mutilation associated with encephalitis. He was also poorly aware of his surroundings.

VEE usually have a consistently elevated temperature during the disease.

- Other non-specific signs such as lethargy and stiffness are seen during the viremic phase. As the disease progresses clinical signs of neurological disease become more evident with the severity of signs dependent on the virus involved and the extent of CNS lesions.
- EEE and WEE usually have a similar initial clinical appearance with ataxia, somnolence, conscious proprioceptive deficits, stiff neck and compulsive walking or chewing. WEE does not usually progress beyond non-specific initial signs or less seldom mild CNS signs such as those above. EEE typically progresses to severe CNS deficits that occur secondary to diffuse cerebrocortical disease. Signs associated with more severe disease in EEE include apparent blindness and circling, excitement and aggressive behavior, laryngeal, pharyngeal and tongue paralysis and signs of brainstem dysfunction such as head tilt, nystagmus, strabismus and pupil dilation.
- VEE may also cause inapparent infections, signs similar to other encephalitis viruses or produce signs such as epistaxis, pulmonary hemorrhage, oral ulcers and diarrhea that may be unrelated to CNS damage.

America. However, epizootics have extended as far north as Texas. *Aedes* and *Psorophora* mosquito species transmit epizootic subtypes, in association with many different vertebrates leading to high mortality in both humans and horses. Unlike EEE and WEE, horses with VEE develop a sufficient viremia to act as an amplifier of the disease.

Clinical signs

- Infection with alphaviruses is associated with an initial incubation period of approximately 1 week in which a biphasic viremia takes place, although the first fever spike may not be noticed. Horses with

- Seizures can occur with any of the alphavirus infections and sudden death may also occur despite seemingly insignificant clinical signs.

Diagnosis

- Establishing a definitive diagnosis is important to allow implementation of control measures, but can be challenging. Clinical signs are usually not useful for diagnosis as they are non-specific or similar to other encephalitides.
- Serologic testing with a four-fold rise in antibody titers is diagnostic. However, a four-fold rise may not be detected as antibody levels rise rapidly after infection and a delay in taking the acute sample frequently results in sampling during the peak antibody titer. Another problem frequently encountered with serologic testing is that horses with EEE often do not live long enough for comparison of paired samples.
- High immunoglobulin M (IgM) titers suggest recent exposure to EEE virus and may be detected with an antibody-capture enzyme linked immunosorbent assay (ELISA).
- Definitive ante-mortem diagnosis can also be made based on viral isolation or identification of viral nucleic acid by reverse transcriptase-polymerase chain reaction (RT-PCR). EEE, WEE or VEE viruses can be isolated from brain tissue of infected horses via Vero-cell culture or mouse. Virus isolation from serum is usually unsuccessful. RT-PCR is a sensitive and specific test for detection of viral nucleic acid in CNS tissue or CSF.
- Other non-specific findings are peripheral leukocytosis and increased cellularity and elevated protein concentration of CSF.

Treatment and prevention

- There is no specific treatment available and current therapy is based on supportive care. Anti-inflammatory drugs and DMSO are commonly used to reduce CNS inflammation in addition to good nursing care, monitoring of hydration status and protection from self-induced trauma.
- Prevention is based on vaccination and limiting exposure to vectors which involves efforts to eliminate mosquitoes or their habitats. Recommendations vary on the region, with vaccination 2–4 times annually recommended in temperate areas where vectors may survive all year round. In areas bordering's Central America or for horses traveling to endemic areas twice-yearly vaccination with VEE is recommended. Foals from vaccinated dams are generally protected for 6–7 months. Vaccination of foals against EE should be started at 4 months of age in endemic areas and repeated at 6 and 12 months of age (Wilson 1999).

West Nile virus

West Nile virus (Flavivirus) is a mosquito-borne disease that affects a broad range of animals including birds, cats, dogs, horses and humans and causes a meningoencephalomyelitis. It is now widespread across the United States, most of Europe, Africa, west and central Asia, Oceania and the Middle East. The virus cycles between bird reservoir hosts and mosquitoes. Competent bird reservoir hosts sustain an infectious viremia for 1–4 days following exposure and then develop lifelong immunity. Susceptible birds may become ill or die from myeloencephalitis. Humans, horses and other mammals are considered dead-end hosts as they do not develop a sufficient viremia to complete the cycle. Many species can develop an immune response to the virus without demonstrating signs of disease (Saville et al 2003). Cases are commonly seen in association with vector seasons. All ages and breeds can be affected. Less than 30% of infected horses show clinical signs.

Viremia in horses occurs 3–5 days following infection, with signs seen 6–10 days after infection. These signs vary from mild peripheral neuritis to encephalitis. Signs include pyrexia in approximately one-third of cases, although many may have had a previous unnoticed pyrexic episode, ataxia which is most prominent in the hindlimbs (71%), obtundation (43%), muscle fasciculations and muzzle twitching (45%) and hypersensitivity to touch (18%) (Saville 2003, Steinmann 2002). Other signs seen include blindness, compulsive walking, dog-sitting, head pressing, seizures and thoracic limb collapse. Lethargy is associated with subclinical cases.

Diagnosis

- WNV encephalomyelitis should be suspected in any horse showing signs of neurological disease in an area where WNV activity has been documented.
- Confirmation of a positive case of WNV infection has been based on IgM-capture enzyme-linked immunosorbent assay (MAC-ELISA) of serum or CSF. A MAC-ELISA revealing serum titers greater than or equal to 1 : 400 suggests recent exposure to the virus. This test is not affected by prior vaccination. It should be noted that confirmation of WNV infection may not always be consistent with a diagnosis of West Nile encephalitis.
- Plaque reduction neutralization test (PRNT) of serum can be affected by prior vaccination and as such is not recommended in horses with a history of vaccination. At necropsy viral isolation and PCR performed on brain tissue can confirm a diagnosis of West Nile encephalitis.
- Cytologic examination of the CSF shows a wide variety of changes in cell count and protein concentration.

Treatment, prognosis and prevention

- Similar to the Alphavirus encephalitides there is no specific treatment and therapy is based on supportive care.
- Approximately 30% of horses with neurological disease die or are euthanized 3–4 days after the onset of clinical signs. Euthanasia is warranted in cases that are unable to stand because of hindlimb paralysis or when signs of cerebral lesions (such as seizures or coma) are present. The 70% that recover usually have a complete resolution of clinical signs in weeks to months.
- Prevention is also based on limiting exposure to mosquito vectors and vaccination.
- A killed vaccine is available and has proved to be both safe and efficacious (Ng et al 2003).

Other arboviral diseases

Equine encephalosis (EE) is an acute arthropod-borne viral disease caused by the equine encephalosis virus which is classified in the genus orbivirus of the family Reoviridae. It is endemic in most parts of South Africa, with *Culicoides* spp. as the presumed vector of the disease. Most infections are subclinical with clinical cases developing ataxia, stiffness and facial swelling that is similar to African horse sickness. Infected horses are viremic for 4–7 days and can be infective for vectors during this time. There is no evidence that horses become carriers of the disease.

Equine infectious anemia is another arboviral infection of horses that may result in neuropathological change. The most common neurological sign seen is symmetric ataxia of the trunk and limbs. Other neurological signs reported are circling, gait alterations and behavioral changes. Hydrocephalus has also been found at necropsy. These signs may rarely occur alone but usually are present with clinical signs related to hemolymphatic dysfunction.

Other than those discussed above there is a variety of neurotropic arboviruses that have been reported to infect horses, leading to seroconversion and occasional disease. These include louping ill, Japanese B, St. Louis, Murray valley, Semliki forest, Russian spring-summer, Powassan and Ross River encephalitis viruses, which are all members of the family Flaviviridae. Members of the family Bunyaviridae such as Main Drain viruses and California group viruses may also cause neurological disease in horses.

Rabies (Figs. 11.70 & 11.71)

Rabies (Lyssavirus (Rhabdoviridae)) is a predominantly fatal neurological disease of warm-blooded animals. The rabies virus is highly neurotropic with strain differences in pathogenicity and host range. Rabies has been diagnosed in horses in most parts of the world. The presentation can be highly variable and should be considered as a differential in any horse showing neurological signs in an endemic area. Rabies has two classic cycles, canine (urban) rabies and wildlife (sylvatic) rabies, which includes bats in South America. The majority of wildlife vectors are small to medium-sized omnivores, such as skunks and raccoons in the United States. Domestic animals which are generally regarded as dead-end hosts may become infected as a result of contact with the wildlife vectors. Rabies is most commonly transmitted by salivary contamination of a bite wound. The incubation period varies from 2 weeks to several months depending on the

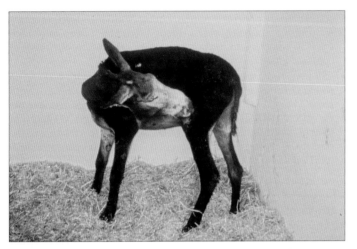

Figure 11.70 Aggression and self-mutilation signs in a donkey with rabies.

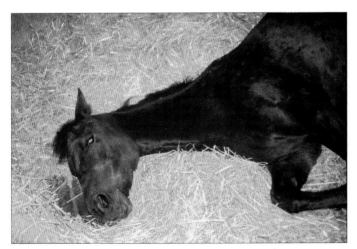

Figure 11.71 Recumbency and obtundation in a horse with rabies.

Differential diagnosis:
Other conditions with signs of gray matter disease such as polyneuritis equi, herpesvirus myeloencephalitis
Protozoamyeloencephalitis
Sorghum/Sudan grass poisoning
Other differentials include cerebral diseases such as hepatoencephalopathy, leukoencephalomalacia, alphavirus encephalitides, occupying masses, meningitis.

site of inoculation, dose and pathogenicity of the viral strain. Following inoculation the rabies virus replicates locally and after several days attaches to peripheral nerve receptors. The virus is then passed to the CNS via retrograde axoplasmic transport. Rabies virus has a predilection for replication in the cell bodies (gray matter) of the CNS with subsequent dysfunction of these neurons leading to behavioral changes and abnormalities of the cranial and peripheral nerves. The cause of death may be respiratory paralysis as a result of infection of the medulla. Shedding of the virus in nasal and salivary secretions has been shown to predate the onset of clinical signs by up to 29 days.

The presenting signs and clinical course are extremely variable (Green 1993). Reported signs have included any of the following: anorexia, depression, blindness, mania, hyperesthesia, muscle twitching, lameness, paresis, ataxia, colic, urinary incontinence and sudden death. The most commonly reported signs in horses are hyperesthesia, recumbency and aggressive behavior. The disease is normally rapidly progressive once signs are seen and results in death in 3–10 days.

Differentiation of rabies from other encephalitides on the basis of clinical signs is impossible.

Diagnosis

- A presumptive diagnosis in an endemic area on the basis of clinical signs is frequently made. Although not reliable such a diagnosis may be important in the light of possible human consequences.
- The gold standard for diagnosis is an indirect fluorescent antibody test using slices of brain which accurately diagnoses 98% of clinical cases. Intracerebral inoculation of mice is also considered an accurate method of diagnosis. Microscopic examination of hematoxylin-and-eosin-stained brain sections may reveal non-suppurative encephalitis and negri bodies which are diagnostic.
- CSF findings are usually non-specific and can include moderate increases in protein, mononuclear cells and occasionally neutrophils. An antigen-capture enzyme immunodiagnostic technique is available for ante-mortem diagnosis using salivary gland specimens but has not gained widespread clinical use (Perrin et al 1986).

Treatment and prevention

- Other than recovery in a presumptive case of experimentally produced rabies in a donkey (Ferris et al 1968), the disease has been reported as invariably fatal and suspected cases should be euthanized.
- The disease must be reported in many countries and managed in conjunction with public health officials.
- Inactivated annual vaccines are used for protection of horses in endemic areas.
- Foals in endemic areas should be vaccinated at 4–6 months of age with two doses given 3–4 weeks apart and followed by a booster at 1 year of age. If a vaccinated animal is bitten by a suspected rabid animal, it can be given three booster immunizations over 1 week and quarantined for at least 90 days.
- Exposed, unvaccinated animals of low economic value should be euthanized immediately. If the animal is valuable, confinement and close observation for at least 6 months is necessary.
- Primary immunization can be administered 1 month before release from quarantine.

Equine herpes virus myeloencephalopathy
(Fig. 11.72)

Equine herpes virus myeloencephalopathy (EHM) is a common cause of central nervous system (CNS) disease in the horse. Equine herpes virus (EHV) 1 is predominantly associated with neurological disease although there have been a number of isolated cases associated with EHV4 infection. EHM has been described in many countries and can occur with or without other EHV signs. Viremia results from

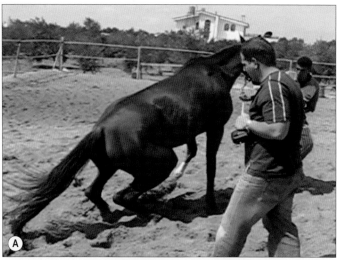

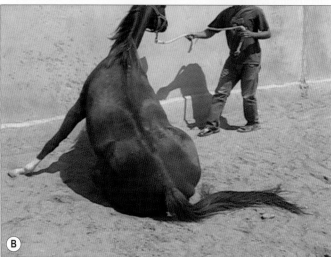

Figure 11.72 (A, B) This Arabian mare was presented for sudden onset of hindlimb weakness, decreased anal and tail tone, and urinary incontinence. She was confirmed to have EHV myeloencephalopathy.

Differential diagnosis of posterior paralysis:
• Rabies
• Traumatic/space-occupying lesion in cord
• Equine degenerative myeloencephalopathy
• Equine protozoal myeloencephalitis
• Vertebral osteomyelitis (e.g. tuberculosis)
• Secondary neoplasia (e.g. squamous cell carcinoma)
• Bracken fern (*Pteridium aquilinum*) poisoning
• Bilateral/generalized myopathy.

inhalation of virus and infection of respiratory epithelium or recrudescence of latent viral infection. Subsequent infection of CNS vascular endothelium results in thrombosis and ischemic myeloencephalopathy. Immune system involvement has been implicated by the lack of clinical signs in foals that have not been previously infected with EHV.

Clinical signs
• Cases may be sporadic and individual or multiple horses in a herd can be affected. The history often includes contact with horses demonstrating signs of herpesvirus disease.
• The onset of neurological signs is usually preceded by 1–6 days by fever, lethargy and inappetence of 1–3 days duration.
• Not all horses that become infected will demonstrate neurological signs. The signs that are most frequently seen are symmetric

hindlimb ataxia and paresis, bladder atony, fecal retention and recumbency. Many other signs have been reported and there is a wide range in the severity of signs seen.
• If recumbency occurs, it is usually within the first 24 hours and is associated with a much poorer prognosis. Those horses that remain standing show stabilization of signs in 24–48 hours and then slowly improve over the following weeks to months.

Diagnosis
• A presumptive diagnosis of EHM is often made on the basis of characteristic neurological signs, related history and characteristic CSF findings.
• Confirmation of the diagnosis can be difficult and requires either isolation of the virus from nasopharyngeal swabs and buffy coats or demonstration of a four-fold rise in serum-neutralizing, complement-fixing antibody or ELISA titers between acute and convalescent samples taken 7–21 days apart.
• Isolation of the virus from CNS tissue is difficult and differentiation between antibodies to EHV-1 and EHV-4 is also difficult, making a definitive diagnosis difficult to achieve. Complement fixation antibody titers are preferable as many horses have high levels of virus-neutralizing antibody, which is long-lived. Many cases have high levels of complement fixation antibodies (>1 : 160) at the onset of clinical signs.
• CSF frequently shows an increased total protein with little or no change in nucleated cell count. Xanthochromia (associated with red cell breakdown) is also frequently noted. Attempts to isolate the virus from the CSF have been largely unsuccessful. It is important to note that the changes seen in the CSF bear no correlation to the severity of clinical signs and cannot be used as a prognostic indicator (Donaldson 2003).

Treatment
• Supportive care including good nursing is the mainstay of treatment.
• Other controversial therapies include corticosteroid administration and administration of antiviral agents. The use of corticosteroids has been based on the theory that there may be an immune component to the neurological manifestations. This is still a controversial issue and evaluating the efficacy of corticosteroids is difficult given the natural course of the disease.
• Antiviral agents such as acyclovir and penciclovir have not yet been effectively evaluated in horses, although evidence suggests that they may lack suitable efficacy.
• Other treatments which are recommended by most authors are flunixinmeglumine (1.1 mg/kg IV q 12 h) for treatment of vasculitis and dimethyl sulfoxide (DMSO) for platelet inhibition and scavenging of free radicals.

Prevention
• Prevention is difficult as many asymptomatic horses have latent infections and vaccines which are currently used to prevent EHV-1 respiratory disease and abortion do not offer protection against myeloencephalopathy. Routine vaccination may, however, reduce exposure to the virus by reducing the incidence of other EHV-1 diseases.
• Vaccination during an outbreak has been controversial in the past but recent studies have not shown an increase in the number of clinical cases associated with vaccination during an outbreak.
• Management practices are important in helping to prevent the introduction and subsequent dissemination of EHV-1 infection; isolating new animals for 3 weeks and maintaining distinct herd groups according to age, gender and occupation. Pregnant mares

should not have access to the general population and stress should be minimized.

Listeriosis

Listeriosis in horses is rare and can be manifested as septicemia, abortion or meningoencephalomyelitis. The neurological form has signs referable to brainstem and cauda equina involvement. Infection has been associated with immunosuppression and ingestion of improperly prepared corn silage.

Diagnosis and treatment

- Blood cultures for *L. monocytogenes* have been positive in clinical cases but CSF analysis has not been reported (elevated protein levels and pleocytosis are likely based on the ruminant disease).
- Antibiotic treatment early in the course of infection should be effective.

Meningoencephalomyelitis (Figs. 11.73 & 11.74)

Meningitis in the horse is most often bacterial in origin and commonly occurs in one of three ways:

- Hematogenous spread from other sites
- Direct extension of a suppurative process in or around the head
- Secondary to penetrating wounds.

Septic meningitis results in profound neurological signs due to involvement of the superficial parenchyma and nerve roots of the brain and spinal cord. As the condition progresses secondary CNS edema and obstructive hydrocephalus may lead to a worsening of clinical signs (Webb & Muir 2000). Bacterial meningitis is most common in foals as a complication of bacterial septicemia and thus the bacteria involved are those that are commonly encountered in neonatal septicemia. α-Hemolytic streptococci, *Actinobacillus equuli*, *Escherichia coli* and staphylococci are most frequently encountered in young foals (Koterba et al 1990). *Salmonella* spp. meningitis can be seen in older foals.

Clinical signs

- Meningitis in foals should be regarded as a clinical emergency and early confirmation of the diagnosis is essential.
- The initial clinical signs such as aimless wandering, depression, loss of affinity for the dam and abnormal vocalization are not specific for meningitis, although specific for neurological involvement. These signs are typical of those seen in hypoxic ischemic encephalopathy in young foals and can cause misdiagnosis in the early stages.

- As meningitis progresses other signs such as hyperesthesia, muscular rigidity, blindness, cranial nerve deficits, ataxia and paresis of all limbs are seen. Without treatment, recumbency, coma, seizures and death can occur.
- CSF analysis demonstrates bacteria or increased numbers of inflammatory cells with high-protein and low-glucose concentration.
- Culture and cytology of CSF in addition to blood culture and culture of any other available septic sites should be performed in an attempt to isolate the causative organism.

Treatment

- Without bacterial isolation and sensitivity patterns or identification of an organism on cytology, treatment with broad-spectrum or combination antimicrobials is required. Commonly used treatments include aminoglycoside and penicillin combinations, potentiated sulfonamides, third-generation cephalosporins and chloramphenicol. Meningeal inflammation considerably improves penetration of drugs into the CSF.
- Duration of antimicrobial therapy should be a minimum of 14 days with therapy continuing for 7 days after the resolution of clinical signs.
- Other therapies aimed at reducing cerebral edema and nursing care are vital, especially in foals which are recumbent.
- Approximately 50% of foals with bacterial meningitis die despite appropriate treatment.

Borreliosis (Lyme disease)

Borrelia burgdorferi may occasionally cause brainstem encephalitis in horses. Transmission to horses is known to occur during feeding activity of adult female ticks in the summer, fall or late winter. Serological studies have demonstrated that a large number of horses are seropositive.

Clinical signs of Lyme disease in horses are variable with the most common signs including low-grade fever, stiffness and lameness in more than one limb, swollen joints, hyperesthesia, lethargy and

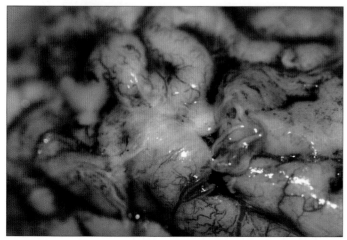

Figure 11.73 Suppurative meningitis.

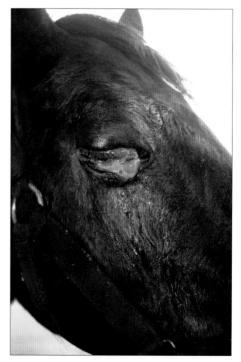

Figure 11.74 Marked exophthalmus in this young horse secondary to meningitis.

behavioral changes (divers). Neurological dysfunction and panuveitis have also been reported.

Diagnosis

- Diagnosis is based on endemic area, clinical signs, ruling out other causes for the clinical signs, and finding a high (>300 KELA units) enzyme-linked immunosorbent assay (ELISA) titer or a positive Western blot (WB) for *B. burgdorferi*.
- The time from infection to seroconversion is 3–10 weeks with the great limitation of serological tests being that they are unable to distinguish between active infection and subclinical exposure.
- Development of newer tests to detect the spirochete and its antibodies are active areas of research.

Treatment

- Treatment consists of intravenous tetracycline or oral doxycycline.
- Treatment is often continued for a month but this is empirical. Recurrence of clinical signs is often reported after treatment is discontinued.
- Other supportive treatments including chondroprotective agents and non-steroidal anti-inflammatories (NSAIDs) should also be considered.
- Prevention in endemic areas involves the prevention of tick exposure, prolonged tick attachment and early antimicrobial treatment following *Ixodes* exposure. Insecticidal sprays are not approved for use in horses and there is no commercially available vaccine at this time, although ponies have been protected against experimental infection by the use of a vaccine (Chang et al 2000).

Equine protozoal myeloencephalitis

(Figs. 11.75 & 11.76)

Equine protozoal myeloencephalitis (EPM) results in a diverse range of clinical signs. *Sarcocystis neurona* appears to be the causative agent in most cases, although some cases have been linked to *Neospora hughesi*. The Virginia opossum *(Didelphis virginiana)* is the only definitive host for *S. neurona* in the United States while a related opossum *(Didelphis albiventris)* carries *S. neurona* in South America. Armadillos and raccoons have been identified as natural intermediate hosts. The

disease occurs in areas in which the causative organism and its host are found, i.e. North and South America. Cases have occurred all over the world in horses which have been exported, often many months to years after arrival. The seroprevalence of the disease has been reported at 26–60% but the incidence of new disease has been reported up to 0.51% indicating that horses which are naturally infected are quite resistant to the development of EPM. A number of risk factors have been associated with the development of clinical disease including racing or showing. It is more common in horses <4 years of age and >13 years of age. There may be a seasonal increase in incidence associated with increased opossum activity. EPM is noted for the diversity of clinical signs that it can cause as a result of lesions of varying size and severity in any part of the CNS. The onset of signs may be insidious or acute. Spinal cord involvement occurs in most cases with related signs while only 5% of cases are reported to show evidence of brain disease. Other than neurological signs there are no other syndromes associated with EPM. The disease course is also highly variable, with progression over hours or years possible, or a waxing and waning of signs over extended periods.

Signs of spinal cord disease that are seen include gait abnormalities (toe-dragging, cross cantering, interference between limbs, asymmetry of stride length), weakness and ataxia in the limbs or trunk but usually most prominent in the pelvic limbs and abnormal proprioception. Signs are usually asymmetric and a small proportion of cases, 5–10%, will demonstrate severe neurogenic atrophy of muscles of the trunk or limbs. The spectrum of clinical signs reported has also included cauda equina syndrome (paralysis of the bladder, rectum, anus and penis, sensory loss of the tail and perineum), sweeney, stringhalt and a radial-nerve-type syndrome.

Signs of brain disease are usually one of three forms. The first ones are acute-onset asymmetric brainstem disease commonly involving dysfunction of cranial nerve VII (facial) and cranial nerve VIII (vestibular). Thus these horses demonstrate signs of vestibular disease with head tilt/turn, circling in one direction and abnormal eye positions and nystagmus. Other cranial nerve can be affected with associated clinical signs. The second manifestation of brain disease that is seen is atrophy of the lingual or masticatory muscles. This is usually of an insidious onset and may appear as a singular syndrome. These

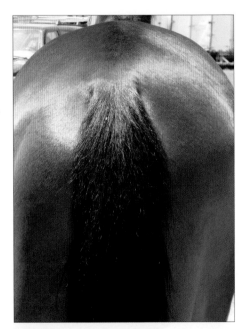

Figure 11.75 EPM. Note the atrophy of the right sided semimembranosis and semitendinosis muscles.

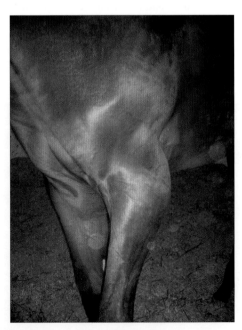

Figure 11.76 EPM. Local wastage of the deltoid muscle.

cases do not normally progress beyond the complete and permanent atrophy of the muscle affected. The third manifestation that is seen is a cerebral syndrome with horses showing signs of dysfunction of the visual or sensory centers, such as blindness or facial hypalgesia. Other less frequent signs that have been recorded are head-pressing, demented behavior or seizures.

Diagnosis

- As EPM may mimic almost any other neurological disease, the list of diagnostic rule-outs is extensive. A definitive ante-mortem diagnosis cannot be achieved by clinicopathological means and most often a diagnosis of EPM is reached based on an accumulation of data. Important considerations in reaching a diagnosis are relevant history and compatible clinical signs, clinical progression, response to treatment, laboratory and other diagnostic aids and exclusion of other differentials.
- Laboratory and other diagnostic aids have been divided into three categories:
  - Positive immunoblot for *S. neurona* antibodies, which supports the diagnosis. A positive serum immunoblot is also only indicative of exposure and not necessarily reflective of active disease;
  - Negative immunoblot, which tends to exclude the diagnosis; and
  - Tests that support alternative diagnoses and thus indirectly exclude a diagnosis of EPM.
- Due to the poor specificity of the serum and CSF immunoblot tests, many clinicians use other criteria such as a response to treatment to allow them to make a retrospective diagnosis.

Treatment

- Antiprotozoal drugs are the most important feature of therapy. Other treatments which may be considered in individual cases are anti-inflammatories, antioxidants, biological response modifiers and physical therapy. Traditional treatment has centered around the use of combinations of pyrimethamine and sulfonamides. These sequentially inhibit folic acid synthesis in the protozoa. Originally pyrimethamine was administered with trimethoprim-sulfonamide tablets but many compounding pharmacies now produce sulfadiazine-pyrimethamine solutions/suspensions.
- Diclazuril, toltrazuril and ponazuril are triazine-based coccidial agents that are effective against coccidia in birds and mammals. These compounds are also noted to be efficacious for *S. neurona*. These compounds target a chloroplast-like organelle within the *S. neurona* which may be responsible for electron transfer reactions and fatty acid synthesis. The triazine compounds have been used to treat AIDS patients with *Cryptosporidium* and *Isosporiasis*. Toltrazuril and diclazuril are licensed in Canada but are not currently licensed in the United States. Ponazuril (Marquis®) is a metabolite of toltrazuril and is currently approved in the United States for the treatment of EPM at a dose rate of 5 mg/kg PO SID for 28 days.
- Nitazoxanide (NTZ) has been approved for the treatment of EPM in the United States (32% Nitazoxanide Navigator®). The antiprotozoal activity of NTZ is believed to be due to interference with the pyruvate:ferredoxinoxidoreductase (PFOR) enzyme-dependent electron transfer reaction which is essential to anaerobic energy metabolism. It is a 28 day titrating+ treatment starting at 25 mg/kg PO SID for days 1–5 then 50 mg/kg PO SID for days 6–28.
- The comparative effectiveness of the ponazuril and NTZ is not objectively known with the subjective opinion of many clinicians being that they have similar efficacy. Whichever therapy is chosen, the manufacturers' recommendations should be followed and monitoring for signs associated with long-term therapy with folic acid inhibitors should be performed on a regular basis (Witonsky et al 2004).

Trypanosomiasis

Trypanosomes are bloodborne protozoa that cause disease in many species, including horses. There are many species with different modes of transmission and strains with differing virulence. Tsetse-transmitted trypanosomes cause disease in Africa. *Trypanosoma evansi* is transmitted by hematophagus flies and vampire bats resulting in surra, an important disease of economic importance in Asia and South America. Dourine is caused by *T. equiperdum* in Asia, South Africa, India and the Russian Federation. This is the only trypanosome that is vertically transmitted. This disease has been eradicated from North America. Clinical signs of trypanosomiasis are variable but include pyrexia, anemia, weight loss, lymphadenopathy and often death. Signs of meningoencephalomyelitis that can be seen include muscle atrophy, facial nerve paralysis, limb ataxia and weakness that is worse in the pelvic limbs.

Treatment involves the use of various trypanosomides but resistance may be encountered. Treatment of animals with dourine is not recommended as they may become carriers.

Botulism (Fig. 11.77)

Botulism is a neuromuscular disease characterized by flaccid paralysis that is caused by neurotoxins produced by strains of *Clostridium botulinum*. Horses are one of the most susceptible species, with both individual and group outbreaks reported.

C. botulinum is a Gram-positive, spore-producing anaerobic bacillus. Spores are found in the soil throughout most of the world with the distribution of strains dependent on temperature and soil pH. Seven serotypes of botulinum neurotoxin exist and are labeled A, B, C_1, D, E, F and G, all of which have similar toxicity. In North America, botulism in horses is most often caused by type B toxin and less often by toxin types A and C_1. Botulinum neurotoxins bind to presynaptic membranes at neuromuscular junctions, irreversibly blocking the release of the neurotransmitter acetylcholine resulting in flaccid paralysis.

Botulinum toxin can be absorbed from wounds infected with *C. botulinum*, or from the gastrointestinal tract after ingestion of feed

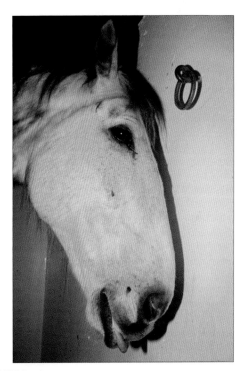

Figure 11.77 Botulism.

contaminated with the bacteria or preformed toxin. Ingestion of spores that develop into bacteria and colonize the gut can also result in the production and absorption of toxin. Toxicoinfectious botulism (bacterial infection of the gastrointestinal tract with subsequent toxin production) typically occurs in foals as the normal gastrointestinal flora in adults prevents colonization of *C. botulinum*.

Type B (and less commonly type A) botulism is associated with the feeding of spoiled hay or silage. Silage with a pH greater than 4.5 is favorable for sporulation and toxin production. This is known as 'forage poisoning'. It has also been suggested that birds may be able to carry preformed toxin from carrion to the feed of horses. Type C botulism is associated with ingestion of feed or water contaminated by the carcass of a rodent or other small animal.

The clinical picture of symmetrical flaccid paralysis is consistent, with the onset and rate of progression dependent on the amount of toxin that is absorbed. The mortality rate has been reported to be as high as 90%, with death occurring within hours to weeks of the appearance of signs. Recovery may take weeks or months but is complete if it occurs.

The initial clinical signs include dysphagia with apparent excess salivation, weak eyelid tone, weak tail tone and exercise intolerance. Affected animals also spend increased amounts of time resting due to generalized muscle weakness, which is also associated with tremors, carpal buckling and ataxia.

Pharyngeal and lingual paralysis causes marked dysphagia and predisposes to aspiration pneumonia. Paralysis of the diaphragm and intercostal muscles results in an increased respiratory rate and decreased chest wall expansion. Severely affected animals die from respiratory paralysis and cardiac failure.

Diagnosis

- Botulism should be suspected in animals with flaccid paralysis displaying the above clinical signs. Botulinum toxin does not affect the central nervous system but does affect the cranial nerves; thus symmetrical cranial nerve deficits in an animal with normal mentation can help differentiate botulism from other disorders.
- Definitive diagnosis can be achieved by the mouse inoculation test. However, horses are extremely sensitive to the toxin and this test is often negative.
- Detection of antibody titers in a recovering unvaccinated horse is also evidence for the diagnosis of botulism.
- Demonstration of spores in the intestine is not diagnostic, as they can be ingested and observed as contaminants.

Treatment and prognosis

- In most cases botulism is fatal. Immediate treatment with a polyvalent antitoxin prevents binding of the toxin to presynaptic membranes. However, antitoxin cannot reactivate neuromuscular junctions that have already been affected. Thus, antitoxin administration may have little effect in animals that are severely affected. Generally, only one dose of antitoxin is needed and provides passive protection for up to 2 months.
- Antibiotics should be administered if toxicoinfectious botulism is suspected or if there are secondary lesions such as aspiration pneumonia or decubital ulcers. Antibiotics that can cause neuromuscular blockade and possibly exacerbate clinical signs such as aminoglycosides should be avoided and neurostimulants such as neostigmine should not be used.
- Good nursing care, including the provision of a deep bed and a quiet environment, are essential. Frequent turning of recumbent animals, nasogastric feeding and fluid support for animals with pharyngeal and lingual paralysis, frequent catheterization of the

urinary bladder, application of ophthalmic ointments and ventilatory support may all be required.

- Prognosis varies with the amount of toxin absorbed and the severity of clinical signs. Mildly affected animals may recover with minimal treatment while severely affected animals that become recumbent have a poor prognosis.

Prevention

- Type B toxoid is available and should be used in areas in which type B botulism is endemic.
- An initial series of three vaccinations a month apart followed by annual boosters should be given.
- Pregnant mares should receive a booster 4 weeks prior to foaling to ensure adequate antibody levels in colostrum.
- Type B vaccine only provides protection against type B toxin; there is no cross-protection against type C toxin and type C toxoid is not licensed for use in North America.

Ehrlichiosis

Horses infected with *Anaplasma phagocytophilia* often have transient truncal and limb ataxia. These animals may also display weakness. The weakness and ataxia seen can be severe and these animals may fall and sustain serious injuries. Inflammatory vascular or interstital lesions have been reported in the brain of affected animals and histologically there is inflammation of small arteries and veins, primarily in the subcutis, fascia, nerves of the legs and reproductive organs.

Tetanus (Figs. 11.78–11.80)

Tetanus is a highly fatal, infectious disease caused by the exotoxin of *Clostridium tetani*. The most common route of infection is by wound contamination with *C. tetani* spores. The organism exists largely in highly resistant spore form and is commonly found in the intestinal tract and feces of animals and in soils rich in organic matter. Under conditions of low oxygen tension such as depths of puncture wounds, or wounds with considerable necrosis, bacterial proliferation and elaboration of toxin occur. The incubation period is generally 1–3 weeks but can be several months. There is a wide variability between the time of wound contamination and onset of signs of tetanus as the spores are viable for many months and may germinate long after a wound has apparently healed, if the conditions are appropriate such as re-injury. This exotoxin is water-soluble and reaches the CNS hematogenously and by passage along peripheral nerves. The main action of the toxin is to block the release of inhibitory neurotransmitter. Thus, reflexes normally inhibited by descending

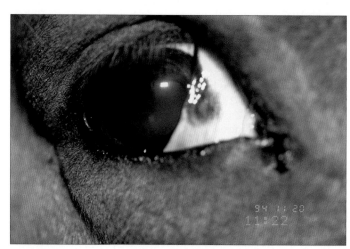

Figure 11.78 Tetanus. Prolapse of third eyelid.

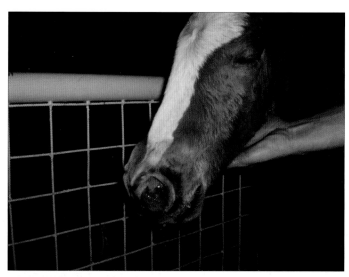

Figure 11.79 Tetanus. Persistent nostril flare.

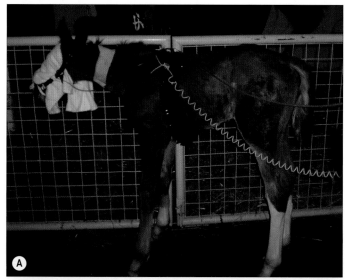

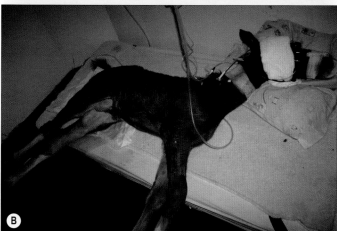

Figure 11.80 (A,B) Tetanus in young foals. (A) Note the pricked ears and raised tailhead. (B) Note the marked stiffness of the limbs; it was not possible to flex the limbs to place the foal in sternal recumbency.

inhibitory motor tracts or by inhibitory interneurons are greatly facilitated, resulting in tetanic contractions of muscle following normal sensory stimuli.

Clinical signs and diagnosis

- The severity of signs and rate of progression of the disease depend on the dose of toxin and the size and age of the animal but are characterized by muscular rigidity, hyperesthesia and convulsions in horses of all ages (Green et al 1994).
- Initial signs include a stiff gait and hyperesthesia.
- Spasm of the muscles of mastication results in difficulty opening the mouth and results in the term 'lockjaw'.
- Facial muscle spasm results in an anxious expression with retracted lips, flared nostrils and erect ears.
- Extraocular muscle contraction causes retraction of the eyeball with resulting prolapse of the nictitating membranes.
- A tap on the forehead or other stimuli frequently results in marked spasm of cervical, facial, masticatory and extraocular muscles.
- The striated muscles are progressively affected causing rigid extension of the neck, limbs and tail (saw-horse stance).
- If an affected mature horse falls, it is usually unable to rise due to rigid extension of the extremities, and further muscle spasms as a result of attempts to rise. Foals that fall may be assisted to stand.
- Death usually occurs in 5–7 days due to aspiration resulting from spastic paralysis of respiratory muscles, laryngospasm or aspiration pneumonia.
- Other complications of recumbency and intense muscle spasm such as fractures can also be lethal.
- In rare cases of recovery, there are no residual signs but the animal is not protected from further episodes.

Treatment

- Treatment is based on the knowledge that the toxin–gangliosides bond is irreversible and that gradual replacement of altered gangliosides by normal metabolic processes will lead to recovery. With this in mind, treatment is primarily symptomatic and supportive. The primary objectives of therapy are:
  - Destruction of *C. tetani* organism. Destruction of the organisms involves administration of large doses of penicillin, metronidazole and wound debridement. In human studies there has been a better outcome in patients receiving metronidazole alone than those receiving penicillin.
  - Neutralization of unbound toxin, Neutralization of unbound toxin involves IV, IM, SC or intrathecal administration of large amounts of tetanus antitoxin (TAT). The dose that is given should be based on the history of the case and influenced by factors such as delay in treatment of several hours after injury, lack of aggressive debridement or no history of vaccination. In addition to TAT administration, tetanus toxoid should also be administered as protective humoral immunity is not induced by natural disease. In severe cases in which wound debridement is not possible it may be necessary to administer TAT a number of times daily as ongoing production of toxin will result in consumption of available antitoxin.
  - Control of muscle spasm and general supportive care.
- Symptomatic and supportive care includes chemical control of muscle rigidity and spasms, placement in a darkened, quiet stall to minimize stimuli, and nutritional care including feeding via a nasogastric tube where necessary (Rie & Wilson 1978).
- Adult horses which are presented in lateral recumbency have little chance of recovery and euthanasia should be considered. Foals may

respond better to therapy as due to their size nursing and supportive care is more easily administered.

Prevention

Horses should receive two vaccinations 3–4 weeks apart followed by annual vaccinations; although there is evidence that protective titers persist for up to 4 years after the first booster. Unvaccinated horses are commonly given tetanus antitoxin (TAT) after injury but it is reasonable to administer tetanus toxoid rather than antitoxin to an animal that has sustained an injury, but has been vaccinated with tetanus toxoid in the previous year.

Circulating tetanus antitoxin may interfere with the immune response to later tetanus toxoid administration and for this reason any foals that have received colostrum from mares that have been vaccinated within 30 days of foaling or alternatively received 1500 IU TAT at birth should not be vaccinated until 3–6 months of age.

Current recommendations are administration of tetanus toxoid at 3, 4 and 6 months of age followed by annual vaccination.

Cerebral abscess (Fig. 11.81)

Cerebral abscesses are rare and sporadic. They are most commonly associated with *Streptococcus equi* infection but can also occur secondary to local disease processes. Signs become apparent with sufficient compression of cerebral tissue; the onset being insidious or acute, depending on the rate of growth of the abscess. The clinical course is often characterized by marked fluctuations in the severity of signs. Behavioral changes such as depression, wandering or unprovoked excitement are most obvious. Contralateral impaired vision, deficient menace response and decreased facial sensation are consistent early findings. Affected horses frequently circle or stand with the head and neck turned toward the side of the lesion. Progression leads to recumbency, unconsciousness, seizures and signs of brainstem compression such as asymmetric pupils, ataxia and weakness.

Diagnosis

- Diagnosis is based on history of a previous Strep. equi episode and clinical signs, although other causes of asymmetric cerebral disease should be ruled out.
- Computed tomography has also been used for diagnosis.
- Hematology findings of hyperfibrinogenemia, hyperglobulinemia and leucocytosis are not consistent.

- Changes in the CSF depend on the degree of meningeal or ependymal involvement. Most cases exhibit xanthochromia and a moderate elevation of CSF protein levels reflective of cerebral damage and compression.

Treatment

- If the signs are acute, severe and rapidly progressive, it is likely that brain edema is also present and corticosteroids should be repeatedly administered until the signs stabilize.
- Prolonged antibiotic administration, although this has not always been successful in horses.
- Surgical evacuation of the lesion is another approach which has been used successfully.
- The prognosis is regarded as poor and horses that recover may have residual deficits, such as impaired vision.

Vertebral osteomyelitis (Fig. 11.82)

Vertebral osteomyelitis (spondylitis) is an infectious or inflammatory degenerative disease of one or more vertebrae. When an adjacent intervertebral disc is involved the condition is termed discospondylitis (Adams & Mayhew 1985). These are rare but serious conditions of the horse. It has been related to hematogenous spread of infectious agents in the newborn and has extension from local wounds (Markel et al 1986, Sullivan 1985). Progression of the vertebral infection leads to paravertebral abscess, meningitis, vertebral collapse and spinal cord compression. Many pathogens have been isolated including *Rhodococcus equi* in foals (Chaffin et al 1995).

Clinical signs and diagnosis

- The initial signs of localized spinal pain usually go unnoticed. Fever, stiffness and sensory deficits with variable paresis are the signs that are noted. This may rapidly progress to recumbency.
- Diagnosis is based on clinical signs, history and positive findings on radiography, scintigraphy, computed tomography or ultrasonography.

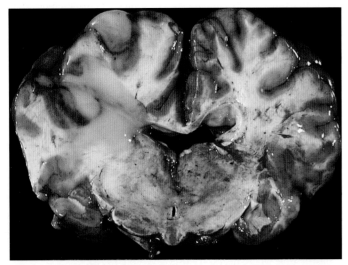

Figure 11.81 Multiple cerebral abscesses. The location and size of abscess(es) determines the clinical signs that are seen. Reproduced from McAuliffe SB, Slovis NM (eds), *Color Atlas of Diseases and Disorders of the Foal* (2008), with permission from Elsevier.

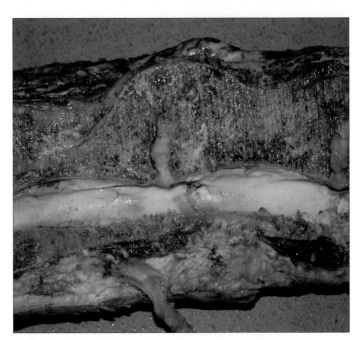

Figure 11.82 Vertebral osteomyelitis. Note the area of osteomyelitis in the center of the vertebral body and associated changes in the cord immediately below. Many of these cases may present acutely recumbent.

Hematology findings are usually consistent with inflammation and CSF analysis may be normal or consistent with spinal cord compression (Hahn et al 1999).

Treatment
- It is important to try to isolate the etiological agent prior to commencing therapy.
- Cultures of blood and feces should be performed in addition to cytology and culture of a fine-needle aspirate.
- Other clinical signs and possibly useful tests should be borne in mind in animals with other clinical signs; for example tracheal wash cultures and cytology in foals suspected of *R. equi* infections.
- Long-term antibiotic therapy is required (3–6 months) and relapses are common.
- The success of treatment also depends on the severity of signs at presentation and intercurrent disease.

Fungal granulomas (Figs. 11.83 & 11.84)
Intracranial fungal granulomas are rare findings. When they occur they may be an extension of local fungal infection, e.g. guttural pouch mycosis or be as a result of systemic spread.

Diagnosis is generally made at necropsy and treatment is generally aimed at the primary lesion.

Parasitic diseases

Verminous meningoencephalomyelitis
Verminous meningoencephalomyelitis is rare and sporadic and caused by the aberrant migration of parasites through the CNS. Due to the variable etiology there is a spectrum of clinical signs that may be seen depending upon the area of the CNS involved. Several parasites have been reported, including *Strongylus*, *Hypoderma*, *Habronema*, *Draschia*, *Halicephalobus* and *Setaria* species. Transmission of *Halicephalobus gingivalis* from mare to dam has been reported (Wilkins et al 2001). *Strongylus vulgaris* thromboarteritis may rarely lead to embolic showering of the cerebrum. Diagnosis is usually based on clinical signs and necropsy findings. CSF changes are not specific or consistent, with some hemorrhage and an increased number of inflammatory cells such as eosinophils and neutrophils to be expected. Therapy should include the use of anthelmintics and anti-inflammatories. However, avermectins may not be effective because of the drug's gamma aminobutyric acid (GABA) inhibiting method of destroying parasites. It is also theoretically toxic to mammals due to the GABA inhibition if it crosses the blood–brain barrier.

Prominent cervical scoliosis with minimal ataxia in adult horses has been described in the north-eastern United States. This syndrome appears to be due to *Parelaphastrongylus tenuis* (meningeal worm of white-tailed deer) entering the cervical spinal cord via the dorsal nerve roots and causing a selective myelitis in the dorsal gray columns. There are no localizing signs of motor or sensory loss and no denervation muscle atrophy associated with this syndrome. The scoliosis may be the result of disafferentiation of cervical musculature. The signs are permanent.

Neoplastic disorders

Neoplasms of the central nervous system of the horse with the exception of the pituitary adenoma (see Chapter 6, p. 229) are extremely rare and in the cases that have been reported, fatal.

Primary neoplasms of the nervous system are very rare and in a survey of North American university veterinary hospitals, all nervous tissue tumors found in horses involved peripheral nerves. Neurofibromas and neurofibrosarcomas were the most common, with neurofibromas frequently being found cutaneously in the pectoral region, neck, face and abdomen.

Secondary neoplasms may reach the nervous system by vascular spread, growing through osseus foramina or penetration of the cranial vault or vertebrae. Lymphosarcoma is the most common secondary tumor affecting the nervous system of horses and has been found in the epidural space as a cause of compressive myelopathy, in the brain and olfactory tracts, and infiltrated into various peripheral nerves. Melanomas most commonly seen in white or gray horses occasionally invade the CNS and have been found in the epidural space following contiguous spread from melanomatous sublumbar lymph nodes. Cutaneous melanomas have also metastasized to spinal meninges, spinal cord and brain.

Other reported secondary nervous system tumors in horses are: hemangiosarcomas, adenocarcinomas, osteosarcoma and plasma cell myeloma.

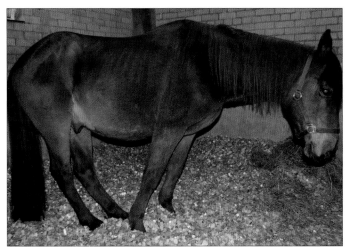

Figure 11.83 Intracranial fungal infection. These cases may be difficult to diagnose ante-mortem and can present with non-specific and bizarre neurological signs. Note the depression and abnormal posture in this mare.

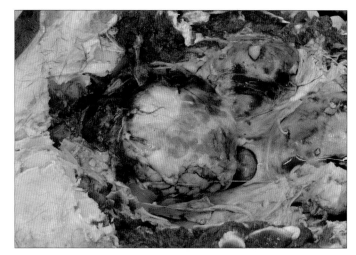

Figure 11.84 Fungal granuloma. This 20 year old pony presented with altered mentation, head pressing, circling, generalized weakness and weight loss of several months duration. An increased protein concentration of cerebrospinal fluid was the only laboratory abnormality detected. Due to deterioration in his neurological condition, the pony was euthanised. At necropsy this fungal granuloma and related compression of the cerebrum were found.

The clinical signs that are seen are usually related to the area of the brain or spinal cord involved and are most often due to compression from the expanding tumor mass.

Tumors involving structures adjacent to the brain such as those in the paranasal sinuses and nasal cavity may affect the cranium. Generally these do not extend into the meninges or brain itself and their significance is in their space-occupying nature. Space-occupying lesions within the cranium exert a wide variety of effects but where they are slow-growing and impinge on the cerebrum there may be no detectable effect but conversely there may be a range of neurological abnormalities including epileptiform convulsions, blindness and defects of gait and posture.

Secondary tumors in the spinal cord are more common than those in the brain itself, and most arise from direct, contiguous spread from adjacent tissues such as the bone of the vertebral body or from invasion of the epidural space. Melanomas are the commonest form of metastasis into the cord. Hematogenous spread into central nervous tissue is extremely rare.

Diagnosis

- Ante-mortem diagnosis is notoriously difficult unless the lesion is very large and is detectable radiographically or by scintigraphy or computer-assisted tomography.
- Abnormal electrical activity may be detectable but a diagnosis of intracranial neoplasia often relies on secondary effects such as loss of thermoregulation, visual deficits and the presence of convulsions.

References and further reading

Adams, R., Mayhew, I.G., 1985. Neurologic diseases. Vet Clin North Am Equine Pract 1 (1), 209–234.

Aleman, M., Katzman, S.A., Vaughan, B., et al., 2009. Ante-mortem diagnosis of polyneuritis equi. J Vet Intern Med 23 (3), 665–668.

Elliott, C.R., McCowan, C.I., 2012. Nigropallidal encephalomalacia in horses grazing *Rhaponticum repens* (creeping knapweed). Aust Vet J 90 (4), 151–154.

Mayhew, G., 1989. Large Animal Neurology. A Handbook for Veterinary Clinicians. Lea & Febiger, Philadelphia, PA, USA.

McAuliffe, S.B., Slovis, N.M., 2008. Color Atlas of Diseases and Disorders of the Foal. WB Saunders, Philadelphia, PA, USA.

Reed, S.M., Bayly, W.M., Sellon, D.C., 2009. Equine Internal Medicine, third ed. WB Saunders, St. Louis, MO, USA.

Rivas, L.J., Hinchcliff, K.W., Robertson, J.T., 1996. Cervical meningomyelocele associated with spina bifida in a hydrocephalic miniature colt. J Am Vet Med Assoc 209 (5), 950–953.

Robinson, N.E., Sprayberry, K.A. (Eds.), 2009. Current Therapy in Equine Medicine, sixth ed. WB Saunders, St. Louis, MO, USA.

Rose, R., Hodgson, D.R., 1993. Manual of Equine Practice. WB Saunders, Philadelphia, PA, USA.

Sanders, S.G., Tucker, R.L., Bagley, R.S., Gavin, P.R., 2001. Magnetic resonance imaging features of equine nigropallidal encephalomalacia. Vet Radiol Ultrasound 42 (4), 291–296.

Scrivani, P.V., 2011. Advanced imaging of the nervous system in the horse. Vet Clin North Am Equine Pract 27 (3), 439–453.

Silva, M.L., Galiza, G.J., Dantas, A.F., et al., 2011. Outbreaks of Eastern equine encephalitis in northeastern Brazil. J Vet Diagn Invest 23 (3), 570–575.

Reproductive disorders

CHAPTER CONTENTS

1 The mare

Clinical examination of the mare

(Figs. 12.1–12.2)

A thorough history of the mare's breeding life should occur prior to any examination or evaluation. This will provide insight into the areas of concern and focus. Then a general physical examination should be conducted to include body condition score.

During examination of the reproductive tract adequate restraint, preferably the use of an examination stock or crush, is advisable so that undivided attention can be more safely given to the examination. It may be necessary to tranquillize some mares but a quiet, unhurried approach will often allow the initial examination to be made. The external genitalia should be assessed, recognizing length and position of the vulva relative to the rectum and the brim of the pelvis. Perineal body mass and angles should be noted. The perineum should be cleaned and the urogenital tract examined.

Manual palpation and ultrasonographic examination per rectum of the uterine body, horns, ovaries and cervix should follow. A speculum exam aids in identifying stage of the estrous cycle as well as the presence of hyperemia, exudate, urine, and traumatic injuries such as adhesions, scars and tears in the vaginal vault and cervix. Manual palpation provides further evaluation of the vaginal vault and during diestrus any cervical defects. Further evaluation of the reproductive tract can include endometrial culture and cytology, clitoral culture, endometrial biopsy, hysteroscopic evaluation and color Doppler studies.

The estrous cycle (Figs. 12.3–12.20)

The estrus cycle in the mare may be regarded as the period between the ovulation of a mature follicle through to the ovulation of the next mature follicle. This is usually a period of approximately 21 days in

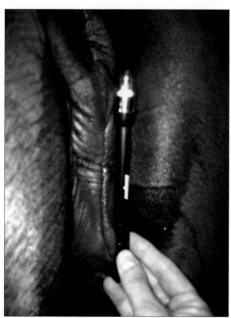

Figure 12.1 Excellent perineal conformation. Note that the anus is directly in line with the vulva lips. Vulva lips are tight and the majority positioned below the brim of the pelvis.

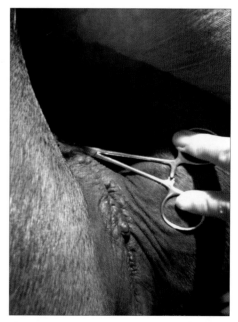

Figure 12.2 Very poor perineal conformation. The anus is sunken in cranial to the vulva lips. Note the hemostats are sitting on a shelf parallel to the ground along with the opening to the vulva. Feces will sit on the shelf and contaminate the vestibule and vagina

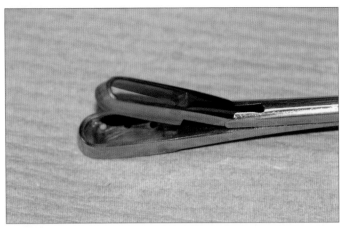

Figure 12.3 Endometrial biopsy punch. Histological examination of the endometrium provides prognosis for pregnancy and helps to indicate treatments for any underlying disease.

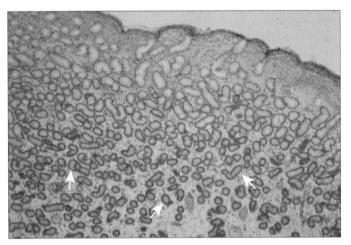

Figure 12.4 Normal endometrial biopsy demonstrating numerous normal endometrial glands (arrows). Note the lack of abnomal features such as nesting or glandular dilation.

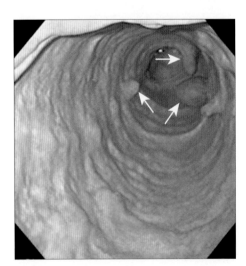

Figure 12.5 Hysteroscopy can be a useful part of the breeding soundness examination, as it allows visual examination of the contents of the uterus, such as exudates, foreign bodies or cysts. Note in this case the endometrial cysts present protruding into the lumen (arrows).

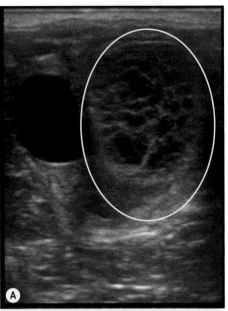

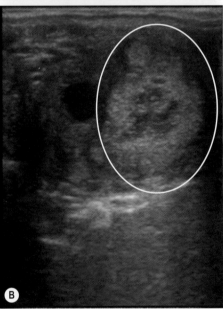

Figure 12.6 Two different yet normal types of corpus luteum (circles). (A) has a spider web appearance and (B) a homogenous parenchyma.

Thoroughbred mares and up to 25 days in pony mares. The period between ovulations may be conveniently divided into separate identifiable periods which reflect changes in behavior and in ovarian function. Estrus display and acceptance of the stallion begins before ovulation and normally lasts for 24–48 hours post ovulation. Thereafter the mare loses receptivity.

The luteal phase commences with the formation first of the corpus hemorrhagicum, which then matures into a corpus luteum. The corpus luteum is responsible for progesterone production, which peaks at approximately the sixth day after ovulation. If maternal recognition of pregnancy does not occur, prostaglandin (PGF2α) is released from the endometrium and luteal regression follows. Follicular waves continue through diestrus and the follicles that do not become atretic continue to enlarge from mid to late diestrus. With luteal regression and progesterone decreasing, these follicles

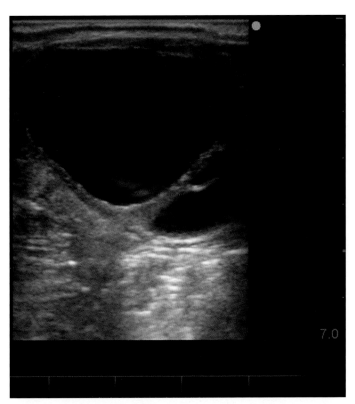

Figure 12.7 A large dominant follicle evident by transrectal ultrasonography.

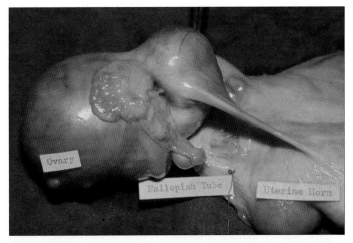

Figure 12.8 Normal ovary. The ovulation fossa lies in the concave area of the kidney-bean-shaped ovary (arrow). Usually the fimbrae of the oviduct covers the area so the ovum will be caught.

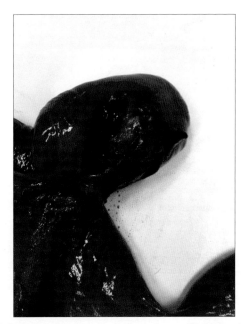

Figure 12.9 Normal ovary. Note the ovulation fossa and fimbrae with a newly formed corpus hemorragicum.

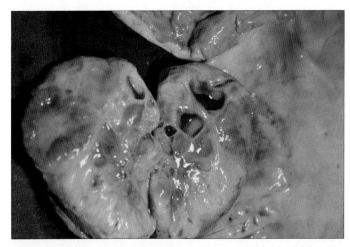

Figure 12.10 The ovary has a corpus luteum present with a few small follicles but mostly parenchyma.

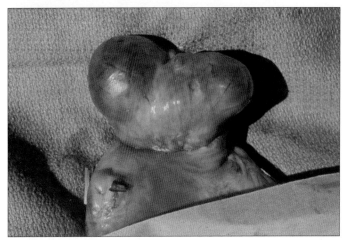

Figure 12.11 Large mature follicle protruding off the surface of the ovary.

(16–20 mm diameter) are stimulated by follicle-stimulating hormone (FSH). One or two dominant follicles will undergo final maturation with the remainder regressing. The growing follicles produce increasing amounts of estrogen bringing the mare into physiological and behavioral estrus. Luteinizing hormone from the anterior pituitary rises, inducing ovulation and the luteal phase commences.

The dimensions of mare ovaries, on average, are 50 mm × 28 m × 33 mm, and the average weight is 120 grams. Pony mares have smaller ovaries with an average weight of only 43 grams. Equine ovaries have distinctive differences from other species. There is a relatively small palpable ovulation fossa with the ovarian stroma having a very fibrous appearance. Large areas of the surface are usually devoid of follicles. Mature follicles may be as large as 70–80 mm and

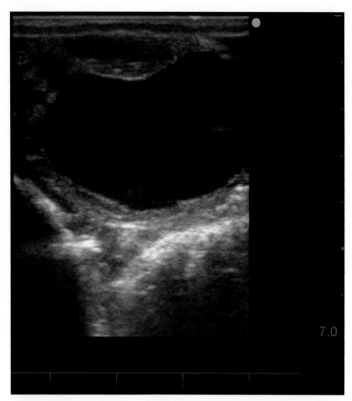

Figure 12.12 Softening dominant follicle changing shape from spherical to non-spherical.

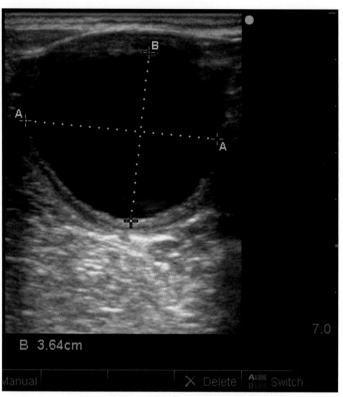

Figure 12.14 Increased echogenicity of the granulose layer with increased demarcation of the anechoic layer peripheral to the granulose layer.

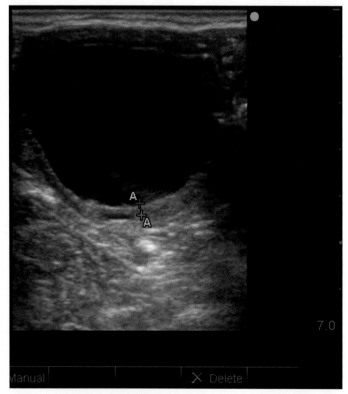

Figure 12.13 Thickening of the dominant follicle wall (A) associated with impending ovulation.

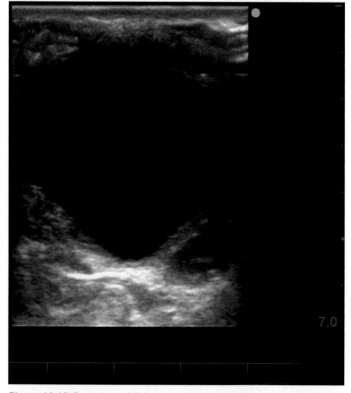

Figure 12.15 Preovulatory follicle on transrectal ultrasonographic examination that is changing shape and has increased echogenic particles within the follicular fluid.

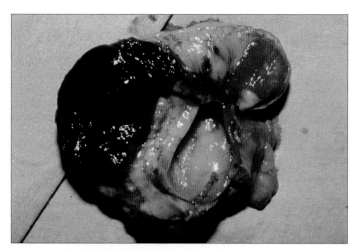

Figure 12.16 Normal ovary. Newly formed corpus hemorrhagicum evident by the blood clot, 24 hours after ovulation.

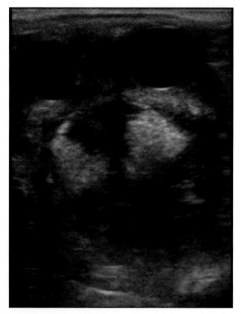

Figure 12.17 Normal ovary. Ultrasonographic appearance of a newly formed corpus hemorrhagicum.

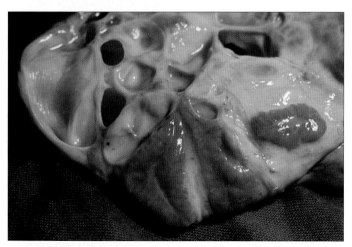

Figure 12.18 Normal ovary (showing mature corpus luteum pinkish/yellow, smaller corpus luteum and atretic follicles).

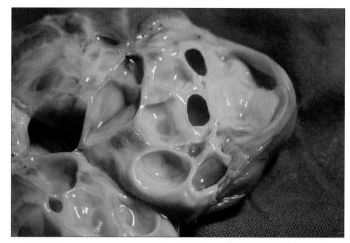

Figure 12.19 Normal ovary. Numerous small atretic follicles with a few medium follicles developing.

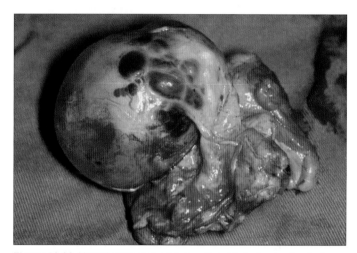

Figure 12.20 Normal ovary of an aged mare. Note: Marked varicosity of veins.

may be numerous. A palpably large follicle (>70 mm) should be carefully evaluated as this may, especially in Thoroughbreds, be due to the presence of more than one mature follicle, an anovulatory follicle or hematoma. Up to 40% of Thoroughbred mares may have a double ovulation. As ovulation approaches the dominant follicle with maximum mean size of 40–45 mm becomes softer and more tender on palpation. Ultrasonographic examination shows changes in shape going from spherical to non-spherical with thickening of the follicle wall (theca layer, basal lamina and granulose layer), and increased echogenicity of the granulosa layer with increased demarcation of an anechoic layer peripheral to the granulose layer. Color-flow Doppler ultrasonography can assess changing perfusion to the dominant follicle to predict if and when ovulation may occur. The presence of increased echogenicity within the follicular fluid can also indicate impending ovulation. Once collapse of the preovulatory follicle and release of the oocyte occurs, a large corpus hemorrhagicum, approximately 70% of the size of the preovulatory follicle, develops. This may often be difficult to differentiate manually (except for its meaty consistency) as it becomes smaller and is progressively luteinized. The primary corpus luteum, which on section has a yellowish hue, develops at the site.

Variations from this cycle of events include ovulation in the luteal phase in approximately 9% of mares, and this can be responsible for a prolonged luteal phase (diestrus). Estrus, service and pregnancy

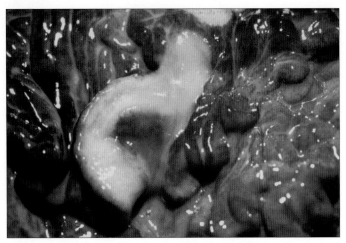

Figure 12.21 Normal uterus showing endometrial cups (50 days gestation).

can, rarely, occur in this period, but more often, the mare remains unreceptive.

Small atretic follicles occur in the mare during a phase in the maturation process when the preovulatory follicle becomes dominant at 23–25 mm early in estrus; the preovulatory follicle's growth rate increases relative to the subordinate follicles that will eventually regress and become atretic. Follicular cystic degeneration which occurs in other domestic species does not occur in mares. It is frequently diagnosed clinically but cannot be substantiated on gross or histological examination. Mares may exhibit a long transitional phase from winter anestrous to spring estrus, with estrus cycles up to 40 days being recorded. Typical ovaries show numerous slow-growing follicles to be present, leading to the erroneous belief that this represents a cystic condition. Other causes of multiple small follicles should additionally be ruled out such as granulosa cell tumor.

Prominent vessels are often present on the surface of the ovary and in some normal aged mares, may display even more marked varicosity.

Following conception, the developing embryo descends into the uterus 5–6 days post ovulation. At or around day 36, implantation of the girdle cells of the trophoblast occurs within the uterine mucosa, usually at the base of a uterine horn. These cells create the endometrial cups (see Fig. 12.21) which produce equine chorionic gonadotrophin (ECG). ECG has and ovulatory and luteinizing effect on the follicles present in the ovaries which form secondary and accesory corpora lutea. There is wide variation in their number between different mares. In the majority of mares regression of the endometrial cups occurs by day 150 of gestation, however cases of retained endometrial cups for up to 2 years post foaling have been documented. Both the primary and supplemental corpus luteum begin to regress and are usually completely atrophic by about 210–220 days. From this stage forward, the ovaries of pregnant mares show little follicular activity.

The ovary

Developmental disorders

Embryological abnormalities of the reproductive organs include **intersexes, cystic aberrations of the genital tract, teratoma of the gonads** and **malformations of the tubular portions** of the system. Fetal and placental abnormalities are complicated by lack of sufficient knowledge of their embryological development.

Normal sexual development proceeds providing the embryo carries the normal karyotype which is expressed by the chromosome pattern 64.XX and the male as 64.XY; the sex chromosomes XX or XY being the principal determinant of the eventual physical and reproductive capacities of the individual horse. Chromosomal sex (either XX or XY) is determined at the time of fertilization.

Defects of individual chromosome structure and of chromosomal numbers may be of a very minute character but almost always have extremely serious consequences on future reproductive ability, leading in most instances, to reduced if not complete infertility. Mares having a history of poor reproductive performance with chronic and primary infertility, having small ovaries, a flaccid uterus and cervix, a hypoplastic endometrium, which fail to cycle regularly (or at all), are prime suspects for some type of chromosomal abnormality.

The most common abnormalities affecting mares are X monosomy (X0) or Turner's syndrome, sex chromosome mosaics and sex reversal syndrome. Sex chromosomal abnormalities can cause the reproductive organs to not develop or function normally or cause gametes to have abnormal chromosome composition. Other chromosomal abnormalities causing infertility in the mare or embryo abnormalities leading to loss have been identified due to partial X chromosome deletions or autosomal duplications and translocations.

Turner's syndrome (63X0)

Mares present with very small ovaries and a flaccid underdeveloped uterus and cervix. The ovaries lack follicular activity and fail to cycle appropriately (or at all). Mares with this condition are often slightly undersize, and while they may have complete genital systems, they often have vestigial ovarian tissue which is difficult to palpate rectally. Angular limb deformities and poor conformation may also be evident.

XY sex-reversal syndrome (64X0)

This condition can occur as a result of failure of formation of testes (Sawyer syndrome, XY gonadal dysgensis) due to a deletion of the sex-determining region (SRY gene) on the Y chromosome, underdevelopment of androgen-producing cells in the testes, enzymatic defects in testosterone biosynthesis or insensitivity of genital tissues to androgens (Androgen insensitivity syndrome—AIS).

Clinical signs

- These mares have a female phenotype but a male karyotype. They can display a wide range of physical appearances. Some mares have been noted to be of normal or even large size.
- For XY gonadal dysgenesis there is a failure of formation of active gonads. The inactive gonads are comprised of primarily fibrous tissue.
- A flaccid cervix and uterus are present with normal external genitalia. Serum testosterone levels are minimal. Androgen insensitivity syndrome or testicular feminization is where tissues are completely or partially insensitive to androgens. This deficiency lies in the androgen receptor gene on the X chromosome which affects responsiveness or sensitivity of the fetus's body tissues to androgens. Most commonly the external genitalia are female with the cervix and uterus lacking. Testes in the inguinal canal labia or abdomen are present with normal or increased testosterone production. With partial resistance both male and female physical characteristics may be present with stallion-like behavior observed.

Autosomal chromosome abnormalities (Figs. 12.22–12.24)

These rare disorders include deletions, duplications or rearrangements of the autosomal chromosomes.

These mares usually appear phenotypically normal but exhibit irregular estrous cycles with or without ovulation or may experience early embryonic death.

Diagnosis of chromosomal abnormalities

- Karyotyping is a biological means of determining the gene status of that individual with the ability to identify abnormalities. Aseptic

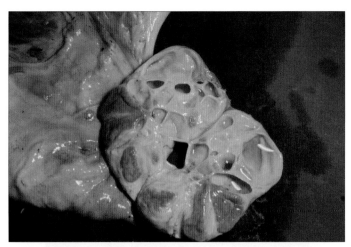

Figure 12.22 Normal ovary (45 days gestation) with numerous small secondary corpora lutea.

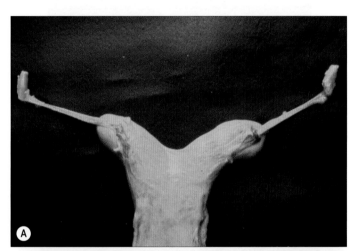

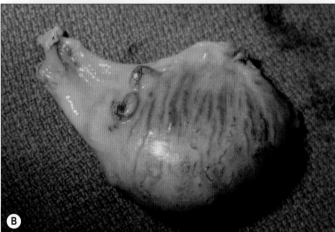

Figure 12.23 (A) Chromosomal abnormality (63XO) Very small ovaries and under-developed uterine horns and body. (B) Intersex ova-testis.

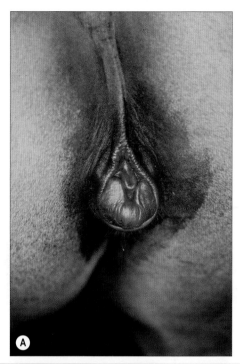

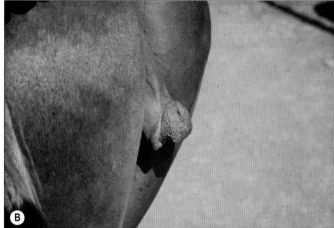

Figure 12.24 (A) Female hermaphrodite. Vestigial opening of the vulva lips, with an enlarged clitoral body. (B) Pseudo-hermaphrodite. Male horse with vestigial vulva and penis.

peripheral blood lymphocytes are cultured for 64–72 hours and then processed to eventually allow electron microscopic examination and comparison of 31 paired chromosomes plus one pair of sex chromosomes; differences are determined and so allow the identification of chromosomal abnormalities.

- **Abnormalities of the gonads** where intersexuality occurs may be classified according to their morphology. **True hermaphrodites** have one or both gonads containing both ovarian and testicular tissue, or may have one male and one female gonad. **Pseudo-hermaphrodites** have the gonads of one sex and the accessory genitalia of the other. A female hermaphrodite has ovaries and male accessory reproductive organs (and the male hermaphrodite the reverse). Ovarian tissue may be extremely small or even absent. Predominant external features of equine hermaphrodites are ventral displacement of the vulva with an enlarged clitoris or a short, backward-projecting penis. Testes may be present with mammary tissue and teats. Testes, epididymis and vesicular glands are usually present abdominally as well as a poorly developed uterus. The genetic nature of this abnormality is uncertain but recorded cases indicate that individual stallions may sire intersex foals from different mares.

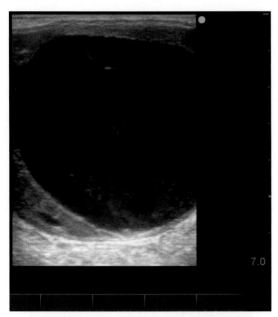

Figure 12.25 Ultrasonographic image of an anovulatory follicle that has luteinized.

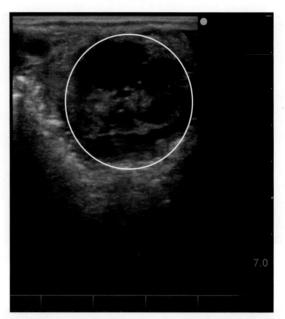

Figure 12.26 Ultrasonographic image of a small inactive anestrus ovary (circle). Note the lack of follicular development.

Diagnosis and treatment

- Measurement of testosterone may be beneficial if intra-abdominal testes are present, as well as ultrasonographic or laparoscopic evaluation of the abdominal cavity.
- Histological evaluation of gonadal tissue may confirm tissue origin.
- There is no known treatment. Castration is recommended.

Non-infectious disorders

Anovulatory follicles (Fig. 12.25)

Ovulation failure occurs in approximately 8.2% of estrous cycles during the physiological breeding season. The follicles may be large (5–15 cm in diameter) and may persist for extended periods of time resulting in a prolonged interovulatory interval. Suggested causes include: insufficient estrogen production from the follicle; insufficient pituitary gonadotrophin stimulation to induce ovulation; decreased gonadotrophin receptors on the follicle; and hemorrhage into the lumen of the preovulatory follicle.

Diagnosis

- Ultrasonographic monitoring of the progression of the dominant follicle should be done during estrus.
- Initial indication of a problem may be the thickening of the follicle wall or the detection of echogenic particles within the follicular fluid, potentially progressing to fibrous strands traversing the lumen or the homogeneous appearance of hemorrhage.
- Some follicles may luteinize and produce low levels of progesterone while others do not and may persist for long periods of time. Uterine edema will usually subside and the mare behaviorally will be neither receptive nor unreceptive.

Treatment

- If the anovulatory follicle luteinizes then prostaglandin therapy will result in lysis and follicular regression. However, in the absence of progesterone and luteinization, initiating estrus will depend on when the regression of the anovulatory follicle occurs.
- A subsequent follicular wave may be initiated in the presence of a regressing anovulatory follicle with behavioral estrus, uterine edema and subsequent ovulation of the new dominant follicle.

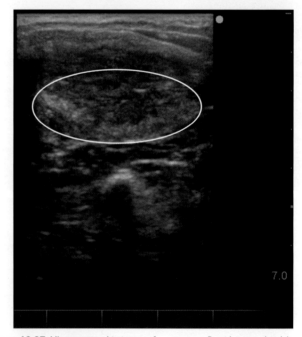

Figure 12.27 Ultrasonographic image of an anestrus flaccid uterus (circle). Note the absence of edema and roundness on cross-section.

- Human chorionic gonadotrophin (HCG) and deslorelin (a GnRH agonist) are generally not effective in inducing ovulation of the affected follicle.

Lack of follicular development (anestrus) (Figs. 12.26 & 12.27)

Seasonal anestrus occurs in most mares, however some mares may be placed under lights for 60 days and still have no follicular development. Mares may come off the race track to be bred and either seem to have a large follicle waiting to ovulate or have small inactive (anestrus) ovaries.

Clinical signs

- Small inactive ovaries may be present with 10–15 mm follicles to no follicular activity present.

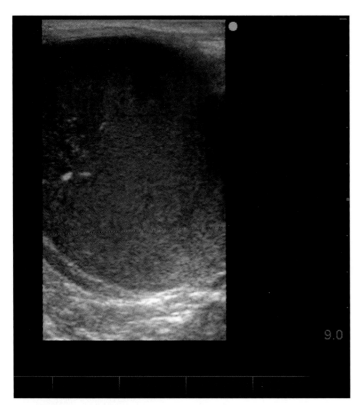

Figure 12.28 Ultrasonographic image of a large hemorrhagic anovulatory follicle that could turn into a hematoma.

Table 12.1 Induction of cyclicity

Drug	Mechanism of action	Dose
Domperidone	DA₂ dopamine receptor antagonist	1.1 mg/kg PO sid–bid
Reserpine	Rauwolfian substance	0.01 mg/kg PO q 24 hour
Sulperide	Selective DA₂ dopamine receptor antagonist	3.3 mg/kg/day
Deslorelin	GnRH agonist	62.5 μg IM, q 12 h
Buserelin	GnRH agonist	12.5 μg IM, q 12h
eFSH	FSH	12.5 μg IM, q 12 h until a 35 mm follicle present; then coast for 24 hours, give hCG and breed in another 24 hours

- The uterus is flaccid and the cervix is wide open and pale due to lack of progesterone and estrogen.

Diagnosis and treatment

- Rectal palpation and ultrasound help to identify the size of the ovaries and the follicular activity.
- Presence or absence of uterine edema aids in determining if the mare is truly anestrus/transition or coming out of transition.
- There are many different drugs and protocols to help induce cyclicity (Table 12.1).

Ovarian hematoma (Figs. 12.28 & 12.29)

Ovarian hematomas result from excessive hemorrhage into the follicular lumen following ovulation or may be the result of a hemorrhagic anovulatory follicle. As one of the common differentials for an enlarged unilateral ovary it is imperative to differentiate it from neoplastic disease (i.e. granulosa cell tumors).

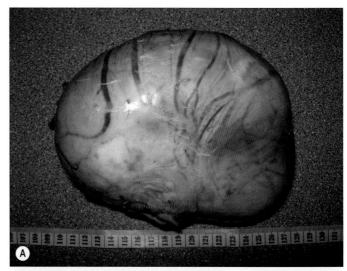

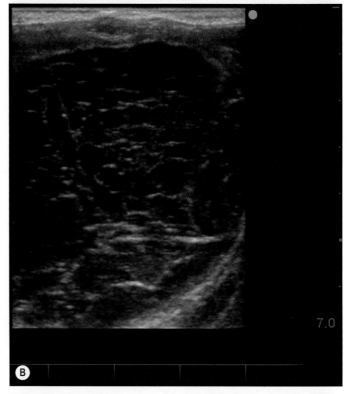

Figure 12.29 (A) A large ovarian hematoma that if incised would release fibrin, organized clots or serosanguinous fluid. (B) Ultrasonographic image of a large ovarian hematoma. Note the fibrous strands and spider web appearance.

Diagnosis and treatment

- Ultrasonographic evaluation of the enlarged ovary reveals hyperechogenic homogeneous blood within the lumen of an extremely large follicle, or a multicystic appearance due to fibrin strand formation spanning the diameter of the structure. The affected ovary has a clearly identifiable ovulation fossa on rectal palpation. The contralateral ovary on examination is of normal size and function and mares continue to cycle normally. Endocrine profiles and behavior are normal.
- Regression of the hematoma should occur over time, during which a normal interovulatory period will occur.

- If the hematoma becomes excessively large it can destroy the remaining normal parenchyma of the ovary and ovarian removal may be necessary because the ovary is left non-functional.

Ovarian tumors (Figs. 12.30 & 12.31)

Granulosa cell tumors (GCT) are the most common ovarian tumor in the mare. GCTs are usually extremely large or small and are usually steroid-producing, slow-growing, benign and unilateral. The opposite ovary is usually inactive probably due to the inhibin produced by the tumor's granulosa cells suppressing the release of pituitary follicle-stimulating hormone. An elevated level of testosterone occurs in about 54% of mares due to the presence of a significant number of thecal cells within the tumor (granulosa thecal cell tumor). Behavioral changes can include aggressive or stallion-like behavior, nymphomania with persistent estrus or long periods of anestrous. Colic signs may occur if the ovary becomes so large that it pulls on the broad ligament lying ventrally in the abdominal cavity. Tumors vary in size from 6–40 cm diameter. Pregnancy may not be affected by the development of the tumors after conception and can be found post foaling on routine examination. Tumor-bearing ovaries are often grossly enlarged with a smooth thickened capsule but sometimes give an impression of follicular structures being present. On section, early

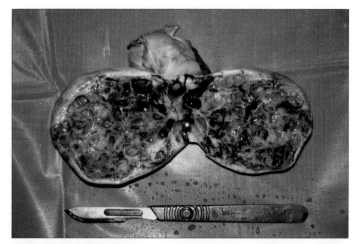

Figure 12.30 Small granulose cell tumor. Note the small cystic areas throughout the ovary.

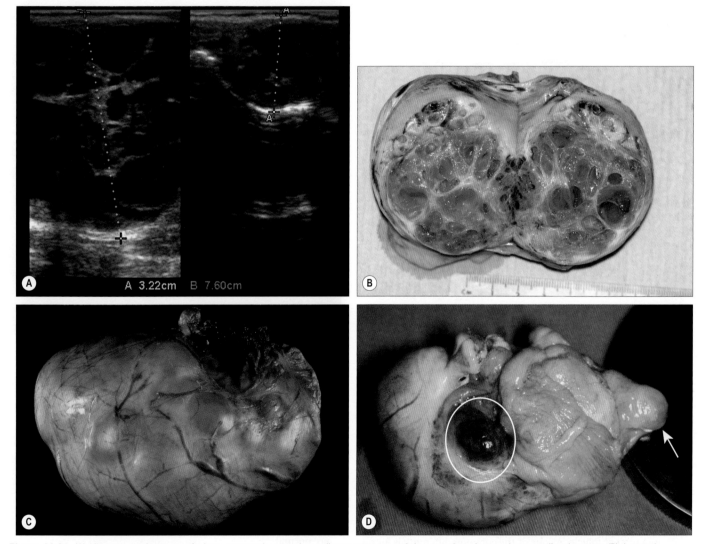

Figure 12.31 (A) Ultrasonographic image of a large ovary with a granulosa cell tumor present and the contralateral ovary that is small and inactive. (B) A typical granulosa cell tumor. Note the yellow cyst-like structures that are encapsulated. (C) Ovarian cyst adenoma. Multiple follicle-like cysts throughout the ovary. (D) Ovary with epoophoron cyst (arrow). The dark spot is a 4-day-old corpus hemorrhagicum protruding into the ovulation fossa (circle).

tumors show multiple cysts with a thin stroma; older tumors show marked thickening of the stroma and may on occasion be filled with blood.

Germ cell tumors are very rare but **dysgerminomas** may be associated with hypertrophic osteopathy of the lower limb, loss of condition and stiffness when walking. They are reported to vary in size but appear to metastasize early to the regional lymph nodes.

Teratomas have also been reported in equine ovaries which are enlarged and the mass contains fluid and an amorphous material with hair-like structures.

Other **mesenchymal tumors**, such as hemangiomas, leiomyoma, fibroma and lymphoma, have been described but appear to be extremely uncommon.

Diagnosis and treatment

* Behavioral changes as described above in combination with lack of an ovulation fossa on rectal palpation, ultrasonographic imaging and serum hormone levels aid in diagnosis. Ultrasonographic appearance of GCTs can vary from enlarged multicystic, honeycomb appearing firm ovaries to a single large cyst or blood-filled structure.
* Differentiation between 'autumn' or anovulatory follicles and ovarian hematomas is imperative. The contralateral ovary is usually small with no to minimal follicular activity.
* Clinical diagnostic assays should include serum antimullerian hormone, inhibin, testosterone and progesterone. These, however, may be equivocal and ascertaining if continued growth with time or regression with hormone therapy (progesterone and estradiol) may be necessary.
* Removal of the affected ovary. This can be done via a flank laparotomy, midline or paramedian approach. Return to normal estrous cycles by the contralateral ovary may take 8–12 months.

Cyst adenoma (Fig. 12.31C)

Epithelial cell tumors are rare and reports are confined to cyst adenoma. These may be identifiable per rectum as large cystic masses; fertility of the other ovary appears to remain normal and pregnancy may be uninterrupted following the surgical removal of the tumor. Affected ovaries are large and enclose multiple, large cysts containing clear, yellow fluid; these masses probably originate from the epithelial cells of the ovulation fossa. Usually these tumors are not hormonally active.

Treatment

Surgically remove the ovary.

Pituitary Pars Intermedia dysfunction (PPID)

Reproductive abnormalities such as abnormal estrous activity, estrous suppression and reduced fertility have been described in mares with PPID. This may be due to the hypertrophy, hyperplasia or adenoma in the pars intermedia of the pituitary destroying or impinging on the gonadotrophic cells of the anterior pituitary or suppression of the gonadotrophin secretion due to elevated levels of androgens or glucocorticoids produced in response by the adrenal cortex. The mare's ovaries are usually small to normal size, however they are firm on palpation with multiple small follicles that are observed on ultrasound deep within the ovarian parenchyma. The ovulation fossa is palpable.

Diagnosis and treatment

* Blood serum assays for glucose, insulin, adrenocorticotrophic hormone (ACTH), and cortisol levels can be indicative as well as abnormal responses to the dexamethasone suppression, ACTH stimulation and thyrotropin-releasing hormone (TrH) tests.
* See treatment for PPID.

Epithelial inclusion cysts

Epithelial inclusion cysts are multiple and occur in close proximity to the ovulation fossa increasing both in size and number with advancing age and these may interfere with ovulation. The other ovary usually continues to function normally and pregnancy may also occur.

Other structures occurring near the ovary include cysts of the mesonephric tubules; **epoöphoron cysts** and **paroöphoron cysts**. These slowly enlarge with time and consequently are more frequently found in aged mares. Epoöphoron cysts can reach up to 7 cm diameter and, on manual palpation, may be mistaken for part of the actual ovary. Paroöphoron cysts are smaller and less common.

The oviduct

Diagnosis and characterization of oviduct disease is difficult because the oviduct is not always palpable per rectum or visible on ultrasonographic examination. Therefore diagnosis often occurs after all other possible causes of infertility have been ruled out. Pathology within the oviduct would prevent the passage of the oocyte, spermatozoa or embryo into the uterus. Abnormalities affecting the oviduct can be categorized as inflammatory (salpingitis) or structural (blockage).

Salpingitis

Inflammatory disease of the oviduct or salpingitis is not common in the mare unlike other species due to the tight muscular sphincter around the uterine ostium (papillae). This tight utero-tubal junction appears to prevent the ascent of endometritis. The special anatomical position of the uterus of the mare in which the oviducts are in the dorsal part of the abdominal cavity above the uterus, rather than lying ventrally also aids in the prevention of inflammation. Salpingitis in the mare appears to be a widespread infiltrative, non-occlusive, and generally non-exudative process. Many cases however, have no identifiable pathogenic (or other) organism. Unilateral adhesions of the oviduct or fimbrae may also affect fertility by distorting the oviduct's position relative to the ovary impairing passage of the oocyte. The cause of both the inflammatory changes and the adhesions is not clear.

Diagnosis and treatment

* This condition is difficult to diagnose unless visually evident on laparoscopic examination or laparotomy. Culture of the oviduct during the procedure.
* Treatment can be attempted based on antibiotic sensitivity testing.

Oviduct blockage (Fig. 12.32)

Blockage of the oviduct may occur due to malformation in younger mares or occlusions or plugs most commonly found in older mares. Abnormal development of the oviducts as with cystic oviducts or the absence of an oviduct lumen hinders movement of the oocyte, spermatozoa or embryo. It has not been clarified if oviduct plugs in the older mare form due to collagen-type masses or inspissations of degenerated oocytes and oviduct secretions, however infertility can be a consequence.

Diagnosis

* Cannulation of the oviductal fimbrae via flank laparoscopy in the standing mare, with infusion of fluorescent microsphere beads will allow for the direct visualization of oviduct anatomy and indirect assessment of oviduct patency by performing a uterine lavage at 24 and 48 hours post surgery to identify the microspheres. If the microspheres are not found in the lavage fluids it is assumed the oviduct is not patent.
* A ventral midline exploratory laparotomy will also allow for visualization of the ovaries and oviducts for anatomical defects. This may

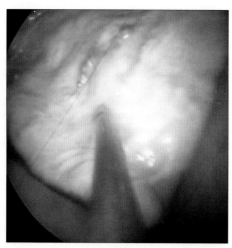

Figure 12.32 Placement of prostaglandin E on the oviduct via laparoscopy.

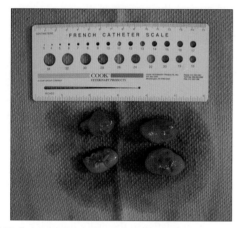

Figure 12.33 Endometrial cysts that have been removed.

be difficult however in maiden mares whose mesovarians and broad ligaments have not been stretched. Infusion of a sterile 5% new methylene blue dye in normal saline through a catheter into the oviduct and detection of the dye within the uterus will determine patency.

Treatment

- Movement or passage of the blockage through the oviduct can be done using two different techniques, the first of which is flushing the oviducts either via ventral midline laparotomy or standing flank laparoscopy.
- The second and less invasive or detrimental to the oviduct is placement of prostaglandin E2 (PGE2) on the surface of the oviduct using a flank laparoscopic approach. The PGE2 potentiates muscular relaxation of the oviduct allowing movement of the oviductal plugs into the uterus.

The uterus

The uterus is comprised of two uterine horns and the uterine body.

Developmental disorders

Congenital abnormalities of the uterus are rare in the mare but the finding of a bifid placenta without avillous areas suggests that bifid uterus may occur, although this has not so far been described. Anatomical abnormalities can be related to chromosomal disorders (see section Ovarian developmental disorders).

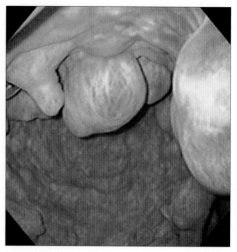

Figure 12.34 Endometrial cysts protruding into the uterine lumen on hysteroscopic examination.

Non-infectious disorders (barren mares)

Endometrial cysts (Figs. 12.33–12.37)

Endometrial cysts are not a cause of infertility, but a sign of lymphatic blockage and decreased uterine clearance, which have been shown to affect fertility. Uterine cysts are fluid-filled structures that can occur anywhere in the endometrium. They usually project outward or away from the surface of the endometrium. The incidence of endometrial cysts in the general mare population has been reported to be 1–22%, while in subfertile and older mares as high as 55%. It has been shown in some cases that the presence of numerous or large endometrial cysts (2.5 cm) can impede mobility of the embryonic vesicle and restrict the ability of the early conceptus to prevent luteolysis after day 10, thereby blocking maternal recognition of pregnancy. Additionally, by having the yolk sac or allantois in contact with a cyst versus the endometrium, absorption of nutrients may be prevented, resulting in early embryonic death.

Both lymphatic and glandular cysts occur in the endometrium of the mare. Lymphatic cysts are most common. They arise from collections of lymphatic fluid in the endometrium or myometrium, usually due to obstructed lymphatic channels or perhaps by gravitational effects of a pendulous uterus. Multiparous mares with uteri that have undergone fibotic changes are most prevalent, with size varying from a few millimeters up to 15 cm in diameter. Lymphatic cysts are cylindrical or spheroidal structures that can be pedunculated or sessile. They are usually thin-walled, round, elongated and may be individual or multilobular, divided by septa. Glandular cysts are a distension of uterine glands caused by periglandular fibrosis. They are usually microscopic to a few millimeters in diameter, are embedded in the endometrium and can be found in any area of the uterus.

Diagnosis

- Lymphatic cysts can be diagnosed through transrectal palpation, by direct intrauterine palpation via the cervix, through hysteroscopic examination, and endometrial biopsy, but most commonly by transrectal ultrasonography.
- The increased use of transrectal ultrasonography has enhanced the practitioner's ability to differentiate early embryonic vesicles from endometrial cyst. In mares that have a few small cysts, ultrasounding the mare pre or post breeding or ovulation and mapping of endometrial cysts can aid in pregnancy diagnosis by comparing ultrasonographic images. Mares that have numerous clusters or multilobular cysts may need repeat examinations before determination of a pregnancy by increasing vesicular size or a visible heart beat can be established.

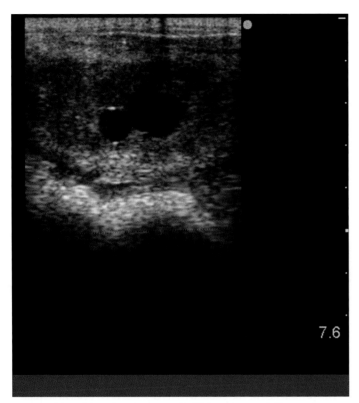

Figure 12.35 Ultrasonographic image of a 12-day pregnancy (left) next to an endometrial cyst.

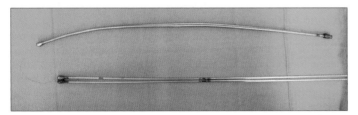

Figure 12.36 Double lumen steal mare catheter that can have wire inserted through. Lateral view (above) and dorsal view (below).

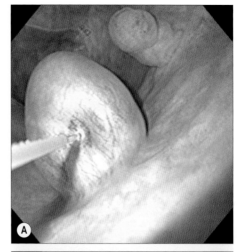

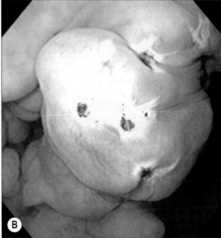

Figure 12.37 (A) Lasering an endometrial cyst. (B) Reduced endometrial cyst with laser burns evident.

Treatment

- Most cysts do not cause a problem, but are usually a sign of an underlying one. These mares are usually older mares with poor uterine clearance and benefit tremendously by simply using uterine lavage and oxytocin in their breeding regimen. Where cysts create a problem is in the distinction or recognition from a pregnancy, however this is more of an inconvenience than a problem. Cyst removal therefore should be delegated to those mares with poor reproductive histories that have large cysts that may obstruct embryo movement or those mares with numerous small cysts that may prevent early embryonic growth or severely compromise the placenta.

- Various treatments have been proposed to include: endometrial curettage, puncture by uterine biopsy, aspiration, or lasering during hysteroscopic examination, snare electrocoagulation via hysteroscopy, repeated lavage with warm saline or ablate manually. Large pedunculated cysts are removed when the mare is in heat, by manually snaring the cyst with a gigli wire introduced through a steal double mare catheter. Once the snare is around the base a gradual sawing motion will cut the cyst from the endometrium. This can usually be accomplished without rupturing the cyst with minimal removal or damage to the underlying endometrium. Care must be taken not to remove more than the epithelial lining. A minimal amount of hemorrhage is associated with this procedure and it is recommended to lavage the mare's uterus for the proceeding couple of days. Smaller more numerous cysts are usually removed via hysteroscopic laser. This technique has not been determined to be satisfactory for large cysts, since so much heat is generated in order to destroy the cyst that there is increased risk of damage to or tearing of the uterus. Smaller cysts, however, are easy to find and destroy. Lasering the cyst at the thinnest section until complete penetration through the wall has been made releases the fluid contents with immediate visible shrinkage. Care must be taken not to laser blood vessels on the cyst's surface making visibility difficult.

Persistent endometrial cups (Figs. 12.38–12.40)

Around days 35–36 of gestation the chorionic girdle starts to invade the maternal endometrium and the endometrial cups are formed. These produce equine chorionic gonadotrophin (eCG). eCG has biological activities similar to FSH and LH. The LH component causes luteinization and/or ovulation of follicles, forming secondary and accessory CLs, and continues to produce progesterone until days 100–120 of pregnancy. eCG stimulates primary and secondary CLs to form and continue to produce progesterone until days 100–120 of pregnancy. Endometrial cups regress as the placenta forms and progestagens are produced. Most endometrial cups have regressed by 150 days of gestation, however there is increasing evidence that persistent

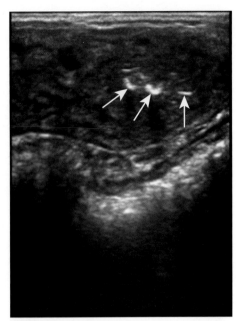

Figure 12.38 Ultrasonographic image of endometrial cups. Note: they are hyperechoic crest-shaped structures (arrows).

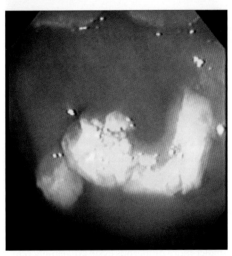

Figure 12.39 Endometrial cups viewed during a hysteroscopic exam. Their size and density depends on age and function.

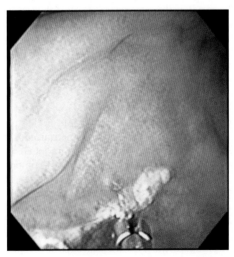

Figure 12.40 A biopsy punch attempting to remove endometrial cup tissue.

endometrial cups in post foaling, post abortion or post embryonic loss after 45 days should be considered when mares fail to cycle properly within the expected time period.

Persistent endometrial cups should be considered when mares fail to show regular estrus activity. Mares will show behavioral estrus but instead of having a normal estrus period leading to ovulation, small multiple follicles will luteinize or hemorrhage forming the spider web appearance associated with secondary CLs (visible on ultrasound examination).

Diagnosis

- Positive blood serum eCG levels. Care must be taken with some commercial kits since they can cross react with LH.
- Transrectal ultrasonography can identify hyperechogenic spots in the base of a horn if the endometrial cups are large and able to be visualized.
- Hysteroscopic examination may reveal the circle of peanut-shaped cups in the base of a horn. These will vary in size and color depending on their activity and longevity.

Treatment

- Different treatments have been attempted to help regress existing endometrial cup tissue. These include laser, biopsy and kerosene endometrial curettage. Unfortunately, kerosene is the only treatment to be looked at critically in three mares and it is still questionable whether treatment is to no avail. Regression therefore finally occurs over time.
- The persistence of the endometrial cups has been evident in mares up to 2 years post foaling and post 45 day embryonic loss.

Non-infectious disorders (pregnant mares)

Uterine torsion (Figs. 12.41 & 12.42)

Uterine torsion is an infrequent complication of pregnancy, reported in 5–10% of all mares that have serious equine obstetric problems. Uterine torsion occurs in middle to late gestation and causes great risk to both mare and foal. The cause is unknown, although it has been postulated that uterine torsion may develop secondary to rolling as a result of gastrointestinal problems or trauma, or the righting reflexes and vigorous movements of the fetus, during the later stages of gestation.

Mares display signs of abdominal discomfort and colic, most commonly with mild intermittent episodes responsive to anti-inflammatories and analgesics. Eventually, inappetence and lethargy ensue. Severity of signs is dependent on degree of rotation, level of vascular or fetal compromise and intestinal involvement. Torsion of the uterus greater than 360° interferes with blood flow to and from the uterus and can result in local anoxia, congestion, fetal death and rupture of the uterus. Chronic oxygen deprivation to tissue and serosal injury further promote adhesion formation in the abdominal cavity.

Diagnosis

Physical examination can be within normal limits, with the problem evident only on rectal palpation of the broad ligaments. Torsion of the uterus can occur clockwise, to the right: the left broad ligament is stretched horizontally over the top of the uterus and the right broad ligament courses tightly ventrally or vertically under the uterus toward the opposite side. The uterus may also torse in a counter-clockwise direction, to the left: the right broad ligament is palpable as a dorsal sheet of tissue going to the left side and the left broad ligament is pulled ventrally, toward midline. Rotation can range from 180° to 360°. Unlike cattle, in the mare, the cervix and cranial vagina are usually not involved unless the degree of rotation is severe or fibrous tissue has formed.

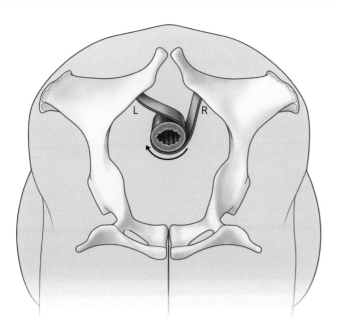

Figure 12.41 Right (clockwise) uterine torsion.

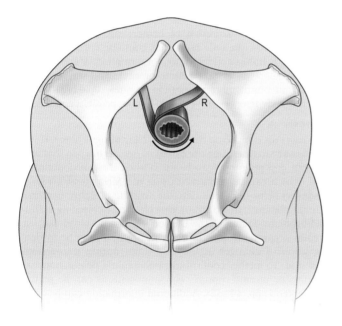

Figure 12.42 Left (counter clockwise) uterine torsion.

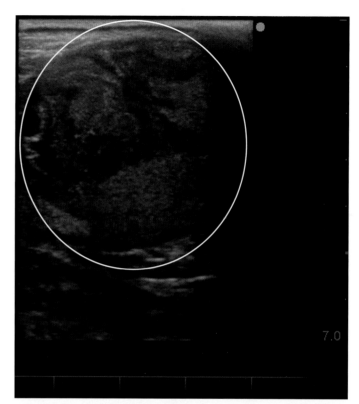

Figure 12.43 Ultrasonographic appearance of hematoma within the broad ligament (circle).

Transrectal and transabdominal ultrasonography can aid in assessment of uterine compromise by enabling determination of uterine wall thickness, placental integrity, vascular distension, fetal viability and condition of the fetal fluid.

If there is concern about intestinal involvement, abdominocentesis may be performed to aid in determining the appropriate mode of replacement or prognosis.

Treatment

- Many methods have been used to correct uterine torsion in the mare. The most common are rolling the anesthetized mare and laparotomy via standing flank or ventral midline incision. Although non-surgical methods such as rolling are less expensive, this technique may predispose to separation of the placenta from the endometrium with subsequent abortion, premature birth or death of the fetus. Uterine rupture and tearing are severe complications associated with this procedure. Evaluation of uterine and intestinal compromise is not possible.

- Standing flank laparotomy has been more popular than the ventral midline approach and is especially easier earlier in gestation; in addition, general anesthesia is not necessary. The uterus should be palpated for signs of edema, congestion and hematomas. This method carries risks: the mesometrium is under considerable tension, and if the horse is standing during laparotomy, this can lead to perforation of the uterus and injuries to the mesometrium during manual retorsion.

- A ventral midline approach allows quick and clear access to the abdominal cavity, visual assessment of uterine wall viability, correction of concomitant gastrointestinal tract problems, and performance of hysterotomy if indicated. Continued monitoring is necessary for systemic compromise and laminitis. Prognosis for fetal survival is good with improvement as gestational age lessens.

Peripaturient hemorrhage (Figs. 12.43–12.46)

Hemorrhage from the middle uterine, external iliac, utero-ovarian and vaginal arteries has been described in late pregnancy and after parturition and accounts for 40% of peripaturient deaths in mares. Most cases occur in older, multiparous mares, but it is becoming an increasing problem in younger primiparous mares from 5–24 (median, 14) years of age. The etiology for rupture has not been definitively ascertained, although at least three hypotheses have been proposed:

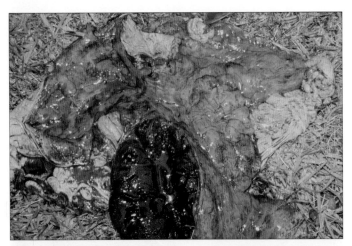

Figure 12.44 Gross appearance of a hematoma within the broad ligament.

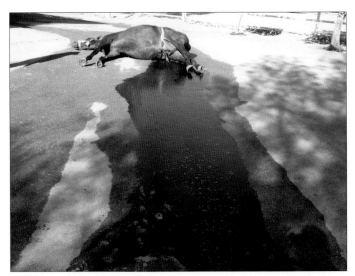

Figure 12.46 This mare foaled 6 weeks previously and at that time had an episode of colic associated with what was diagnosed to be a uterine artery hemorrhage contained within the broad ligament. At 6 weeks post-foaling she had another severe per-acute episode of colic and died. At necropsy it was found that there had been an adhesion between the small intestine and broad-ligament which had become detached; this disrupted the clot that had formed and the mare had another uterine artery hemorrhage that now extended into the abdominal cavity and resulted in her rapid death.

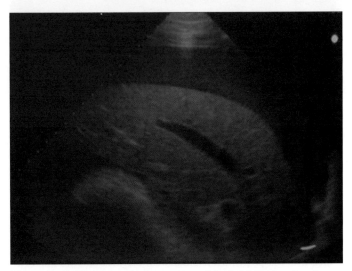

Figure 12.45 Ultrasonographic image of intra-abdominal fluid. Note the spleen floating in the flocculent fluid.

1) Middle uterine a arterial rupture usually occurs on the right side of the mare's uterus, possibly as a result of the cecum displacing the uterus and increasing tension on the right uterine artery in addition to additional direct pressure by the cecum on the artery
2) Normal age-related vascular degeneration
3) Copper deficiency interfering with elasticity of the vessels.

Mares with discomfort or colic in the middle or late stages of gestation or 24–72 hours after parturition should be considered to be potential hemorrhage candidates. In some instances, mares are simply found dead because of acute arterial hemorrhage. More often, however, mares develop signs within 24 hours of parturition, and most are associated with rupture of the right uterine artery.

Three clinical scenarios can occur. In the first, the hemorrhage is confined to the broad ligament. Although this type of hemorrhagic episode is usually self-limiting because containment within the ligament enhances hematoma formation, it can be incredibly painful, and most mares lie down and get up repeatedly, lie on their side or look frequently at their belly. Mucous membranes can be normal to pale, depending on the extent of hemorrhage. The second scenario occurs when the mare hemorrhages into the uterus. This is usually a postpartum event, unless there has been traumatic injury to the uterus. Finally, the most detrimental scenario is seen with rupture within the

broad ligament and extension of hemorrhage into the abdomen. When this occurs, the only border for containment is the abdomen itself, which is not as conducive to clot formation. Mares may lie on their sides, adopt a sternal position, or circle and stagger; and will have pale mucous membranes, high heart rates, rapid breathing, cold sweat, low body temperature (96–98°F) and, possibly, acute death.

Diagnosis
Often diagnosis is made on the basis of clinical signs alone. However, it is necessary to determine the extent of hemorrhage so that optimal treatment and prognosis can be established. Transabdominal ultrasound (which can be performed using a 5-MHz linear array rectal transducer) helps to differentiate the swirling of active hemorrhage free in the abdomen from intrauterine bleeding or bleeding within the broad ligament. Filling of the uterine horns with blood can lead to placental separation, and intrauterine trauma may be evident by observation of changes in the fetal fluids during transabdominal ultrasound. To further confirm intra-abdominal hemorrhage versus peritonitis or uterine rupture, abdominocentesis can be performed (see Chapter 1, pp. 34–35). Additional information can be obtained from blood work (with total protein and albumin concentration decreasing prior to a decrease in hematocrit). These findings can help determine which therapeutic regimen to use.

Treatment
• Mares should be treated for shock secondary to hemorrhage, however a fine line is walked between providing enough support to maintain sufficient blood flow to vital organs and avoiding increasing blood pressure to the point of interfering with clot formation and hemostasis. The ultimate treatment has obviously not been found to exist, and many protocols have been reported. The most important initial consideration is to improve perfusion and keep the mare quiet and warm to promote clot formation. Various drugs have been used, including acepromazine, xylazine, butorphanol and diazepam, to keep the mare as comfortable as possible while other treatments are being initiated. Care must be taken when using sedatives since many decrease blood pressure and can further

accentuate hypovolemic shock and decrease blood flow to vital organs. With the goal of keeping the mare as quiet as possible, it is probably prudent to leave the foal with the mare, as long as the mare's movements do not cause harm. If the foal must be removed from the stall, it should be kept in close view of the mare. Further therapy to reverse shock and control hemorrhage can include the following:

- Hypertonic saline: the hyper-osmolality of the solution rapidly increases intravascular volume improving perfusion.
- Regular isotonic intravenous fluids: provide replacement for intravascular volume expansion, buffering, and dispersal to intercellular space.
- Colloids plasma: helps maintain intravascular volume and provides clotting factors; whole blood expands oncotic blood volume while providing increased oxygen carrying capacity, clotting factors and platelets.
- Aminocaproic acid: inhibits fibrinolysis via inhibition of plasminogen activator substances and anti-plasminogen activity.
- Yunnan baiyao: an oral hemostatic Chinese herbal medicine, used originally by soldiers in the Vietnam war to stop bleeding.
- Naloxone: pure opioid antagonist used to improve circulation in refractory shock by binding endogenous opioids hypotension is reduced, cardiac work decreased and pulmonary vascular resistance is lowered. Care should be used when given with butorphenol since they will negate each other.
- Formalin: is believed to cross link proteins potentially altering platelet or endothelial cell surface, proteins resulting in activation of platelets or decreased endothelial permeability; recent studies have discourage its use (Sellon, D 1999 AAEP proceedings).

- Surgical intervention has been attempted in a small number of cases, but the compromised status of the mare and the difficult location of the source of the hemorrhage makes the survival rate poor. One of the first case studies reported on periparturient hemorrhage in mares indicated that prepartum hemorrhage accounts for only 14% of periparturient hemorrhage. In addition, treatment of periparturient hemorrhage at the clinic was aimed at restoring cardiovascular volume, enhancing coagulation, controlling pain and reducing the effects of hypoxemia, as mentioned previously. In that study, 61 of 73 (84%) mares survived, with 16% dying or being euthanized. Regarding mares' future potential to foal without recurrent hemorrhage, 26/53 (49%) mares produced one or more foals after recovering. It was concluded that treatment was associated with a good prognosis for survival and a reasonable prognosis for future fertility.

Vestibulo/vaginal varicosities (Fig. 12.47)

Probably the most common form of prepartum hemorrhage is not severe or life-threatening but manifests more as a chronic trickle of blood. This is associated with the varicosities in the vestibular-vaginal sphincter (hymen) in old mares.

Clinical signs

Mares show intermittent or chronic vaginal bleeding, which is not necessarily (or even usually) related to mating or parturition. Most incidents, however, occur during the last month of pregnancy and may be mistaken for impending abortion or parturition. It is rare for more than 50–100 ml of blood to be lost but an occasional case may develop severe enough chronic bleeding to lower the mare's packed cell volume (PCV) and total protein. Blood can be seen on the vulva lips or between the hind legs.

Diagnosis and treatment

- Diagnosis can be made by speculum examination, during which large varicosities associated with hemorrhage will be evident.

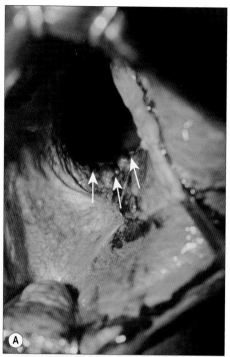

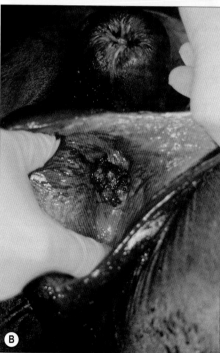

Figure 12.47 (A) Vaginal varicosity. Veins bleeding with clots of blood overlying veins (arrows). (B) Small hemorrhagic 'grape-like' varicose veins.

Additional blood can be seen in the cranial aspect of the vagina depending on the effects of conformation and gravity.

- Confirmation that the origin of hemorrhage is indeed varicosities and not placental in origin can be obtained by performing transrectal ultrasonography and confirming that the cervix is closed and that the placenta and fetal fluids appear normal.
- The volume of blood lost is usually not severe enough to warrant supportive intravenous fluids, but administering preventative antimicrobials (blood is an excellent bacterial growth medium),

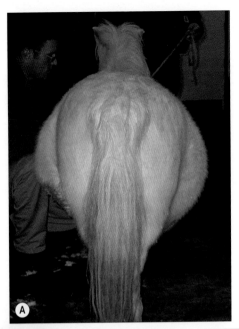

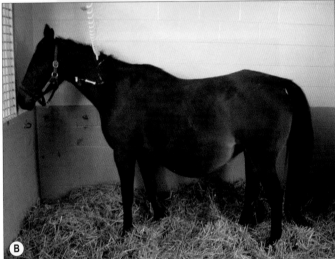

Figure 12.48 (A) Miniature mare presented for hydrops allantois. Note her papple-shaped abdomen. (B) Large pendulous abdomen in a mare at 8 months of gestation. Note that the abdomen is disproportionately large for the stage of gestation.

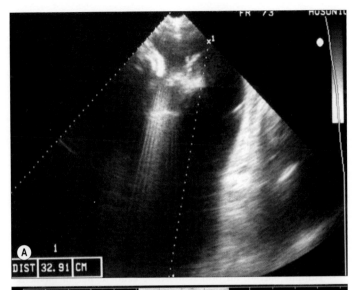

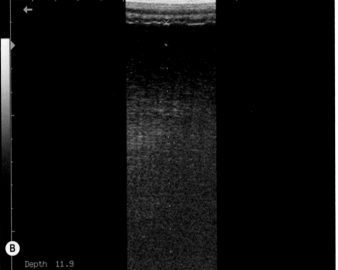

Figure 12.49 (A,B) Transabdominal ultrasonographic image of increased amount and depth of the allantoic fluid.

altrenogest (to help ensure that the cervix is tight) and yunnan baiyao (to promote hemostasis) may be prudent.

- Monitoring the mare's hematocrit can aid in screening for excessive hemorrhage. If the mare does not stop bleeding after parturition, the vessels can be ligated.

Hydrops allantois/hydrops amnios (Figs. 12.48–12.51)

Hydroallantois, a sudden increase in the volume of allantoic fluid during a period of 10–14 days, is more common than hydroamnios, an excessive accumulation of amniotic fluid in the amniotic cavity. Hydroamnios, unlike hydroallantois, develops gradually over several weeks to months during the second half of gestation. It is often associated with a deformed fetus with a facial, genetic or congenital abnormality. Although swallowing in the fetus plays a role in the maintenance of fetal fluid balance, other mechanisms may be important. The normal volume of amniotic fluid in mares near term is 3–7 l and is composed of secretions of the amnion and the nasopharynx of

the fetus, fetal saliva, transudation from maternal serum and fetal urine (late in pregnancy). Whether the problem arises because of an increase in secretion or decrease in resorption or both is not clear. It has been suggested that the fetus might actively regulate the volume and composition of the amniotic fluid by deglutition, and the prevention or impairment of swallowing may lead to hydramnios. The normal volumes of allantoic fluid in the near-term mare have been reported to be 8–15 liters. The pathophysiology of hydroallantois in the mare remains unknown. Some authors have suggested that the increase in fluid is a placental problem caused either by increased production of fluid or decreased transplacental absorption. Others have proposed that the etiology is related to placentitis and heritability.

Clinical signs

- In both hydroallantois and hydroamnios, mares present with abnormally increased abdominal distension for the duration of gestation.
- Mares may be anorexic, have high heart rates, be depressed and may have severe ventral edema/plaques, abdominal discomfort, and labored breathing caused by hydraulic pressure on the diaphragm.

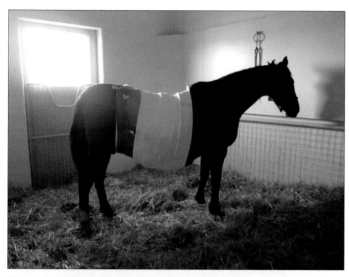

Figure 12.50 A belly band as abdominal support in a mare with a rupture of the prepubic tendon. The same type of abdominal support can be used in mares with hydrops of the fetal fluids.

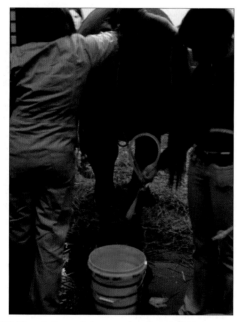

Figure 12.51 Slow drainage of the excessive allantoic fluid.

- Mares may have great difficulty walking, and many mares prefer to remain recumbent, especially with hydroallantois.
- Mares in advanced stages of hydropsic conditions may have evidence of ventral abdominal wall herniation or prepubic tendon rupture.
- Early management is aimed at preventing these body wall tears, which improves the mare's prognosis, since obtaining a live foal has not been reported with hydroallantois and has been reported only once with hydroamnios.

Diagnosis

- Rectal palpation is diagnostic and reveals a huge, taut, fluid-filled uterus. The fetus cannot be felt, and the uterus is usually tightly distended.

- Transrectal ultrasound reveals an excessive volume of hyperechogenic (speckled) fluid. Differentiation between an increase in allantoic verses amniotic fluid can sometimes be difficult.
- Transabdominal ultrasound will confirm the presence of excessive volumes of fluid and help differentiate between the two cavities as well as permit evaluation of fetal viability.
- Ultrasonography of the abdominal walls for evidence of edema or separation of musculature is necessary to monitor impending body wall tears, especially prepubic tendon rupture, which is a common sequela with hydroallantois and can dramatically change the prognosis for the livelihood and reproductive value of the mare.

Treatment

- Once diagnosis of hydroallantois is confirmed, fetal viability and udder development is determined and milk electrolytes can be assessed to estimate the level of fetal maturity in late gestation.
- Gestational age and fetal viability determine the treatment method of choice. Mares evaluated earlier (5–7 months) in gestation may undergo elective termination of pregnancy. Later in gestation or in mares with profound abdominal enlargement and large volumes of fluid in the uterus require controlled drainage of the fluid before delivery of the fetus.
- Support of the abdomen may help lessen the pressure on the abdominal musculature and prepubic tendon.
- Controlled drainage is essential because of the alteration of total body fluid balance. Sudden loss of this large volume of fluid may result in shock. Slow siphoning of the allantoic fluid can be accomplished by using a chest drain tube, inserting the protected sharp end of the tube through the cervix (following cervical dilation) and through the placenta with sterile extension tubing attached to control the flow rate. Concurrent large volumes of intravenous fluids should be administered to prevent hypovolemic shock.
- Fetal death may occur as a result of fetal asphxia, fetal infection secondary to contamination of the placental fluids or membranes during drainage or uterine contraction from prostaglandin release.
- Close monitoring for impending parturition is necessary; these mares may have poor cervical dilation and uterine contractility (inertia) as a result of the chronic uterine stretching and may require assistance with delivery.
- In most situations, the fetus can usually not be saved, but prompt intervention yields the best prognosis for physical recovery as well as for future fertility of the mare.
- Conservative supportive management of mares with hydroamnios can result in the birth of a live foal. Mares should be monitored for signs of weakness in the prepubic tendon and abdominal wall, while the fetus and placenta are monitored for signs of stress and pending abortion. Like with hydroallantois, hydroamnios has the potential complications of hypovolemic shock and cardiac arrhythmias that can be addressed by supportive care (large-volume crystalloid infusion).
- When the abdominal wall weakens or there is no viable foal, induction of parturition or cesarean section surgery (with fetal malformations) may be necessary.

Ruptured prepubic tendon or abdominal hernia (Fig. 12.52)
Two types of body wall tears occur in the late term pregnant mare: abdominal wall hernias and prepubic tendon tears or rupture (see ch 8 pg 301). These injuries are seen in inactive or older mares that lack muscle tone.

Clinical signs

- Abdominal wall hernias manifest with clinical signs of colic; mares do not strongly resist walking, have progressive abdominal

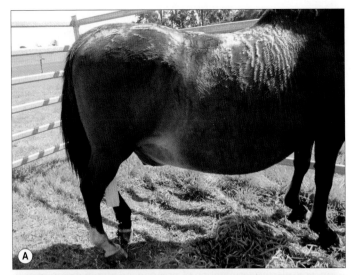

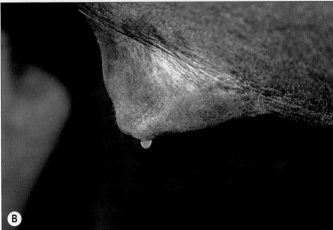

Figure 12.52 (A) Tears of the abdominal musculature frequently occur in association with tears of the prepubic tendon in older mares in late pregnancy. Due to the associated swelling and edema, it may be difficult to differentiate between muscle tears or combined muscle/tendon tears based on clinical examination alone, and frequently ultrasonographic examination is required to define the extent of the injury. This mare has both tearing of the prepubic tendon and both recti. Note the cranial position of the mammary gland which is a common feature of prepubic tendon tears (the mare died shortly after this image was taken due to massive hemorrhage). (B) Bleeding into the mammary tissue with subsequent presence of blood in mammary secretion can be seen with muscle tears, but is a common feature of prepubic tendon tears.

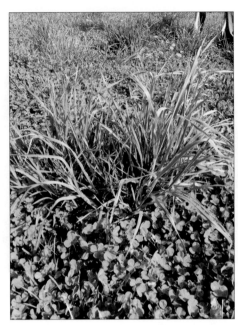

Figure 12.53 Tall fescue, a perennial grass infected with *Neotyphodium coenophialum*.

distension and develop ventral edema. In contrast, mares with prepubic tendon rupture have significant abdominal pain, progressive ventral body wall edema, stretched mammary glands, and elevation of the tailhead and ischial tuberosity (resulting in a sawhorse-like stance).

- Potential predisposing factors to body wall defects cited in the literature include hydrops allantois, hydrops amnion, traumatic injury, twins and fetal giants.
- These conditions must be carefully differentiated from the more common, benign, subcutaneous edema of the ventral abdominal wall which is due to circulatory changes caused by the weight of the foal.

Diagnosis

- Transcutaneous ultrasonographic examination identifies disruption of the tendon fibers immediately cranial to the pubis in

prepubic tendon rupture, compared with the finding of discrete tears within muscle fibers in defects in the abdominal walls.
- In addition, evidence of herniation or displacement of the abdominal wall cranial to the pubis can be identified during rectal examination of the caudal abdominal floor.

Treatment

- Options include induction of parturition to help decrease the weight on the floor of the abdomen and prevent additional tearing from excessive weight of the fetus; application of a belly band to provide abdominal support for the pendulous abdomen with stall rest; prosthetic repair once the acute stage of abdominal wall break down has passed; elective cesarean section or euthanasia of the dam.
- Because these abdominal defects are not resolved post-partum, recommendations should be made that the mare not carry future pregnancies to term.
- In breeds in which use of assisted reproductive techniques is acceptable, mares could serve as embryo donors and remain reproductively useful.

Fescue toxicosis (Fig. 12.53)

Tall fescue (*Lolium arundinaceum* (Schreb.)) a perennial grass is infected with the endophyte *Neotyphodium coenophialum* which produces toxins that when ingested cause severe adverse effects in late-term pregnant mares.

Clinical signs

- Reproductive abnormalities include prolonged gestation, late-term abortion, premature placental separation, dystocia, traumatic injury to the reproductive tract, thickened placentas, retained placentas and agalactia.
- A high incidence of foal mortality results from prolonged gestation, dystocia with anoxia, dysmaturity, weakness, starvation, failure of passive transfer and septicemia.

Treatment and prevention

- Treatment should start at least 30 days prior to parturition or as soon as possible if knowledge of continued grazing on endophyte-infected fescue.

- Removing the mare from endophyte-infected pasture or hay is imperative and attending the parturition is important due to increased risk of dystocia.
- Dopamine (D2) antagonists (such as domperidone, pre-foaling, or reserpine and fluphenazine, post-foaling) can be used to aid in reversing the endophytes' effects.

Non-infectious disorders (post-partum mares)

Retained placenta (Figs. 12.54–12.56)

In the mare placental separation from the endometrium occurs during the third stage of labor. Post-partum uterine contractions along with the decreased blood supply from the fetal placental vessels and endometrium allow maternal crypts to relax and shrinkage of the chorionic villi. The progression of the chorioallantois into the vaginal vault through the cervix stimulates continued release of oxytocin and placental delivery. The cause of a retained placenta is unclear. However it is the most common post-partum complication with an incidence of 2–10.5%. A higher incidence has been reported in draft mares, increased age, prolonged gestation, hydrops, abortion, stillbirth, twinning, dystocia, placentitis and cesarean. A placenta is generally considered 'retained' if it is still attached to the endometrium 3 hours after parturition. The non-pregnant horn is more commonly retained than the edematous pregnant horn. Early treatment is essential so metritis, endotoxemia with laminitis and death do not occur.

Clinical signs

- The fetal membranes may be either visible and partly expelled or they may be totally contained in the uterus. Commonly, the mare becomes clinically ill before this is detected if the placenta is not completely examined post expulsion.
- Turning the placenta so the chorioallantoic surface is on the outside and laying it in an 'F'-shaped pattern allows for the body and both horns including the tips (identified by the avillus area of the oviductal opening) to be examined completely.
- One of the most common types of retention of fetal membranes is where the chorioallantois attached within the non-pregnant horn is broken off and retained in the uterus.

Diagnosis

- The placenta may be protruding from the vulval lips in some situations, however most retained placentas can be identified by manual uterine examination. If the tip is retained and the uterus is very big, identification may be difficult but should be considered if there is a moderate to large amount of fetid thick fluid present. Quite often, the placenta will become lodged in the tip of the tube when a uterine lavage is being performed.
- If gross examination of the placenta lacks a horn or is shredded, examination of the uterus is imperative. Transabdominal and transrectal ultrasonography can also aid in detection of placental presence.

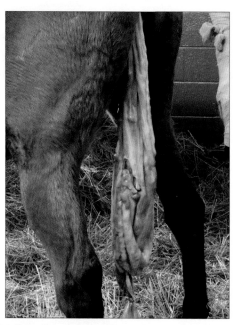

Figure 12.54 Retained fetal membranes.

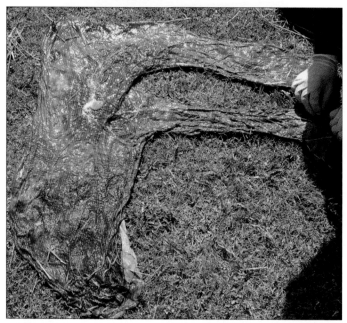

Figure 12.55 Examination of the placenta should be performed by placing it in 'F' or reverse 'F' position. Consistency in placement facilitates the identification of missing parts.

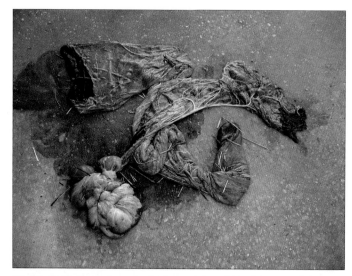

Figure 12.56 Placental examination is especially useful in determining if all the placenta has been passed. In this case the tip of the non-pregnant horn has been retained and is obviously missing during the placental examination.

Treatment

- Different regimens using oxytocin and fluids with calcium borogluconate have been documented to be effective in providing placental release. Manual removal is not recommended if the membranes are firmly attached, due to potential of endometrial hemorrhage, tear, contamination, retention of the tip of a placental horn, uterine tip invagination, permanent endometrial damage and delayed uterine involution.
- The uterus during parturition is naturally contaminated with bacteria, therefore after 8 hours of retention with autolysing retained fetal membranes an environment is produced that is conducive to exponential bacteria growth. The increased number of bacteria and inflammatory products can produce a metritis allowing absorption of bacteria and toxins causing septicemia, endotoxemia and laminitis. Further treatment should therefore focus on removal of inflammatory debris and bacteria by intrauterine lavage with large volumes of saline or dilute povidone iodine solution. Flushing should continue until the solution is the same color going in as coming out. This procedure may need to be done twice a day depending on the amount, consistency and smell of the intrauterine fluid. If the chorioallantois is still intact, infusion of the sac with saline allows distention of the uterus with subsequent placental release (a technique first described by Burns et al in 1977). The fluid needs to be kept in the sac by holding the membranes tightly around the nasogastric tube. Membrane expulsion usually occurs in 5–30 minutes. Supplemental broad-spectrum antibiotics such as procaine penicillin and gentamicin as well as anti-endotoxemia/laminitis therapy consisting of flunixin meglamine (0.25 mg/kg), pentoxyphilline (8.5 mg/kg) are essential and should be initiated to help prevent complications. Administration of intrauterine antibiotics is controversial due to their potential irritation to the uterus and inactivation by autolysed tissue and bacteria.
- One of the most important aspects of treating retained fetal membranes is recognition of their presence. Not all retained placentas are visible and unless a placenta has been examined for completion it may not be discovered until the mare presents depressed, febrile, anorexic, tachypnic and toxic with bounding digital pulses. Therefore it is imperative to stress the importance of placental evaluation by whomever is present at delivery. Examination of the fetal membranes ascertains completeness, in addition to any other abnormalities, i.e. placentitis, which can allow the veterinarian to gain time and incite the treatment of potential problems.

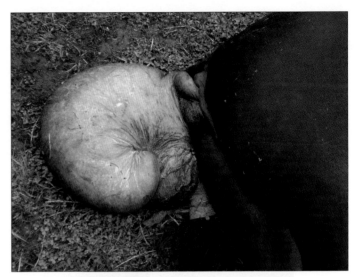

Figure 12.57 Uterine prolapse.

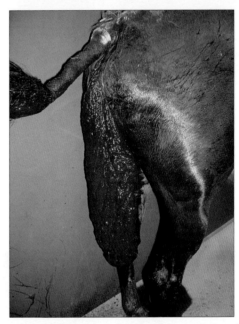

Figure 12.58 Prolapsed uterus (followed prolonged dystocia). From McAuliffe SB, Slovis NM (eds) (2008) *Color Atlas of Diseases and Disorders of the Foal.* Elsevier, Oxford (with permission)

Uterine prolapse (Figs. 12.57 & 12.58)

Uterine prolapse does not commonly occur in the mare due to cranial attachments of the broad ligaments. However, dystocia and retained placental membranes have been associated with an increased incidence. This may be a result of decreased uterine involution following delivery (atony), administration of large doses of oxytocin or hypocalcemia.

Clinical signs and diagnosis

- Clinical signs can be mild, to include restlessness, pain, anxiety, tenesmus, increased pulse and respiration rate, or more severe with weak pulse, rapid shallow breathing, pale mucous membranes, recumbency and death.
- Diagnosis is made by observing the everted organ protruding through the vulva as a red corrugated mass that should not be mistaken for a portion of the chorioallantois filled with fluid. Usually most of the exposed surface is uterine body with occasionally a uterine horn present. Prolapse of the uterus causes a decrease in venous return and allows exposure to air and dirt, producing an edematous, contaminated and possibly lacerated organ.

- Possible complications include internal hemorrhage, incarceration and ischemia of intestines and/or bladder resulting in hypovolemic or endotoxic shock.

Treatment

- Replacement of the uterus as quickly and as cleanly as possible with minimal trauma is optimum. This may be accomplished by first controlling the straining, by either administering sedatives, a caudal epidural or inducing general anesthesia depending on how tractable the mare is, and the environment and facilities available. Epidural anesthesia may reduce the amount of reflex straining provoked by vaginal manipulation, however it will not eliminate the mare's abdominal press. Mares showing signs of endotoxic or hemorrhagic shock should be stabilized while uterine replacement occurs. If incorporation of viscera in the prolapse is suspected rectal palpation before uterine replacement should aid in determining if an exploratory celiotomy is necessary to assess the viability of the entrapped organs. Conversely, if hemorrhage is suspected rectal palpation may cause further instability in any potential clot formation. Elevation of the uterus and placement of the mare with her hind end higher than the front will aid in restoring circulation, reduce congestion and edema and decrease traction on the uterine ligaments, facilitating correct anatomical replacement. Warm water and non-detergent soap or mild disinfectant such as dilute povidone-iodine solution can be used to clean the exposed surface of the uterus, while others advocate a sulfa-urea powder to help remove the edema or applying sugar or dextrose to the endometrium. While these substances provide a good environment for bacterial growth, they appear to aid in fluid loss, and decrease the size of the prolapse making it easier to reduce. Deep endometrial lacerations should be closed with absorbable suture. By exerting pressure on the uterus with the palm of your hand only or a closed fist as it is kneaded into the vagina, further trauma to the friable uterus can be prevented.

- Once the uterus has been replaced into the abdomen, rectal palpation can confirm both horns are in the correct anatomical position. Partial eversion of one horn will promote continued pain and straining with subsequent recurrence of the prolapse. Infusion with sterile saline or a warm antiseptic solution will distend the uterus replacing the invaginated horn. A uterine relaxant such as acetylepromazine or buscopan may be warranted to allow the encompassing horn to relax with release of the tip as fluid is infused. Once the fluid has been removed low doses of oxytocin can then be administered to help uterine involution. This regimen may also be used when invagination of a uterine horn occurs due to prolonged tension and weight of a retained placenta. Evaluation of the invaginated horn for necrosis and vascular compromise may be necessary depending on duration. Systemic antibiotics, prophylactic treatment for potential endometritis/metritis, septicemia, endotoxemia and laminitis should be initiated. This should probably include intrauterine treatment.
- Future fertility is dependent on uterine damage.

Uterine tear (Figs. 12.59–12.61)

Uterine rupture most commonly occurs as a sequelae to dystocia, uterine torsion, hydroallantois, fetotomy or uterine lavage. A mare can, however, sustain a uterine tear after an apparently normal delivery as a result of a foal's foot piercing the wall of a uterine horn.

If the tear is small, either full and partial thickness and dorsal, recognition may not occur for a few days, until the mare presents depressed, anorexic, febrile with mild to moderate colic, +/– toxic depending on duration and extent of peritonitis. Large uterine tears may be associated with severe hemorrhage and peritoneal contamination. These mares are critical with the interval from occurrence to diagnosis and initiation of treatment being important factors in prognosis for survival. Clinical presentations can include signs of hemorrhage, severe colic, peritonitis (depression, fever, anorexia) and endotoxic shock.

Diagnosis

- Confirmation of a tear can be made by palpation of the uterine tear either via the vagina/uterus or transrectally, although in some instances the lesion cannot be located until surgery.
- Care should be taken not to turn a partial- into a full-thickness tear. It has been suggested that thickness may be best determined by simultaneous rectal and uterine palpation. Complete blood count can aid in diagnosis.

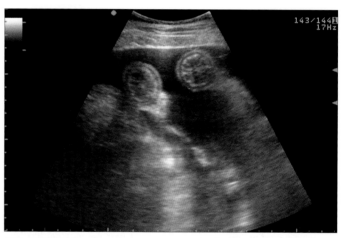

Figure 12.60 Transabdominal ultrasound of a mare with peritonitis. Notice the increased amount and echogenicity of the free peritoneal fluid. This can be differentiated from hemorrhage by the lack of swirling of the fluid and analysis of abdominal fluid. Notice also the small intestine with marked edema that can be seen floating within the abdominal fluid.

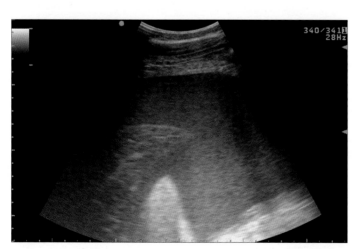

Figure 12.59 Ultrasonographic image of the ventral abdomen demonstrating a large amount of echogenic fluid. This echogenicity is indicative of fluid with a high cell count. This image is consistent with peritonitis or hemorrhage.

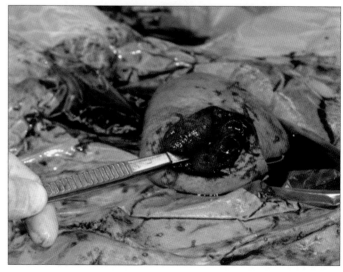

Figure 12.61 Tear at the tip of the uterine horn.

- Transabdominal ultrasound is an excellent tool that can be used easily in the field to diagnose peritonitis and aid in differentiating it from hemorrhage. There would be an excessive amount of peritoneal fluid often flocculent in appearance with or without evidence of fibrin deposition depending on duration.
- Further evidence can be identified by abdominocentesis (see Chapter 1, p. 34–35).

Treatment

- Small lesions may heal without surgical repair, however aggressive medical treatment should be initiated to prevent further peritonitis, endotoxemia and laminitis. Peritoneal lavage may be indicated.
- Surgical intervention via a ventral midline celiotomy with peritoneal lavage is indicated for large tears with extensive peritonitis. Postoperatively uterine lavage, and oxytocin can be added to the treatment regimen to help control hemorrhage and aid in involution and emptying of the uterus.
- The effect on fertility depends on the presence of adhesions on both serosal and luminal surfaces, chronic infection and the degree of permanent damage to the uterus.

Infectious/inflammatory disorders (non-pregnant)

Infectious and inflammatory conditions of the uterus include persistent post-mating-induced endometritis, chronic infectious endometritis, chronic degenerative endometritis (endometriosis) and sexually transmitted disease (STD).

Persistent post-mating-induced endometritis

(Figs. 12.62 & 12.63)

Transient inflammation is a normal physiological response to breeding. Normal, fertile mares clear the inflammation from their uterus within 12 hours of insult. Mares susceptible to persistent, post-mating endometritis have an intrinsic inability to evacuate uterine contents following breeding. Prolonged uterine inflammation following breeding ultimately leads to non-pregnant mares or early embryonic loss. A uterus that is located ventral to the pelvis contributes to the problem. Numerous studies indicate that decreased uterine contractility is a primary defect in the susceptible mare. It is not known if the defect is a structural defect in the muscle cell itself, or is due to an abnormal response to hormonal or neural signaling. The persistence of inflammatory debris within the uterine lumen results in accumulation of neutrophils, immunoglobulins and protein in the uterine lumen. This initiates a vicious cycle of fluid accumulation, interstitial edema and endometrial irritation. The longer the process continues the higher the likelihood the endometrium will be damaged, enabling bacteria to attach to the epithelium. Excessive interstitial edema may result from either prolonged inflammation or elastosis of the arteriole walls. The lymphatics may become overwhelmed from the excessive edema and may not be able to drain the tissues of the edema and cellular matter.

Pluriparous mares older than 14 years of age with poor perineal conformation are most prone to persistent postmating endometritis. Maiden mares (either old or young) may develop endometritis because the cervix does not open sufficiently during estrus. The cause for this cervical malfunction is not known.

Clinical signs and diagnosis

- The principal clinical sign is fluid accumulation present within the uterine lumen 24–48 hours after breeding. This may be manifested by a uterine discharge noted at the vulva lips or along the caudal aspect of the hind legs.
- Ultrasonography of the uterus 24–48 hours after breeding reveals fluid within the uterine lumen and in more severe cases intramural edema after ovulation. The fluid is not palpable via the rectum.
- Presumptive diagnosis may also be made due to past history.

Treatment

- Treatment should be delayed until 4 hours after breeding to ensure that viable sperm are not prematurely removed from the uterus. Treatment should be conducted before 8 hours because the uterine inflammatory response in reproductively normal mares is greatest between 8 and 12 hours after breeding. The longer the seminal by-products remain in the uterine lumen, the greater the inflammatory response and the greater the endometrial damage. Therefore, treatment is directed at rapid removal of debris and fluids.
- Sterile uterine lavage using warm saline or lactated ringer's solution in conjunction with administration of oxytocin aids in removal of inflammatory products.

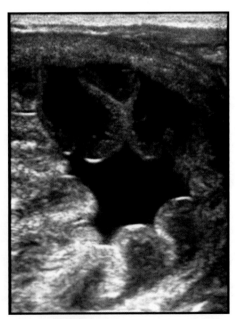

Figure 12.62 Ultrasonographic image of intralumenal uterine fluid and excessive edema post-mating and ovulation.

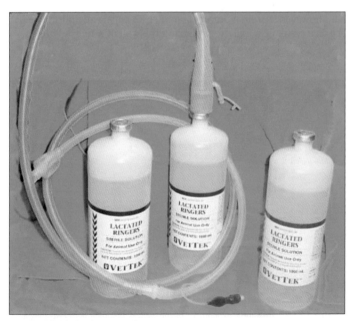

Figure 12.63 Sterile uterine lavage.

- Mares that have dilated lymphatic lacunae in addition to persistent postmating-induced endometritis may be treated with a combination of oxytocin treatment between 4 and 8 hours after breeding, and cloprostenol prior to ovulation.
- Cloprostenol should not be given after ovulation, as it will adversely affect corpus luteum formation and pregnancy rates.

Chronic endometritis (Figs. 12.64–12.68)

The reproductive history of the mare and a physical examination may provide the most productive information for determining the cause of endometritis. Poor perineal conformation is a significant factor allowing fecal, urinary and air contamination. These mares have a history of long-standing inflammatory changes. Their reproductive histories may include: repeat treatments with intrauterine antibiotics, repeat breedings per season, poor perineal conformation, incompetent cervix and persistent post mating induced endometritis. The mares are susceptible to endometritis because they have a breakdown in uterine defense mechanisms that allow contamination of the uterus with subsequent development of persistent endometritis. The most common organisms found in endometritis are *S. zooepidemicus*, *Escherichia coli*, *K. pneumoniae* and *P. aeruginosa*, yeasts and fungi (*Candida*

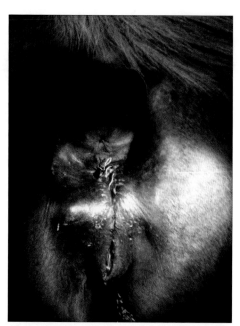

Figure 12.64 Poor perineal conformation allowing air and feces to enter vestibule, vagina and uterus.

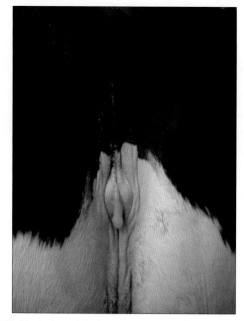

Figure 12.65 Uterine/vaginal discharge, evident at the vulva lips.

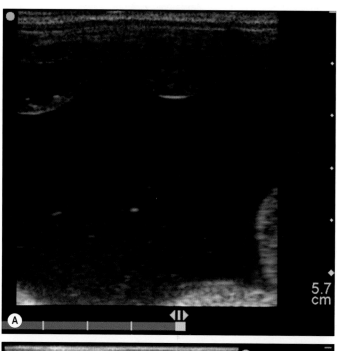

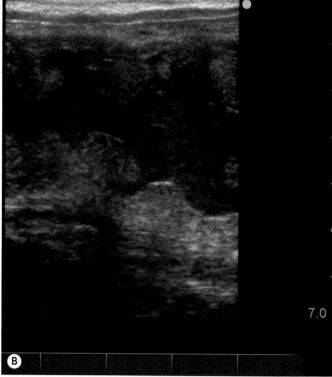

Figure 12.66 (A,B) Large amount of uterine intralumenal flocculent fluid seen on transrectal ultrasonographic examination.

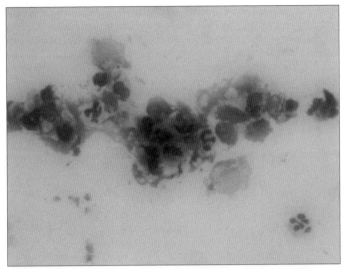

Figure 12.67 Endometrial cytology. Note the presence of large endometrial cells and neutrophils; this is an abnormal finding associated with endometrial inflammation (the presence of endometrial cells indicates a representative sample).

spp. and *Aspergillus* spp.) (Table 12.2). Anaerobes have also been described as possibly playing a role. In addition, the unique property of *S. zooepidemicus* enables it to physically adhere to the endometrium in susceptible mares. Dormant *S. zooepidemicus* have also been identified on biopsy using fluorescent in situ hybridization within the endometrial tissue. Poor conformation allowing contamination of the reproductive tract from the environment, repeated/lengthy intrauterine antibiotic treatment and excessive reproductive manipulation have all been implicated as potential causes of yeast and fungal invasion of the uterus.

Diagnosis

- Diagnosis of uterine inflammation due to persistent infection is based on history, physical examination, speculum examination, ultrasonography of the uterus, uterine cytology and culture and uterine biopsy. Uterin exudate (discharge) may be evident within the uterus, in the cervix or vaginal vault, and externally as a vulvar discharge.
- The vaginal vault and cervix appear hyperemic on speculum examination with or without the presence of exudate. Rectal palpation may reveal a large relaxed uterus while on transrectal ultrasonography there may be flocculent intraluminal fluid accumulation, the extent of which is dependent on the causative agent and severity.
- Endometrial cytology provides direct evidence of the presence of neutrophils in the uterine lumen. Any mare that has >5 neutrophils per high-powered field confirms active inflammation. Cytologies can be acquired by: a guarded endometrial swab; collecting cells from the cap of a calajan culturette; a small sterile guarded atraumatic brush or small-volume uterine lavage.
- A guarded uterine culture or sterile low-volume lavage confirms the causative organism, and the antibiotic sensitivity pattern helps direct the treatment.
- Endometrial biopsy for culture has been shown to be the best method for identifying the infectious agent, while histology provides the severity of the inflammation and prognosis.
- For fungus or yeast, diagnosis can be made most successfully by endometrial cytology revealing branching fungal hyphae or budding yeast in the presence of inflammatory cells. Endometrial cultures plated on blood or sabouraud's agar can also aid in identification.

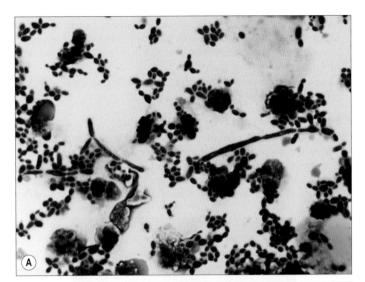

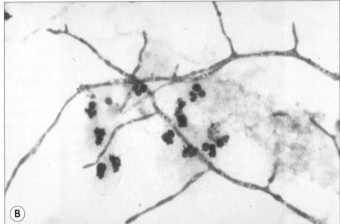

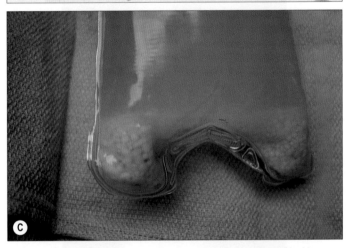

Figure 12.68 (A) Endometrial cytology illustrating large numbers of budding yeast. (B) Endometrial cytology illustrating fungal hyphae and neutrophils. (C) Uterine lavage from a mare with a yeast infection. Note the readily evident conidia which have formed a sediment in the lavage fluid.

Treatment

- The goal of therapy for bacterial endometritis is to remove the offending bacteria and enhance uterine defense mechanisms, thereby decreasing the inflammatory process within the uterus. This has been accomplished with intrauterine infusions of antibiotics, antiseptics, and plasma; uterine lavage; ecbolics and systemic antibiotic therapy.

Table 12.2 Common organisms found in endometrtis (Hagyard Equine Medical Institute Laboratory 2011 breeding season)

Uterine	Amikacin	Ampicillin	Ciprofloxacin	Chloramphenicol	Gentamicin	Imipenem	Naxcel	Nitrofurantoin	Penicillin G	Polymyxin B	Timentin	Trimethoprim Sufla	Doxycycline
Escherichia coli (240 iso'd)	98	32	92	81	70	100	93	100	0	100	81	33	
beta Strept species (209 iso'd)	0	100	0	100	0	100	100	100	100	0	100	97	86
Pseudomonas aeruginosa (85 iso'd)	96	0	100	0	62	100	0	0	0	100	89	0	determined
Staphylococcus aureus (47 iso'd)	98	20	100	100	70	100	100	100	20	38	98	77	from 14
alpha Strept species (30 iso'd)	20	100	70	97	57	100	100	87	93	53	100	50	isolates only
Actinobacillus equuli (28 iso'd)	75	89	100	96	86	100	96	100	89	93	96	71	
Pseudomonas putida (20 iso'd)	95	0	95	0	55	95	5	10	0	100	0	0	
Enterobacter aerogenes (19 iso'd)	95	0	100	95	58	95	79	74	0	100	32	42	
Klebsiella pneumoniae (18 iso'd)	89	6	100	83	83	100	83	78	0	89	83	50	
Enterobacter cloacae (17 iso'd)	100	6	94	53	82	100	94	41	0	100	76	47	
Enterococcus faecalis (15 iso'd)	0	100	47	33	0	93	0	100	100	0	33	0	
Acinetobacter baumannii (10 iso'd)	60	20	60	30	60	100	20	20	10	100	60	40	
Acinetobacter lwoffi (10 iso'd)	80	50	80	70	90	100	90	40	40	80	100	40	
Pasteurella haemolytica (8 iso'd)	50	100	100	100	88	100	100	100	100	75	100	100	
Citrobacter freundii (7 iso'd)	71	0	57	43	0	100	100	71	0	100	14	0	
Staphylococcus aureus, MRSA (6 iso'd)	67	0	100	100	0	0	0	100	0	0	0	0	
Pantoea agglomerans (6 iso'd)	100	100	100	100	100	100	100	100	17	100	100	100	
Citrobacter koseri (5 iso'd)	60	0	100	100	60	100	100	100	0	100	60	20	
Streptococcus pneumoniae (5 iso'd)	0	100	80	100	20	100	100	100	100	100	100	100	
Flavimonas oryzihabitans (5 iso'd)	100	60	100	80	100	100	80	20	0	100	80	80	
Proteus mirabilis (2 iso'd)	100	0	100	100	0	100	100	50	0	50	50	0	

12 Yeast species isolated
14 Fungus species isolated

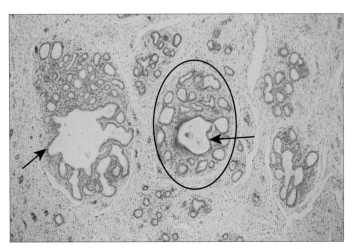

Figure 12.69 Histology of an endometrial biopsy. Note the large number of dilated endometrial glands (arrows) within a nest (circle), and the increased number of nests present due to fibrosis.

- Mucolytic agents that break down excessive mucous as well as agents that diminish debris and breakdown biofilms are believed to help with the inflammatory process and bacterial agents.
- To decrease fungal and yeast numbers, treatment has been attempted using uterine lavage in conjunction with DMSO, vinegar (2%) or dilute betadine (0.05%). Antifungal and yeast agents such as clotrimazole (500–700 mg), amphotericin B (100–200 mg), fluconazole (100 mg) and nystatin ($0.5–2.5 \times 10^6$) can also be used. For chronic infections, identification and sensitivity of the yeast of fungus yields are the best treatment options.

Endometriosis (Fig. 12.69)

Endometriosis is a chronic degenerative condition of the endometrium. It occurs in older mares that have been exposed to repeated inflammatory conditions or ageing. These severe changes can be a sequela of vescicovaginal reflux (urine pooling), chronic bacterial contamination or delayed uterine clearance with inflammatory byproducts remaining in the uterine lumen.

Diagnosis and treatment

- Reproductive history is an important piece of the puzzle. Endometrial culture and cytology aids in determination of the presence of chronic inflammation.
- Endometrial biopsy reveals chronic inflammatory changes to include endometrial gland fibrosis and nesting as well as degenerative changes of the vasculature.
- Unfortunately the process has been found to be irreversible and untreatable and those mares that do get in foal have a harder time maintaining the pregnancy to term.
- Pharmaceuticals (such as acetylcylic acid or pentoxyphilline) that potentially increase blood flow to the uterus may improve the outcome.

Contagious equine metritis (CEM) (Figs. 12.70 & 12.71)

CEM is a highly contagious venereal disease of horses. The disease may be spread by fomites, instruments and gloves in addition to coitus and is caused by *Taylorella equigenitalis*.

Clinical signs and diagnosis

- Clinically mares show a muco-purulent white discharge between 2 and 10 days post-infection. The discharge may persist for up to 3 weeks and shortening of the estrus cycle is a common finding in affected animals. Experimentally infected mares showed mild, bilateral salpingitis.

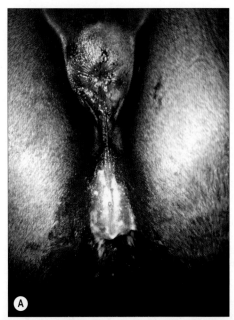

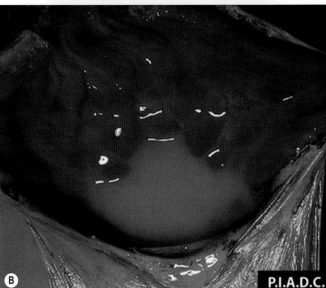

Figure 12.70 (A) Mucopurulent discharge noted at the vulvar lips characteristic of clinical CEM. (B) Mucopurulent exudate present in the uterus associated with CEM.

- The inflammation is most severe at approximately 14 days after infection. There have, however, been no recorded erosions or hyperplasia of any of the glandular portions of the uterus.
- Diagnosis is confirmed by microaerophilic incubation of cultures of the uterus, cervix and clitoral sinus and fossa. A special media (chocolate or Amies agar) must be used due to the slow growth of these bacteria. Small moist swabs should be used to enter the clitoral sinus so the bacteria can be isolated from this small space more readily.
- The disease is important because of its venereal nature and its deleterious effect on fertility. Numerous serologic tests have been developed to detect antibodies to CEM in serum.
- The enzyme-linked immunosorbent assay (ELISA) and passive hemagglutination tests are superior for detection of infected mares. Antibodies can be detected by 14 days post exposure using a complement fixation test.

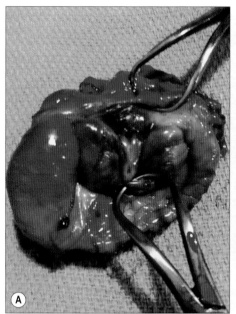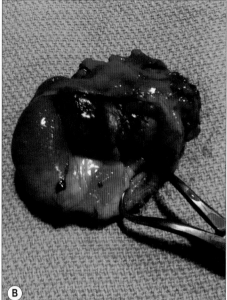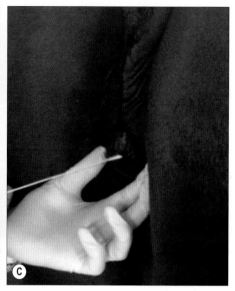

Figure 12.71 (A) Excised clitoris. Note the tiny clitoral sinus where the organism causing CEM-*Taylorella equigenitalis* likes to reside; the use of a small head swab is necessary to enter the sinus appropriately for culture. (B) Excised clitoris. Note the large clitoral fossa where *Taylorella equigenitalis* grows as it is dark and damp; as the space is larger, this area can be cultured with a larger tipped swab. (C) A small tipped culturette capable of fitting into the clitoral sinus to isolate the CEM organism *Taylorella equigenitalis*.

Treatment

- Intrauterine infusion of antibiotics combined with thorough cleansing of the clitoris, clitoral fossa and clitoral sinuses is the treatment of choice in mares. Daily intrauterine infusions for 5–7 days with appropriate antibiotics such as penicillin, ampicillin, neomycin, and nitrofurazone have been reported to be successful. The clitoral fossa and sinus must be thoroughly flushed then scrubbed daily for 5 days with chlorohexidine solution and packed with nitrofurazone or chlorohexidine ointment. If infection persists clitoral sinusectomy may be recommended.

Other sexually transmitted bacterial infections

Other bacteria, including some strains of *Klebsiella* spp. or *Pseudomonas* spp. can also be regarded as contagious and are usually the result of poor hygiene, allowing their establishment within the genital tract. In the case of *Pseudomonas* spp. the use of antiseptics prior to service as a control measure for other venereal infections, may allow, and even encourage, its proliferation and spread. Mares infected after service by stallions contaminated with *Pseudomonas* spp. may show ulceration and erosion of the clitoris and vagina.

Most mares affected by any of these opportunist pathogens, show early return to service, mucopurulent discharges after coitus with inflammation of the cervix and a cervico-uterine discharge; isolation of organisms from uterine swabs must always be related to active clinical infection. Routine isolation of potentially pathogenic organisms from clinically normal mares must be interpreted carefully before prolonged antibiotic treatment is commenced.

Infectious/inflammatory disorders (pregnant)

Placentitis (Figs. 12.72–12.77)

Placentitis, an inflammation of the placenta, is usually caused by an infectious agent, most commonly bacteria. These organisms gain access to the placenta and potentially the fetus by three characteristic mechanisms:

1) Ascending infection: this occurs when the pathogen gets past the vulva lips and the vestibulo-vaginal sphincter (hymen) and enters

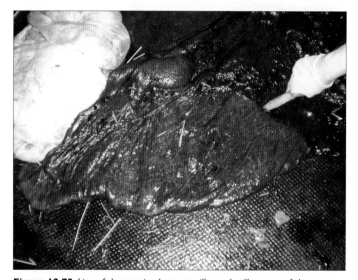

Figure 12.72 Line of demarcation between villus and avillus areas of the placenta in a mare with an ascending placentitis.

the cervix. The bacteria proceed to destroy the microvilli preventing gas and nutrient exchange in that area. The lesion and bacteria spread from the cervical star region moving cranially to the body of the uterus and towards the fetus. A clear line of demarcation can be seen where the avillus and villus areas meet. Abortion is due to fetal death from septicemia, placental insufficiency or the inflammatory process causing the uterus to contract. The most common pathogens in ascending placentitis include *Streptococcus* spp., *Escherichia coli*, *Pseudomonas* spp., *Klebsiella* spp., *Staphylococcus* spp., and the fungus *Aspergillus*. Differentiation between bacterial and fungal lesions is not normally possible by visual observation of the placenta.

2) Hematogenous infection: this occurs when a mare is systemically sick or bacteremic and the organism seeds within the vasculature

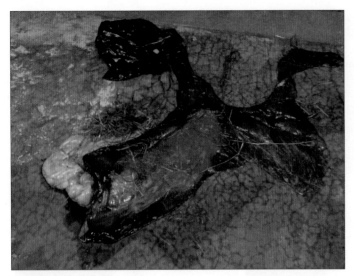

Figure 12.73 Placentitis of ascending origin associated with a fungal infection (*Aspergillus* spp.).

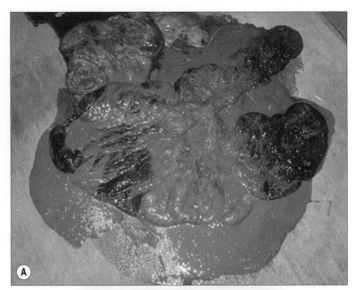

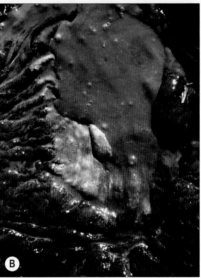

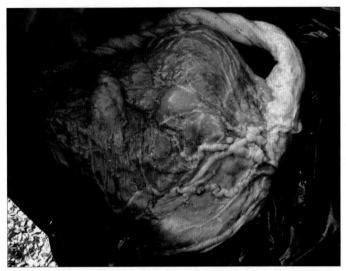

Figure 12.74 Placentitis associated with a hematogenous origin. Note the lesion within and on the vasculature of the fetal membranes.

Figure 12.75 Nocardioform placentitis associated with avillus areas at the base of the horns. Note the thick mucoid exudates associated with this type of placentitis. (A) Severe case of *Crossiella equi* spp. resulting in abortion. (B) Small focal lesion of *Amycolatopsis* in a mare that delivered a normal foal.

of the uterus/placenta and fetus. *Leptospirosis* spp., *Klebsiella pneumoniae*, *Pseudomonas aeruginosa*, *Staphylococcus*, *Streptococcus* and *Salmonella abortus equi* are bacteria that can enter by this mechanism.

3) The last means is unidentified and has been attributed to a gram-positive branching bacillus and described as a mucoid or nocardioform placentitis. *Crossiella equi* spp. and *Amycolatopsis* spp. are the two most common organisms identified to produce the characteristic lesions. They produce an extensive and severe exudative placentitis focused at the most dependent part of the uterus, producing an avillus area in the placental body and horns rather than at the cervical star. This sticky brown mucus lies above a well-defined avillus area of the placenta. How these organisms gain acess to the uterus and placenta is not known.

Clinical signs and diagnosis

- Signs of placentitis include vaginal/vulvar discharge and premature mammary gland development. Ascending infections may show

one or both of these signs whereas hematogenous and mucoid usually only show premature lactation. *Leptospirosis* spp. may only be identified post abortion unless isolated on screening titers since mares do not usually get systemically sick or show other evidence of this disease.

- A diagnosis of ascending or nocardioform placentitis can be determined using transrectal and/or transabdominal ultrasound in combination with a culture if a vaginal discharge is present. The culture can identify the infective organism and provide antibiotic sensitivity to help with treatment. Measurements of maternal progestagens and total estrogen can help corroborate the placental and fetal well-being.

- Transrectal ultrasonographic evaluation of the caudal reproductive tract has become a routine diagnostic tool for placentitis with measurement of the combined uterine and placental thickness (CUPT) and comparison to established normal values in mares throughout gestation (Table 12.3). Since ascending infections are most common and initiated at the cervical star, ultrasonographic

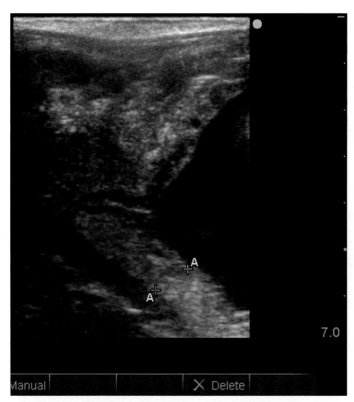

Figure 12.76 A normal transrectal ultrasonographic image of the cervix, internal os, uterine vessel and combined thickness of the utero-placental unit (0.84 cm). Note there is no CTUP thickening; the cervix is closed with no placental edema or separation.

Table 12.3 Evaluation of CTUP of nine normal mares throughout gestation

Month of gestation	Mean CTUP, mm	95% confidence interval, mm
4	3.98	3.81–4.47
5	3.58	3.50–3.81
6	3.84	3.78–4.04
7	3.91	3.86–4.07
8	4.33	4.21–4.69
9	4.38	4.28–4.66
10	5.84	5.53–6.77
11	7.35	6.93–8.54
12	9.52	8.51–11.77

From Renaudin et al 1997.

examination of this area is warranted. Transabdominal ultrasonography evaluates fetal viability and placental abnormalities.

- Although placental thickening is difficult to consistently interpret via transabdominal ultrasound due to the stretching and contracture of the different regions of the pregnant uterus, separation of the chorioallantois from the endometrium and the presence of exudate as seen with mucoid or hematogenous placentitis may be identified.
- Volume and echogenicity of the fetal fluids can be evaluated transabdominally, as well as fetal heart rate, tone, activity and size.
- *Leptospirosis* spp. can be demonstrated post-abortion in the allantochorion, umbilical cord or fetal kidneys by fluorescent antibody tests (FAT), silver staining or immunohistochemistry (IHC). Exposure usually occurs 2–4 weeks before abortion therefore the affected

mares have high serological titers. Serology in the mare and fetus is based on ELISA and microscopic agglutination tests. Positive diagnosis in mares occurs with serum titers of $\geq 1:6400$. Positive PCR has been validated on urine samples, however the sample needs to be aquired in the middle of the stream during the second void after the administration of lasix. Culture is not a practical method for diagnosis since it takes 6 months for *Leptospirosis* to grow. Shedding of *Leptospirosis* spp. can occur in the urine of mares for long periods of time post abortion. If identification within the urine via PCR or staining is not possible, it has been suggested (University of Kentucky Livestock Disease and Diagnostic Center) that decreasing titers by half correlates with cessation of shedding of the organism.

Treatment

- Therapies are directed at resolving microbial or spirochete invasion, decreasing inflammation and uterine contractions. Systemic treatment can include antibiotics, exogenous progestagens, anti-inflammatories, tocolytic agents and medications that improve uterine perfusion.
- In mares that are considered high risk (those that have a history of previous feto-placental compromise, cervical incompetency/lacerations, chronic disease, old age, poor reproductive conformation), routine placental ultrasonographic evaluations, in conjunction with fetal viability assessments and serial hormonal evaluations, allow early determination of placental and fetal problems.

Herpes virus (Fig. 12.77D)

After respiratory infection or reactivation of latent herpes 1 virus, uterine infection occurs via viremia. Transplacental spread of virus then occurs at sites of uterine infarction after endometrial vasculitis and thrombosis, allowing infection of placental trophoblasts, whereby cell to cell spread or infected leucocytes transmit virus to intravillous endothelium and to fetal organs.

Clinical signs and diagnosis

- A feature of spontaneous EHV1 abortions in mares is the often sudden and explosive nature of the event, the fetus being expelled without warning and still enveloped within the fetal membranes. No premature mammary gland development is noted.
- Diagnosis routinely includes the detection of EHV1 in the aborted fetus. However some may go undiagnosed because the fetus is not available for examination.
- Diagnosis can be made with PCR of fresh fetal tissues and paraffin-embedded placenta. Since the virus is transmitted by close contact via aerosol exposure, respiratory secretions, fetal tissues, placenta and uterine fluids from mares that have aborted need to be disposed of and the mare isolated. Virus can be transmitted via organic material on clothes, shoes and material inside stalls, trailers, water buckets or feed.
- Horses that have been exposed to infected horses but have not developed any clinical signs within 21 days of the potential exposure are unlikely to do so.
- On necropsy gross pathological lesions of the fetus or stillborn foal include icterus and generalized petechial and ecchymotic hemorrhages. Livers are enlarged, mottled and discolored yellow. Edema is evident in the kidney with pale white radiating streaks in the cortex and medulla.

Treatment

- Preventative vaccination has decreased the incidence of abortion storms dramatically, with most affected mares exposed coming from naïve herds.

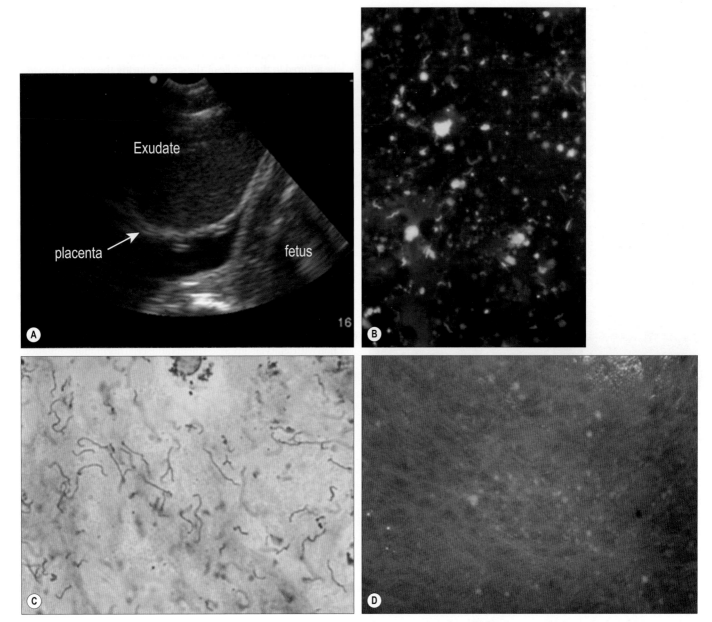

Figure 12.77 (A) Transabdominal ultrasound image revealing utero-placental separation due to mucoid exudates. (B) Fluorescent antibody test for *Leptospirosis* spp. (C) Silver staining for *Leptospirosis* spp. (D) Gross examination of a herpes virus abortion reveals yellow/white micro-abscesses in the liver.

- Initial recommendations to reduce the risk of abortion from EHV1/4 included vaccination with Pneumobort K at 5, 7, 9 months of gestation.
- Recently increasing the frequency to every 2 months year round has been suggested on farms with large movements of mares or that have had endemic problems.
- Immunity to the virus only lasts 4–6 months so repeated abortions can occur in successive seasons.

Equine viral arteritis (EVA)

The causative agent of the respiratory and abortagenic disease equine viral arteritis is a small single-stranded RNA virus (Togavirus). Infection is believed to occur by direct contact via nasal droplet spray during the acute phase of infection and by infected stallions, semen. Susceptible mares that are then bred to shedding stallions acquire the disease.

Clinical signs and diagnosis

- Can vary ranging from subclinical disease (only recognized by sero-conversion), to acute illness and abortion. Signs include: pyrexia, depression, anorexia, edema of scrotum, ventral trunk and limbs, conjunctivitis, lacrimation, serous nasal discharge and respiratory distress.
- Adult horses usually make an uneventful recovery after a viremic phase which can persist for up to 40 days after infection.
- The incidence of abortion is up to 50% of exposed mares. Abortion may occur with or shortly after infection due to myometrial necrosis and edema leading to placental detachment and fetal death.
- EAV can be isolated from both fetus and placenta by virus isolation, especially from placenta, fetal spleen, lung and kidney and fetal/placental fluids.
- Semen samples with sperm-rich fraction should be collected for virus isolation of suspected infected stallions.

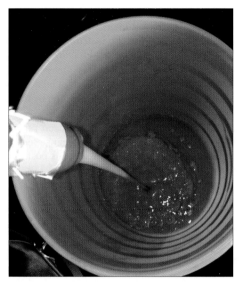

Figure 12.78 Uterine exudate flushed from a mare's uterus with severe metritis.

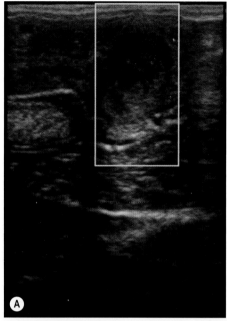

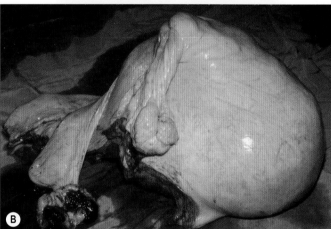

Figure 12.79 (A) Transrectal ultrasonographic image of an intramural uterine mass. Note the density of the mass within the uterine wall. (B) Leimoyosarcoma.

- Antibodies to EAV can be demonstrated by complement fixation and virus neutralization tests.

Treatment and prevention
- Previously infected horses are immune to re-infection with virulent virus for up to 7 years.
- A modified live virus vaccine is registered for use in some states in the USA. The use of the MLV does not produce any side effects apart from a short-term abnormality of sperm morphology and a mild fever with no overt clinical signs.
- Virus can be sporadically isolated from the nasopharynx and blood for up to 7–32 days post-vaccination, so horses vaccinated initially should be isolated for 1 month. Subsequent vaccination should only require 10–14 days of isolation.
- Vaccinated mares bred by positive stallions are protected from clinical infection, however able to shed the virus by the respiratory route for 21 days post exposure.

Infectious/inflammatory disorders (post-partum)
Metritis (Fig. 12.78)
Metritis is an inflammation of the deeper layers of the uterus which is usually associated with inflammatory and infectious processes immediately after parturition. Metritis most commonly occurs when a retained placenta is present, which provides a good media for bacterial growth.

Mares that are unable to get out and move around due to sick foals or lameness issues may be more prone to metritis since clearance of post partum lochia and contamination is not as easily achieved. This again produces an environment conducive to bacterial growth with subsequent inflammation and uterine compromise.

Clinical signs and diagnosis
- Affected mares present depressed, febrile, anorexic, tachypnic, and may be toxic with bounding digital pulses. A thick yellow/tan vaginal discharge may be noted.
- Systemic involvement can progress to endotoxemia, septicemia and laminitis.
- The mortality amongst these mares is high.

- A diagnosis can usually be reached from the presenting clinical features and vaginal and uterine examinations, during which an obvious, fetid uterine discharge is detected.
- The uterus can be pendulous with poor uterine involution.

Treatment
Treatment is aimed at removing the placenta if present as well as uterine fluid, bacteria and inflammatory products. This includes: frequent large volume uterine lavage, appropriate systemic and intra-uterine antibiotics, anti-inflammatories and measures to prevent laminitis such as icing feet and vasodilators or rheostatic agents (pentoxyphilline, isoxoprine).

Neoplastic disorders (Fig. 12.79)
Neoplasms of the uterus of the mare are not common. Leiomyoma is probably the most common, however leiomyosarcoma, adenocarcinoma, fibroleimyoma, lymphosarcoma and rhabdomyosarcoma have been reported emanating from the uterine wall.

Leiomyoma (Fig. 12.79B)
This type of uterine tumor may sometimes be misdiagnosed as a pregnancy but the solid pendulant nature of the mass is typical. They are

usually small, however they can grow large enough to occlude the uterine lumen. They are usually benign but may hemorrhage causing a persistent endometritis.

Clinical signs and diagnosis

- Usually these tumors are an incidental finding when small. If hemorrhage occurs a bloody vulvar discharge may be noted. Infertility is usually not a presenting complaint.
- Transrectal ultrasound examination reveals a dense mass associated with the endo- or myometrium.
- Hysteroscopic examination can confirm protrusion into the uterine lumen or maintenance within the wall.
- Histopathology post removal confirms tumor type.

Treatment

- None. If large, removal from the uterine wall through a small incision made in the serosal surface of the uterus via flank laparotomy.
- Laparoscopy can also be performed. Prognosis for future fertility is excellent.

The cervix

The cervix is subject to physical trauma principally during parturition. This may show as slight to severe bruising, adhesions or more serious injury where full thickness tears can occur.

Cervical lacerations (Fig. 12.80)

Cervical lacerations are most commonly produced during a dystocia with an oversized fetus, obstetrical chains or fetotomy wire, although they are also seen after what appears to be a normal parturition. Minor lacerations to the external os that do not interfere with closure of the cervix during diestrus are of no consequence, while those that interfere with the competency of the cervical canal warrant attention. Failure of the cervix to properly close promotes susceptibility to chronic endometritis and loss of maintenance of pregnancy.

Diagnosis and treatment

- Examination of the cervix is best done manually during diestrus or under the influence of exogenous progesterone; this allows palpation of the entire circumference of the external os, the cervical canal, mucosa, musculature and internal os. Speculum examination can be unreliable.

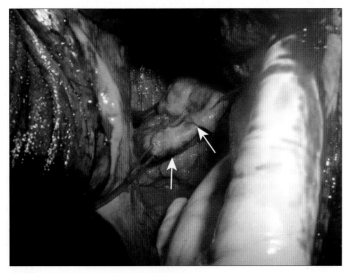

Figure 12.80 Cervical laceration visualized on speculum examination.

- Healing of the cervix must occur prior to cervical repair so the tissue is not friable and able to withstand suturing. Manual break down and blunt dissection with an instrument may be necessary if adhesions are present prior to cervical repair.
- Subsequent breeding may occur 30 days after repair with artificial insemination the method of choice, although breeding shed awareness and use of a roll will allow less penetration by the stallion with a decreased likelihood of further trauma.
- Pregnancy rates after surgical repair have been reported as being 75%. Care must be taken during foaling because recurrence of the tear is probable and repair on an annual basis post foaling may be necessary.

Cervical adhesions (Fig. 12.81)

Adhesions can be a sequela to lacerations, preventing the cervix from opening, occluding the lumen, or producing anatomical abnormalities between the cervix and vagina.

Diagnosis and treatment

- Evidence of adhesions can be seen during visual speculum examination; however manual assessment again is optimum. This may be complicated by chronic endometritis.
- Adhesions between opposite sides of the cervix may cause complete closure and lead to a closed pyometra and complete infertility.
- Surgical reduction of adhesions can be done by blunt dissection or by breaking them down with scissors carefully. Use of a duck bill speculum to expose the cervix and vaginal vault is recommended.
- Treatment of the area with topical creams post surgery is recommended to maintain patency and prevent adhesion formation again.

Failure of cervical relaxation

Failure of the cervix to relax can be seen in older maiden mares that have had years of estrous cycles without breeding or foaling and/or mares that have had repeated assisted reproductive techniques such as embryo transfer performed.

Clinical signs and treatment

- Both situations reveal pre breeding intralumenal free fluid on transrectal ultrasound. Manual examination of the cervix shows a lack of normal cervical relaxation for the appropriate stage of estrus.
- Transrectal ultrasonography post breeding again identifies free fluid within the uterine lumen.
- Manual cervical dilation has been attempted in both situations however is more successful in maiden mares verses older mares with tight cervix due to fibrous changes in the cervical tissue.
- Pre and post breeding uterine lavage can help in reducing intralumenal fluid and removing spermatozoa and inflammatory debris post mating. Cervical dilation may be enhanced using prostaglandin E_2 or Buscopan[R] cream applied to the cervical area.

The vagina, vestibule and vulva

Developmental disorders

Very few developmental defects occur in this region in the horse. True hermaphrodites often have rudimentary anatomical features and some mares have a complete hymen which results in failure of intromission, complete infertility and, often, gross accumulation of uterine and vaginal secretions behind the membrane.

Non-infectious disorders

Immunological conditions affecting the vulva rarely occur (see Uterine diseases of the pregnant mare). **Bullous pemphigoid**, a vesico-bullous ulcerative disease which occurs at muco-cutaneous

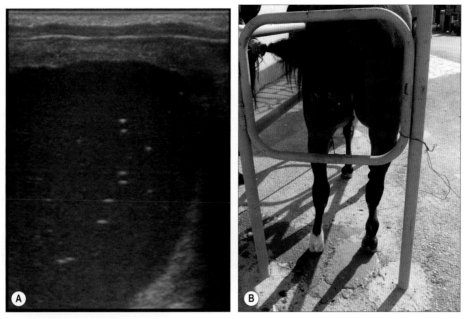

Figure 12.81 (A) Closed pyometra due to cervical adhesions. Note the uterus distended by flocculent fluid on transrectal ultrasonographic examination. (B) Pyometra. Note the markedly purulent vaginal discharge.

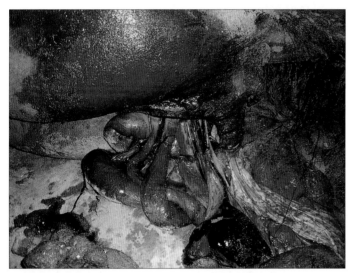

Figure 12.82 Intestines prolapsed through a vaginal tear post foaling.

junctions, may affect the vulval-skin junction where ulceration with epidermal collarette formation may be seen.

Depigmented vulval and perineal skin (**vitiligo**) occurs following traumatic damage from service and foaling injuries or from viral and bacterial infections.

Mating and foaling accidents (Figs. 12.82 & 12.83)

The mare is notoriously unpredictable with respect to foaling dates and times. Some mares run milk for several days (or sometimes weeks) prior to foaling, others have a normal udder or even no mammary gland development up to delivery, yet foal normally without any pre-monitory signs. Normally, parturition passes through the three stages of labor, often with minimal need for either interference or assistance. However the second stage of labor in the mare is particularly rapid, and usually so short that the equine obstetrician has little time for delay if a live foal is to be delivered. Correction of malpresentation should be done as soon as it is evident. Failure to do so may lead to

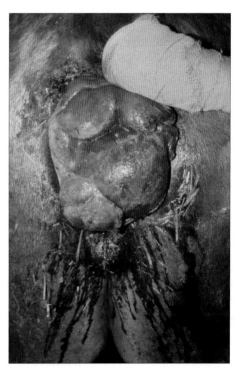

Figure 12.83 Rectal prolapse.

death of the foal and/or perineal lacerations or vaginal and uterine tears. Other severe post partum injuries concerning other body systems include prolapse and eversion of bladder or prolapse intestine through the vaginal wall, or rupture of the mesocolon and/or small colon wall due to rectal prolapse.

Trauma to the vagina during foaling

Mares are frequently bruised during foaling but this resolves quickly. Where trauma is more extensive, adhesions and fibrosis of the vaginal wall may occur leading to vaginal scarring and loss of elasticity. Some degree of urine pooling in the anterior vagina (with or without pneumovagina) is relatively common. Subsequent fertility may be reduced in these cases. Extensive vaginal tearing may occasionally result in extensive vaginal adhesions which may even occlude the vagina.

Diagnosis and treatment

- Speculum examination reveals bruising of the cervix as well as any adhesions. Manual examination can give additional information as to severity and thickness of the abnormalities.
- If bruising of the cervix due to trauma is evident, giving the mare time to heal will aid in decreasing the inflammation of the area and allow for better future fertility.
- If vaginitis is present, the extent should be ascertained and then emollients applied so adhesions do not occur. If adhesions are already present, then they should be broken down manually or by blunt dissection, and emollients applied to avoid recurrent formation.

Trauma to the vagina during breeding

The vagina may also be traumatized during service, resulting in bruising of the cervix and vaginal vault in mild cases, to actual rupture of the dorsal vaginal wall, above or adjacent to the cervix.

Clinical signs and diagnosis

- Affected mares strain vigorously and persistently after service and may show a blood stained discharge. Where contamination of the peritoneal cavity occurs as a result of both bacterial and seminal fluid, low-grade peritonitis results, causing fever, anorexia and depression.
- Diagnosis is done through visual or manual examination.

Treatment

Most cases respond to medical treatment and, only when the injury and peritonitis are associated with traumatized bowel, do mares commonly die following this injury. The complications arising from herniation of bowel through the vaginal tear can be avoided in most cases by preventing the mare from lying down or suturing the tear closed.

False cover

A term used to indicate that a stallion has served the mare rectally and not vaginally may result in severe straining and (temporary) **rectal mucosal prolapse**. Some stallions become particularly adept at this and the stallion handler of such horses must be alert to prevent its continuing occurrence. Only rarely do mares show severe inflammatory damage and it is rarely fatal unless full-thickness rectal tears have occurred. Great care must be taken as the mucosa is frequently bruised or torn and the defect may develop into a full thickness tear if rough manual examination follows the injury.

Vaginal prolapse (Fig. 12.84)

This occurs infrequently in the mare and is generally the result of persistent irritation or inflammation of the vaginal walls, bladder problems or impending abortion. A reddish mass of mucosa usually protrudes from the vulval lips and careful clinical assessment must be undertaken to differentiate this from a prolapsed bladder or a bladder eversion.

Vesico-vaginal reflux (urine pooling) (Fig. 12.85 & 12.86)

Vesico-vaginal reflux or urine pooling is the retention of incompletely voided urine in the vaginal vault. If the mare is not in heat (diestrus), then the cervix is closed and the urine remains in the vagina producing a vaginitis and cervicitis. However if the mare is in estrus the cervix opens and allows the urine to enter the uterus leading to endometritis. This causes reduced conception rates due to chronic irritation and inflammation of the endometrium with subsequent premature lysis of the corpus luteum; changes in the luminal PH

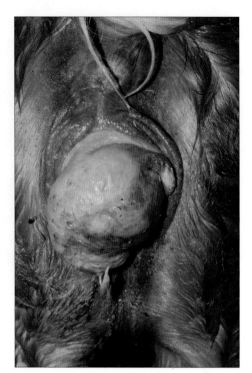

Figure 12.84 Vaginal prolapse.

which may be toxic to spermatozoa; and periglandular fibrosis of the uterus leading to poor nutrition of the developing fetus. Pooling of urine results from decreased vaginal muscle tone and elongated ovarian ligaments facilitating poor suspension of the reproductive tract and allowing the vagina to fall below the level of the pelvic floor. This occurs more commonly in aged multiparous mares. Abnormal conformation of the perineal region, where the vulvar labia are at an angle of less than 80 degrees to the pelvic floor, also allows the urethral orifice to fall cranial to the ischium and pneumovagina to occur. Relaxation of the reproductive tract during estrus and excessive episioplasty (Caslick's procedure) also contribute to urine retention. Obstetrical trauma, incomplete uterine involution and urethral sphincter paralysis should also be investigated as a cause of vesico-vaginal reflux.

Clinical signs and diagnosis

- Mares may show varying signs ranging from none, to urine staining or crystals below her vulva extending down between her legs or urine squirting through her vulva when the mare moves or runs.
- Diagnosis can be made by identifying urine at the vaginal fornix during speculum examination. The condition may be intermittent with mares being more likely to pool urine during estrus than diestrus due to increased relaxation of the reproductive tract under the influence of estrogen.
- Hyperemia of the vaginal vault may be present without evidence of urine and culture of the endometrium can be negative if bacterial contamination from the vaginal vault has not occurred. Endometrial cytology, with or without the presence of bacteria, reveals inflammatory cells and frequently urine crystals.
- Ultrasonographic examination can be used to detect fluid in the cranial vagina and in the uterine body. Endometrial biopsy is recommended before treatment is initiated to ascertain the chronicity and severity of the disease by the fibrotic and inflammatory changes. This will provide the owner with a realistic idea of whether or not the mare will be able to carry a foal to term if she does become pregnant.

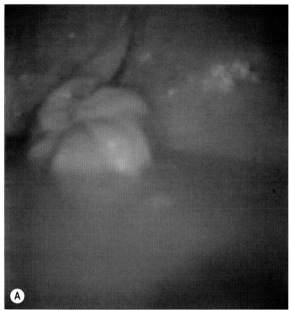

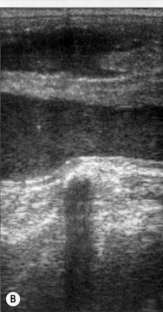

Figure 12.85 (A) Urinary pooling. (B) Urovagina as seen on transrectal ultrasonographic examination. Note urine in the bladder (below) and in the vagina (above).

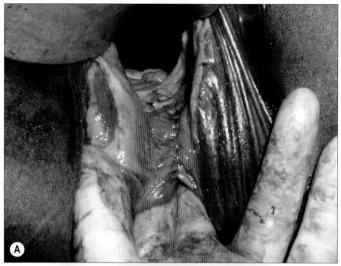

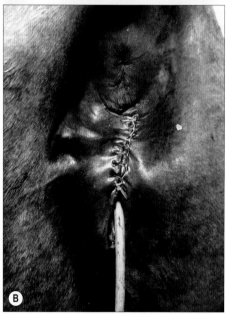

Figure 12.86 (A) Urethral extension. (B) Urinary catheter in place after a urethral extension procedure has been performed. Note also the Caslick's procedure which has been performed to prevent air entering the vagina.

Treatment

- Treatment can be divided into medical, acupuncture and surgical. In mares that exhibit minimal pooling mainly during estrus, oxytocin use with lactated Ringers uterine lavage pre and post breeding, in conjunction with breeding and inducing ovulation early in estrus has produced successful pregnancies.

- In more severe cases acupuncture can be added to the regime, and then finally surgical intervention.

- Surgical corrections include vaginoplasty, more commonly a urethral extension and perineal body reconstruction.

- Vaginoplasty and perineal body reconstruction is generally unsuccessful in mares with severe vaginal tilting.

- For good surgical results to occur with urethral extensions, fistula formation must be avoided.

Pneumovagina

A condition which is closely related to poor perineal conformation, is characterized by the ballooning of the entire vaginal vault with air, a blanched mucosa and, in severe cases, the presence of fecal and other particulate matter in the vagina. Where the condition is chronic, the vaginal walls and cervix may be inflamed. Affected mares often make flatulent noises when trotting. Racing fillies which have this condition are often poor-performers on the track, showing intermittent, low-grade, colic-like signs, 'cramps', straddling and frequent attempts to urinate after exercise.

Clinical signs and diagnosis

- Normal mares with good perineal conformation rarely exhibit pneumovagina. However where the abdominal organs sink, due to a stretched or aged abdomen, they draw the rectum and anal sphincter cranially and, in so doing, progressively change the angle of declination of the vulva.

- Diagnosis can be done by identifying poor vulvar conformation, hearing the 'wind sucking' into the vagina or via transrectal

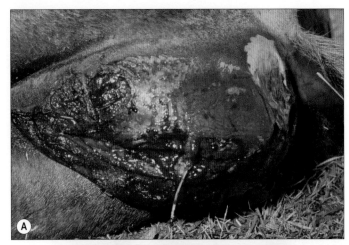

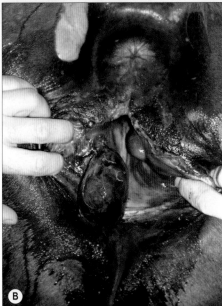

Figure 12.87 (A) Vulval bruising and laceration 12 hours post foaling. Mare had showed complete foaling paralysis, never regained her feet and was euthanized. (B) Hematoma and bruising of the vestibule post dystocia.

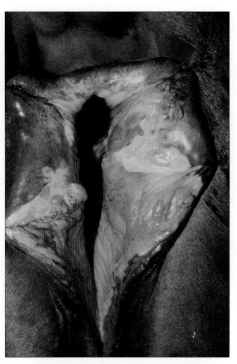

Figure 12.88 Third-degree perineal laceration. Seen after 6 weeks; granulated sufficiently for preparation for surgical repair.

ultrasound on which air can be identified either in the vagina or both vagina and uterus.

Treatment

- Mares with vulval angles of less than 30–40° are most amenable to surgical treatment with Caslick's operation (vulvoplasty). Extremely poor conformation associated with vulval angles of over 70° are very difficult to repair and while being assisted by surgery, these mares are never fully corrected and so they have a permanently reduced fertility.
- Surgical correction (Caslick's operation (vulvoplasty) or Pouret's operation for perineal reconstruction) are the only satisfactory solutions for most mares. Following Caslick's operation all mares require surgical episiotomy immediately prior to foaling if perineal lacerations are to be avoided.

Physical injury to the vulva (Fig. 12.87)

This occurs principally at parturition and may result in bruising of the vulval lips. With difficult foaling, vulval tearing and hematoma formation occurs, while more severe and prolonged dystocia or grossly oversized foals may cause very deep bruising and contusions to the

vulva. Trauma as a result of kicking by other horses can also cause hematomas and swelling of the vulva and perineum but this has a different appearance.

Perineal lacerations (Fig. 12.88)

Perineal lacerations can occur as a result of malpositioning of the fetus with the forefeet traumatizing the vestibule or perineum, stretching as the foal's poll and shoulders emerge through the vulva, delivery of an oversize fetus or from overzealous assistance during foaling. A higher incidence occurs in primiparous mares or mares that have had previous perineal surgery.

Clinical signs

- First-degree lacerations involve the mucosa of the vestibule and skin of the dorsal commissure of the vulva lips. Second-degree lacerations include the vestibular mucosa and submucosa, dorsal vulva commissure and the perineal body musculature. Both of these categories may be repaired by performing a caslick (vulvoplasty) either immediately, if edema is minimal, or after healing of the mucocutaneous surface in the absence of infection.
- A third-degree laceration involves the forelimb of the foal penetrating the dorsal vaginal and ventral rectal walls, continuing to destroy the perineal body and the anal sphincter as parturition progresses.
- If the foal should change position or assistance is present when the forelimb is evident through the rectum, the forelimb may be replaced within the vagina before complete destruction of the perineal region occurs resulting in a rectovaginal fistula.

Treatment

- Surgical repair is recommended 4–6 weeks after the third-degree perineal laceration or rectovaginal fistula to allow inflammation to resolve, wound margin epithelialization and wound contracture. Repair of these injuries immediately is usually temporary and frustrating.
- Surgical preparation and post-operative instructions should include stool softeners, since surgical success depends on fecal consistency.

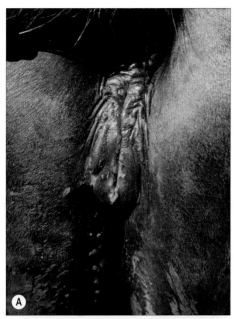

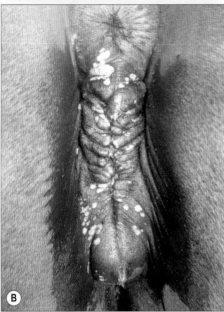

Figure 12.89 (A) Equine herpes virus-3 infection. Coital exanthema. Lesions are approximately 10 days after service. (B) Coital exanthema lesions that have healed leaving depigmented areas on vulvar lip.

Post-repair pregnancy rates have been shown to be 75%, justifying a good prognosis.

- Mares with previous surgical repairs should be monitored closely towards the end of gestation so assistance can be rendered as necessary.

Infectious disorders (Fig. 12.89)

Infectious processes in the vagina are usually related to events already described such as concurrent metritis or endometritis or infected, traumatized mucosa from service or parturition. Most such infections are bacterial or fungal in origin. While **infectious vulvo-vaginitis** has been reported in mares, specific causal organisms have not been consistently demonstrated. Gross contamination of the vagina with fecal material (where either rectovaginal fistula or third-degree perineal lacerations are present) or urine (where poor vulval, vestibular, vaginal or perineal conformation results in urovagina) inevitably results in bacterial infection of the vagina (and in most cases of the uterus). The organisms involved in these cases are usually mixed contaminants and are seldom specific pathogens.

Infectious diseases affecting the vulva are principally of viral and bacterial origin.

Viral diseases

Viral disease such as **coital exanthema** which is caused by equine herpes virus-3, manifests as short-lived vesicles which rapidly progress to yellow-pigmented papules and, within 5 days, to crusty erosions of the perineal skin. The disease is usually venereally transmitted but can be spread by fomites, gloves and gynecological instruments. Usually spread of this virus requires the vulval or vaginal mucosa to be abraded. Affected mares should not be bred in the active stages of the infection; however no residual infertility has been found in mares recovering from the disease. Once healing has occurred the affected areas have depigmented flat spots as residual evidence.

Bacterial diseases

The clitoral sinuses which fill with smegma are excellent repositories for **contagious equine metritis** (*Taylorella equigenitalis*). *Klebsiella* spp., *Pseudomonas* spp. in carrier mares and other diseases such as streptococci can also contaminate these sinuses to readily re-infect a mare causing chronic endometritis or contaminate or infect the stallion during service. Swabs taken for routine or clinical reasons are obtained from the clitoris, clitoral sinuses, smegma pea, if present, and the urethral opening.

Generalized diseases such as **bastard strangles** occasionally cause abscesses in and around the vulva. Such infections are frequently responsible for leukoderma and leukotrichia around the vulval lips.

Protozoal diseases

Dourine is a venereal disease of equidae, caused by *Trypanosoma equiperdum* is spread by sexual contact. The disease has been known and recorded since 400 AD and it is thought to have originated in North Africa and spread to other parts of Africa, Asia, Europe, USSR, Indonesia and the Americas. Currently it has been eradicated from parts of Africa, USA and Western Europe.

Clinical signs

Edematous vulval swelling occurs 8–14 days post contact with a variable dirty mucopurulent discharge from the vulva, but these signs are not pathognomonic and the organism responsible is often difficult to detect. Irritation of the vulvovaginal mucosa leads to frequent attempts to urinate with the mare showing discomfort by leg stamping, tail twitching and rapid blinking of the vulval lips and clitoris. Severe swelling of the vulva and perineum can occur with a cloudy red vaginal discharge. Chronic lesions appear after the acute phase with raised circular to oblong urticarial plaques ('dollar plaques') in the vulva and adjacent skin. These may disappear and be replaced by others within hours or days. Later, the same area may show areas of depigmentation of skin and clitoris. Characteristically with this disease, weakness and ataxia of the hindquarters occurs with stumbling and knuckling of the lower limb joints. Terminal stages of the disease show anemia, cachexia, intermittent irregular fevers, severe nervous signs such as posterior paralysis, hyperesthesia and hyperalgesia. Signs of disease may persist for up to 2–4 years, although most cases progress over 1–2 months.

Diagnosis and treatment

- The disease may be diagnosed by complement fixation tests and identification of the organism from vaginal discharges. Abortion may occur in pregnant mares.

- Few horses recover from the disease either being destroyed or die.

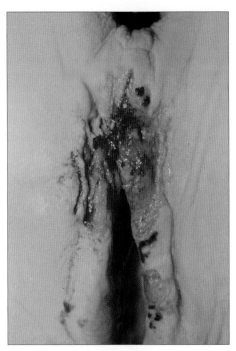

Figure 12.90 Squamous cell carcinoma of the vulvar lips and vestibular mucosa.

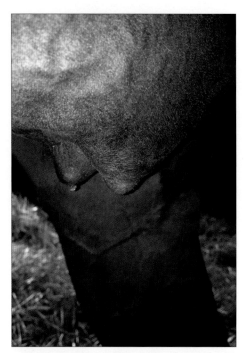

Figure 12.92 Pregnant mare mammary gland with normal appearance of wax.

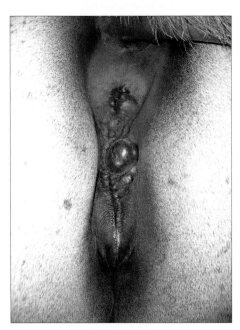

Figure 12.91 Melanoma of the vulva and rectum.

Neoplastic disorders (Figs. 12.90 & 12.91)

Neoplasms occur on the wall of the vagina and may even protrude from the vulval lips. **Hemangiomas** are occasionally found on the vaginal wall but have little particular significance.

Pale skinned horses, with white or non-pigmented skin around the vulva are liable to develop **squamous cell carcinoma** at this site. This may extend into the walls of the vagina. The tumor is most common in areas where high levels of ultraviolet light are present, such as the tropics.

Perineal melanotic masses frequently occur in gray mares and often offer a mechanical obstruction to service or foaling. Traumatic

damage of these masses during foaling or service can lead to discharge of black, gelatinous, amorphous material. Occasionally, **melanosarcoma** is involved in this area and surgical removal appears to stimulate metastases to the spinal cord, leading to posterior paralysis.

Mammary glands

Developmental disorders

Congenital abnormalities are uncommon; most mares have at least two ducts in each teat, but may not produce equal quantities of milk through each duct. The mare has a lactiferous sinus which is less likely to become blocked than are cow's teats. There is a marked variation in size of teats, both in length and diameter. Maiden mares may have relatively short teats set close on the mammary gland, making it difficult for foals to suck, particularly if the foal is weak; equally, some mares have excessively large teats which can also be difficult for weak foals to suckle.

Non-infectious disorders (Figs. 12.92 & 12.93)

Although proximity to foaling is often indicated by the presence of 'wax' adherent to the teat orifice some mares may have premature mammary gland development or run milk for up to 6 weeks prior to foaling, and others may show no waxing and no mammary development prior to foaling. Premature mammary gland development prior to foaling may be related to placentitis, death of one twin foal, or impending abortion. This is often manifested as milk stains on the back legs and, when this occurs, it should be a warning of problems with the foal or placenta and further investigation is warranted. If the mare 'runs milk' for more than a few hours prior to foaling, she may have lost a lot of her good colostrum and the foal should be supplemented with tested high-quality colostrum or plasma. Before the foal nurses the mare's colostrum IgG concentration should be determined.

Because of the protected anatomical location of the mare's mammary gland it is much less commonly affected by trauma than in the cow or goat. Occasionally gross edema, urtical reactions and even serum exudation occurs during allergic reactions to drugs or

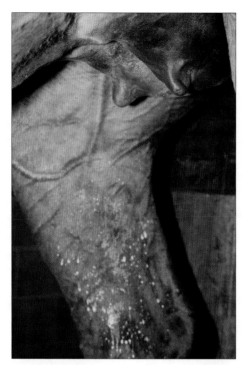

Figure 12.93 Pregnant mare that is 'running milk' or losing her colostrum down her legs. This foal will need supplementation with good-quality colostrum.

Table 12.4 Treatment of fescue toxicosis

Drug	Mechanism of action	Dose	Foaling
Domperidone	DA$_2$ dopamine receptor antagonist	1.1 mg/kg PO sid–bid	Pre/post
Reserpine	Rauwolfian substance	0.01 mg/kg PO q 24 h	Post
Fluphenazine	DA$_2$ dopamine antagonist	25 mg IM one time IM decanoate	Pre
Sulperide	Selective DA$_2$ dopamine receptor antagonist	3.3 mg/kg/day	Pre

Table 12.5 Induction of lactation in non-foaling mares (Protocol 1)

1 Days 1–7; 3 cc (150 mg progesterone + 10 mg estradiol) P+E intramuscular once daily
2 Day 8; 5 mg (1cc) Lutalyse (prostaglandin F$_2$ alpha)
3 Day 8; Begin sulpiride injections 0.5 mg/lb twice daily IM
4 Day 9; Begin milking (5 times per day) giving 5 IU oxytocin 2 minutes before milking

(P. Daels)

Table 12.6 Induction of lactation in non-foaling mares (Protocol 2)

1 Days 1–7; 3 cc (150 mg progesterone + 10 mg estradiol) P+E intramuscular once daily
2 Day 8; 5 mg (1 cc) Lutalyse (prostaglandin F$_2$ alpha)
3 Day 1–10; Sulpiride 500 mg IM twice daily
4 Day 1 of treatment place one foal with the non-pregnant mare to supply suckle stimulus to the mare (in place of the five times per day milking). Supplement foal with mares' milk or mares' milk replacer
5 Oxytocin at 5 IU per injection occasionally as needed for milk let-down
6 Replace foals as needed depending on the aggressiveness of the foal
Using the above protocol, maximum milk production is obtained after 10 days of treatment with sulpiride. This protocol worked in approximately 80% of mares treated

(Adapted from P. Daels by J. Steiner)

other allergens. Swelling and pain in the udder area results in a stiff gait and obvious discomfort. Most cases presenting with these signs are, however, due to infectious mastitis.

Agalactia
Agalactia or the lack of the production of milk/colostrum and development of the mammary gland can occur prior to foaling and continue post foaling. The cause may be unknown or most commonly due to fescue toxicosis (see Fig. 12.54).

Clinical signs and diagnosis
- A lack of mammary gland development within 2–3 weeks prior to foaling as well as minimal colostrum or milk production post foaling is present.
- Grazing on endophyte-infected fescue pasture is not recommended for pregnant mares. Physical examination will reveal lack of development of the mammary gland. If there is question to whether the mare is producing enough milk post foaling, muzzling the foal for an hour to determine the amount of milk produced can aid in identification of decreased milk production.

Treatment
- Removal of the mare from endophyte-infected fescue pastures 60 days prior to foaling. Starting on domperidone 14–30 days prior to foaling. Domperidone a DA$_2$ dopamine receptor antagonist will increase levels of prolactin aiding in increased mammary gland and milk production.
- Post-foaling, domperidone or reserpine (a rauwolfian substance) can aid in mammary gland development. Care must be taken when using reserpine that it is used orally at a dose of 2.5 mg once daily to prevent side effects as seen with injectable such as diarrhea in the mare and sleepiness in the foal.
- See Table 12.4 for treatment of fescue toxicosis.
- Other drugs and protocols used to induce lactation in non-foaling mares (i.e. nurse mares) can be found in Tables 12.5 and 12.6.

Infectious disorders
Acute, chronic and indurative mastitis (Fig. 12.94)
The most common organisms involved are *Streptococcus* spp. and *Staphylococcus* spp.

Clinical signs
Acute cases are febrile, stiff in the hind quarters and the glandular edema may extend into the perineum caudally and anteriorly with obvious enlargement of the transthoracic veins. Where the gland remains hard after weaning, and does not return to its normal contracted state, a chronic fibrotic induration may have occurred. This may be due to inflammation of the gland tissue related to overfeeding of the mare during weaning and may resolve in time, or it may be related to persistent fibrosis from chronic, low-grade mastitis.

Diagnosis and treatment
- Culture and cytology of the mammary gland secretions is needed for diagnosis.
- The condition is treated with appropriate systemic and local antibiotic therapy, anti-inflammatories and hot packing.

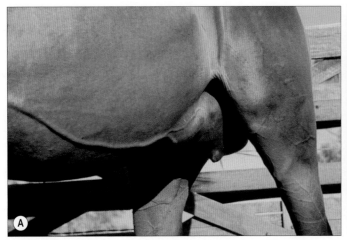

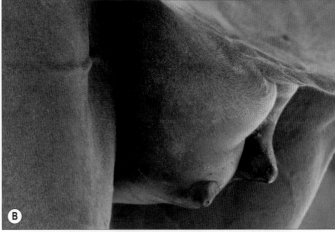

Figure 12.94 (A) Mastitis. Enlarged asymmetrical mammary gland. This can be uncomfortable enough to make mares hesitant to walk. There is obvious engorgement of the transthoracic vein. (B) Mastitis (chronic). A weaned mare showing enlarged mammary gland due to fibrous tissue decreasing functional normal lactation.

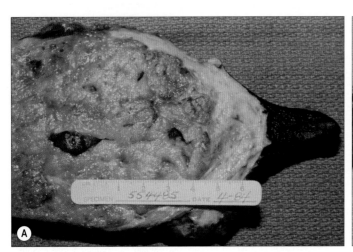

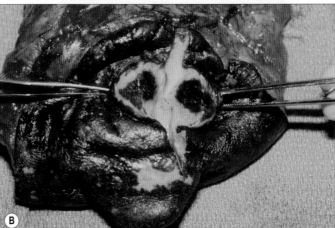

Figure 12.95 (A) Mammary gland adenocarcinoma. (B) Mammary gland melanoma. Melanosarcoma and melanin deposits in mammary tissue above lactiferous sinus.

Neoplastic disorders (Fig. 12.95)

Mammary tumors are not common, but verrucose, fibroblastic and nodular sarcoids are found on the skin overlying the gland.

Very rarely, **primary adenocarcinoma** affects the glandular tissue and the size, progression and high propensity to metastasis make the clinical syndrome more dramatic than most other swellings of the gland. Early gross enlargement of the iliac lymph nodes may be detected per rectum.

Secondary melanoma and **melanosarcoma** occur occasionally in aged gray mares and are associated with mammary enlargement.

2 The stallion and gelding

Clinical examination of the stallion (or gelding) (Figs. 12.96–12.99)

Any previous breeding or other history pertinent to the genital tract examination should be collected and assessed.

Examination of the male horse should include thorough observations of the horse in a totally relaxed state to observe the natural state of prepuce, scrotum and the number, relative size and shape of the testes. Without undue excitement, the stallion should be allowed to

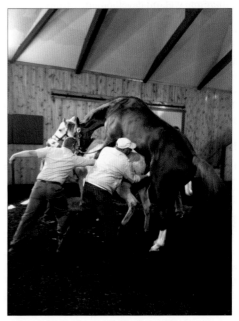

Figure 12.96 Natural mating allows assessment of mating behavior, libido and demeanor.

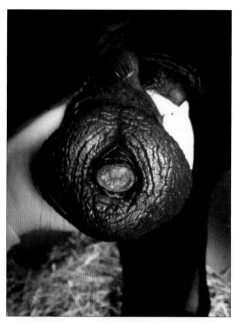

Figure 12.97 Careful inspection of the prepuce, penis and urethral sinus and process.

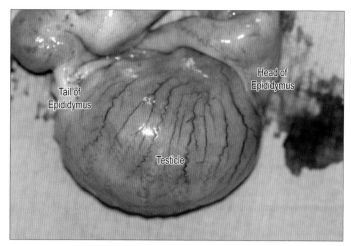

Figure 12.99 Anatomy of the testis: the gonad and epididymis.

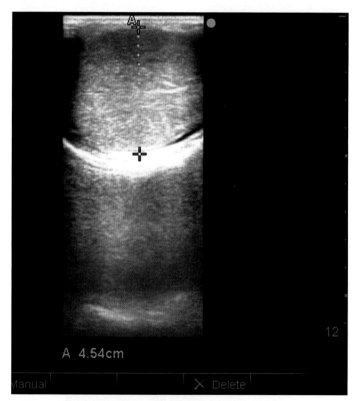

A 4.54cm

Manual | X Delete

Figure 12.98 Ultrasonographic image of a testicle demonstrating normal parenchyma and width measurement.

approach mares, again if possible, to allow natural tumescence of the penis, rather than full erection, to occur. This permits examination for defects, skin abnormalities or infective processes to be quietly observed before any manual examination of the genital tract is carried out.

The next step in the examination is the actual process of mating; assessment of mating behavior, libido and demeanor towards the mare and the handlers. Evaluation of the prepuce, penis and distal urethra is also possible at this time.

For a full and complete semen examination, two collections (using an artificial vagina) should be made 1 hour apart to acquire a representative sample. Wherever changes or abnormalities are encountered, these should be further explored as necessary for the completion of the examination.

Detailed palpation of the external genitalia, and particularly the scrotum and both inguinal canals, should be made. Ultrasonographic examination of the scrotum, testicles, epididymis and spermatocord allows recognition of abnormalities as well as precise measurement of the testicles. Great care must be taken and the use of stocks is recommended for thorough examination of the internal accessory glands per rectum. Ultrasonography of the accessory glands and bladder should be performed under sedation if necessary.

The male equine reproductive system includes the testes and spermatic cord, penis, prepuce and accessory sex organs. The testes descend just prior to, or at birth in normal horses. Anatomically each testis is comprised of the gonad and the attached spermatic cord and epididymis. When the normal testis is transected, the cut surface bulges, and where this does not occur, severe degenerative changes of the seminiferous tubules have occurred. The normal color of the cut testis varies, tending to be darker in older horses.

The appendix testis, which is the homologue of the infundibulum of the uterine tube, is a common normal structure to be seen on the surface of the testis. It always occurs on the surface of the stallion's testis adjacent to the head of the epididymis. It may be flat or rounded and is usually only a few millimeters across. The appendix epididymis is a vestigial remnant of the mesonephric duct origin and is occasionally found as a cystic structure located between the head of the epididymis and the body of the testis, or just adjacent to this area.

Aggressive behavior in the stallion often occurs from many causes such as bad handling, poor or insufficient exercise, over-feeding and poor management (including persistent use as a teaser without subsequent service). It may also be a characteristic behavior in some blood lines but may be related to either overwork or underwork in stud duties. Clinically, it may take the form of aggression towards the handler, the mare or other horses in general. Among the more common causes are over-use in 2-, 3- and 4-year-old stallions in their first season, and it is for this reason, if no other, that 2-year-old colts are better not mated at all. Any serious disturbances to normal mating habits which occur in these young horses may affect mating behavior for the rest of their breeding life.

The testis, scrotum and spermatic cord

(Figs. 12.100–12.103)

Developmental disorders

Vascular malformations of the spermatic cord are uncommon but varicosity has been observed in the spermatic vein and the pampiniform plexus. As the plexus plays a very important role in the thermoregulation of arterial temperature to the testis, any abnormality such as this might easily result in reduced fertility or sometimes even in complete infertility

Congenital absence of one testis is extremely rare and extra testes are even rarer (and probably do not occur). A suspected polyorchid horse is almost always found to be either an incomplete abdominal cryptorchid, or has cystic structures on the cord which have been mistaken for an extra testis. Fusion of the left testis and spleen has been reported in cryptorchids and ectopic adrenocortical tissue has been found in the lower segments of the spermatic cord, adjacent to the head of the epididymis, and in the mediastinum testes. Congenital absence of the cremaster muscle may be found in horses having no ability to lift the testicle. The scrotum of affected horses may have a pendulous nature but it is more usually found incidentally.

Rotation of the testis is not uncommon in racing horses. Opinions are divided as to the pathological significance of this state, but it may be a normal variation. In other cases surgical correction has been performed. The condition can be recognized by the abnormal (anterior) positioning of the tail of the epididymis; attempts to re-locate are successful only as long as the testis is restrained in the normal position; release leads to an immediate return to the original dislocated position. More severe rotation leads to torsion of the spermatic cord, which leads to dramatic vascular compromise, abdominal pain and edema of the scrotum with an enlarged, very firm and extremely painful testis.

Cryptorchidism

Probably the most common abnormality relating to the testes is the cryptorchid testis when one (or both) testes fail to descend completely into the scrotum.

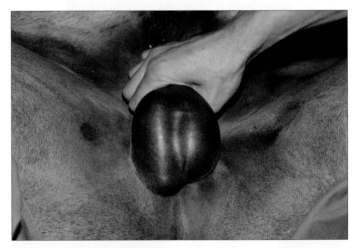

Figure 12.102 180 degree torsion of the left testicle.

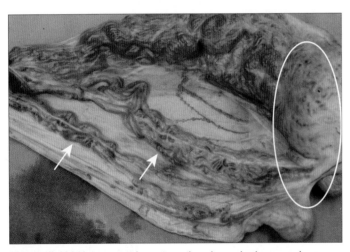

Figure 12.100 Varicose testicle causing unilateral scrotal enlargement due to a secondary venous system (arrows), by-passing the pampiniform plexus; testis (circle) was smaller and firmer than normal.

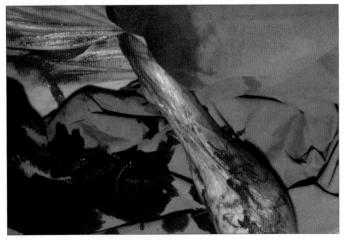

Figure 12.101 Developmental absence of the cremaster muscle.

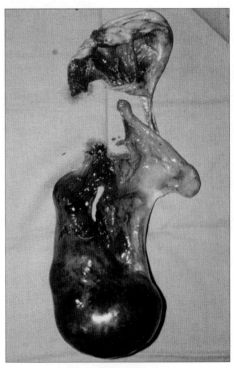

Figure 12.103 Testicle removed due to 360 degree testicular torsion leading to severe vascular compromise, which resulted in pain and swelling of the scrotum.

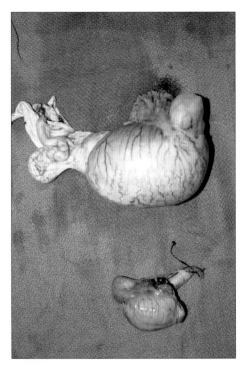

Figure 12.104 A descended and intra-abdominal testicle. Note the large difference in size with the normal descended testicle a lot larger then the retained intra-abdominal one.

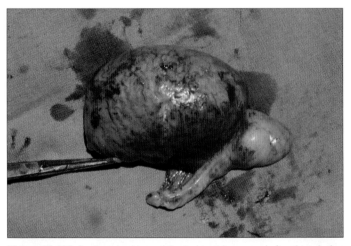

Figure 12.105 Small retained intra-abdominal testicle removed after the tail of the epididymus and body had previously been removed.

Clinical signs (Figs. 12.104–12.106)

A temporary, usually unilateral (the right-side testis is most commonly involved), inguinal retention is relatively common amongst ponies with small testicles. Permanent inguinal retention occurs in all types of horse, and is recognized when the testis is lodged within the inguinal canal. The affected testis (usually unilateral but either can be involved) may be palpable and may be misshapen. Abdominally retained testicles may be freely mobile within the abdomen and may, furthermore, be found in a wide variety of locations. Usually, however, they are to be found deep to the internal inguinal ring. The abdominally retained testicle is commonly very much smaller than the descended one although in some cases, and particularly those in which teratomatous changes are present, they may be considerably larger than the normal one and are then often 'flabby' in consistency. Incomplete abdominal retention occurs when the tail of the

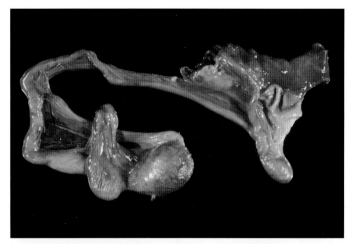

Figure 12.106 Long epididymus associated with a retained testes.

epididymis is in the inguinal canal while the body of the testicle lies at or above the internal inguinal ring. The gross appearance of a cryptorchid testicle is often abnormally dark and where there has been a previous attempt to castrate the animal the epididymis may be removed in the mistaken belief that it is the testicle. The anatomical structure and relationship between the tail and body of the epididymis of the cryptorchid testis to the rest of the testis is often changed with elongated epididymal bodies up to 30 cm long being present which often leads to inexperienced surgeons removing these portions, leaving the testis and the balance of the epididymis in the abdominal cavity. A simple confirmatory test to avoid this error is to cut the tail of the epididymis or body transversally and examine for the coiled tubes of vas deferens rather than testicular tissues.

Diagnosis and treatment

- Palpation and ultrasonography can help to identify the retained testes in the inguinal canal or transrectally in the abdomen. Resting testosterone levels can differentiate geldings from stallions (if bilateral cryptorchidism is suspected) about 89% of the time.
- Another test that will help identify those in the gray zone is the hCG stimulation test. The administration of hCG increases synthesis and secretion of testosterone by Leydig cells in the stallion. The injection of hCG is followed within 1–2 hours by an elevation of testosterone to a level much higher than the normal episodic changes. Elevation can be seen up to 3 days after the injection of 6 000–12 000 IU of hCG.
- Surgery can be performed for either unilateral or bilateral castration.
- Immunization against LH-releasing hormone (LHRH) can also be used as a method of chemical castration for a variable length of time.

Other developmental abnormalities

These include herniation of the small intestine through the inguinal canal which appears to have a slightly higher incidence in Standardbred and Quarterhorses than in other breeds. Inguinal and scrotal hernias are frequently present at birth, causing gross enlargement of the scrotum. This most often resolves within a few days and does not require intervention. The defect is sometimes large enough to warrant manual reduction over the first few days after birth, with subsequent surgical intervention if the reduction is not maintained. Acquired hernias with accompanying swelling, pain on palpation and reluctance to move occur idiopathically or as a result of accidents due to kicks, or falls when horses become caught over rails. In older horses, herniation can be encountered at castration if a large inguinal canal remains patent.

Non-infectious disorders

Where stallions are unable to exercise due to painful hindleg conditions such as fractures, there can be excessive weight-bearing on the other normal leg, leading to edema of the scrotum only, and unless this quickly resolves, it may cause future infertility. A similar appearance is often presented by stallions in which there is gross accumulation of peritoneal fluid (ascites) with consequent hydrocele in the tunica vaginalis.

Testicular hematoma or abscess (Fig. 12.108)

Physical trauma to the scrotum and testicle of the horse occurs from kicks and injuries acquired by hanging over rails, but may also occur where horses are ridden or driven through spiky, awned grasses,

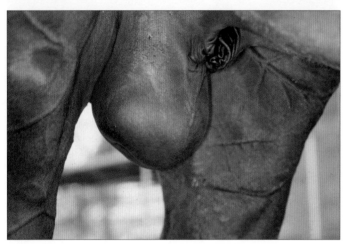

Figure 12.107 Scrotal edema: severe edema due to lack of movement associated with a fractured pastern and stall rest.
Differential diagnosis:
- Hydrocele/hematocele
- Inguinal/scrotal hernia, testicular torsion
- Orchitis, ascites
- Uroperitoneum, hemoperitoneum, varicose testicle, testicular neoplasia, trauma.

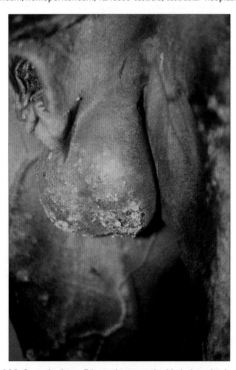

Figure 12.108 Scrotal edema: Edema due to embedded plant thistles.

thistles or shrubs. Thistle spikes may penetrate the skin of the legs, lower abdomen, scrotum and testicles causing exudate of serum, crusting and gross edema of the scrotal skin.

Clinical signs and diagnosis

- Clinical signs include enlarged, warm and painful scrotum or testicle; stiffness or pain when moving.
- The scrotum should be examined carefully in all cases where there is swelling in order to establish the cause. Some such conditions are very serious while others are less so in the short term but all may result in temporary (or sometimes permanent) infertility as a result of temperature changes, adhesions or vascular compromises of one (or both) testicle(s).
- Ultrasonography can help identify where and what is the cause of the swelling. Fibrin tags and adhesions may also be present as the lesion persists.

Treatment and prognosis

- Anti-inflammatory drugs, cold hydrotherapy, stall rest and appropriate antibiotics.
- If the loss of testicular parenchyma is excessive due to pressure necrosis and fibrous tissue formation unilateral orchiectomy may be indicated.
- Prognosis for future fertility depends on size of the hematoma and degree of fibrous tissue formation.

Orchitis (Fig. 12.109)

Inflammation of the testis may be initiated by either trauma, infection, parasites or autoimmune disease. Occasionally, it occurs as a result of racing and may be due to a more-pendulous-than-normal scrotum, leading to physical injury. In other cases it may be a result of infection, particularly from *Streptococcus* spp.

Clinical signs

The accompanying edema causes enlargement of the affected testis and, almost always, the scrotum. In acute cases, the affected testis is enlarged, hot and often very painful, and unless the condition is quickly relieved, irreversible damage occurs, leading to a testicular atrophy and fibrosis. Systemic signs can include fever, leukocytosis and hyperfibrinogenemia.

Diagnosis and treatment

- Examination of the scrotum and its contents with the help of ultrasonography can be useful in establishing the true nature of scrotal swellings and an accurate diagnosis dramatically improves the chances of returning the animal to normal reproductive function.

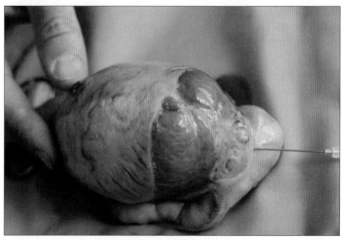

Figure 12.109 This horse initially had orchitis and was treated with antibiotics, however the testicle atrophied and showed marked degenerative changes.

- A semen collection and evaluation may identify leukocytes in addition to providing a culture and sensitivity.
- Systemic antibiotics, anti-inflammatories and cold hydrotherapy can aid in eliminating the bacteria and inflammation.
- If only one testicle is affected then unilateral orchidectomy can be performed.

Testicular degeneration

Testicular degeneration may or may not be accompanied by an obvious reduction in testicular size and weight. There are many causes, the most common being thermal injury. Normal spermatogenesis occurs at a slightly lower temperature than the general body temperature and any condition that results in an elevation of the scrotal temperature will necessarily impair the normal fertility and result in testicular atrophy.

Vascular changes as a result of impaired heat-exchange mechanisms in the vessels of the spermatic cord and pampiniform plexus and fluid (blood, serous or peritoneal fluid) accumulations within the *tunica vaginalis*, as well as any condition that causes edema and inflammation of the scrotum have harmful effects upon spermatogenesis.

Age, systemic infections or even prolonged exposure to high ambient temperatures have also been associated with testicular atrophy and consequent infertility. Equine viral arteritis has been specifically implicated as a cause of testicular atrophy. Furthermore, testes that have reduced blood supply as a result of cord torsion, scrotal and inguinal hernia and varicocele of the spermatic vein may be affected similarly.

The effects of malnutrition, ingestion of toxic plants and physical obstruction to the epididymis can all cause degenerative changes. Administration of exogenous androgens, autoimmune disease, sperm outflow obstruction and neoplasia have also been identified as causing testicular degeneration.

Clinical signs and diagnosis

- Clinical signs include decreased fertility, decreased testicular size and declining semen quality.
- Clinical assessment can be done by manual palpation of the testes, measurement of the testicles by ultrasonography, examination of semen, and, ultimately, test mating.
- Histopathology from a testicular biopsy or removed testicle will provide a definitive diagnosis.

Treatment

- None. If the cause can be identified, cessation of the underlying problem may arrest future progression of the disease.
- *Testicular atrophy* may be encountered after 10–12 years of age in some specific genetic lines. The onset can be very sudden with an abrupt onset of complete infertility. No satisfactory explanation has been found to date, although degenerative vascular lesions have been seen in some testes. Testicular biopsy is a technique for sampling but its use can be hazardous and may cause further degenerative changes to occur.
- *Hypertrophy* may occur in one testis due to injury and atrophy of the other and is commonly encountered where one testis has been previously removed. In the case of cryptorchids used as stallions, increase in size of the undescended testicle may occur. Frequently, where an undescended testicle has been left in situ for a long period, hypertrophy can be found on removal.

Epididymitis

Epididymitis is a rare condition in stallions and is poorly documented. Infection with *Salmonella abortus equi* and *Streptococcus zooepidemicus*

have been recorded as being initially related to trauma, orchitis or infections of the accessory sex glands.

Clinical signs and diagnosis

- Clinically there is both pain and swelling of the scrotal area that, if associated with orchitis, quickly becomes edematous and tight, causing difficulty in palpation of structures within the scrotum.
- Ultrasonographic examination can be used very effectively to establish the nature of this (and many other) scrotal problems.

Complications arising from castration (Figs. 12.110–12.115)

Many different surgical procedures are used for castration including the use of open and closed methods. The closed methods are usually performed on a recumbent horse under general anesthesia and under these circumstances it is possible to pay particular attention to hemostasis and primary wound healing of the scrotal incision is usual. Open castration (in which the *tunica vaginalis* is incised) is frequently

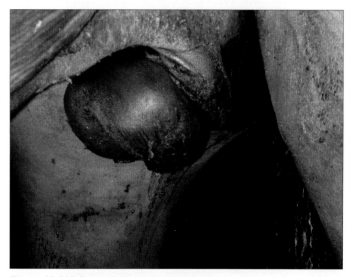

Figure 12.110 Prepucial edema post castration.

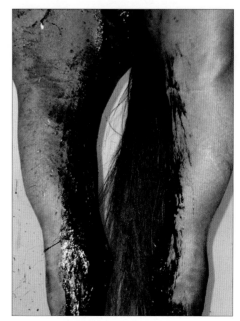

Figure 12.111 Extensive hemorrhage following an open castration.

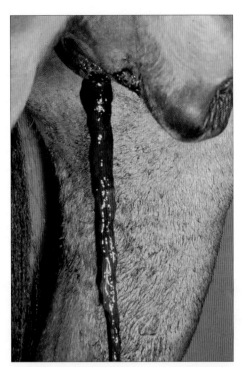

Figure 12.112 Herniation of omentum through the inguinal ring post castration.

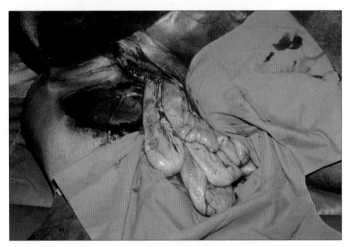

Figure 12.113 Eventration of intestines through the inguinal ring post castration.

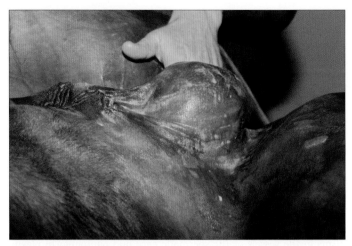

Figure 12.114 Enlarged scrotum due to seroma formation post castration.

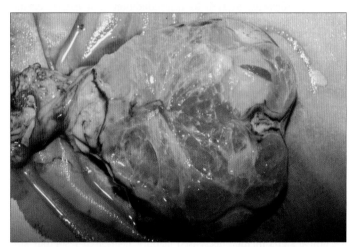

Figure 12.115 Scrotal seroma opened visualizing multilobulated pockets of serous fluid and fibrin strands.

performed in the standing horse under local anesthesia. The resulting scrotal wound is usually left open to allow drainage and second intention healing. Where no (or minimal) infection or post-surgical hemorrhage occurs, there is usually only minor swelling and a slight amount of serous fluid. Occasionally, however, significant scrotal swelling, with edema of the prepuce and ventral abdomen, develops over the first few days after surgery. This is generally due to the presence of variable-sized blood clots retained in the scrotum or to fluid accumulation and gravitation. It may be related to poor hemostasis, poor drainage (possibly as a result of an inadequate scrotal incision) or lack of appropriate post-operative exercise.

Occasionally, following castration, a 'tail' of red-colored tissue may be seen to hang from the scrotum. This is almost always omentum and very occasionally may precede herniation of small intestine. Fortunately, the latter complication is particularly unusual. Herniation of small or longer lengths of small intestine is an unfortunate and extremely serious complication of castration. Open castration in horses having wide or patent inguinal canals and those with inguinal or scrotal hernias seems particularly likely to predispose to this disorder. Closed castration may also be complicated by herniation of small intestine into the scrotal sac, resulting in severe and intractable colic associated with strangulating small intestinal obstruction. Standing, open castration of a horse with an inguinal or scrotal hernia is almost bound to lead to dangerous herniation of intestine.

Accumulation of lymph or serum around the remnants of the spermatic cord leads to the formation of a sterile **seroma**. These are often non-painful, warm swellings that develop over the first few days post operatively. The seroma is made up of a multiloculated mass of clotted blood and fibrin strands. Improved drainage of the operative site or surgical excision of the mass is usually followed by a rapid and full recovery.

Infectious disorders (Figs. 12.116–12.119)

The testicle is seldom directly involved with infectious processes but many systemic virus and bacterial infections exert considerable harmful effects upon spermatogenesis through their febrile nature and the consequent thermal inhibition (and possibly hypoplasia) of the testicular tissue. **Equine viral arteritis, African horse sickness** and some other virus infections may cause orchitis. **Orchitis**, as a result of direct sequestration of bacteria (particularly,

Staphylococcus spp., *Streptococcus* spp. and *Brucella* spp.), is rare in the horse but may cause severe painful swelling of one (or both) testis(es). The condition is indistinguishable from traumatic orchitis. The long-term effects upon fertility are considerable with many affected horses becoming infertile following even relatively minor episodes of infective or traumatic orchitis. A diagnosis may be supported, in the acute stages, by examination of the scrotum and its contents using ultrasonography. Testicular biopsy is an effective, but a somewhat risky, technique for a definitive diagnosis. It is usually reserved for advanced cases because of the increased risk of reduced fertility.

Botryomycosis of the spermatic cord (see Chapter 9, p. 328) is due to infection from *Staphylococcus aureus* and clinically shows as a chronic granulating thickening of the cord stump. The lesion shows miliary small or minute abscess foci and, similar to other scirrhous cords, may show a persistent discharging sinus.

Occasionally in warm weather, even in temperate climates, scrotal wounds can become 'fly-struck' (**myiasis**). This can be due to *Lucilia* spp. flies. In tropical areas where the screw worm fly (*Callitroga* spp.) occurs, umbilical cords and scrotal wounds are frequently affected.

Scirrhous cord (Figs. 12.116–12.118)

Scirrhous cord

An infected operative site following castration causes hot painful swelling and the persistent discharge of serosanguineous or purulent material from the affected side(s) (see Figs. 12.116 & 12.117).

Clinical signs

- Affected horses are often systemically ill, being febrile and innappetent. Serious infection usually develops after 5–10 days and may be particularly difficult to control. In some cases little or no apparent discharge will be encountered for up to 6 weeks, but it will be noticed that the wound fails to heal and slight or moderate local swelling persists.
- Infected castration sites may persist for years, particularly when the site is infected by *Staphylococcus* spp. bacteria.
- Where castration is accompanied by cord ligation there is an added opportunity for local reaction and persistent infection.
- The use of non-absorbable suture material, string or non-surgical wire has been commonly associated with persistent infection and draining sinuses from castration sites. Evidence for all of these unpleasant and debilitating complications of castration may be very difficult to obtain as some cases have little local swelling and the surgery may have been performed years previously. Usually, however, the clinical signs include gross swellings of the scrotum, prepuce and abdominal wall, pain on movement, loss of appetite, elevated temperature and the presence of a draining serosanguineous to purulent discharge.

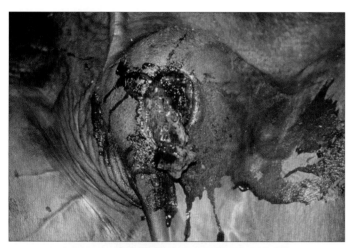
Figure 12.116 Infected castration site.

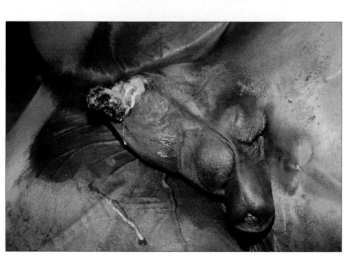
Figure 12.117 Scirrhous cord.

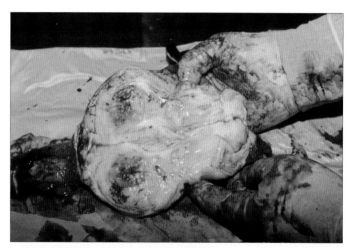
Figure 12.118 Abscess of the cord remnant.

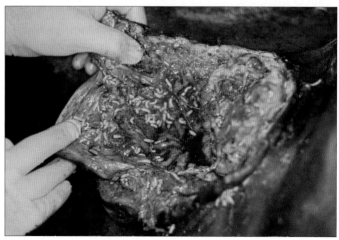
Figure 12.119 Scrotal wound infected with fly larvae (myiasis commonly found in tropical areas).

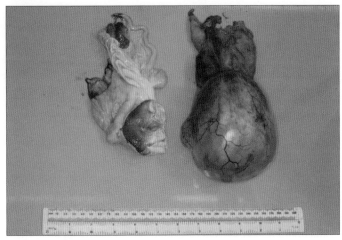

Figure 12.120 Testicular teratomas. Right: large fluid-filled cystic teratoma; Left: teratoma containing cartilage and bone.

Treatment

- Surgical drainage, antibiotics and exercise usually remedy the early post-castration problems. However, where infection slowly becomes established, the scrotal incisions may heal and swelling regresses temporarily for short to long periods.
- Lesions of dense fibrous tissue and chronic, multiloculated or focal abscess of the cord remnants are found during surgical exploration, which is the only effective way of diagnosing the extent of the problem.

Neoplastic disorders (Fig. 12.120)

Tumors of the testes are not common; however two types do occur more frequently than others. Retained testes quite frequently show **benign teratomatous changes**. These may be found to contain cartilage, bone, fibrous tissue and cysts, which may contain hair, glandular tissue and other amorphous material. Testicular teratomas occur predominantly in young cryptorchid stallions and may well be congenital neoplasms.

Seminomas (Figs. 12.121 & 12.122)

This type of tumor occurs in older stallions; they are slow growing and may reach considerable size. Usually, only one testis is involved.

Clinical signs, diagnosis and treatment

- The tumor mass has an obvious, nodular appearance and while some are single and large, others are multiple and smaller. Seminomas become clinically apparent when the affected gonad increases markedly and rapidly in size.
- Metastasis into the spermatic cord, inguinal and lumbar lymph nodes is not uncommon in this condition.
- Ultrasonography can help differentiate a tumor from other causes of testicular enlargement. Biopsy or unilateral orchiectomy will be definitive.
- Treatment is based on unilateral orchiectomy.

Interstitial cell tumors

These tumors are commonly recorded in old stallions and may be easily overlooked as they have very little effect on the size of the gonad.

Other types of neoplasms have been recorded in stallions but are of very low incidence. This may only reflect the fact that the majority of male horses are castrated at a young age.

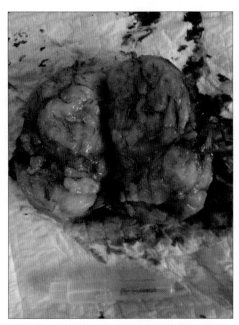

Figure 12.121 Seminoma (yellow tissue) that has obliterated most of the normal parenchymal tissue.

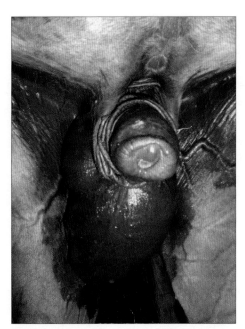

Figure 12.122 Enlarged testicle due to seminoma.

The penis and prepuce (Figs. 12.123 & 12.124)

Developmental/congenital disorders

Normal anatomical features of the penis and prepuce of the stallion include the urethral process, head (glans penis), body of the penis and the prepuce. Congenital abnormalities are not common, but can include constriction or stenosis of the preputial ring, short or retroverted penis, dysgenesis or aplasia of the corpus spongiosum glandis, hypospadia or epispadia, and deviations of the penis in stallions. Such stallions have obvious difficulty serving mares without assistance. Diagnosis is made by observation, the inability to protrude the penis, urine scalding or lack of appropriate orientation or flow. Treatment

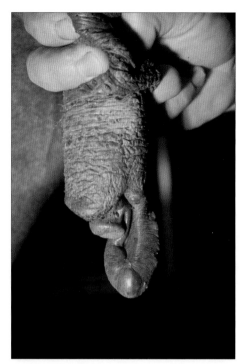

Figure 12.123 Developmental deformity of caput glandis.

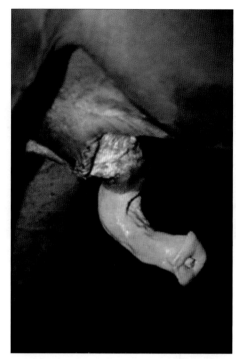

Figure 12.125 Spiral and lateral deviation of the penis. (Courtesy of Dr Alessandra Rota.)

- The gonads are testes, however they are usually intra-abdominal. Aggressive stallion-like behavior can be present due to testicular production of testosterone.

Diagnosis and treatment

- Observation of external and internal genitalia to include ultrasonographic examination or laprascopic evaluation of the abdominal cavity.
- Measurement of testosterone may be useful. Histological evaluation of gonadal tissue may confirm tissue origin.
- There is no treatment available for this condition, so castration is recommended.

Non-infectious disorders

The penis of the neonatal foal may be seen to hang from the prepuce for the first day or two of life but this normal occurrence usually resolves within the first 2 weeks as increasing retractor strength develops. In some foals the opposite occurs when the penis is not relaxed during urination and urine scalding of the sheath and hind legs is a further temporary complication. In the adult horse urination is accompanied by appropriate posture and penile relaxation.

Traumatic damage to the penis (Figs. 12.126 & 12.127)

This is a serious condition in the horse. Physical injury may arise from kicks, accidents caused by falls on fences or even by tail hairs of mares during service. Damage to the urethral process occurs most commonly when natural (paddock) mating occurs and the sharp hairs of the mare's tail are pulled across the erect glans penis. Minor bleeding from the area may be noted immediately after service and, while a single such episode is unlikely to cause any long-term ill-effect, repeated trauma may result in localized fibrosis and urethral infection. Accidental tears to the urethral process and fossa glandis may lead to hemorrhage following service. Where this occurs, there is usually lowered fertility or even infertility until hemorrhage ceases, or is controlled and healed. Clinically, semen samples show pink discoloration due to the presence of blood (hemospermia).

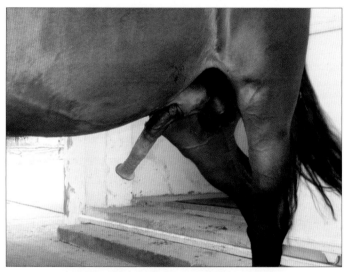

Figure 12.124 Lateral deviation of the penis. (Courtesy of Dr Dickson Varner.)

depends on the abnormality from dilation of the preputial ring, transection or castration.

Intersex

The two most common defects are true hermaphrodism in which there is the presence of both male and female external genitalia with ovatestis, or male pseudohermaphrodite with an exaggerated penile-like clitoris.

Male pseudohermaphrodite

Clinical signs

- An exaggerated clitoris that has a sinus area that protrudes like a vestigial penis may be present anywhere within the perineal region. There is usually an increased distance from the rectum to this structure than normal distance of the rectum to the vulva. Vaginal structures may be normal or abnormal.

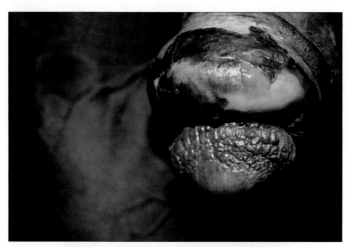

Figure 12.126 Swelling of the penis and prepuce due to trauma during breeding.

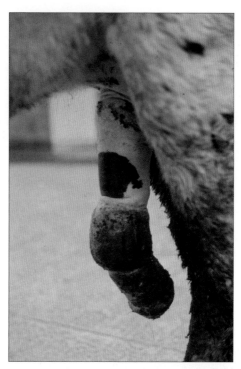

Figure 12.128 Stallion kicked during breeding with swelling that was untreated and now with permanent paraphimosis.

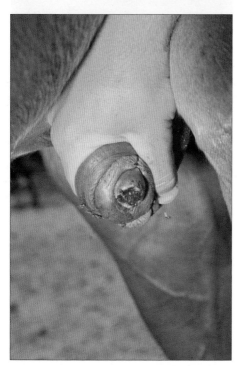

Figure 12.127 Trauma to the urethral process that occurred during pasture breeding.

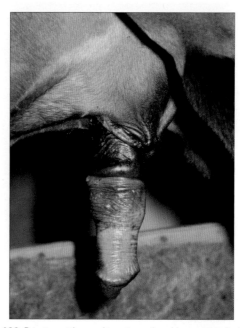

Figure 12.129 Priapism with paraphimosis produced by excising the base of the penis during castration.

Paraphimosis (Figs. 12.128–12.130)

Painful constriction of the glans penis by a phimotic preputial ring or the inability to withdraw the penis into the preputial cavity occurs from a variety of causes. Trauma from kicks, or **priapism** due to debilitation, or the use of some types of tranquilizers are possible causes. **Priapism** with subsequent **paraphimosis** has also occurred as a result of surgical error during castration where the root of the penis is incised instead of a testicle.

Penile prolapse is also a possible secondary complication of disease conditions in other organs, including malabsorption, lymphosarcoma and debilitation. Paralysis of the penis may also be of neurological origin, with spinal cord or sacral, or polyneuritis equi, resulting in a loss of retractor ability.

Clinical signs and treatment

- The acute swelling associated with these conditions and with accident-related paraphimosis should be treated as an emergency.

The penis should be catheterized, pressure bandaged and supported under the horse's abdomen to prevent progressive edema and undue tension on the retractor muscles.

- A number of these cases are incurable, failing to respond to any treatment and partial posthioplasty or amputation may be the only recourse, and as it occurs almost exclusively in stallions the potential consequences of failure to resolve are considerable.

Penile/preputial hematoma (Figs. 12.131–12.136)

Direct kicks to the erect penis of stallions are particularly serious conditions, which commonly result in **hematoma formation.** A kick

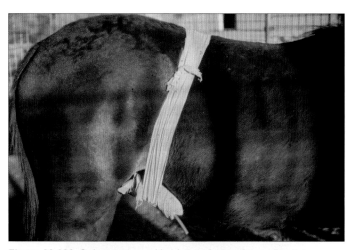

Figure 12.130 Catheterization and bandaging of a paraphimosed penis to reduce inflammation and allow urination.

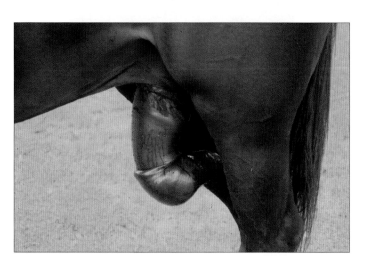

Figure 12.131 Hematoma of the penis after being kicked during natural breeding.

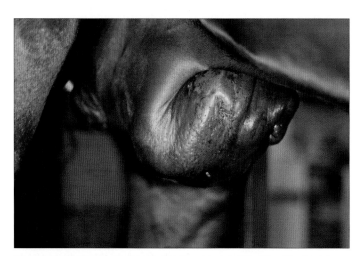

Figure 12.132 Severe local swelling of the prepuce and non-erect penis.

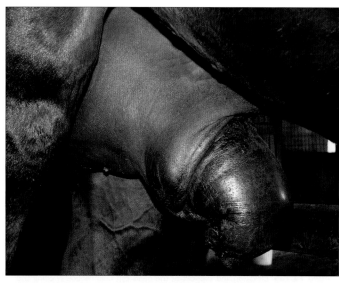

Figure 12.133 Penis and prepuce have dependent swelling due to blood and edema post trauma making it difficult to retract the penis completely.

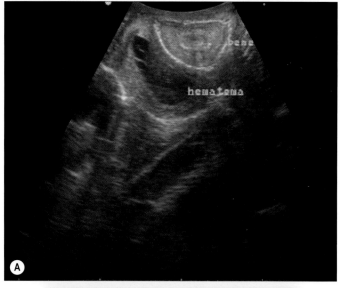

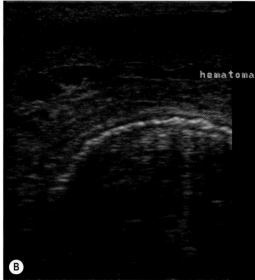

Figure 12.134 Ultrasonic images of the penis: (A) shows the presence of a large recent hematoma; (B) shows an organizing hematoma.

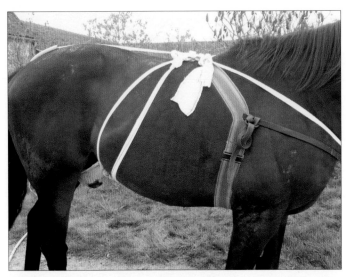

Figure 12.135 Elevation and support of the penis can help reduce swelling and improve venous return.

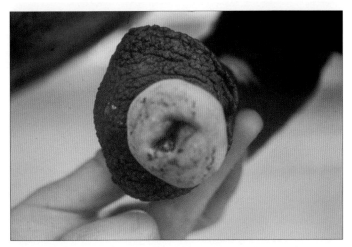

Figure 12.136 Enlarged urethral process due to chronic infestation of habronemiasis.

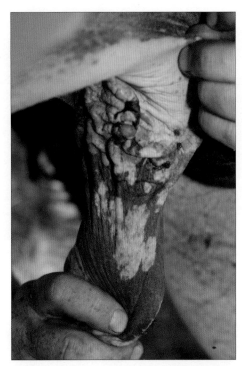

Figure 12.137 Precancerous changes indicative of developing squamous cell carcinoma.

Treatment and prognosis

- Most of these injuries will resolve if treatment is initiated immediately. Cold therapy including icing or hydrotherapy can aid in reducing edema and swelling. Compression of the hemorrhaging tissue by bandaging may aid in cessation with elevation and support of prepuce and penis by a sling to the body wall, preventing dependent swelling formation. Local emollients help to keep the penis or preputial skin malleable so drying and cracking from the skin pressure and stretching are minimized.
- Replacement of the penis within the prepuce should be done if possible. Systemic nonsteroidal anti-inflammatories and antibiotics should be initiated. If severe and/or lack of response to medical treatment, surgery is indicated.
- Untreated hematoma of the penis may lead to fibrosis of the site and the development of permanent paraphimosis.
- Some affected stallions, while able to mount mares, cannot attain a full erection, but providing sensory innervation is still present, may be able to ejaculate into an artificial vagina.

Occlusion of the urethra (Figs. 12.136–12.138)

Contusions to the penis with swelling due to hemorrhage and edema of the injured tissues or inability to pass small cystic calculi may cause occlusion of the urethra cause and/or urinary retention which, if untreated, leads to colic and, even, rupture of the bladder. Poorly fitted stallion rings may also cause occlusion and, in severe cases, lead to sloughing of the glans penis. Urethral injury may result from kicks, laceration to the glans or urethral process during coitus from tail hairs of the mare, or acute or chronic *Habronema* spp. infestation.

In the adult male horse, where urination occurs without penile relaxation, or where phimosis (narrowing of the opening of the prepuce) occurs following injury, infection due to *Habronema* or neoplasia (such as squamous cell carcinoma or melanoma), urination within the prepuce frequently leads to **scalding** and increased smegma formation within the sheath. In white-skinned or colored

to the prepuce and non-erect penis may cause severe local swelling but seldom affects the penis directly.

Clinical signs

Usually these injuries result in hemorrhage from the rich plexus of veins outside the tunica albuginea; rupture of this, such as occasionally occurs in bulls, probably does not occur in the horse. The penis may become very heavy with blood and edema and its dependent nature serves only to aggravate the condition. Gross preputial swelling usually has more effect upon urination and the inability to retract the penis back into the swollen prepuce, which commonly shows difficulty in resolving naturally.

Diagnosis

- A general physical examination should be performed to rule out any other ailments or potential sources for edema and swelling (i.e. protein loss, emaciation). Manual palpation and ultrasonography examination can help differentiate edema from a hematoma.
- Aspiration initially is not recommended due to the potential to contaminate a sterile environment that is conducive for bacterial growth.

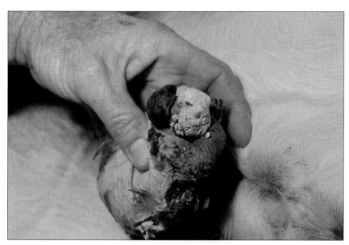

Figure 12.138 Smegma accumulation in the urethral fossa.

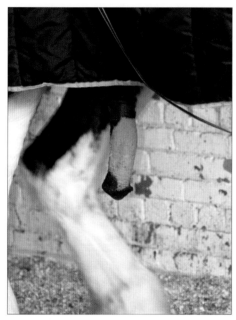

Figure 12.139 Semi-erect penis associated with administration of a phenothiazine.

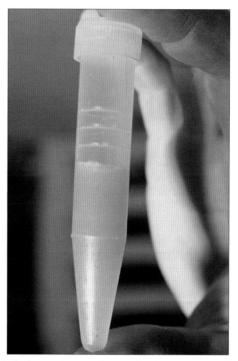

Figure 12.140 Pink discoloration of semen due to the repsence of blood (Hemospermia). The hemospermia in this case was due to a urethral injury that resulted in bleeding during service.

Diagnosis and treatment
- Early diagnosis is imperative so appropriate treatment can be initated. History and visual recognition with physical examination is important.
- Administration of benztropine mesylate has been associated with resolution of priapism if induced by phenothiazine administration. Non-steroidal anti-inflammatories, support with slings, massage, hydrotherapy and diuretics have shown little effect.
- Lavage of the corpus cavernosum to remove clots and sludged blood should be considered in acute cases if chemical reversal is not successful.
- Surgical correction producing a shunt between the corpus cavernosum and corpus spongiosum has been documented as well as castration with subsequent penile amputation recommended if resolution does not occur.

Hemospermia (Fig. 12.140)
Vascular defects in the genital tract result in hemospermia, which may occur as a result of bleeding from sites in the accessory sex glands, bladder, urethra and glans penis. Consequently, it may be difficult to positively identify the exact point of hemorrhage.

Clinical signs
The ejaculate may be pink, due to small amounts of blood, or may contain obvious blood clots, or may be overtly hemorrhagic with several hundred milliliters of blood being discharged on dismount after service. Most stallions become sub-fertile until the condition is remedied.

Diagnosis and treatment
- Careful evaluation of the external genitalia and accessory sex glands by palpation and ultrasonography can help identify the source of hemorrhage, as well as fiberoptic examination of the urethra, bladder and openings of the accessory glands. A rent or tear in the urethra is one of the most common differentials.

horses, this often leads to pre-cancerous skin changes occurring on both prepuce and penis. Accumulation of dried smegma occurs particularly in the urethral fossa in old geldings and may lead to occasional low-grade inflammatory changes such as frequent urination or straining to pass urine.

Priapism (Fig. 12.139)
Defects in the vascular, nervous control and musculature of the penis lead to serious and sometimes permanent changes to the use and carriage of the penis. Priapism (persistent abnormal erection of the penis) may occur either as a fully or semierect condition.

Clinical signs
A semierect penis occurs in conjunction with a variety of other diseases including injuries and inflammation of the spinal cord, purpura hemorrhagica, complication of castration and the use of some phenothiazine tranquilizers (either alone or in combination with other drugs).

- Treatment is determined by origin and cause of the hemorrhage. For tears or defects in the urethra, sexual rest is recommended until healed.

Infectious disorders

Disease of the penis and prepuce may occur subsequent to trauma, dourine, coital exanthema and habronema, with bacterial infections caused by *Pseudomonas* spp., *Klebsiella* spp. or *Taylorella equi genitalis* (CEM).

Coital exanthema

Clinically important viral infection of the penis and prepuce is restricted to equine herpes virus-3, which in maiden stallions occurs after contact with a clinically affected or carrier mare.

Clinical signs

The disease initially appears as blisters over the penis and preputial mucosa, which rapidly rupture, leaving a yellowish necrotic area, which exudes serum, forming small encrusted sores on the preputial reflection. This site corresponds with the longest duration point of contact with the vulval region of carrier mares.

Diagnosis and treatment

- Viral isolation can be performed from early lesions and paired sera using both complement fixation and serum neutralization tests.
- The condition is often transient provided that the stallion is rested until the condition has healed completely. Non-steroidal anti-inflammatories can aid with inflammation and pain.

Bacterial urethritis (Figs. 12.141)

Bacterial urethritis occurs in the stallion, usually from extension of infection from the urethral process and may cause erosion of the mucosa at any point along the urethra.

Diagnosis

Endoscopic examination shows superficial and sometimes deep erosions of the mucosa which may be hemorrhagic and lead to hemospermia and infertility. *Pseudomonas* spp. is the organism most commonly isolated from such infections.

Bacterial infections

The bacterial fauna of the prepuce is usually fairly diverse and involves a number of species which when in normal numbers are regarded as normal commensal organisms. Overzealous hygiene measures taken in stallions (particularly the use of strong disinfectants and antiseptics) may result in a difficult and persistent inflammation of the penis and preputial lining with over-production of smegma.

Frequently, the stallion remains free of clinical signs of infection, but may continue to transmit bacterial infections caused by *Pseudomonas* spp., *Klebsiella* spp. or *Taylorella equi genitalis* (CEM) to mated mares. Serial samples for bacterial culture should be taken from the prepuce, diverticulum, urethral fossa (fossa glandis) and free portion of the penis. The urethral orifice both pre and post ejaculation can be cultured as well as the smegma from the fossa glandis which may yield a pure culture of pathogenic organisms.

Contagious equine metritis

Contagious equine metritis is caused by the organism *Taylorella equi genitalis* and transmitted sexually between mares and stallions (see p. 473). The stallion is considered an asymptomatic carrier.

Clinical signs

Since the stallion is an asymptomatic carrier, it is usually the mares with which they have been bred that are diagnosed with a severe endometritis , which then leads back to identification in the stallion.

Diagnosis and treatment

- Bacterial isolation from the fossa glandis, urethral orifice, penis and prepuce. Serological evaluation is not a good means of identification in the stallion since there is no immune response unlike the mare.
- Sometimes the organism is not identified on stallion culture and test breeding of a mare with subsequent identification is necessary. Special media that is a chocolate agar with 10% horse blood and antibiotics to inhibit other bacterial growth is necessary for culture.
- Washing the erect penis and prepuce with a 4% chlorhexidine soap followed by coating the dried penis with an antimicrobial ointment should be done for at least 5 days. Sexual rest until reculture negative is imperative.

Pseudomonas aeruginosa and Klebsiella pneumoniae

Pseudomonas is a Gram-negative rod that is found in warm damp locations, while *Klebsiella*, also a Gram-negative rod, is found in soil and on bedding. There are pathogenic and non-pathogenic or environmental strains, differentiated as pathogenic in *Pseudomonas* by the production of hemolysins, while *Klebsiella* is classified by its capsule type. There are seven capsule types with K1, K2, K5 associated with equine metritis and K7 andK5 most likely to be found in the stallion. Frequent washing of the stallion's penis destroys the normal flora and predisposes to persistent colonization with these organisms.

Clinical signs

Both *Pseudomonas* and *Klebsiella* can be identified on the stallion's penis without causing pathological conditions; however, if there is mucosal damage or increased numbers, these bacteria become opportunistic and can become highly infective and difficult to treat. Stallions that are mated to infected mares continue to transmit the organisms to other mares.

Diagnosis and treatment

- Aerobic culture is used for diagnosis. Identification of pathogenic pseudomonas and capsule type with Klebsiella is important.
- *Pseudomonas* can be quite difficult to eliminate. However, success has been reported using an iodine base surgical scrub followed by application of a 1% silver sulfadiazine cream for 2 weeks.
- Therapy can be monitored with a wood's lamp. A dilute solution of HCl can also be used to rinse the penis for 2 weeks paying attention to the fossa glandis and irritation. *Klebsiella* can be treated with a daily rinse with a dilute solution of sodium hypochlorite for 2 weeks after removal of smegma.

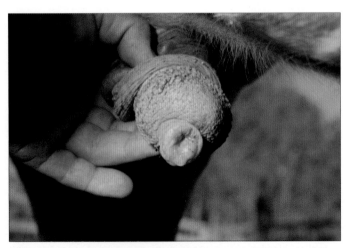

Figure 12.141 Bacterial urethritis. Enlarged urethra, mildly painful and caused occasional inhibition of service.

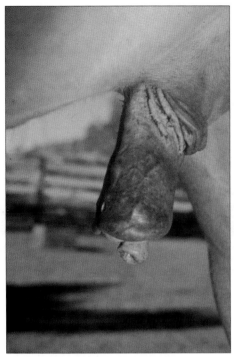

Figure 12.142 Dourine (*Trypanosoma equiperdum*). Edema of the urethral process, prepuce, penis and surrounding skin.

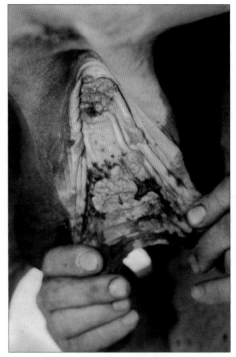

Figure 12.143 Squamous cell carcinoma associated with the preputial ring.

Dourine (Fig. 12.142)

Dourine is a protozoal venereal infection due to *Trypanosoma equiperdum* and probably originated in North Africa, spreading to other parts of Africa, Asia, Europe, Indonesia and the Americas. The disease has been eradicated from North Africa, Western Europe and North America (See also p. 483).

Clinical signs

Early signs in the stallion include edema of penis, prepuce and testes, followed by raised plaques on the penis and prepuce, leading to so-called 'dollar plaques', so-named because the lesions are hardened disc-like masses under the skin the size of a dollar coin. These characteristically appear and disappear over variable intervals of a few hours to a few days, only to be replaced by others. Paraphimosis and penile edema with edema and swelling of the urethral process are commonly present. Depigmentation of the mucosa of the genital tract may occur; paralysis of the hind quarters and cachexia develop and death ensues.

Diagnosis and treatment

- The disease is transmitted by coitus and trypanosomes may be present in seminal fluid, or mucus exudate from the penis. Complement fixation tests can also identify the disease.
- Treatment is not practical, but isolation is imperative while diagnostics are performed.

Parasite infestation

Infections are commonly due to *Draschia megastoma*, *Habronema musca* or *Habronema microstoma*. Larval worms may be deposited into cuts, tears or other areas of broken mucosa or skin where they can induce a granulomatous reaction.

Clinical signs

The lesions are small at first and lead to ulceration of the external surface of the urethral process. Progressively there is enlargement of the urethral process and variable ulceration. It may occur in both geldings and stallions; in the stallion, bleeding occurs during and following mating and may lead to both temporary inhibition due to pain and irritation, and to reduced fertility due to the presence of blood intermixed with ejaculate.

Diagnosis and treatment

- Identification of impression smears, lesion scrapings and biopsy can differentiate parasites from other etiologies.
- Systemic treatment with ivermectin is usually curative, with a follow up treatment a month later. Local treatment with an anti-inflammatory agent and larvicidal drugs may be necessary if lesions are large. Surgical debridement may also be necessary if the urethral process is involved or lesions excessive.

Neoplastic disorders

Neoplasia of the external genitalia is particularly rare in stallions but relatively common in geldings. Smegma has been incriminated as having carcinogenetic properties and this especially applies in horses with poorly pigmented skin such as Appaloosa, and colored horses such as Cremello, Palamino, Pinto and Overo.

Squamous cell carcinomas (Figs. 12.143–12.147)

These tumors are found on the prepuce of geldings of any age, often showing as small granulomatous tumors. The earliest stage of the development of squamous cell carcinoma in geldings is a well-recognized 'pre-cancerous', plaque-like inflammatory change which is most obvious at the preputial reflection but which may affect larger areas of the preputial lining with adjacent lesions on the penis.

Clinical signs

- These pre-cancerous plaques frequently respond to regular washing to prevent smegma accumulation and then may not develop overt

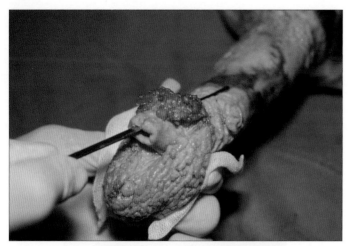

Figure 12.144 Squamous cell carcinoma demonstrating erosion of the penile shaft to urethra.

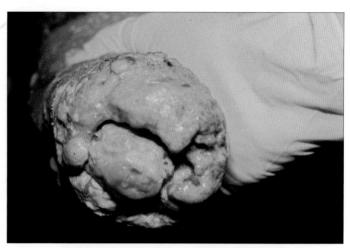

Figure 12.147 Invasive non-proliferative tumor more common in younger horses.

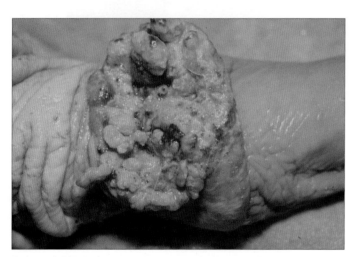

Figure 12.145 Squamous cell carcinoma at the preputial reflection.

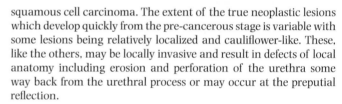

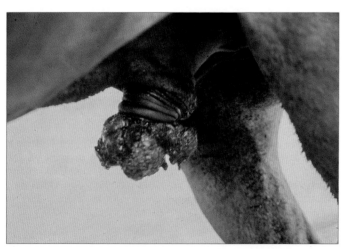

Figure 12.146 Inability to withdraw penis into prepuce due to a squamous cell carcinoma.

squamous cell carcinoma. The extent of the true neoplastic lesions which develop quickly from the pre-cancerous stage is variable with some lesions being relatively localized and cauliflower-like. These, like the others, may be locally invasive and result in defects of local anatomy including erosion and perforation of the urethra some way back from the urethral process or may occur at the preputial reflection.

- In some cases massive proliferative neoplastic lesions develop and may even result in an inability to withdraw the penis into the prepuce (pseudo-paraphimosis). In most cases, and particularly when the condition develops in old horses, the tumor is not highly malignant, growing rather more slowly than might be expected from its nature.
- Spread to local lymph nodes and other remote structures such as the vertebral bodies and lungs does however occur. When it develops in younger horses the outlook is much poorer.
- The more invasive type of penile squamous cell carcinoma which occurs in younger horses is often less proliferative in appearance, but palpation of the penis will identify an irregular firmness occupying a variable length of the free length.
- Metastasis to inguinal and iliac lymph nodes is relatively common in these horses and their life expectancy, even following radical surgery, is much reduced.

Diagnosis and treatment

- Clinical signs are diagnostic with confirmation by histopathological examination of a biopsy.
- Treatment of small lesions can be attempted using chemotherapy such as 5-fluorouracil ointment. Radiation therapy with radon or iridium seed implant or teletherapy have also been documented in addition to systemic non-steroidal anti-inflammatory drugs.

Melanoma

Melanoma occurs relatively commonly in gray horses and occasionally are found affecting the preputial ring where they may cause phimosis.

Nodular and fibroblastic sarcoids (Fig. 12.148)

These commonly occur on the preputial skin. Multiple lesions are commonly encountered although single (or few) nodular lesions are also common. Only very rarely do these masses occur on the preputial skin and they are only rarely found on the free part of the penis.

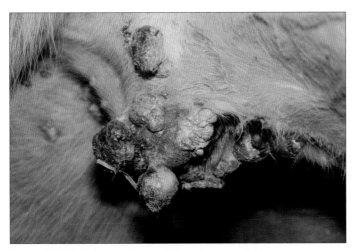

Figure 12.148 Multiple nodular sarcoids on the preputial skin.

3 The placenta

The placenta (Figs. 12.149–12.162) is the physiological unit made up entirely of fetal tissues, which lies in contact with the endometrium of the mare and is responsible for the exchange of nutrients and waste matter between the foal and the dam. Any factor or condition that alters this relationship has the potential to cause changes to the foal, which may lead to death, resorption, abortion, deformity or infection of the neonate. Such a wide-ranging set of conditions can be encountered that it behooves the reproductive clinician to undertake a careful study of every placenta at parturition. A great deal of useful information can be gleaned, concerning not only the placenta, but also the endometrium, to which it was attached during the pregnancy, and the potential status of the foal. Indeed it is possible that in many cases of abortion, more may be learnt from the placenta than from the aborted fetus itself. A careful examination of the placenta may furthermore provide useful information regarding future pregnancies.

Abortion represents a traumatic event for the mare and the fetus (and indeed the mare owner), and few events occur which cause more anguish, recriminations, deceit and poor relationships between owners of mares and stallions. It is a time for particular tact on the part of the veterinarian who should exert the greatest possible effort to reach a conclusive diagnosis, and hopefully establish a definitive etiology.

The fetus and placenta should be thoroughly examined both externally and internally in a situation where the risks of contamination to other mares and the surroundings is minimal. Laying the placenta in an 'F' shape allows full evaluation of the horns, tip of the horns and body. The chorionic and allantoic surface should be viewed. A full examination is performed, specimens taken, and the fetus and placenta properly disposed of. Measurement of the foal's crown-rump length should be made and it should be examined for the presence (or otherwise) of hair on the mane, muzzle, eyelids and coronet (Table 12.7). These will provide a reasonable estimate of the gestational age and this may be compared with the computed gestational age derived from accurate service dates. A full range of samples, including liver, lung, kidney, thymus, lymph node and adrenal gland, should be taken and preserved in 10% formal saline and stomach contents placed in a sterile, iced, sealed bottle. Fresh specimens of all the above organs should also be taken on ice and despatched to the laboratory immediately for virus, bacterial and fungal isolations. Where delay in transit may occur, viral samples may be frozen until suitable transport can

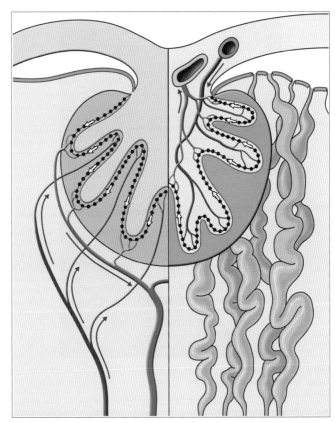

Figure 12.149 Depiction of the microvilli association with the endometrium and the vascular components that allow nutrient and gas exchange.

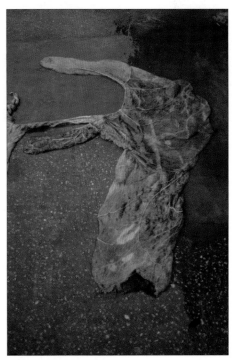

Figure 12.150 Normal placenta laid out in a reverse 'F' for examination with the chorionic surface exposed.

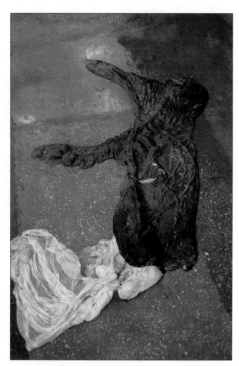

Figure 12.151 Normal placenta laid out in reverse 'F' for examination with the allantoic surface exposed.

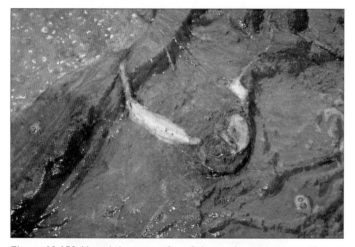

Figure 12.152 Normal chorionic surface of placenta demonstrating an avillus area consistent with a fold in the placenta. This is a normal finding.

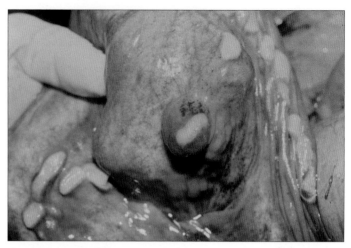

Figure 12.153 Endometrial cups day 70. Normal ring of endometrial cups with one developed on top of an endometrial cyst.

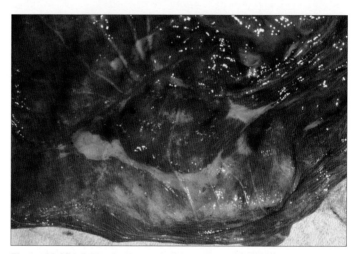

Figure 12.154 Full-term placenta showing evidence of where the endometrial cups had been.

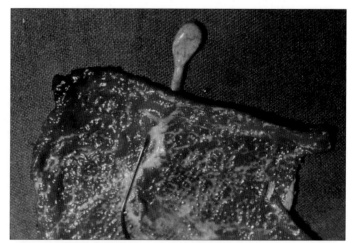

Figure 12.155 Endometrial scar on chorionic surface due to the formation of an endometrial pouch noted on a stalk on the allantoic surface.

be arranged. If a diagnostic laboratory is close by submission of the complete placenta and fetus is most useful.

Portions of placenta (allanto-chorion) should be taken, for both microbiological examination and histopathology, from the region of the cervical star and any other areas where discoloration or thickening is detected. Samples from the allanto-amnion for bacterial and fungal culture complete the range of specimens needed for a full investigation.

Visual examination of the placenta will also often provide indicators as to the future fertility of the mare and potential septic problems, which may develop in the neonatal foal. Culture of the mare's uterus post abortion can also help identify early the causative agent. In order to gain familiarity with this important organ, it is necessary to have a good knowledge of the anatomy, function and normal variations of the placenta.

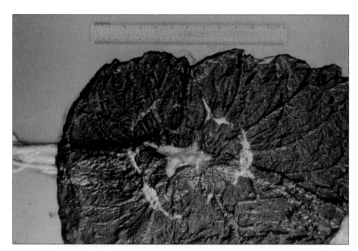

Figure 12.156 Scar from the endometrial cups in a circle and the central avillous area where blood vessels originate on the allantoic surface.

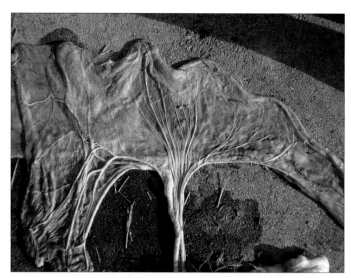

Figure 12.158 Normal placenta with the attachment of the umbilical cord in the pregnant horn.

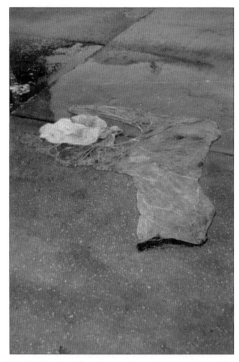

Figure 12.157 Umbilical cord originating from the non-pregnant horn.

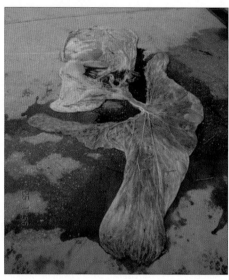

Figure 12.159 Normal placenta with the attachment of the cord centrally between the uterine horns.

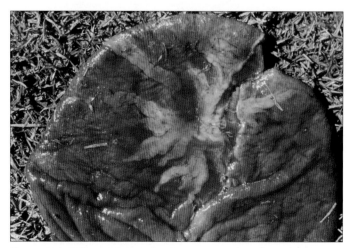

Figure 12.160 Normal placenta showing tear in the cervical star, through which the foal was delivered.

It is beyond the scope of this book to describe the early embryonic changes that occur in the fetus and placenta, apart from some aspects of endometrial cup formation and their recognition as part of the embryological development of the structure found in the mature placenta. Embryologically, the chorionic girdle cells of the conceptus invade the maternal endometrium to cause implantation after about 35 days. This leads to the formation of distinctive irregular plaques of tissue, the endometrial cups, which form a disconnected ring of tissue at the point of implantation.

Due to the developmental relationship of the girdle cells to the allantoic stalk, the umbilical cord is always located at the center of the ring of cups. Physiologically the endometrial cups consist of trophoblast cells derived from the girdle cells, and are responsible for the production of (equine) chorionic gonadotropin. While the endometrial cups occupy much of the endometrial stroma in the area of

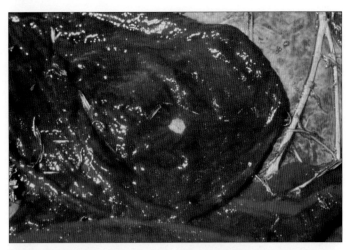

Figure 12.161 Normal placenta showing the avillous area of the oviductal opening in the pregnant horn. Note the edematous, thickened appearance of the tip of the pregnant horn.

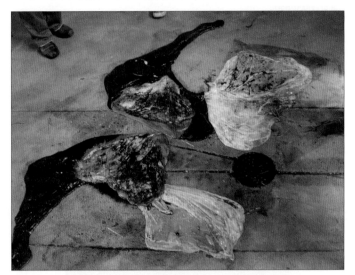

Figure 12.162 Large avillus areas of twin placentas where they are in contact with one another. From McAuliffe SB, Slovis NM (eds) (2008) Color Atlas of Diseases and Disorders of the Foal. Elsevier, Oxford (with permission).

Table 12.7 Equine gestational age crown-rump length

Days	Body weight (kg)	Crown-rump length
140–159	2.15 + 0.79	43.14 + 4.3
160–179	3.76 + 2.55	46.43 + 9.25
180–199	6.43 + 1.27	59.42 + 5.40
200–219	9.25 + 1.95	70.10 + 5.43
220–239	13.91 + 2.86	77.40 + 6.36
240–259	20.03 + 4.00	89.37 + 5.4
260–279	26.85 + 4.08	98.88 + 4.8
280–299	32.59 + 7.97	104.33 + 10.2
300–310	39.41 + 6.52	109.56 + 7.63
320–339	50.00 + 6.99	117.77 + 6.17
340–359	50.82 + 6.04	120.00 + 5.43

implantation, they do not destroy the underlying endometrial glands and indeed, may in some cases even implant on structures such as endometrial cysts without any other detectable abnormalities or deficiencies. The endometrial cups gradually become less recognizable as they regress, usually from about days 130–150 of gestation. Their regression however does leave remnants and scars in the placenta and in some cases the resultant sloughed endometrial surface forms the core of allantoic pouches, which frequently project into the allantoic cavity. Examination of the placenta in the area of attachment characteristically shows a ring of cup remnants surrounding a central avillous area (caused by the remains of the yolk sac).

Embryologically, the placental circulation gradually takes over the function of the yolk sac circulation from about day 60. The allantois, which becomes visible from about day 20, grows rapidly to assume the major blood supply to the chorion at about day 30. The fused chorion and allantois (the allanto-chorion) then attaches to the endometrium to form the placenta.

The gross anatomical features of the placenta may be visualized best by placing the easily identified body and the two uterine horns in the form of an 'F' configuration on an open flat surface. Normal structures which can then be observed from the inverted allanto-chorion are the thickened (edematous) pregnant horn, the much thinner, smaller, non-pregnant horn, the body, the umbilical cord, and the attached allanto-amnion.

The placement of the umbilical cord may be close to the non-pregnant horn or the pregnant horn or may be located at some place intermediate between these two locations. The variation in this location is related to the transuterine migration of the fetus, which occurs in some mares after implantation occurs. There is no migration of the point of implantation over the surface of the endometrium.

Examination of the chorionic surface is extremely important since it helps identify pathology. The normal placenta shows normal avillous structures such as the cervical star. This area is the site of rupture during normal parturition, and represents the point of contact between the avillous cervix and the chorionic surface of the placenta. The avillous imprint of the opening of the oviduct is usually also obvious. Also, folds in the chorion appear as avillous areas of varying size and location. A particular and very important situation occurs with twinning, where one developing chorion abuts against the other, resulting in the development of a relatively large avillous area. This deficit can usually be identified no matter what stage of pregnancy has been reached before absorption, abortion or full time delivery occurs and its recognition is of paramount importance to the equine obstetrician.

Non-infectious disorders

Twinning (Figs. 12.163–12.169)

Twinning in horses is widely feared amongst breeders and a variety of permutations can be encountered. One apparently normal twin and the placental remnant of the second fetus, or abortion of a resorbing twin with a dead premature foal may be detected. Alternatively, there may be a full term delivery of twins, either both alive, one alive or both dead. (Triplets are exceptionally rare and are not viable.)

The placentas of all types of twinning are very characteristic and show marked abscence of villi at the common site of contact. Care should always be taken to examine both sides of the placenta, as viewing of a twin placenta from the allantoic side only could be misleading if only one placenta and foal had been found. It is certainly true that almost all twin foals that are born alive (either at full term or before term) are handicapped by having a decreased placental surface area. Most experienced equine obstetricians consider that all twins are dysmature regardless of their gestational age.

With the increased use of ultrasonography 14–15 days post ovulation, the number of abortions, loss or birth of twins has decreased. There are different methods to reduce twins to a singleton depending on the stage of gestation. The best method having the greatest success is still rupturing an embryonic vesicle manually prior to day 16 post-ovulation. The remaining embryonic vesicle continues to grow

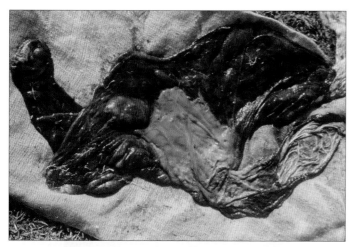

Figure 12.163 Twin pregnancy with avillus area.

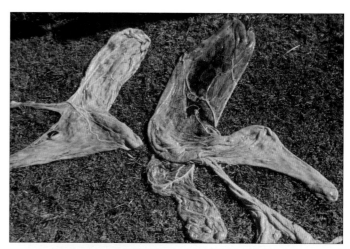

Figure 12.166 Same placenta as Fig. 165 viewed from the allantoic surface.

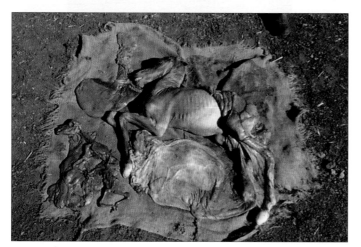

Figure 12.164 Twin abortion with the large fetus and a resorbing mummified small fetus.

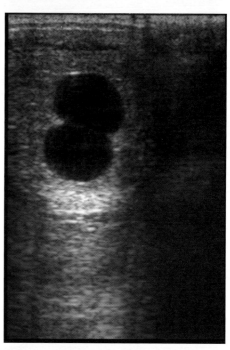

Figure 12.167 Twin at 14 days pregnancy viewed on transrectal ultrasonographic examination. Notice their orientation on top of each other and the similar size.

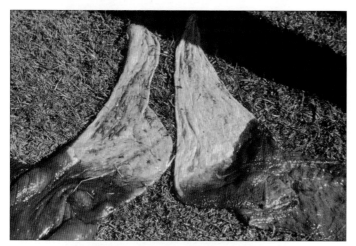

Figure 12.165 Well demarcated avillus areas at the point of contact between twin placentae.

normally and a normal sized viable foal is present at birth. Other methods of reduction prior to 60 days of gestation include transvaginal ultrasound guided injection or aspiration of one of the vesicles. This procedure has varying results dependent on clinician, time of gestation when the procedure is performed and whether the vesicles

are unilateral or bilateral. Reduction in feed intake has also been tried, with lesser success. Between 65–120 days of gestation cranio-cervical dislocation can be performed, in which the cranium of the least viable fetus is separated from the cervical vertebrae. This procedure can be done transrectally or through a flank laparotomy intra-abdominally and has the best success rate next to manual crushing producing a normal sized healthy foal. The last procedure that has been described is transabdominal ultrasound guided fetal injection. This procedure is performed later in gestation (>150 days) so that the foal born is usually smaller and more compromised due to the decreased surface area of the placenta. Clinician and fetal position is also a factor in the success rate.

Placental defects (Figs. 12.170–12.176)

The presence of specks of material known as '**amnionic pustules**' are frequent findings on the umbilical cord and amnion. There is no

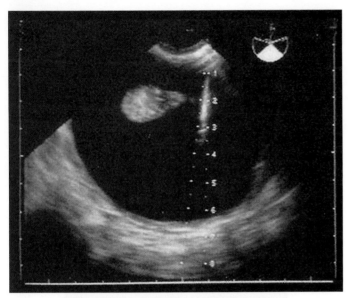

Figure 12.168 Transvaginal ultrasound-guided aspiration of a twin.

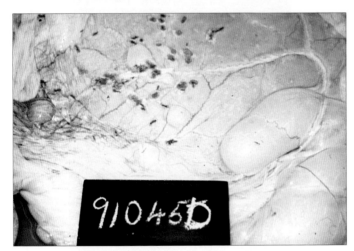

Figure 12.170 Normal mineralized deposits on the surface of the amnion. (Courtesy of Irish Equine Centre).

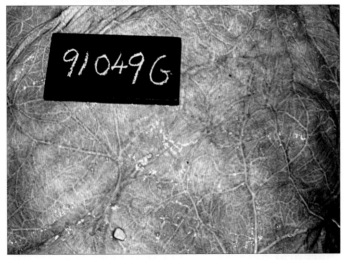

Figure 12.171 In this image small pieces of hippomane have become attached to the allantoic surface. While this is an unusual finding it is not associated with any pathological change in this case. (Courtesy of Irish Equine Centre).

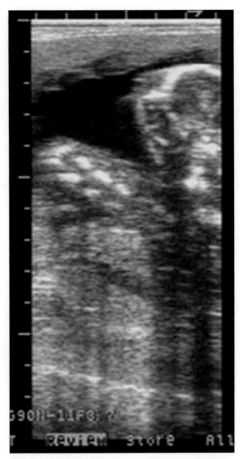

Figure 12.169 Transrectal ultrasonographic examination of a twin after cranio-cervical dislocation had been performed. Note the space between the cranium and the cervical vertebrae.

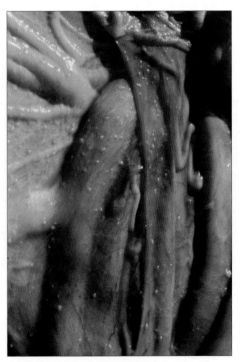

Figure 12.172 Amnionic pustules exhibiting normal deposits of urinary salts in the amnion.

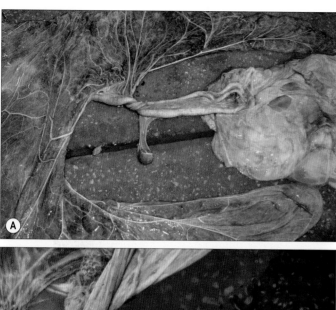

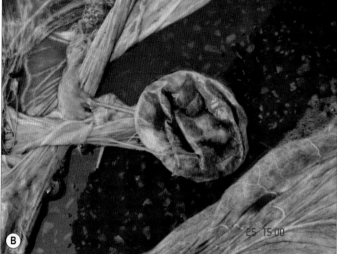

Figure 12.173 Calcified yolk sac remnant originating from the umbilical cord. This is often confused as a twin but location is the differentiating factor as well as contents of the sac.

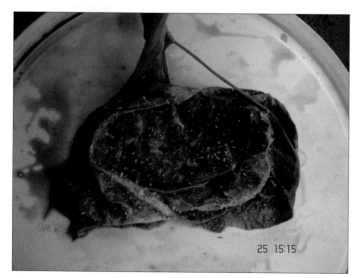

Figure 12.174 Large calcified yolk sac. These can twist around the umbilicus causing vascular compromise and abortion.

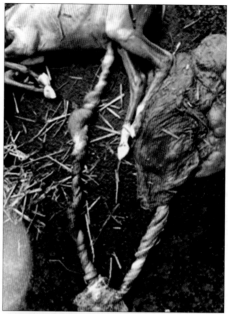

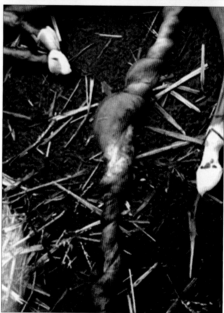

Figure 12.175 Urachal cysts. Compression and torsion of umbilical cord can lead to sacculation of the urachus and urachal cysts.

evidence to suggest that these are in fact pustules or have any inflammatory origin and are probably normal depositions of urinary salts.

Serious, and sometimes even minor, defects in the development of the placenta (and/or its individual components) almost always results in abortion but some embryological structures may remain and become calcified, such as a **yolk sac remnant** found in the infundibulum. Deposition of calcium salts in plaques in various locations on the urachus and amnion may become twisted and further calcified, leading to quite large calcified structures. These are often mistaken for fetal remnants. Dilatations of the urachal vessel to the allanto-amnion can give rise to urachal cysts.

A bifid, non-pregnant horn is an unusual developmental defect of the placenta. Both segments of the apparently divided horn are fully villous, with no avillous areas present, such as would be seen with abutting twin placentas. This situation suggests that there might be a

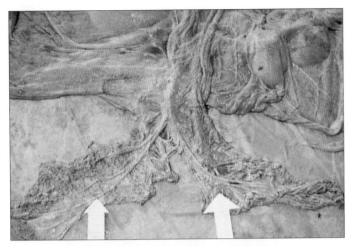

Figure 12.176 Bifid non-pregnant horn abnormality (viewed from the amnionic surface). Shows distribution of blood vessels in the divided chorioallantois.

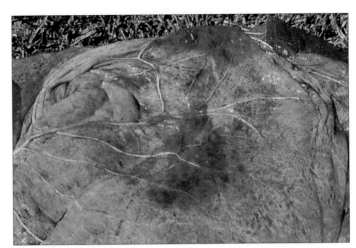

Figure 12.178 Mild intramural hemorrhage caused by the foal kicking. This led to perforation of the mare's uterus.

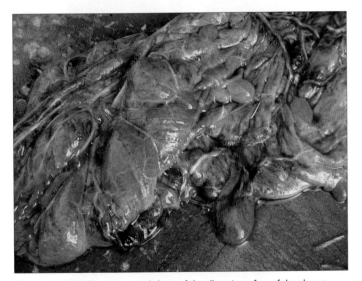

Figure 12.177 Chorionic cysts/edema of the allantoic surface of the placenta.

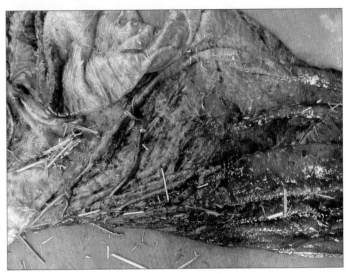

Figure 12.179 Moderate placental hemorrhage. The foal was lethargic, slow to rise and suckle, however improved with treatment over the next 3 days.

bifid uterine horn in these mares but such an anatomical abnormality has not been described.

Physical disorders of the placenta

(Figs. 12.177–12.186)

A wide variety of physical changes may be detected in the placenta. Edema of the inside surface of the chorion (with cyst-like formation) is most frequently seen in placentas from premature deliveries or in apparently normal, pre-term placentas from mares which are examined after death for other reasons. The significance of the 'defect' is equivocal but it would seem likely that circulatory and inflammatory factors may be involved in some cases while in others it may be an entirely incidental (normal) occurrence.

Severe foal struggling or abnormal pressure within the uterine wall-allanto-chorionic interface due to uterine contractions causes **hemorrhage into the allanto-chorion**. This may be mild, more extensive or severe and life-threatening to the foal. Large **hematomas** may develop at the site of such hemorrhage. Other indications of fetal stress related to malpositioning include tears through the body of the allanto-chorion other than at the cervical star, and the presence of meconium staining of both the foal and the placental contents. In all these circumstances the placental (or fetal) findings are indicators of

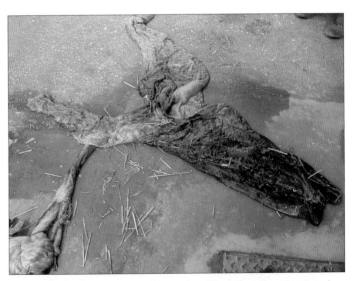

Figure 12.180 Extensive placental hemorrhage. The foal was born anemic and weak and required therapy for 5–6 days post partum.

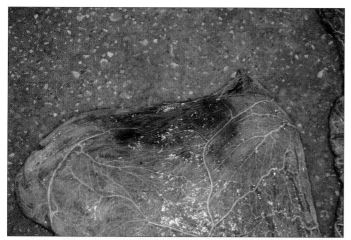

Figure 12.181 Cervical area of placenta showing marked hemorrhage. This can be consistent with fetal stress or thickening of the placenta. This finding should alert the veterinarian to the potential of hypoxic injury to the foal.

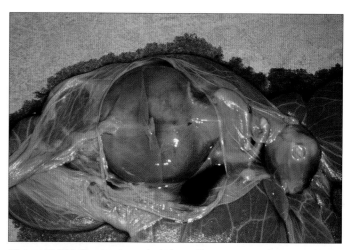

Figure 12.184 Abortion due to fetal abnormality.

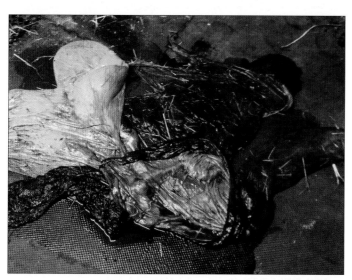

Figure 12.182 Meconium staining of the placenta. Release of meconium before or during parturition is a sign of fetal stress and should alert the practitioner to potential problems including aspiration of meconium and hypoxia. Notice also the marked hemorrhagic appearance of this placenta.

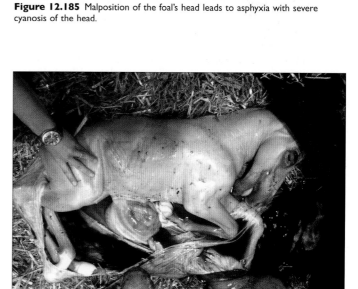

Figure 12.185 Malposition of the foal's head leads to asphyxia with severe cyanosis of the head.

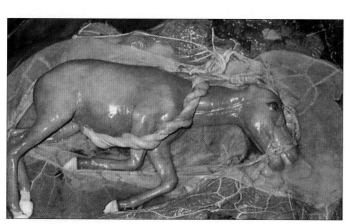

Figure 12.183 Normal twisting of the umbilical cord.

Figure 12.186 This clone foal was delivered by terminal C-section at 315-days of gestation due to death of the mare. The picture shows not only a defect of the abdominal wall, with small intestine evident outside the abdominal cavity, but also a marked immaturity for the stage of gestation associated with marked placental abnormalities.

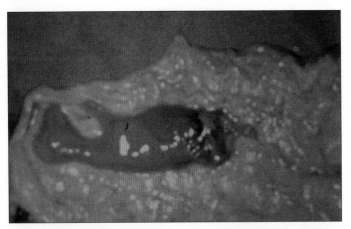

Figure 12.187 Fetal resorption at 80 days. The aborted membranes revealed this autolysed fetus.

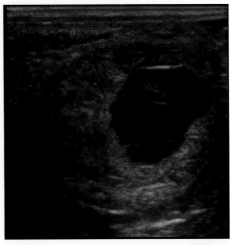

Figure 12.188 Fetal resorption at 30 days. Notice lack of organ definition.

excessive fetal movement, which is possibly due to fetal stress. Any of these may be found associated with abortion or sometimes with normal delivery of foals, which are slow to adapt and may be affected by the neonatal maladjustment syndrome (see Fig. 11.11). Careful placental examinations may provide some effective indicators of impending problems and provide the clinician with an opportunity to take appropriate preventive measures.

The umbilical cord is normally twisted on its length. Up to 6–9 twists may be observed in normal foals in utero and it is unlikely that these are of any significance with respect to umbilical efficiency. These normal twists are usually evenly distributed and the cord lacks obvious constrictions in its length.

The length of the umbilical cord is variable. In the Thoroughbred, normal length is approximately 85 cm at term and has 6–9 twists as previously mentioned. Longer cords may have a greater tendency to have increased number of twists as the fetus moves, potentially producing pathological areas of passive congestion in the umbilical vessels; this causes fetal compromise and usually abortion. Foals with shorter cords appear to be more at risk to fetal stress syndromes immediately prior to and during delivery, when early vascular occlusion may occur; in these cases, the fetus will become stressed due to hypoxemia and death may ensue if action is not taken quickly.

Other physical events that may terminate pregnancy are travel, galloping by heavily pregnant mares, fetal death/resorption and forced service in pregnant mares. A detailed history and examination of the foal and the placenta usually establishes the relevant unusual features of management or behavior.

Fetal resorption (Figs. 12.187–12.189)
Fetal resorption is a frustrating and expensive problem encountered in many mares. It may be related to many conditions associated with the immediate uterine environment, physical well-being of the mare, and embryonic factors (genetic and nutritional components):

- Uterine abnormalities: endometritis, endometriosis, glandular abnormalities, vascular degeneration.
- Mare: Age, endocrine disorders, lameness/arthritis, perineal and physical conformation, nutritional deficiencies.
- Embryonic: chromosomal abnormalities, mare/stallion mismatch, nutritional/placental (twins).

Resorption can occur at any stage of early gestation. For mares that undergo pregnancy loss prior to endometrial cup formation, re-breeding that season is an option, although the cervix will be more tight than usual and fluid pre- and post-mating will be evident.

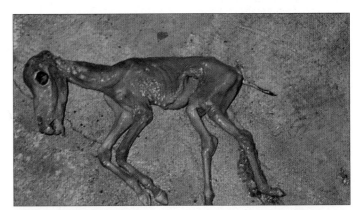

Figure 12.189 Twin resorption with advanced autolysis resulting in abortion at 7 months.

Identification of fetal resorption can vary from no-pregnancy present, to abnormal amount or flocculence of fetal fluids, lack of heart beat or definition of the fetus on transrectal ultrasonography.

Body pregnancy (Figs. 12.190 & 12.191)
Body pregnancy (fetal development within the uterine body instead of either of the uterine horns) almost always has marked effects upon the development of the fetus. These terminate either in abortion, or a premature foal (gestational age of less than 320 days) or a dysmature foal (a foal born after a normal gestational period but with characteristics of prematurity). The placentas of these cases characteristically show placental horns of equal size and density and the allantoic surface frequently shows edema and cystic formations.

Premature placental separation (Fig. 12.192)
Premature placental separation is a very serious complication of parturition. It may cause death of a full term fetus as a result of serious hypoxia if delivery is delayed at all. As the term implies, separation of the placenta occurs before normal delivery of the foal, thereby depriving the foal of adequate gaseous exchanges. It is, furthermore, uncommon for the placenta to separate over limited areas only. More usually the entire placenta separates within a short period of time, making delivery all the more urgent. The condition can be recognized by the appearance of the cervical star at the vulva and the enclosed legs of the fetus, the so-called 'red-bag' delivery. In normal placental separation, the placenta ruptures at the cervical star and this remains within the vagina following delivery of the foal, but with premature

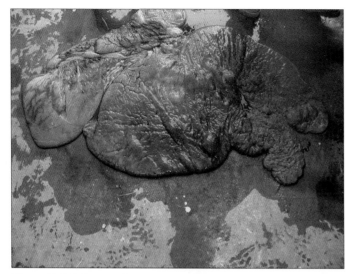

Figure 12.190 Placenta of a mare with a body pregnancy. The chorionic surface displays two equal size and density horns. This mare also had extensive placentitis, which resulted in generalized thickening of the placenta.

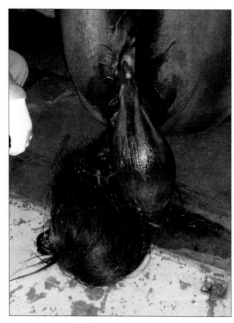

Figure 12.192 Premature placental separationd or 'red bag' delivery reveals the intact cervical star and chorioallantoid extruded on top of the foal at parturition.

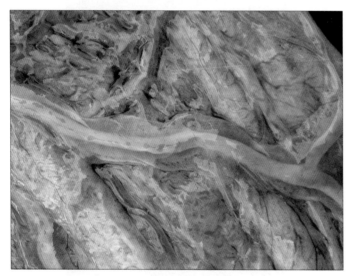

Figure 12.191 Marked perivascular edema of the chorionic surface of a placenta from a body pregnancy. Such edema is frequently associated with placental abnormalities and dysfunction.

separation, the placenta continues to be expelled with, eventually, either complete or incomplete tearing of the placenta in the mid-body, with delivery of the foal. All foals that are delivered under these conditions are compromised to some extent and many are born dead. It is imperative that this particular problem of parturition is recognized and acted upon immediately, by rupturing the membranes and delivering the foal.

Infectious diseases (see Placentitis)

Viral diseases

Infection with **equine herpes virus-1** is capable of causing respiratory disease, posterior paralysis and is a particularly common cause of abortion. Foals which are infected in utero are usually born dead or very weak, succumbing early to a progressive pneumonia (and other organ failure). Abortion may occur at any time between 7 months and full term, and usually occurs without any sign of illness in the mare. The disease is spread by ingestion of the virus

from contaminated food or water, or from contact with an infected placenta, fetus or uterine discharges from an aborted mare. The nasal discharges from infected horses are particularly liable to transmit the condition, which is highly contagious. Abortion may occur singly or as a 'storm', involving several (or more) mares under the same management and severe losses have been reported, even in vaccinated mares. When abortion occurs, there is rapid separation of the placenta within the uterus. The fetus is often delivered within the placenta, with the chorionic side of the placenta still on the outside (the so called '**red-bag' abortion**). Some pregnancies may continue to full-term, but the foals are usually weak and most die from intractable virus pneumonia and/or hepatic and adrenal collapse within 10 days. The fetus may show any number of gross lesions such as subcutaneous edema, jaundice, increased body fluids and an enlarged liver with varying numbers of 1 mm diameter, whitish-yellow, necrotic foci. The placenta is either normal in appearance and consistency, or the chorion has a much-thickened, edematous, red appearance. It is either delivered immediately with the foal, or shortly afterwards. Retention of fetal membranes under these conditions is particularly unusual.

Abortion is a very common clinical sign associated with **equine viral arteritis** and usually occurs within a few days of the onset of clinical signs. Mares may be infected via the respiratory tract or venereally. There are no remarkable lesions of either placentas or aborted foals in case reports of this disease. Experimental infections have suggested that abortion is due to fetal anoxia caused by myometrial vessel compression, which is in turn due to edema in the uterine walls.

Systemic bacterial diseases (Figs. 12.193 & 12.194)

Systemic bacterial infection causing inflammatory changes to the blood vessels has been found in some mares. The appearance of the placenta in these infections is variable and related largely to the species of organism involved and the duration and route of infection. Infections associated with *Klebsiella* spp. produce a characteristic diffuse and often severe, inflammatory change along the placental blood vessels while that due to *Streptococcus* spp. tends to be less severe but more extensive, involving blood vessels over almost the entire placental surface. Bacterial infection of the embryonic **yolk sac** also

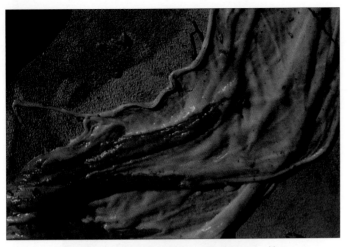

Figure 12.193 Placentitis associated with *Klebsiella pneumoniae*. Hematogenous spread with involvement of the blood vessels.

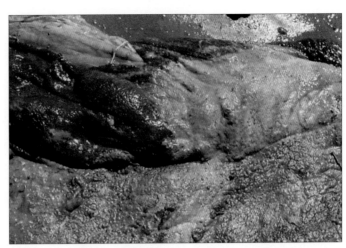

Figure 12.195 Fungal placentitis due to *Aspergillus* spp. The cervical star shows a gray-brown infected leathery placenta.

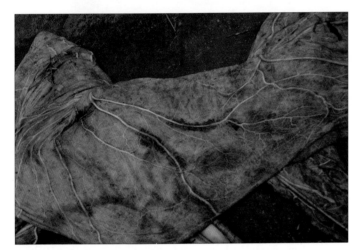

Figure 12.194 Placentitis due to B-hemolytic *Streptococcus* distributed hematogenously.

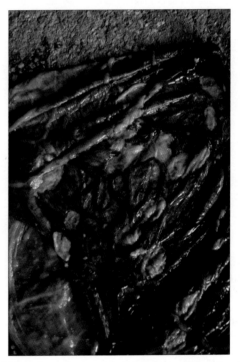

Figure 12.196 Small multifocal necrotic lesions due to a fungal placentitis.

occurs and is usually found as a result of an abortion investigation. Bacterial infection causing abortion may also present a normal yolk sac area with green coloration of the entire allantois, probably as a result of concurrent placental hemorrhage and consequent hemoglobin breakdown.

Fungal diseases (Figs. 12.195–12.197)

Fungal placentitis is not common but occurs under similar circumstances and in similar locations as the bacterial infections. While it is more commonly located in the region of the cervical star, suggesting that the likely route of infection is via the cervix, it may occur in other locations, such as uterine body or horns via hematogenous route. Clinically the lesions appear as thickened, leather-like areas around the cervical star or edematous avillous areas, with a tenacious exudate of brownish mucus in other areas of the placenta. These areas of avillous necrosis often lead to poor intra-uterine nutrition for the foal and commonly lead to abortion, with a severely malnourished foal; lesions may also be present in the foal, and therefore, stomach contents should always be taken for a microbiological study. *Aspergillus* spp. are the most common isolates both from placenta and fetus. A touch prep cytology can help differentiate fungal from bacterial or nocardioform.

Mare reproductive loss syndrome
(Figs. 12.198 & 12.199)

In April and May 2001 central Kentucky experienced a tremendous number of early and late fetal losses, birth of weak, critically ill foals and increased number of cases of pericarditis and panophthalmitis. The outbreak was termed 'mare reproductive loss syndrome (MRLS)'. At the same time an overwhelming number of eastern tent caterpillars (ETC) emerged into the environment.

Clinical signs

- Mares present with premature placental separation or 'red bags', foal standing, and have expulsion of fetuses and stillbirths. Fetal lesions include pneumonia and inflammation of the umbilical cord (funisitis).

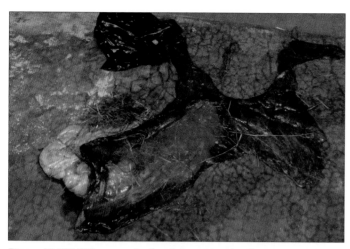

Figure 12.197 Diffuse ascending fungal placentitis with avillus area covered with a tenacious exudate. Note the lesion extends from the cervical star to the body.

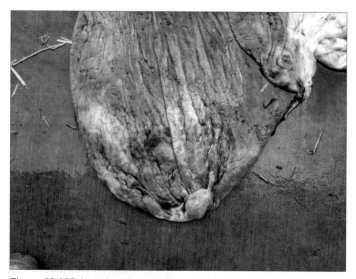

Figure 12.198 Ascending placentitis. This image shows the cervical star area with marked thickening of the placenta and a thick tenacious exudate.

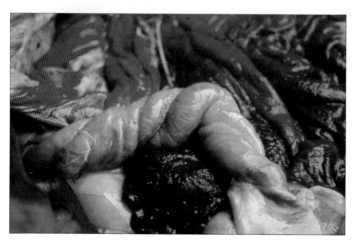

Figure 12.199 Funisitis associated with late fetal loss and MRLS.

- Cultures of fetal and placental tissues grow non beta hemolytic *Streptococcus* or *Actinobacillus*. These however are not considered the primary problem but secondary opportunistic contaminants.
- Foals that are born alive are incredibly weak and severely dehydrated usually developing neurological problems.

Diagnosis and treatment

- Early fetal loss (EFL) can be identified by transrectal ultrasonography during examination at around days 45–60 of gestation. There is an increase in abnormal echogenic, flocculent fluid around the fetus; some of the fetuses will have decreased movement, heart rate or can be dead. Changes can occur within 24 hours.
- Mares can also be found empty after their fetus is expelled. An initial survey of farm managers in early May documented a 20% rate of EFL.
- Two other presentations of this disease can occur, pericarditis and unilateral panophthalmitis. Lesions occur in yearling and adult horses with eye lesions being unresponsive to normal treatment; most horses will loose vision in the affected eye. Pericarditis usually responds to treatment in cases that are identified early.
- It has been found that the setae of the eastern tent caterpillar can penetrate the gut (as found on histological sections) which can carry potential pathogens from the oral cavity into the circulation, and the uterus.
- Treatment is based on supportive care.

References and further reading

Allen, W.E., 1988. Fertility and Obstetrics in the Horse. Blackwell Scientific Publications, Oxford, UK.

Burns, S.J., Judge, N.G., Martin, J.E., et al, 1977. Management of retained placenta in mares. In Proc AAEP 43;381–390.

Cox, J.E., 1987. Surgery of the Reproductive Tract. Liverpool University Press, Liverpool, UK.

Daels, P.F., 2006. Induction of lactation and Adoption of the Orphan Foal. Proc AAEP, Annual Resort Symposium, Rome, Italy.

Jubb, K.V.F., Kennedy, P.C., Palmer, N., 1985. A Pathology of Domestic Animals, third ed. Academic Press, Philadelphia, PA, USA.

McKinnon, A.O., Squires, E.L., Vaala, W.E., Varner, D.D., 2011. Equine Reproduction, second ed. Wiley–Blackwell Publishing, Chichester, UK.

Renaudin, C., Troedsson, M.H.T., Gilis, CL, et al, 1997. Ultrasonographic evaluation of the equine placenta and transabdominal approach in pregnant mares. Theriogenology 46:559–573.

Robinson, N.E., 2005. Current Therapy in Equine Medicine, fifth ed. WB Saunders, Philadelphia, PA, USA.

Rose, R.J., Hodgson, D.R., (eds), 2000. Manual of Equine Practice, second ed. WB Saunders, Philadelphia, USA.

Rossdale, P.D., Ricketts, S.W., 1980. Equine Stud Farm Medicine. Ballière Tindall, London.

Samper, J.C., Pycock, J.F., McKinnon, A.O., 2007. Current Therapy in Equine Reproduction. Saunders, Elsevier, St Louis, USA.

Sellon, D.C., Taylor, E.L., Wardrop, J., et al, 1999. Effects of intravenous formaldehyde on hemostasis in normal horses. Proc AAEP 45;297–298.

Steiner, J.V., 2006. How to Induce Lactation in Non-Pregnant Mares. Proc AAEP 52;259–269.

Varner, D.D., Schumacher, J., Blanchard, T.L., Johnson, L., 1991. Diseases and Management of Breeding Stallions. American Veterinary Publications, Coleta, USA.

INDEX

Page numbers followed by 'f' indicate figures, 't' indicate tables, and 'b' indicate boxes.